MEDICINE IN THE MEDIEVAL NORTH ATLANTIC WORLD

KNOWLEDGE, SCHOLARSHIP, AND SCIENCE IN THE MIDDLE AGES

VOLUME 5

Medicine in the Medieval North Atlantic World

Vernacular Texts and Traditions

Edited by
DEBORAH HAYDEN AND
SARAH BACCIANTI

BREPOLS

British Library Cataloguing in Publication Data.
A catalogue record for this book is available from the British Library.

D/2025/0095/20
ISBN 978-2-503-61333-8
E-ISBN 978-2-503-61334-5
DOI 10.1484/M.KSS-EB.5.141319

ISSN 2736-7150
e-ISSN 2736-7169

Printed in the EU on acid-free paper.

In memory of James E. Hayden, Sr.
(31 August 1946–27 December 2020)
D. H.

To my brother, Padre Didier Pietro Maria Baccianti,
OP, for patiently answering all my questions on religion
S. B.

Table of Contents

Part III
Charms and Rituals

Contributors

Sharon Arbuthnot (sja50@cam.ac.uk) is based at the University of Cambridge and has recently returned to the Electronic Dictionary of the Irish Language (eDIL) project, on which she was employed as a researcher and editor between 2009 and 2020. In the intervening years, she worked as a lexicographer and, subsequently, as Director of Faclair na Gàidhlig, the historical dictionary of Scottish Gaelic. She has published on vocabulary specific to the domains of technology, sex, wildlife and the supernatural, as well as medicine, and has a particular interest in medieval Irish texts concerned with wordplay and 'Isidorian' etymology. She is the author of a two-volume edition of *Cóir Anmann*, a Middle-Irish collection of etymological explanations of personal names, and is in the final stages of editing work on the early glossary, *Dúil Dromma Cetta*.

Sarah Baccianti (sarah.baccianti@nationalmuseumsni.org) is the Research Manager at National Museums NI. Before moving to the museum sector, she lectured in Old English and Old Norse literature at the University of Oxford, Université de Lausanne, University College Cork, and Queen's University Belfast. She obtained her doctorate at the University of Oxford where she researched the narrative structure of chronicles and *historiae* written in Old Norse, Old English, and Anglo-Latin. Her research project, funded by the British Academy Newton International Fellowship, explored the reception and transmission of scientific and medical knowledge in medieval Denmark and Iceland. Although the funding period has ended, she continues to pursue this research independently.

Siobhán Barrett (siobhan.barrett@mu.ie) is a post-doctoral researcher in the Department of Early Irish, Maynooth University, working on the Research Ireland-funded project *LEIGHEAS: Language, Education and Medical Learning in the Premodern Gaelic World*. Her research interests are medieval Irish medical herbal remedies, plant names, and medical glossaries.

Caroline R. Batten (battenc@english.upenn.edu) is Assistant Professor of English at the University of Pennsylvania. They received their D.Phil from the University of Oxford and have published widely on sickness and health, gender and sexuality, and somatic emotion in Old English and Old Norse literature, with a particular focus on medical charms. They are the author of *Health and the Body in Early Medieval England* (Elements in England in the Early Medieval World, Cambridge University Press, 2024).

Erin Connelly (erin.connelly@warwick.ac.uk) is an Assistant Professor in the School of Life Sciences, University of Warwick. Her main focus of research pertains to interdisciplinary collaboration across a range of applications, including the investigation of natural products.

Ranke de Vries (rdevries@stfx.ca) is Ben Alder Professor of Celtic Studies at St Francis Xavier University, Nova Scotia, Canada. Her research interests include medieval Irish and Welsh language and literature in general; medieval Irish medical knowledge (particularly as represented in pre-fourteenth-century saga literature); and textual editing.

Conan Doyle (conant.doyle@gmail.com) graduated with a PhD in Anglo-Saxon, Norse and Celtic from Cambridge University in 2018. He is an assistant professor of medieval English at the Faculty of Humanities, Charles University in Prague. His research interests include the medieval reception of classical medicine, and classical literature more generally. He is currently publishing his first monograph: *The Reception of Latin Medicine in Early Medieval England: Evidence from Old English Texts*.

Christian Etheridge (christian.etheridge@nationalmuseum.se) is chief researcher on the Berit Wallenberg Foundation funded project: *Fragments of the Past: The Legacy of Carl Nordenfalk and the Collection of Manuscript Cuttings held at the Nationalmuseum in Stockholm* hosted at the Nationalmuseum in Stockholm. He has written on the history of science, art history, manuscript studies and the transmission of ideas in the Middle Ages. He is the author of *Danish Mendicant Sponsorship of the Fourteenth Century Wall Murals in Birkerød Church* (Gambier OH, 2022). Together with Michele Campopiano, he is the editor of *Medieval Science in the North: Travelling Wisdom, 1000-1500* (Turnhout, 2021).

Joseph Flahive (j.flahive@ria.ie) is Assistant Editor to the Dictionary of Medieval Latin from Celtic Sources at the Royal Irish Academy, Dublin, and co-editor of its *Non-Classical Lexicon of Celtic Latinity*. He is a medievalist with expertise in the languages, manuscripts, and literatures of Britain and Ireland. His areas of interest include Celtic and Hiberno-Latin. He researches in Latin lexicography; Insular palaeography; and early Irish literature, with focus on the relationship between Latin and the vernacular, particularly in regard to *fianaigheacht*. He is the author of *The Fenian Cycle in Irish and Scots-Gaelic Literature* (Cork, 2017).

Deborah Hayden (deborah.hayden@mu.ie) is Professor in Medieval Irish and Celtic Studies at Maynooth University. She has published and taught widely on aspects of the intellectual and literary culture of medieval Ireland and the Insular world in its European context, and has particular interests in the history of linguistic thought and education in classical and medieval tradition, premodern Irish medical writing, early Irish lexicography, medieval Irish and Welsh legal tradition, and translation literature. She is Lead Editor of the peer-reviewed journal *Language & History* and Principal Investigator of the project *LEIGHEAS: Language, Education and Medical Learning in the Premodern Gaelic World*, funded by a Consolidator Laureate Award from Research Ireland (2022–2026).

Viktoriia Krivoshchekova (viktoriia@celt.dias.ie) is a post-doctoral researcher and an O'Donovan Scholar at the Dublin Institute for Advanced Studies, School of Celtic Studies. Her research explores ideas on the relationship between mind and language in early medieval Ireland. Viktoriia's research interests include philosophy of mind, philosophy of language, cognitive linguistics, early Irish grammar and exegesis.

Katherine Leach (kate.leach-2@dartmouth.edu) received her PhD in 2020 from the Department of Celtic Languages, Harvard University. Her dissertation focused on pre-modern Welsh charms for healing. Research interests include pre-modern Welsh charms and rituals, medieval notions of magic and superstition, medieval medicine, and pre-modern healers in Wales, Scotland, Ireland, and England. Currently, Kate is Assistant Dean of Undergraduate Students at Dartmouth College.

Christina Lee (christina.lee@nottingham.ac.uk) is Associate Professor in Viking Studies at the University of Nottingham. Her research interests are in the perceptions of health and healing in Early Medieval England and she also is part of a cross-disciplinary group ancientbiotics which considers how medieval remedies may inform modern science. She has published on disability, leprosy, and trauma.

Brigid Mayes (mayesbrigid@gmail.com) is a medical herbalist with a practice in Co. Westmeath, Ireland. Her interest in the history of plant medicine led her to a study of the *Materia Medica* compiled in 1415 by Gaelic physician Tadhg Ó Cuinn. This work was the subject of her dissertation for a Master of Arts in the History of Welfare and Medicine at University College Dublin (2018).

Laura Poggesi (laura.poggesi@edu.unige.it) is adjunct professor of Germanic Philology at the University of Genoa. In 2024 she was post-doctoral research fellow at the University of Florence, where she has worked on Middle English sermons. In 2022 she gained a PhD in Germanic Philology at the Universities of Pavia and Bergamo. For her PhD Dissertation she provided the first edition and Italian translation of the Middle English medical recipes contained in Cambridge, Trinity College Library, MS R.14.32. Her research interests include textual criticism, translation practices in medieval England, and the transmission of medical texts in Middle English.

Elisa Ramazzina (e.ramazzina@qub.ac.uk) completed her PhD in Germanic Philology, specializing in Old English, at the University of Pavia. Currently, she is a Lecturer in the Earliest English Writings at Queen's University Belfast. Prior to her current position, she taught Old English at various levels at H. M. Classics Academy in Belfast and worked as a Research Assistant at the University of Oxford, contributing to the ERC-funded project 'CLASP: A Consolidated Library of Anglo Saxon Poetry'. During her role as a Marie Curie Fellow at Queen's University Belfast from 2017 to 2019, Elisa immersed herself in the realm of medieval literature through her project 'Cleansing Water: Water and Baptism in Old English Poetry'. Elisa's research interests primarily focus on the medieval natural world and landscape, with a specific emphasis on water and monster studies. She engages with Old English and Middle English texts, often drawing comparisons with medieval Latin, Old High German, Middle High German, and medieval Italian texts. Embracing an interdisciplinary approach, Elisa also explores Material Philology and Digital Philology methodologies in her scholarly pursuits.

Anne Irene Riisøy (anne.irene.risoy@usn.no) is Professor at the University of South-Eastern Norway, where she teaches pre-nineteenth century history. She holds a PhD from the University of Oslo which was subsequently published by Brill as a monograph on *Sexuality, Law and Legal Practice and the Reformation in Norway* (2009). Riisøy has an ongoing interest in legal history, but since her PhD she has switched focus from the late medieval and early modern periods back to the Viking Age and the transition between the Viking Age and the early medieval period. A postdoctoral project on outlaws and outlawry resulted in several articles. A second key area of interest has been to apply Old Norse Poetry, particularly the Eddic poems, to the exploration of Viking Age law and legal practice. A third area of interest is the earliest Norwegian legal material on manslaughter and wounds and the corresponding rules on compensation to the victim and/or fines to the king.

David Stifter (david.stifter@mu.ie) is Professor of Old and Middle Irish in the Department of Early Irish at Maynooth University (Ireland). His research interests include language variation and change in Old Irish, Early Irish literature, comparative Celtic linguistics (especially Old Irish and Continental Celtic), and language contact in the ancient world and in the early medieval British Isles. He has published widely on Old and Middle Irish language and philology and on the Continental Celtic languages (Celtiberian, Gaulish and Lepontic). His handbook *Sengoídelc. Old Irish for Beginners* (Syracuse University Press 2006) is a popular introduction to Old Irish. His introductions to the language, writing and epigraphy of *Cisalpine Celtic* (2020) and *Ogam* (2022) have been published by Prensas de la Universidad de Zaragoza.

Matteo Tarsi (matteo.tarsi@nordiska.uu.se) is a researcher at the department of Scandinavian languages at Uppsala University. His research interests encompass lexicology, etymology, comparative historical linguistics, and history of linguistics. He is the author of *Loanwords and Native Words in Old and Middle Icelandic* (Brepols, 2022), a study of the coexistence of loanwords and native synonyms in Icelandic up to *c.* 1550.

Eystein Thanisch (eystein.thanisch@gmail.com) has research interests in medieval historiography, concepts of authorship and authority, and the digital representation of medieval texts. His PhD thesis (University of Edinburgh) was on the later medieval and post-medieval reception of the Middle Irish poet and historian, Flann Mainistrech. He subsequently spent four years as one of the Manuscripts Research Fellows working on the development of Faclair na Gàidhlig, the historical dictionary of Scottish Gaelic, based at Sabhal Mòr Ostaig, University of the Highlands and Islands. In this role, he helped transcribe and tag a corpus of Gaelic manuscripts of Scottish relevance, including several medical manuscripts. He has also contributed to IrishGen, an effort to represent the medieval Irish genealogical corpus as a graph database.

List of Illustrations

Figures

Tables

Acknowledgements

Many of the contributions to this volume began life as conference papers read at two separate events. The first of these was a workshop on 'Science and Medicine in the Insular Middle Ages', hosted by Dr Sarah Baccianti at Queen's University Belfast on 7 December 2018, while the second was a conference on 'Medicine in the Medieval North Atlantic World', jointly hosted via Zoom from 13–15 May 2021 by the editors of this volume with the invaluable assistance of Dr Siobhán Barrett and Dr Bernhard Bauer. These conferences were supported by funding for two major research initiatives that were ongoing between 2018 and 2021, namely, Sarah Baccianti's British Academy Newton International Fellowship project on *Scientific Knowledge in Medieval Scandinavia*, based at Queen's University Belfast, and Prof. Deborah Hayden's project *Medieval Irish Medicine in its North-western European Context: A Case Study of Two Unpublished Texts* (MIMNEC), which was funded by a Research Ireland Starting Laureate Award in the Department of Early Irish at Maynooth University.

Although it ultimately took place in the digital realm, it was our original intention to hold the 'Medicine in the Medieval North Atlantic World' conference as an in-person event on the campus of Maynooth University from 19–21 March 2020. Anyone who has ever attempted to organize an academic gathering before — particularly the kind that spans several days and involves multiple international speakers — will know not only how much work is involved, but also how much of that work happens in the last week or so leading up to the first day of papers. For the event organizers, those final few days of preparation can feel like a relentless blur of emails about catering, accommodation, travel, room bookings, and other mundane practicalities, never mind the usual last-minute tweaking of papers and arguments while trying to keep pace with the everyday teaching and administrative demands of academic life. It was particularly heart-wrenching, therefore, to have to make the difficult (but in retrospect very much the correct) decision to postpone the conference just days before it was to begin on account of the outbreak of the COVID-19 pandemic in Ireland, where a full statewide lockdown order came into force on 27 March.

The 'Medicine in the Medieval North Atlantic World' conference turned out to be one of the first dominos in a long chain of scheduled academic events across the globe that were to fall suddenly and quickly at the time, and there was much uncertainty as to whether the event could ever be resurrected at all. Funding for both projects was due to run out by the end of the academic year, when two of the three invited plenary speakers were planning to retire and the third would be moving to another hemisphere; no-one yet knew with any clarity what costs, if any, could be recouped; and three of the four organizing committee members, not to mention many of the speakers, did not know where they would be working in a few months. And then, of course, there was the great uncertainty about just how long and how serious the pandemic situation itself would turn out to be.

It is thus particularly satisfying to not only have been able finally to host the conference via Zoom in May 2021, featuring nearly all the speakers who had committed to the original event plus many more audience members from across the globe, but also to bring to fruition in printed form so many of the papers read at that inspiring and thought-provoking online forum. We wish to express our gratitude to the British Academy and Research Ireland for their continued financial support of the 'Medicine in the Medieval North Atlantic World' conference well beyond the original timeframe envisaged, as well as to Dr Rosie Bonté at Brepols for her unstinting encouragement, assistance, and advice at all stages of the publication process. The final phase of book preparation was supported by further funding from Research Ireland through Deborah Hayden's Consolidator Laureate Award project *LEIGHEAS: Language, Education and Medical Learning in the Premodern Gaelic World* (2022–2026). We are also grateful to the two anonymous peer-reviewers for their many helpful and constructive comments on all the chapters in the volume, and to the Editorial Board members of the *Knowledge, Scholarship, and Science in the Middle Ages* series at Brepols for seeing it through to publication. Most importantly, however, we thank all the contributors for their time, patience, collegiality, and expertise, without which this project would never have seen the light of day. Work on this volume has, for both of the editors, been a great tonic over the course of the last few very challenging years.

Deborah Hayden
Maynooth University, June 2024

Sarah Baccianti
National Museums NI, June 2024

Abbreviations

ACLL	Brepolis, *Archive of Celtic Latin Literature* <clt.brepolis.net/acll/>
AFM	*Annala Rioghachta Eireann: Annals of the Kingdom of Ireland by the Four Masters*, ed. and trans. by John O'Donovan, 7 vols (Dublin: Hodges Smith, 1856) <https://celt.ucc.ie/published/T100005E/index.html>
AND^{2}	*Online Anglo-Norman Dictionary*, 2nd edn <https://anglo-norman.net>
AU	*Annala Uladh: Annals of Ulster otherwise Annala Senait, Annals of Senat: A Chronicle of Irish Affairs from A.D. 431 to A.D. 1540*, ed. by W. M. Hennessy and Bartholomew Mac Carthy, 4 vols (Dublin: Royal Irish Academy, 1887–1901; repr. with new introduction and bibliography by Nollaig Ó Muraíle, Dublin: De Búrca, 1998) <https://celt.ucc.ie/published/T100001C/index.html>
CELT	Corpus of Electronic Texts <https://celt.ucc.ie>
eDIL	eDIL 2019: *An Electronic Dictionary of the Irish Language*, based on the Contributions to a Dictionary of the Irish Language (Dublin: Royal Irish Academy, 1913–1976) <www.dil.ie>
eMGH	*Monumenta Germaniae Historica* <clt.brepolis.net/eMGH/>
ISOS	*Irish Script on Screen – Meamrám Páipéar Ríomhaire* (School of Celtic Studies, Dublin Institute for Advanced Studies) <www.isos.dias.ie>
LLT	Brepolis, *Library of Latin Texts* (*LLT-A* and *LLT-B* databases) <clt.brepolis.net/llta/>
Med.Gal.	Durling, Richard J., *A Dictionary of Medical Terms in Galen*, Studies in Ancient Medicine, 5 (Leiden: Brill, 1993)
NCLCL	*The Non-Classical Lexicon of Celtic Latinity* <journals.eeecs.qub.ac.uk>
OED	*Oxford English Dictionary* <http://www.oed.com>
ONP	*The Dictionary of Old Norse Prose* <https://onp.ku.dk/onp/onp.php?>
PL	*Patrologiae cursus completus, series latina*, ed. by J. P. Migne (Paris, 1844–1890)

RIA Catalogue	*Catalogue of Irish Manuscripts in the Royal Irish Academy*, ed. by T. F. O'Rahilly and others, 8 vols (Dublin: Royal Irish Academy, 1926–1970)
Thes.	*Thesaurus Palaeohibernicus. A Collection of Old-Irish Glosses Scholia Prose and Verse*, ed. and trans. by Whitley Stokes and John Strachan, 2 vols (Cambridge: Cambridge University Press, 1901–1903)

DEBORAH HAYDEN and SARAH BACCIANTI

1. Introduction

Cultural Crossroads and Medical Learning in the Medieval North Atlantic World

This volume explores aspects of medicine and medical ideas in the medieval North Atlantic world, focusing primarily on vernacular texts and traditions from Ireland, England, Wales, and Scandinavia across a chronological range that spans the early to late Middle Ages. On the one hand, the book is a collective effort on the part of scholars of medieval medicine and related fields to respond to a wealth of recent scholarship on the transmission and translation of texts from various genres — particularly historical and literary ones — across the frequently shifting linguistic, political, and national boundaries that have shaped this archipelagic region throughout its history.[1] The volume also seeks to transcend disciplinary boundaries within the field of medieval medicine itself, however, by recognizing that there is much to be gained from fostering dialogue among scholars working on medical texts or themes in the various linguistic traditions of the Insular world.

In the area of medieval medicine, where the focus of so much valuable work has often been directed further south towards Mediterranean Europe and the medieval Islamicate cultures of Spain, North Africa and the Near

1 Some notable recent examples include Allport and others, eds, *Networks in the Medieval North*; Brady, *The Origin Legends*; Busby, *French in Medieval Ireland*; Byrne and Flood, eds, *Crossing Borders*; Edmonds, *Gaelic Influence*; Eriksen, ed., *Intellectual Culture in Medieval Scandinavia*; Etchingham and others, *Norse–Gaelic Contacts*; Griffin and Purcell, eds, *Text, Transmission and Transformation*; Poppe and others, eds, *Celts, Gaels, and Britons*; Sif Rikharðsdóttir, *Medieval Translations*; Sims-Williams, *Irish Influence*; and Jón Viðar Sigurðsson and Bolton, eds, *Celtic–Norse Relationships*. A volume edited by Etheridge and Campopiano, *Medieval Science in the North*, is the first major contribution on the reception and transmission of scientific knowledge in Scandinavia and England and the crucial role that this played in the international network of scholars in the North Atlantic and in continental centres of learning.

Deborah Hayden • Maynooth University; deborah.hayden@mu.ie
Sarah Baccianti • National Museums NI; sarah.baccianti@nationalmuseumsni.org

Medicine in the Medieval North Atlantic World: Vernacular Texts and Traditions, ed. by Deborah Hayden and Sarah Baccianti, KSS, 5 (Turnhout, 2025), pp. 23-52
BREPOLS PUBLISHERS DOI 10.1484/M.KSS-EB.5.143979

East,[2] the very concept of an 'Insular' and remote North Atlantic region separated from the European continent by a body of water may evoke notions of peripherality that is not only geographical but also intellectual in nature, even if the importance of medieval England as a crucial node in the transmission of vernacular medical and scientific learning has been acknowledged in recent years.[3] The less well-explored textual traditions of Ireland, Wales, and Scandinavia have, however, much to contribute to these wider debates about the reception and transmission of European medical learning in the medieval North. As Aisling Byrne and Victoria Flood have recently observed in a discussion of late-medieval literary sources, Britain, Ireland, and Scandinavia have 'long been understood as possessing a particular coherence' as a vibrant, multilingual zone of diverse cultural contacts, and the present volume similarly frames this European periphery in a positive light by viewing it 'as a centre of literary exchange, criss-crossed by a network of varied cultural influences'.[4] It is argued by the present authors that the comparative study of these influences and exchanges has great potential to yield new insights not only into the nature of medieval European medical learning and its transmission across the Insular world, but also into processes of translation and vernacularization that shaped the textual cultures of this region throughout its history.

'Medicine' is a term that is likewise interpreted here as referring not simply to past practices of treating disease in a narrow sense, an approach that risks seeing the historical evidence for this branch of scientific learning as little more than a primitive or inferior precursor of modern biomedicine. Rather, the essays in this volume address a much larger nexus of themes concerning the cultural significance of ideas about the body, mind, health, and illness, including topics such as medical education, theory, and authority; legal tracts on bodily injury; literary representations of cognition and wounds; medical lexicography and translation; the production, dissemination, and audiences of medical texts; and the relationship between faith and ritual healing practices. Collectively, these varied approaches inform not only our understanding of the history of medical learning and practice itself, but also its place within medieval societies and learned discourses more generally. It is, indeed, sobering to reflect on the fact that this volume has taken shape as a deadly pandemic swept the globe, shutting down travel, isolating individuals

2 For a useful introduction to the field, see Siraisi, *Medieval and Early Renaissance Medicine*; on the transmission of Arabic medical learning to western Europe, initially via the Mediterranean regions, see e.g. Burnett and Jacquart, eds, *Constantine the African* and Kwakkel and Newton, *Medicine at Monte Cassino*. On medical learning in late-medieval Spain, see e.g. McVaugh, *Medicine before the Plague*.

3 Examples include Burnett, *The Introduction of Arabic Learning*; Green, 'Salerno on the Thames' and Black, '"I Will Add what the Arab Once Taught"'; see also the chapter by Conan Doyle in this volume.

4 Byrne and Flood, 'Insular Connections', pp. 2 and 17.

from their support networks, and exposing the weaknesses and vulnerabilities of communities. As modern scientists worked long hours in the laboratory to find an effective cure for COVID-19 and terms such as 'contact tracing', 'quarantine', 'social distancing', and 'vaccine' came to form part of the everyday lexicon of the general populace, societies were forced daily to contemplate and confront not just the dangers, fears, and uncertainties associated with sickness and death, but also how interconnected many facets of health and human flourishing are with the environment that surrounds us.

In a recent meditation on what it means to write a 'cultural history of medieval medicine', Iona McCleery noted that what might at first appear to be 'a fairly radical way of opening up the field as it could include everything that might affect well-being' is nonetheless an approach more reflective of the medieval sources themselves.[5] One might consider, for example, the definition of medicine offered by Isidore of Seville (d. 636), an author so revered by Irish scholars of the early Middle Ages that they referred to his *Etymologies* as the 'pinnacle' (*cuilmen*) of learning:[6]

> Ad hanc [medicina] itaque pertinent non ea tantum quae ars eorum exhibet, qui proprie Medici nominantur, sed etiam cibus et potus, tegmen et tegumen. Defensio denique omnis atque munitio, qua [sanum] nostrum corpus adversus externos ictus casusque servatur.
>
> > (To medicine belong not only things practiced by the skill of those properly called physicians [*medici*], but also matters of food and drink, clothing and shelter. Ultimately, it consists of every defense and fortification by means of which our body is preserved [healthy] in the face of external blows and accidents.)[7]

Isidore's definition of the scope of medicine is suggestive of one of the key theoretical frameworks of medical learning evident in many medieval texts, namely, that of the so-called 'six non-naturals'. According to Galenic-Hippocratic tradition, these were external factors, the management of which was considered essential to good health; they included eating and drinking, sleeping, exercising, air, cleansing the body, and the 'accidents of the soul', or passions and emotions.[8] The theory of the four humours, which had appeared as early as *c.* 410 BC in the Hippocratic work *The Nature of Man*, was also fundamental to thinking about medicine in the medieval West from an early period. This held that the constitution of the human body was made up of four vital liquids, or 'humours' — blood, phlegm, yellow bile,

5 McCleery, 'Introduction', p. 2.

6 On the reception and perceived significance of Isidore's *Etymologies* in early medieval Ireland, see Smyth, 'Isidorian Texts' and Ó Máille, 'The Authorship of the *Culmen*'.

7 Isidore of Seville, *Etymologies*, IV.i.2 (ed. by Lindsay, I, p. 165; trans. by Barney and others, p. 109); this passage is also cited in McCleery, 'Introduction', pp. 3–4.

8 Siraisi, *Medieval and Early Renaissance Medicine*, p. 101.

and black bile — the relative balance of which would determine the healthy or diseased state of an individual.[9] Later theorists further explained that all corporeal living things were possessed of a characteristic 'complexion', referring to the combination of the humours with the elemental qualities of hot, wet, cold, and dry. A person's dominant humour could determine their whole physical and emotional disposition, which could vary according to the conditions of life (such as the passage of time) or external circumstances. These underlying physiological frameworks provided a rational link between disease and therapy, since the physician could seek to restore a proper balance of elements in the body by prescribing medications with qualities inverse to those of the afflicted individual.[10]

Another key aspect of medical learning in medieval western Europe was the continually evolving relationship between so-called secular healing on the one hand and Christian ideas about spiritual and physical curative practices on the other. To a large extent, these were not separable categories: throughout the Middle Ages, patients and healers invoked God or other deities to treat illness and disease, and natural medicine based on the principles of rational theory outlined above regularly overlapped with elements associated with the Christian Bible and liturgy, such as prayers (e.g., the Paternoster, Creed, and various litanies) or the use of objects such as the eucharist or holy water. The inclusion of verbal charms, textual amulets, and other kinds of magical practices in remedy collections or other types of sources no doubt often answered to needs of a very practical nature: in other words, they were viewed as more or less legitimate aids those in distress in cases where all other forms of medical help had failed.[11] The connection between faith and medicine went much deeper than this, however, since many writers of late antiquity traced sickness and other evils afflicting human life to the biblical Fall of Man or debated whether the sudden onset of illness could be interpreted as evidence of divine retribution for sin.[12] The metaphor of 'Christ the Physician', healer of both body and soul, is widespread in medical, penitential, and other sources from across the medieval West,[13] and hagiographical works served to emphasize the power of saints as earthly agents of miraculous healing who sometimes worked with, and sometimes against, ordinary medical practitioners.[14] Throughout the Middle Ages, written works from many genres emphasized the perceived

9 On the reception of humoral theory in early medieval England, see the chapter by Conan Doyle in this volume.

10 Siraisi, *Medieval and Early Renaissance Medicine*, pp. 101–02.

11 Olsan, 'Charms and Prayers'. On textual amulets, see Skemer, *Binding Words* and Hindley, *Textual Magic*.

12 For discussion, see e.g. Temkin, *Hippocrates* and (with particular reference to the early medieval Carolingian world) Leja, *Embodying the Soul*, pp. 94–98.

13 See e.g. Arbesmann, 'The Concept of "Christus Medicus"' and McNeill, 'Medicine for Sin'.

14 For discussions of this motif, see e.g. Flint, 'Early Medieval "Medicus"' and Metzler, *Disability*, pp. 138–53.

intersection between health and ethics through texts on medical deontology or the use of figurative language that links medicine to moral behaviour.[15]

Medicine and the Languages of the Medieval North Atlantic

Medical writing in the vernacular is attested from a relatively early stage in the Insular world, where some 300 medical or scientific items in Old English — including astrological and computistical treatises, herbals, and remedy books — survive in manuscripts produced between the ninth and twelfth centuries.[16] The twelfth and thirteenth centuries saw the appearance of remedy collections and other medical treatises in Anglo-French, and Welsh- and Irish-language material is preserved in manuscripts dating to around the end of the fourteenth or the beginning of the fifteenth century onwards. While compilations of herbal remedies and charms predominate in records for the earlier period, the fourteenth and fifteenth centuries also witnessed a significant increase in the production of other types of vernacular medical material. Among the *c.* 8000 such items in Middle English, for example, are numerous academic and surgical treatises.[17] The transmission of scientific and medical knowledge from the continent to Scandinavia is well attested, with scholars from this region studying in France and Italy, as well as Eastern Europe, well throughout the sixteenth century. For instance, the royal physician to the Danish King Erik IV, Henrik Harpestræng (d. 1244) was most probably trained in Italy or France.[18] Three treatises are associated with Harpestræng: the Latin *De simplicibus medicinis laxativis* and the *Liber herbarum*, and the Old Danish *Den danske urtebog*.[19] As observed in Christian Etheridge's contribution to this volume, the continental influences in Harpestræng's medical treatises

15 A recent study of this theme, focusing on the evidence of late-medieval English sources, is Langum, *Medicine and the Seven Deadly Sins*. On the textual tradition of medical deontology, see MacKinney, 'Medical Ethics'.

16 Pahta and Taavitsainen, 'Vernacularisation', p. 9.

17 For this figure, see Pahta and Taavitsainen, 'Vernacularisation', p. 11, whose estimate is based on texts recorded in *Scientific and Medical Writings in Old and Middle English*, ed. by Voigts and Kurtz.

18 See Holck, 'Middeladerens danske lægebog'. Holck argues that Harpestræng must have been part of a network of medical scholars.

19 *De simplicibus medicinis laxativis*, which contains thirty-five herbs arranged in alphabetical order, each accompanied by recipes and advice on storage and use, is extant in only one version found in the fifteenth-century manuscript, Copenhagen, Det Kongelige Bibliotek, MS GKS 1654 4to. The *Liber herbarum* is a herbal containing fifty-three herbs, along with their medical uses and qualities. It is based on the teachings of the Salernitan School. *Den danske urtebog* (The Danish book of herbs) is a reference pharmacopoeia, the main sources of which are Constantinus Africanus' *De gradibus liber* and Floridus Macer's *De viribus herbarum*.

reflect the holdings of scientific and medical manuscripts in twelfth-century Scandinavian cathedral libraries, which included works by Marbod of Rennes and Macer Floridus, as well as the *Antidotarium Nicolai* and Galen's *Microtegni* and *De simplicium medicamentorum*.

The number of medical manuscripts still extant from medieval Scandinavia is small, with many overlapping texts and sources among the surviving manuscripts and fragments. The majority of this corpus, which derives mainly from Denmark and Iceland,[20] is still unedited or in need of revisitation, as is the case for the early twentieth-century editions of Copenhagen, Den Arnamagnæanske Samling 194 8vo and Dublin, RIA, MS 23 D 43. The latter, a manuscript of the late fifteenth century, is the largest surviving Old Icelandic medical manuscript and contains translations into Old Icelandic of the *Liber lapidum*, the *Antidotarium Nicolai* and Harpestræng's *Liber herbarum*.[21] This last item is a leechbook for which an exact source is still to be found, but which shares similarities with other Icelandic and Danish leechbooks (such as Copenhagen, Den Arnamagnæanske Samling, MSS AM 655 XXX 4to, AM 194 8vo, and AM 187 8vo; and Copenhagen, Den Arnamagnæanske Samling, MS AM 434a 12mo).[22] Dublin, RIA, MS 23 D 43 also contains a cookbook that is derived from a Danish original, most probably from the cookbook in fourteenth-century manuscript Copenhagen, Det Kongelige Bibliotek, Ny kgl. Samling 66 8vo.[23] The extant corpus of Norse medical manuscripts and fragments, along with marginalia and literary texts,[24] suggests that the circulation of medical knowledge in Scandinavia precedes the manuscript evidence, depicting the periphery of the medieval North Atlantic world as a place of medical learning and practice that is yet to be fully explored.

In comparative terms, English-language sources have fared somewhat better than medical works in other vernaculars as a subject of enquiry by modern scholars. Since they were first published by Oswald Cockayne in the second half of the nineteenth century, much ink has been spilt on elucidating

20 Norse medical texts from Norway and Sweden have been less researched, mainly due to the limited survival of manuscripts. Of interest here are Oslo, Chr. Kath. Bibliothek, MS NB 8vo 3725, the oldest Norwegian Black Book dated to *c.* 1480 (commonly known as *Vinjeboka*), as well as many scientific and medical manuscript fragments (Etheridge, 'Medieval Scientific Book Fragments') and the Swedish leechbook Linköping, Stiftsb., MS M5 (*c.* 1500).

21 See *An Old Icelandic Medical Miscellany*, ed. and trans. by Larsen.

22 On this last, see *Den islandske lægebog*, ed. by Kålund, and *Norse Magical and Herbal Healing*, trans. by Waggoner.

23 Marginalia in Dublin, RIA, MS 23 D 43 provides evidence that the manuscript was transcribed, or at least held and used in Iceland, with references to sites in the north of Iceland where one could find certain herbs listed in the herbal.

24 For instance, in *Hrafns saga Sveinbjarnarsonar*, Hrafn (d. 1213) — an Icelandic chieftain, pilgrim and doctor — is said to be a descendant of a lineage of doctors which started in 1043; see also Kaiser, *Krankheit und Krankheitsbewältigung*, and the healing miracles in the *Biskupa sögur* (see *Biskupa sögur* I, ed. by Foote, and *Biskupa sögur* II, ed. by Egilsdóttir).

and contextualizing the earliest English compilations of remedies such as *Bald's Leechbook*, *Leechbook* III, and the *Lacnunga*, as well as the so-called *Herbarium* complex, consisting of the herbal attributed to Apuleius Platonicus, Pseudo-Dioscorides' *De herbis feminis*, and various other short texts on the medicinal uses of plants, animals, and minerals.[25] Old English charms and ritual remedies have received particular attention in various edited collections and scholarly monographs, several of which seek to demonstrate the manifold connections between such cures and other aspects of medieval English literary and religious culture.[26] A substantial number of Middle English medical texts have likewise now appeared in modern editions.[27]

Largely thanks to the work of Tony Hunt, a considerable range of medical texts written in Anglo-French has come to light in the last three decades, including a translations of material related to the *Trotula* collection of texts on women's health, treatises on surgery and visiting the sick, and collections of medical remedies in prose and verse form.[28] Many of these works have served as the basis for lexicographical tools and further research on specific semantic domains, such as plant names, or have shed light on connections between different vernaculars of the Insular world.[29] Although some of the surviving medieval Welsh medical texts — which consist largely of remedy collections — were published in the nineteenth and early twentieth centuries, this work has now been superseded by Diana Luft's more modern and comprehensive edition, translation and analysis of those collections, the first instalment of

25 *Leechdoms*, ed. and trans. by Cockayne; for more recent editions and translations of some of these texts, see *The Old English Herbarium*, ed. by de Vriend; *Anglo-Saxon Remedies*, ed. and trans. by Pettit; *Medieval Herbal Remedies*, trans. by Van Arsdall; and *Medical Writings*, ed. by Niles and D'Aronco. A recent monograph on the Old English medical texts within the framework of wider literary culture is Kesling, *Medical Texts*.

26 See e.g. *Anglo-Saxon Magic*, ed. and trans. by Storms and 'The Anglo-Saxon Charms', ed. by Grendon. More recent monograph studies include Jolly, *Popular Religion*; Arnovick, *Written Reliquaries*; and Arthur, *'Charms', Liturgies, and Secret Rites*.

27 The bibliography is too voluminous to list in full here, but useful accounts can be found in Robbins, 'Medical Manuscripts in Middle English'; Voigts, 'Multitudes'; and Pahta and Taavitsainen, 'Vernacularisation'. Examples of edited English medical texts from this later period include 'A Latin Technical Phlebotomy', ed. by Voigts and McVaugh; *Healing and Society in Medieval England*, ed. by Getz; Henry Daniel, *Liber Uricrisiarum*, ed. by Harvey, Tavormina and Star; *A Middle English Medical Remedy Book*, ed. by Alonso Almeida; *Agnus Castus*, ed. by Brodin; *A Late Middle English Remedybook*, ed. by Calle-Martin and Castaño-Gil; *A Leechbook*, ed. and trans. by Dawson; Lanfranc of Milan, *Lanfranck's 'Science of Cirurgie'*, ed. by Fleischhacker; 'Middle English Rimed Medical Treatise', ed. by Garrett; and *The 'Liber de Diversis Medicinis'*, ed. by Ogden.

28 See, for example, Hunt, *The Medieval Surgery*, as well as his editions of texts in *Popular Medicine*, *Anglo-Norman Medicine*, as well as *Three Receptaria*, ed. by Hunt and Benskin.

29 See e.g. Hunt, *Plant Names*. One of the texts published by Hunt (*Popular Medicine*, pp. 217–63), found in BL, Add. MS 15236, is a collection of botanical, medical, and prognostic texts copied around 1300, and which are 'noteworthy for a number of Irish glosses which they contain' (p. 217). On the contribution of vernacular medical texts for online lexicographical tools for Anglo-Norman French and Middle English, see below, p. 35.

which was published in 2020.[30] The availability of this more expansive corpus of Welsh material in a modern edition will allow scholars to build significantly on earlier discussions of Welsh medical tradition, which have sought to situate it within the wider context of the literary culture, translation practices, and legal learning of that region.[31] In the scholarly commentary accompanying her edition, Luft also notes numerous analogues between Welsh, English, and Anglo-French medical learning, thus demonstrating the potential of this material to add to our understanding of cross-linguistic and cross-cultural exchange in Britain during the later medieval period.

Medical manuscripts written in the Gaelic vernaculars far outnumber those which have come down to us from medieval Wales, but the vast majority of this material remains unedited or in need of revisitation in light of more recent scholarship on medical traditions across western Europe. In the medieval and early modern periods, professional medicine in Ireland and Gaelic-speaking Scotland was, like other vocations such as poetry, law and history, the preserve of several learned families who exercised their occupation on a hereditary basis and often received land tenure in exchange for the services they provided to their aristocratic patrons.[32] Medical scholars in this region are also known to have been responsible for the organization and regulation of schools, a primary function of which was to compile texts for educational and reference purposes. The extant corpus of manuscripts produced by these individuals, which comprises more than 120 separate codices, includes works dealing with a wide range of topics such as anatomy, disease, herbalism, and preventive medicine, many of which are translations or adaptations of well-known Latin treatises used in the curricula of the early continental universities. Comments regarding practising physicians found in the colophons and marginalia to the Gaelic-language medical manuscripts also suggest, however, that while some Irish and Scottish doctors evidently travelled to study at centres of learning on the European continent, a medical education received at home was, in at least some cases, regarded as an equally worthwhile accomplishment and in no way an impediment to professional advancement.[33] Such observations raise

30 *Medieval Welsh Medical Texts*, ed. and trans. by Luft. For earlier editions of some of this material, see *The Physicians of Myddvai*, ed. and trans. by Williams and Pughe; *Le plus ancien texte*, ed. and trans. by Diverres; and 'Hafod 16', ed. and trans. by Jones.

31 Morfydd Owen has published several contributions on Welsh medicine, many focusing on aspects of its legal context: see e.g. Owen, 'Meddygon Myddfai'; 'The Medical Books of Medieval Wales'; 'Medics and Medicine'; 'Names for Sicknesses and Disease'; and 'The Doctor in the Laws of Hywel'. Another valuable contribution to the study of medieval Welsh medical writing and translation practices is Parina, 'Medical Texts in Welsh Translation'.

32 Nic Dhonnchadha, 'Medical Writing in Irish', 217; on the role of hereditary medical families in this region, see also the more recent discussions in Ó Muraíle, 'The Hereditary Medical Families' and Sheehan, 'Locating the Gaelic Medical Families'.

33 Nic Dhonnchadha, 'Medical Writing in Irish', p. 217. For examples of Irish medical scholars who received their education in the early continental universities, see Hayes, 'Irish Medical Links with the Continent'.

interesting, but as yet largely unanswered, questions about what the medical texts themselves might reveal concerning the nature of medical education, as well as of Latin and vernacular literacy, in Ireland and Gaelic-speaking Scotland during the late-medieval period.[34]

One of the most prolific scholars to have published in the area of Irish medical learning was Winifred Wulff, who edited the Irish translation of the *Rosa Anglica* by the Oxford physician John of Gaddesden along with several other texts of varying lengths on topics such as plague, surgery, deontology, lovesickness, and gynaecology.[35] In subsequent decades, other scholars published Irish-language renderings of Latin treatises on subjects such as fevers, pharmacy, health regimen, physiognomy, and veterinary medicine,[36] while the Irish medical glossary tradition and a major Irish treatise on *materia medica* have also received attention.[37] The most recent Gaelic-language medical texts to be made available to a modern readership include translations and adaptations of Latin works by known authors on a range of topics, such as anatomy, physiology, skin disease, and surgery,[38] and scholarly studies of some published medical texts have revealed the extent to which their authors compiled and reworked material from various sources to form new treatises, often with practical aims in mind.[39] Significant progress has also been made in the cataloguing of medical manuscripts in the Gaelic languages, many of which are now digitized and easily accessible in open-access databases.[40] In

---

34 For preliminary remarks on this subject, see Harris, 'Latin Learning and Irish Physicians' and Hayden, '*Auraicept na nÉces*'.

35 See e.g. *Rosa anglica*; 'Tract on the Plague'; 'On the Qualitees'; 'De amore hereos' and *A Mediaeval Handbook*, all ed. by Wulff. The manuscript tradition of the Irish *Rosa anglica* has more recently been revisited by Nic Dhonnchadha, 'The Irish *Rosa Anglica*'.

36 See, for example, 'A Treatise on Fevers', ed. by Duncan; *An Irish Version of Gualterus 'De Dosibus'*, ed. by Sheahan; *Regimen sanitatis*, ed. and trans. by Gillies; *Regimen na sláinte*, ed. by Ó Ceithearnaigh; 'Rudimenta physionomiae', ed. by Mac Niocaill; and 'Fragments of Two Mediaeval Treatises on Horses' and 'Fragments of Irish Medieval Treatises on Horses', both ed. and trans. by Ó Cuív.

37 On Irish medical glossaries, see e.g. 'Three Irish Medical Glossaries', ed. by Stokes; these texts were also the focus of a more recent Irish Research Council Postdoctoral Fellowship held at Maynooth University by Dr Siobhán Barrett from 2021–2023 (Grant agreement no. GOIPD/2020/341). An edition and translation of a fifteenth-century Irish treatise on *materia medica* has recently been published online: see Tadhg Ó Cuinn, *An Irish Materia Medica*, ed. and trans. by Ó Conchubhair, and also the chapter by Brigid Mayes in this volume.

38 See e.g. 'Téacs ó scoil leighis' and '"On Stretching and Yawning"', ed. by Nic Dhonnchadha; *Anathomia Gydo*, ed. and trans. by Ní Ghallchobhair; and 'A Text Preserved at the Aghmacart Medical School', ed. by Faerber.

39 See, for example, Nic Dhonnchadha, 'The Irish *Rosa Anglica*' and 'Tráchtas leighis ón 14ú haois' (on a fourteenth-century anatomical treatise based on various Latin sources, including the *Anatomia Galeni [Anatomia Ricardi]*, the *Compendium medicine* of Gilbertus Anglicus, and Galen's *Tegni*).

40 The majority of the Gaelic-language medical manuscripts can now be viewed on ISOS, which also includes digital versions of printed catalogues as well as several new or updated catalogue entries produced by Dr Aoibheann Nic Dhonnchadha of the Dublin Institute

stark contrast to the orientation of much scholarship on the medical traditions of other vernaculars in the medieval North Atlantic world, however, the substantial collections of remedies extant in the Gaelic-language medical manuscripts have been largely neglected, with editions of some of this material only recently appearing in print.[41]

In spite of these important contributions, however, the topic of medical learning has often remained at the periphery of scholarly debates concerning the textual culture of the medieval Gaelic world on the one hand, and of medieval European medicine on the other. Studies of medical practice in Ireland during the pre-Norman period have focused almost exclusively on either a handful of charms and protective spells that survive in early medieval sources or on the contents of medico-legal texts concerning payment for injuries and sick-maintenance that have been dated to the mid-seventh century.[42] In the preface to his 1966 edition of *Bretha Déin Chécht*, an Old Irish law tract on the payments due to a physician for various types of injuries, D. A. Binchy stated that the surviving Irish vernacular written corpus does not preserve 'a single record of pre-Arabic medicine, whether indigenous or borrowed. We have nothing like the Anglo-Saxon leechdoms to throw light on the theory and practice of the earlier medicine, nothing beyond a few fragmentary incantations'.[43] It is worth pointing out, however, that the only extant copies of the seventh-century medico-legal texts which were the focus of Binchy's editorial endeavours are found in a medical manuscript of the fifteenth century (Dublin, NLI, MS G11), most of which is as yet unpublished — leading one to question whether his claim has yet to stand the test of the wealth of as-yet unexamined medical material.[44] Indeed, research published in the last decade has begun to paint a more complex picture of the surviving evidence for this written genre, pointing to the influence on Irish material of medical writing in contemporary vernacular traditions such as English, Anglo-French, and Welsh, as well as to the manifold ways in which Irish-language medical writing was intertwined with vernacular literary production stemming from a much earlier period, including Old

---

for Advanced Studies, as well as Ronald Black's unpublished catalogue entries for medical manuscripts in the National Library of Scotland.

41 For example, 'A Short Tract', ed. and trans. by De Vries, examines a collection of zootherapeutical cures, while Hayden, 'A Sixteenth-century Irish Collection' brings to light a collection of remedies for andrological ailments. On the value of this genre of material more generally, highlighting some correspondences between medicinal remedies in Irish and other vernaculars of the Insular world, see Hayden, 'Textual Transfer'.

42 On the law texts, see 'Bretha crólige' and 'Bretha Déin Chécht', both ed. and trans. by Binchy, as well as his 'Sick-Maintenance in Irish Law'. For recent surveys of scholarship on Irish charms and charming tradition, see Tuomi and others, eds, *Charms, Charmers and Charming in Ireland* and Hayden, 'Old English in the Irish Charms'.

43 'Bretha Déin Chécht', ed. and trans. by Binchy, p. 5. For a similar claim, see Davies, 'The Place of Healing', p. 43.

44 For similar observations, see Hayden, 'Old English in the Irish Charms', pp. 351–55.

Irish hagiographical, liturgical, and penitential texts, grammar and verse composition, legal writing, and narrative literature.[45]

The study of the reception and transmission of medical knowledge in medieval Scandinavia has seen a revival in recent years, mainly through linguistic and manuscript studies that have focused on the provenance of Old Norse medical and nature-related terminology and provided an overview of scientific and medical manuscript holdings in cathedral schools, universities, and in private libraries in Scandinavia.[46] These studies are a welcome addition to the now outdated research that was undertaken in the nineteenth and early twentieth centuries by Finnur Jónsson, Fredrik Grøn, Gustaf Klemming, Kristian Kålund, and Henning Larsen.[47] Since the second half of the twentieth century, scholarship has focused on the portrayal of various illnesses, medicine, and medical practices in Old Norse literature, for instance in *Hrafns saga Sveinbjarnarsonar*, in the *Biskupasögur* and more generally in the *Íslendingasögur*. However, even though this work has been fundamental for opening the doors to reading the sagas through the lens of medical knowledge, it tends to shed light only on general ideas on medicine and medical knowledge in the Middle Ages. The central point of such discussions has been mainly on retrospective diagnosis, or, when dealing with healing charms, on setting them in the context of previous studies relating to magic and the use of medieval *grimoires*.[48] These views have been challenged more recently, highlighting the necessity of revisiting the outdated view that the periphery of Europe was unaware of the medical knowledge being produced and transmitted across the medieval North Atlantic world and the European continent more widely.[49] These new studies have focused on the evidence from other contemporary vernacular texts, as well as recent scholarship on the Islamic and western medical traditions. More research needs to be undertaken and more medical manuscripts and fragments need to be revisited and edited

45 See e.g. Barrett, 'King of Dál nAraide's Salve'; Hayden, '*Auraicept na nÉces*', 'Attribution and Authority', 'Observations on the "Doors of Death"', 'A Sixteenth-century Irish Collection' and 'Three Versified Medical Recipes'; and De Vries, 'Medieval Medicine'.

46 See e.g. Etheridge, 'Transmission and Reception of Science' and 'Medieval Scientific Book Fragments'; Heizmann, *Wörterbuch der Pflanzennamen*; Schwabe, 'Den norrøne legemiddelboktradisjonen'; and Tarsi, 'Loanwords and Native Words'.

47 See e.g. Finnur Jónsson, *Lægekunsten i den nordiske oldtid*; Grøn, *Altnordische Heilkunde*; *Läke- och örte-böcker*, ed. by Klemming; and *An Old Icelandic Medical Miscellany*, ed. by Larsen.

48 See e.g. *Hrafns Saga Sveinbjarnarsonar*, ed. and trans. by Guðrún P. Helgadóttir; Kaiser, *Krankheit und Krankheitsbewältigung*; Ledderose, *Heilkundige Männer und Frauen*; Maraschi, *Similia similibus curantur* and 'Sympathetic Graphophagy'; McDougall, 'The Third Instrument of Medicine'; Mitchell, *Witchcraft and Magic*, 'Leechbooks, Manuals, and Grimoires' and 'Faith and Knowledge in Nordic Charm Magic'; Whaley, 'Miracles in the *Biskupa sögur*'; and Whaley and Elliot, 'Dupuytren's Disease'.

49 See e.g. Arkomani, 'The Best Drink a Girl Can Get'; Brynja Þorgeirsdóttir, 'Humoral Theory in the Medieval North' and '"*Eyrsilfr drukkit, þat gerir bana*"'; Baccianti, 'Guaritori, acqua santa e latte materno' and 'Healing Hands, Holy Water, and Hellish Diseases'.

in order to further understand the movement of knowledge, scholars and manuscripts in Scandinavia.

This necessarily selective summary of the state of research on vernacular medical texts of the medieval North Atlantic world demonstrates that much valuable work has been carried out to date on sources from various linguistic traditions, exploring not only their inheritance from and engagement with Latin source-material, but also aspects of lexicography, intellectual history and literary context. It can be argued, however, that much can yet be gained from approaching these traditions within a more comparative framework. In a discussion of the vernacularization of science, medicine, and technology in European cultures of the later Middle Ages that was published over two decades ago, William Crossgrove observed that 'The compartmentalization of philological traditions by languages and language families unfortunately often leads scholars working in one language to be relatively unaware of work in other traditions'.[50] The same scholar also emphasized, however, the potential for digital resources to facilitate cross-linguistic comparison and thereby move the field forward in exciting ways, noting in particular the need for 'repertoria' of vernacular manuscripts akin to that which had, at the time, only recently been produced for English sources by Linda Ehrsam Voigts and Patricia Deery Kurtz. The so-called 'eVK' was intended as a companion to the electronic version of Lynn Thorndike and Pearl Kibre's *Catalogue of Incipits of Mediaeval Scientific Writings in Latin* (eTK), with the aim of assisting scholars in locating manuscript witnesses to English vernacular medical and scientific texts.[51] It has since been enriched by publication of the electronic corpus of *Middle English Medical Texts* (MEMT), which includes eighty-six texts and 496,322 words from three traditions of medical writing (surgical treatises, specialized texts, and remedy books).[52] Such tools have provided a crucial foundation for further historical and linguistic research, both because they enable the relatively small number of scholars working in this field to investigate much larger manuscript corpora and thereby identify new patterns and questions. A comparable 'electronic repertorium' of Gaelic-language medical sources is currently being produced at Maynooth University under the auspices of the project *Language, Education and Medical Learning in the Premodern Gaelic World* (LEIGHEAS), which runs from 2022–2026.[53] The

50 Crossgrove, 'The Vernacularization', p. 47.

51 Crossgrove, 'The Vernacularization', p. 60, referring to *Scientific and Medical Writings in Old and Middle English*, ed. by Voigts and Kurtz. This resource records information on texts surviving in nearly 2000 manuscripts held in libraries and private collections in 15 countries and has more recently been supplemented by a searchable bibliography and name list of variant spellings of authors' names (eVK2).

52 See *An Electronic Corpus of Middle English Medical Texts*, ed. by Taavitsainen, Pahta, and Mäkinen.

53 Funded by a Consolidator Laureate Award from Research Ireland (grant agreement no. IRCLA/2022/2922; PI Dr Deborah Hayden); see <https://leigheas.maynoothuniversity.ie> [accessed 4 June 2024].

inclusion of citations from vernacular medical texts in electronic dictionaries, as well as continuing work on the digitization of manuscript sources, has also facilitated the study of technical terminology and the identification of connections across different texts.[54]

Overview of Contents

By exploring aspects of the translation, transmission, and cultural significance of medical texts and ideas in English, Celtic, and Scandinavian traditions, the contributions to this volume represent one small step forward in fostering greater dialogue between scholars working on the various vernacular literary traditions of the Insular world. The collection does not purport to be comprehensive, however: it should be noted, for example, that much insight into the development of medical learning in this region can yet be gained by engaging further with specialists working on Anglo-French texts, and indeed several of the contributions to this collection acknowledge their debt to past scholarship in this area. Many chapters also highlight the manifold connections between medical learning evidenced in the vernacular languages of the Insular world and the wider intellectual context from which that learning arose — one that extended far beyond the geographical boundaries of the medieval North to encompass the whole of Europe and the Islamicate world.

The volume is divided into three main sections, with the component chapters of each section arranged in a broadly chronological way but with a view to highlighting both thematic interconnections and cultural contacts across different linguistic traditions. The first section focuses on ideas about medicine and the body manifested in medical texts as well as other written genres, such as narrative literature and law tracts. Conan T. Doyle's chapter is placed first because it explores some of the earliest surviving vernacular evidence for humoral theory, which, as noted above, was one of the core tenets of human physiology upon which medieval medical thought more generally was founded. Focusing on Old English medical texts and their inheritance from Latin medical literature of late antiquity and the early Middle Ages, Doyle demonstrates that the theory of the four humours finds its most explicit early Insular iterations not in texts that are specifically medical in content, but rather in the computistical and natural historical writings of Bede, Byrhtferth of Ramsey, and Ælfric of Eynsham. The Old English medical sources themselves, moreover, rely on epistemologically diverse material, ranging from the folk remedies of Pliny the Elder and Marcellus Empiricus to the encyclopaedic

54 Relevant examples of such lexicographical tools include the *electronic Dictionary of the Irish Language* (eDIL <www.dil.ie>), the online *Anglo-Norman Dictionary* <http://anglo-norman.net>, and the Middle English Dictionary hosted by the University of Michigan <https://quod.lib.umich.edu/m/middle-english-dictionary/dictionary>.

works of Oribasius and the *Practica* of Alexander Trallianus. Doyle argues that the Old English compilation of remedies known as 'Bald's Leechbook' provides the most significant amount of evidence for the study of humoral theory in early medieval England and suggests that this collection presents the framework with a remarkably consistent lexis despite the plurality of sources from which it was compiled.

Elisa Ramazzina's chapter extends the chronological scope of Doyle's study of Old English sources by examining the development of bathing practices in medieval England not only through the lens of remedy collections such as *Bald's Leechbook* and the *Lacnunga*, but also of later treatises such as the Middle English translations of the *Secreta secretorum* and the *Compendium medicinae* by Gilbertus Anglicus. Ramazzina suggests that references to bathing in the earliest extant English medical sources, though they typically appear in a succinct and somewhat schematic form, nonetheless point to knowledge of humoral theory and can be closely linked to ideas about diet as evidenced in texts aimed at a monastic audience, such as the Benedictine *Rule*. She further argues that sources composed in Middle English, which were clearly influenced by sources emanating from continental centres of learning that emerged only in the later Middle Ages, suggest that bathing had come to play an increasingly vital role in healing practices during this period. One result of this development is that, unlike in the earlier works, medical treatises in Middle English are sometimes found to contain distinct sections devoted specifically to baths and their therapeutic virtues.

Anne Irene Riisøy then turns our attention to the legal dimension of medical practice with a discussion of the earliest Norwegian laws concerning compensation for bodily harm. The study of early medieval laws relating to injury and care of the sick is a comparatively well-established method for exploring ideas about medical learning in the medieval North, as has previously been demonstrated, for example, by D. A. Binchy's work on the extant Old Irish medico-legal tracts, noted above, and by studies of comparable material in Welsh and Germanic traditions by Morfydd Owen and Lisi Oliver, respectively.[55] In extending Oliver's work on Germanic regulations for bodily harm to encompass the earliest Norwegian legal material, however, Riisøy introduces further valuable comparanda for our understanding of how bodily injuries were compensated and cared for in various parts of the early medieval world.

Although no Irish medical texts survive in contemporary manuscripts of the early and central Middle Ages, Ranke de Vries argues that we can gain indirect glimpses of the circulation of ideas concerning medieval medical

55 For the Irish material, see 'Bretha Déin Chécht', ed. and trans. by Binchy; 'Bretha crólige', ed. and trans. by Binchy; and 'Di ércib fola', ed. and trans. by McLeod, as well as Binchy, 'Sick-Maintenance in Irish Law'. The Welsh laws pertaining to medicine and medical personnel are treated in Owen, 'Medics and Medicine', while Germanic tradition is discussed in Oliver, *The Body Legal* and Wormald, 'The *Leges Barbarorum*'.

theory in this region by examining medieval Irish saga literature from a medical perspective. Her discussion focuses on three narrative episodes depicting brain injury and its subsequent treatment: the leaking brains of Cormac Cas from the thirteenth-century compilation *Acallam na Senórach* (The conversation of the old men); Conán's head worm, found in the same text; and Cenn Fáelad's loss of his brain of forgetfulness as featured in the late Middle Irish or Early Modern Irish version of the text *Cath Maige Rath* (The Battle of Mag Rath), dated to the thirteenth or fourteenth century. De Vries suggests that, while elements in the Irish tales that contain these injuries may have subsequently been embellished, exaggerated, reinterpreted, or used in an allegorical sense, all three of the examples in question can be found have a solid foundation in European and Arabic medieval medical teaching regarding the anatomy and function of the brain.

The depiction and perception of the human brain in Irish literary evidence is also the focus of Viktoriia Krivoshchekova's chapter, which explores ideas concerning embodied cognition reflected in these sources. Cognition is a comparatively little-studied area of medieval Irish intellectual history, but as Wendy Turner has recently pointed out in a study of this theme from a wider European perspective, medical understanding of the mind formed a key component of medieval theories concerning the physiological care of the brain, the religious implications of thought and legal opinions on intent.[56] Krivoshchekova takes a crucial step in the direction of drawing Irish material into these wider debates on the role of the brain and cognition in medical thought by focusing on the ways in which metaphors of embodiment were used to describe the work of the mind. The first part of her study examines two vernacular poems that represent cognition by means of literary metaphor comparing the mind to a body, while the second traces similar metaphorical mappings in conventional language using a larger corpus of Old Irish texts. Krivoshchekova thus seeks to demonstrate how the methodological insights of cognitive linguistics and complex network theory can be combined in order to shed light on the ways in which Irish texts conceptualize the mind through bodily experiences.

The next three chapters in the first section deal with aspects of *materia medica* and pharmacological learning in manuscripts from England and Ireland. Erin Connelly and Christina Lee examine a selection of nettle remedies in English medical texts from the early to later medieval periods with a view to illustrating how this ingredient was used medicinally across time and in different social settings. They also consider the implications that their case study may have for modern research, where nettles largely are applied in cosmetics and for wound care. Laura Poggesi similarly considers the significance of medical recipes in Middle English sources, focusing on a

56 Turner, 'Mind/Brain', p. 156.

comparison of two mid-fifteenth-century manuscripts that appear to have been made for different purposes: one being an anthology of material from various genres that may have been addressed to a woman, and the other a medical compendium containing more than forty texts on medical and scientific topics that seems to have belonged to a medical practitioner. Poggesi seeks both to interpret the discrepancies found among the recipes shared by the two manuscripts in question on the basis of their supposed target audiences, and to explore the extent to which practical medical knowledge in late medieval England constituted a common heritage shared by both specialists and lay people.

The study by Brigid Mayes offers a useful Irish comparandum for these discussions of pharmacological learning in England, since it focuses on the large collection of *materia medica* compiled by the fifteenth-century Irish scholar Tadhg Ó Cuinn. This work, one copy of which was edited and translated by Mícheál Ó Conchubhair in 1991, consists of 292 chapters explaining the uses and properties of various pharmacological ingredients, the majority of which are plants.[57] Mayes argues that this text, which enjoyed a wide circulation in many other late-medieval Irish manuscripts, was a landmark work in the history of plant-based medicine in Ireland and sheds light on the nexus between theory and practice in that region. Her case study of the text focuses on Ó Cuinn's treatment of two species of Plantago (Plantago major and Plantago minor), known in Irish as *crúach Pádraig* and *slánlus*, both of which have a long and widespread history of medical use. Mayes examines Ó Cuinn's indications for these plants, the ways in which their use is validated by reference to Galenic theory, and the resonances of the text in other traditions and periods.

The first section is brought to a conclusion with Christian Etheridge's in-depth examination of the role of cathedrals in the reception and dissemination of scientific knowledge in medieval Scandinavia. Etheridge demonstrates that, although there were no universities in Scandinavia until the late fifteenth century, it is nonetheless possible to trace the activities of several scholars from this region who studied or taught at universities in England or on the European continent from the thirteenth century onwards, as well as in cathedrals and monastic schools during the twelfth century. Many of these scholars subsequently returned home to Scandinavia, and a small but significant number even wrote their own scientific treatises, some of which were widely dispersed across Europe. Drawing on the evidence of surviving manuscripts, incunabula and booklists, Etheridge's chapter offers a much-needed systematic survey of the evidence for scientific activity in the cathedrals of medieval Scandinavia and of the connections that obtained between this geographically peripheral region and the broader European sphere.

---

57 Tadhg Ó Cuinn, 'An Irish *Materia medica*', ed. and trans. by Ó Conchubhair.

The second section of the volume comprises five papers that explore aspects of the lexicography of medicine and scientific knowledge in the Insular Middle Ages. While an emphasis on Irish material here reflects the philological focus of much past and current scholarship on the Celtic languages more generally, the chapters nonetheless collectively highlight questions concerning multilingualism, translation and the importance of examining parallel developments in technical terminology for our understanding of cultural contacts and textual transmission across a range of languages. Joseph J. Flahive's chapter opens the section by highlighting the usefulness of lexicography as a tool for measuring the circulation of medical knowledge in Ireland during the early medieval period, despite the absence of direct evidence for such learning in the form of extant Old Irish medical texts. His contribution surveys words used in technically medical senses that have been identified in the work of the Dictionary of Medieval Latin from Celtic Sources from the digital *Archive of Celtic Latin Literature* and explores the extent to which this Celtic-Latin medical vocabulary fell within the European mainstream of late antique literature. Flahive also seeks to identify possible sources from which this vocabulary may have been drawn and attempts to analyse the etymological background of non-standard lexemes, while also considering the possible motivations for coining such vocabulary.

Sharon Arbuthnot's chapter complements Flahive's study by offering a preliminary investigation of the methods employed by medieval Irish scholars of the later medieval period to create a serviceable 'medicalese'. Arbuthnot argues that translations of medical texts into Irish are broadly in keeping with those produced elsewhere in Europe between the fourteenth and sixteenth centuries, a point which is evidenced by her examination of a sample of medieval Irish medical terminology that attests to linguistic processes such as borrowing, hybridization, calquing, repurposing, and suffixation. This case study not only highlights a dynamic period of linguistic innovation in the history of the Gaelic languages, but also lays some crucial groundwork for further research into a possible area of interplay between the various vernaculars in use in Ireland in the late Middle Ages.

The theme of cultural contacts evidenced in the realm of scientific lexicography is reprised in the following chapter by Siobhán Barrett, which examines the Irish reflexes of an important sub-genre of medical text: namely, glossaries. Barrett's discussion focuses on an early sixteenth-century medico-botanical glossary, preserved in an Irish medical manuscript now kept at the University of Oxford, that lists the Latin names of *materia medica* alongside synonyms in English and French. Although the Irish language is mainly used in this source to provide descriptions of a given substance or points of clarification, Barrett observes that the absence of Irish names for medicinal substances is a surprising idiosyncrasy in the context of Irish glossary-compilation more generally. She also argues that the text in question sheds light on the meaning of words found in other glossaries and thus provides important evidence for the multilingual environment in which the physicians of medieval Ireland operated.

Matteo Tarsi's chapter turns our attention to medical tradition in late-medieval Scandinavia with an analysis of lexical synonymic pairs from the semantic fields of medical and nature-related terminology found in the extant Icelandic medical manuscripts. After providing an overview of methodology for lexicographic research in this area and a survey of the relevant terminology, he offers a case study that considers an example of lexical corruption in an Old Norse cure for kidney stones drawn from the popular Salernitan medical text known as the *Antidotarium Nicolai*. Eystein Thanisch's chapter then concludes the section on lexicography by exploring how technical terminology relating to science and medicine came to form the basis for structured collections of definitions, propositions and aphorisms that could be used for pedagogical and reference purposes. Thanisch surveys the evidence for such literature in the medical sources of medieval Ireland and Gaelic-speaking Scotland, focusing on two manuscript collections that provide evidence of scribal connections between these regions. The definitions in question establish scientific classifications of concepts and phenomena relevant to medicine, particularly pathology and anatomy, with reference to key ontological categories such as species, genus, and properties. Thanisch argues that such collections of definitions, which have received little attention in previous scholarship on the Gaelic-language medical texts, represented an attempt to encapsulate the essentials of medicine and formed the basis for argumentation in other medical texts, thus making them a valuable source for our understanding of the study of medicine in the medieval Gaelic world.

As noted above, research on the history of medicine has long recognized the wide range of healing practices that formed part of the so-called 'medical marketplace' of both the early and later Middle Ages, where natural medicine based on rational principles was often closely intertwined with Christian spiritual practices. As Peter Murray Jones and Lea Olsan have observed, however, 'There has been a strong temptation in twentieth-century scholarship on medicine to try to separate healing into categories defined as rational (usually scholastic medicine), religious (employing prayer, and the intercessory power attributed to the Virgin Mary and the saints) and magical (amulets, spells, charms)', even though these modern paradigms often do not adequately reflect medieval practices of combining cures belonging to all three categories in textual miscellanies that were often highly pragmatic in nature.[58] Our decision to group together the studies in this volume that are devoted to medical cures that can be variously described as verbal charms, magical spells, textual amulets, or performative rituals is not intended as a dismissal of this important point concerning the nature of medieval medical practice.

58 Murray Jones and Olsan, 'Medicine and Magic', p. 299, drawing on Horden, 'What's Wrong with Early Medieval Medicine?'.

Rather, it seeks to reinforce it by juxtaposing discussion of the transmission and context for vernacular 'magical' and 'ritual' cures in texts from Ireland, Wales, England, and Scandinavia in a manner that highlights not only the common inheritance of these traditions as part of wider medical learning, but also the intriguing ways in which such remedies could be adapted to suit particular target audiences.

The first chapter in this third section, by Caroline R. Batten, examines aspects of the ritualized and incantatory remedies in the Old English medical corpus and demonstrates how such cures operate according to recognisable magical and semiotic principles of similarity ('like produces like') and opposition ('opposites work on opposites'). Batten argues, however, that these principles are employed in unusual and dramatic ways in Old English narrative charms designed to heal disease. The discussion focuses on two particular texts, namely the verse remedies known as 'Against a Dwarf' and 'The Nine Herbs Charm', which can be seen to combat the violation of the human body by nonhuman disease agents by harnessing, coercing, and co-opting ambivalent and monstrous forces to operate against one another, in a striking interpretation of the principle of similarity. Batten suggests that both of the charms in question invoke prelapsarian and eschatological Christian imagery as a source of oppositional power and a reminder that fleshly vulnerability was considered a temporary state for the faithful, ensuring the charmer's triumph over the micro- and macrocosmic forces that threaten the patient's body.

David Stifter then turns our gaze westward with his study of the small body of Old Irish magical texts, comprising healing charms, incantations, and protective spells, that survive in manuscripts of the eighth and ninth centuries. These texts are of particular importance for our understanding of the circulation of medical knowledge and charm traditions among Irish scholars during the early medieval period, but they have received relatively little attention due to the manifold challenges that they pose with regard to reading, translation, and content. Stifter's chapter provides a provisional new edition, based on personal inspection, high-resolution images and multispectral scanning, of the three charms in the Irish sacramentary known as the 'Stowe Missal' (Dublin, RIA, MS D ii 3 [1238]), accompanied by a translation and analysis of each text. He also introduces the four Old Irish incantations found on a single leaf from a manuscript in the monastery at St Gall, Switzerland (Stiftsbibliothek MS 1395, p. 419) and provides a linguistic and rhetorical-structural analysis of two further sources: one an Old Irish protective spell found in a manuscript fragment from Karlsruhe (Badische Landesbibliothek, MS Aug. Fr. 18) and the other an Old Irish incantation in the ninth-century scholar's notebook known as the 'Reichenau Primer' (St Paul im Lavanttal, Stiftsbibliothek, MS 86a/1).

The theme of ritual cures from Irish tradition of the later medieval period is treated in Deborah Hayden's chapter, which focuses on ideas about fertility and conception evidenced in the extant corpus of Irish medical manuscripts written between the fourteenth and sixteenth centuries. While much of this teaching can be connected to broader European learning transmitted in academic circles during this period, including commentaries on the Hippocratic *Aphorisms* and cures from the widely circulated Latin collection of texts on women's medicine known as the *Trotula*, some Irish rituals relating to fertility and conception show evidence of innovation and acculturation. The second half of Hayden's discussion focuses on the transmission and parallels for one particular ritual remedy that can be illuminated by reference to other medical, literary and folkloric sources from England and Wales that are concerned with conception.

Medieval Wales is also the focus of Katherine Leach's chapter, which turns our attention to the little-studied corpus of healing charms recorded in Welsh vernacular manuscripts during the later Middle Ages. While some charms from this tradition can be readily traced to wider, shared European charming traditions, such as the so-called 'Longinus' charm for staunching blood and the *Super Petram* charm for toothache, they also display innovations unique to the Welsh corpus, indicating that their scribes sought to shape certain conventions of the genre to suit specific cultural values and needs. Leach also discusses some Welsh charms that appear to have no direct parallels but nonetheless echo aspects of Latin and Germanic sources, however, such as a cure for scrofula found in at least two manuscripts. Her contribution thus provides an important case study from the Welsh perspective of the complex and multi-faceted ways in which healing charms operated across linguistic, religious and cultural boundaries as they were copied, adapted and disseminated.

Sarah Baccianti's chapter examines the late fifteenth- or early sixteenth-century Norse charm in Reykjavík, Lbs fragm., 14 1^{r}–1^{v}, commonly known as 'Kveisustrengurinn' (The colic leaf/string). This charm against various ailments was written in Old Norse, Latin, and Greek and belongs to the tradition of written charms that were worn for healing and protection from disease. Few prayer rolls that were used as wearable charms have survived from the Middle Ages, and '*Kveisustrengurinn*' is the only example still extant from medieval Iceland. Baccianti offers a discussion of this charm in the context of the corpus of extant healing charms from medieval Iceland and provides a new perspective on Norse medical knowledge that positions Iceland within the contemporary western European medical tradition.

The essays in this volume thus bring a range of perspectives and approaches to the study of the vernacular written traditions of the medieval North Atlantic world, but all centre on questions concerning the nature and scope of medical learning as a key facet of textual culture in that region. There is much work yet to be done on the editing and interpretation of unpublished medieval medical texts in all the vernacular languages in question, as well as on the Latin sources from which they drew. At the same time, many medical texts and works from other literary genres that are already available to scholars will no doubt benefit from revisitation using the comparative framework adopted here. It is hoped that the contents of this collection will help to stimulate further research into this rich and fascinating area of medieval intellectual culture.

Works Cited

Manuscripts

Carinthia, St Paul im Lavanttal, Stiftsbibliothek, MS 86a/1 ('The Reichenau Primer')
Copenhagen, Den Arnamagnæanske Samling, MS AM 187 8vo
Copenhagen, Den Arnamagnæanske Samling, MS AM 194 8vo
Copenhagen, Den Arnamagnæanske Samling, MS AM 434a 12mo
Copenhagen, Den Arnamagnæanske Samling, MS AM 655 XXX 4to
Copenhagen, Det Kongelige Bibliotek, MS GKS 1654 4to
Copenhagen, Det Kongelige Bibliotek, MS Ny kgl. Samling 66 8vo
Dublin, National Library of Ireland, MS G11
Dublin, Royal Irish Academy, MS D ii 3 (1238) ('The Stowe Missal')
Dublin, Royal Irish Academy, MS 23 D 43
Karlsruhe, Badische Landesbibliothek, MS Aug. Fr. 18
Linköping, Stiftsbibliotek, MS M5
Oslo, Christiania Kathedralskoles Bibliothek, MS NB 8vo 3725 ('Vinjeboka')
Reykjavík, Landsbókasafn Íslands, MS Lbs fragm. 14
St Gall, Stiftsbibliothek, MS 1395

Primary Sources

Agnus Castus: A Middle English Herbal, ed. by Gösta Brodin (Uppsala: Uppsala University Press, 1950)
Anathomia Gydo, ed. and trans. by Eithne Ní Ghallchobhair, Irish Texts Society, 66 (London: Irish Texts Society, 2014)
Anglo-Norman Medicine, ed. by Tony Hunt, 2 vols (Cambridge: D. S. Brewer, 1997)
'The Anglo-Saxon Charms', ed. by Felix Grendon, *The Journal of American Folklore*, 22 (1909), 105–237
Anglo-Saxon Magic, ed. by Godfrid Storms (The Hague: Martinus Nijhoff, 1948)
Anglo-Saxon Remedies, Charms, and Prayers from British Library MS Harley 585, The Lacnunga, ed. and trans. by Edward Pettit, 2 vols (Lampeter: Edwin Mellen, 2001)
Biskupa sögur I, ed. by Peter Foote, Íslenzk fornrit, 15 (Reykjavík: Hið íslenska fornritafélag, 2003)
Biskupa sögur II, ed. by Ásdís Egilsdóttir, Íslenzk fornrit, 16 (Reykjavík: Hið íslenska fornritafélag, 2002)
'Bretha crólige', ed. and trans. by D. A. Binchy, *Ériu*, 12 (1938), 1–77
'Bretha Déin Chécht', ed. and trans. by D. A. Binchy, *Ériu*, 20 (1966), 1–66

A Catalogue of Incipits of Scientific Writings in Latin, ed. by Lynn Thorndike and Pearl Kibre (Cambridge: Cambridge University Press, 1963)

'De amore hereos', ed. by Winifred Wulff, *Ériu*, 11 (1932), 174–81

'Di ércib fola', ed. and trans. by Neil McLeod, *Ériu*, 52 (2002), 123–216

An Electronic Corpus of Middle English Medical Texts, ed. by Irma Taavitsainen, Päivi Pahta, and Martti Mäkinen (Amsterdam: John Benjamins, 2005)

'Fragments of Irish Medieval Treatises on Horses', ed. and trans. by Brian Ó Cuív, *Celtica*, 17 (1985), 113–22

'Fragments of Two Mediaeval Treatises on Horses', ed. and trans. by Brian Ó Cuív, *Celtica*, 2 (1952–1954), 30–63

'Hafod 16 (A Medieval Welsh Medical Treatise)', ed. and trans. by Ida Jones, *Études celtiques*, 7 and 8 (1955–1959), 46–75, 270–339 and 66–97, 346–93

Healing and Society in Medieval England: A Middle English Translation of the Pharmaceutical Writings of Gilbertus Anglicus, ed. by Faye M. Getz (Madison: University of Wisconsin Press, 1991)

Henry Daniel, *Liber Uricrisiarum. A Reading Edition*, ed. by E. Ruth Harvey, M. Teresa Tavormina, and Sarah Star (Toronto: University of Toronto Press, 2020)

Hrafns Saga Sveinbjarnarsonar, ed. and trans. by Guðrún P. Helgadóttir (Oxford: Clarendon Press, 1987)

An Irish Version of Gaulterus De dosibus, ed. by Shawn Sheahan (Washington, DC: Catholic University of America, 1938)

Isidore of Seville, *The Etymologies of Isidore of Seville*, trans. by Stephen A. Barney, W. J. Lewis, J. A. Beach, and Oliver Berghof (Cambridge: Cambridge University Press, 2010)

—, *Isidori Hispalensis Episcopi: Etymologiarum sive Originum*, ed. by W. M. Lindsay (Oxford: Oxford University Press, 1911)

Den islandske lægebog: Codex Arnamagnæanus 434 a, 12 mo, ed. by Kristian Kålund, D. Kgl. Danske Vidensk. Selsk. Skr. 6. Række, historisk og filosofisk Afd. VI.4 (Copenhagen: Høst/Bianco Lunos Bogtrykkeri, 1907)

Lanfranc of Milan, *Lanfrank's 'Science of Cirurgie'*, ed. by Robert von Fleischhacker, Early English Text Society, o.s. 102 (London: Kegan Paul, Trench, Trübner & Co., 1894)

Läke- och örte-böcker från Sveriges Medeltid, ed. by G. E. Klemming (Stockholm: P. A. Norstedt och söner, 1886)

A Late Middle English Remedybook (MS. Wellcome 542, ff. 1r–20v): A Scholarly Edition, ed. by J. Calle-Martin and M. Á. Castaño-Gil (Bern: Peter Lang, 2013)

'A Latin Technical Phlebotomy and its Middle English Translation', ed. by Linda E. Voigts and Michael R. McVaugh, *Transactions of the American Philosophical Society*, 74.2 (1984), 1–69

A Leechbook or Collection of Medical Recipes of the Fifteenth Century, ed. and trans. by Warren R. Dawson (London: Macmillan, 1934)

Leechdoms, Wortcunning, and Starcraft of Early England: Being a Collection of Documents, for the Most Part Never before Printed, Illustrating the History of Science in this Country before the Norman Conquest, ed. and trans. by Thomas Oswald Cockayne, 3 vols (London: Longman, Roberts, and Green, 1864–1866)

The 'Liber de Diversis Medicinis', ed. by Margaret Sinclair Ogden, Early English Text Society, o.s., 207 (Oxford: Oxford University Press, 1938)

Medical Writings from Early Medieval England, Volume 1. The Old English Herbal, Lacnunga, and Other Texts, ed. and trans. by John D. Niles and Maria A. D'Aronco, Dumbarton Oaks Medieval Library, 81 (Cambridge, MA: Harvard University Press, 2023)

A Medieaval Handbook of Gynaecology and Midwifery …', ed. by Winifred Wulff, *Irish Texts*, 5 (London: Sheed and Ward, 1934)

Medieval Herbal Remedies. The Old-English Herbarium and Early Medieval Medicine, trans. by Anne Van Arsdall, 2nd edn (London: Routledge, 2023)

Medieval Welsh Medical Texts, Volume 1: The Recipes, ed. and trans. by Diana Luft (Cardiff: University of Wales Press, 2020)

A Middle English Medical Remedy Book Edited from Glasgow University Library MS Hunter 185, ed. by Francisco Alonso Almeida (Heidelberg: Universitätsverlag Winter, 2014)

'Middle English Rimed Medical Treatise', ed. by R. M. Garrett, *Anglia*, 24 (1911), 163–93

Norse Magical and Herbal Healing. A Medical Book from Medieval Iceland, ed. and trans. by Ben Waggoner (New Haven: Troth, 2001)

The Old English Herbarium and Medicina de Quadrupedibus, ed. by Hubert Jan de Vriend (London: Oxford University Press, 1984)

An Old Icelandic Medical Miscellany: Ms. Royal Irish Academy 23 D 43, with Supplement from Ms. Trinity College (Dublin) L-2–2, ed. and trans. by Henning Larsen (Oslo: Dybwad, 1931)

'"On Stretching and Yawning": A Text from the Medical School at Aghmacart, Queen's County', ed. by Aoibheann Nic Dhonnchadha, *Ossory, Laois and Leinster*, 3 (2008), 239–69

'On the Qualitees, Maners and Kunnynge of a Surgean', ed. by Winifred Wulff, *Zeitschrift für celtische Philologie*, 18 (1930), 249–86

The Physicians of Myddvai, ed. by J. Williams and trans. by J. Pughe (Llandovery: D. J. Roderic for the Welsh MSS Society, 1861)

Le plus ancien texte des Meddygon Myddveu, ed. and trans. by Pol Diverrès (Paris: Maurice le Dault, 1913)

Popular Medicine in Thirteenth-century England: Introduction and Texts, ed. by Tony Hunt (Cambridge: D. S. Brewer, 1990)

Regimen na sláinte: Regimen sanitatis Magnini Mediolanensis, ed. by Séamus Ó Ceithearnaigh [James P. Carney], 3 vols (Dublin: Stationery Office, 1942–1944)

Regimen sanitatis: The Rule of Health, a Gaelic Medical Manuscript of the Early Sixteenth Century or Perhaps Older from the Vade Mecum of the Famous Macbeaths, Physicians to the Lords of the Isles and the Kings of Scotland for Several Centuries, ed. by H. C. Gillies (Glasgow: Glasgow University Press, 1911)

Rosa anglica seu rosa medicinae Johannis Anglici: An Early Modern Irish Translation of a Section of the Mediaeval Medical Text-book of John of Gaddesden, ed. and trans. by Winifred Wulff, Irish Texts Society, 25 (London: Irish Texts Society, 1929)

'Rudimenta physionomiae', ed. by Gearóid Mac Niocaill, *Celtica*, 6 (1963), 271–78

Scientific and Medical Writings in Old and Middle English: An Electronic Reference, ed. by Linda E. Voigts and Patricia Deery Kurtz (Ann Arbor: University of Michigan Press, 2000)

'A Short Tract on Medicinal Uses for Animal Dung', ed. and trans. by Ranke de Vries, *North American Journal of Celtic Studies*, 3.2 (2019), 111–36

Tadhg Ó Cuinn, *An Irish Materia Medica* (*interim version*, 1991), ed. and trans. by Mícheál Ó Conchubhair (alias Michael O'Connor) <https://celt.ucc.ie/published/G600006.html>[accessed 14 April 2023]

'Téacs ó scoil leighis Achaidh Mhic Airt', ed. by Aoibheann Nic Dhonnchadha, *Ossory, Laois and Leinster*, 1 (2004), 50–75

'A Text Preserved at the Aghmacart Medical School: Bernard de Gordon's *De prognosticis*, Book II, 9', ed. by Beatrix Faerber, *Ossory, Laois and Leinster*, 7 (2019), 100–22

'Three Irish Medical Glossaries', ed. by Whitley Stokes, in *Archiv für celtische Lexicographie I*, ed. by Whitley Stokes and Kuno Meyer (Halle: Max Niemeyer, 1900), pp. 325–47

Three Receptaria from Medieval England: The Languages of Medicine in the Fourteenth Century, ed. by Michael Benskin and Tony Hunt, Medium Aevum Monographs, New Series, 21 (Oxford: Society for the Study of Medieval Languages and Literature, 2001)

'Tract on the Plague', ed. by Winifred Wulff, *Ériu*, 10 (1926–1928), 143–54

'A Treatise on Fevers', ed. by Lilian Duncan, *Revue celtique*, 49 (1932), 1–90

Vinjeboka. Den eldste svartebok fra norsk middelalder, ed. by Oskar Garsein (Oslo: Solum forlag, 1993)

Secondary Studies

Allport, Benjamin, Rosalind Bonté, and Hans Jacob Orning, eds, *Networks in the Medieval North. Studies in Honour of Jón Viðar Sigurðsson*, The North Atlantic World, 5 (Turnhout: Brepols, 2023)

Arbesmann, Rudolph, 'The Concept of "Christus Medicus" in St. Augustine', *Traditio*, 10 (1954), 1–28

Arkomani, Aliki-Anastasia, 'The Best Drink a Girl Can Get: Skírnismál 35, 6 and a Remedy for Epilepsy', in *Perkensian Rambles: A Collection of Essays in Honour of Richard Perkins*, ed. by Daisy L. Neijmann (London: University College London, Department of Scandinavian Studies, 2005), pp. 23–32

Arnovick, Leslie K., *Written Reliquaries: The Resonance of Orality in Medieval English Texts*, Pragmatics and Beyond, n.s. 153 (Amsterdam: John Benjamins, 2006)

Arthur, Ciaran, *'Charms', Liturgies, and Secret Rites in Early Medieval England*, Anglo-Saxon Studies, 32 (Woodbridge: The Boydell Press, 2018)

Baccianti, Sarah, 'Guaritori, acqua santa e latte materno: alcuni resoconti di pratiche e incantesimi medici nell'Isalanda medievale', *Filologia Germanica-Germanic Philology*, Supplemento, 3 (2022), 33–52

——, 'Healing Hands, Holy Water, and Hellish Diseases: Some Accounts of Medical Performance in Medieval Iceland', in *The Medieval North and its Afterlife: Essays in Honor of Heather O'Donoghue*, ed. by Siân Grønlie and Carl Phelpstead (Berlin: Medieval Institute Publications, 2024), pp. 67–77

Barrett, Siobhán, 'Varia I. The King of Dál nAraidi's Salve', *Ériu*, 69 (2019), 171–78

Binchy, D. A., 'Sick-Maintenance in Irish Law', *Ériu*, 12 (1938), 78–134

Black, Ronald, *Catalogue of Gaelic Manuscripts in the National Library of Scotland* <https://www.isos.dias.ie/libraries/NLS/english/index.html> [accessed 3 August 2022]

Black, Winston, '"I Will Add What the Arab once Taught": Constantine the African in Northern European Medical Verse', in *Herbs and Healers from the Ancient Mediterranean through the Medieval West. Essays in Honor of John M. Riddle*, ed. by Anne Van Arsdall and Timothy Graham (London: Routledge, 2012), pp. 153–85

Brady, Lindy, *The Origin Legends of Early Medieval Britain and Ireland* (Cambridge: Cambridge University Press, 2022)

Brynja Þorgeirsdóttir, '"*Eyrsilfr drukkit, þat gerir bana*": The Earliest Old Norse Medical Book, AM 655 xxx 4to, and its Context', *Gripla*, 34 (2023), 207–40

——, 'Humoral Theory in the Medieval North: An Old Norse Translation of Epistula Vindiciani in Hauksbók', *Gripla*, 29 (2018), 35–66

Burnett, Charles, *The Introduction of Arabic Learning into England* (London: British Library, 1997)

Burnett, Charles, and Danielle Jacquart, eds, *Constantine the African and Ali ibn al-Abbas al-Maǧūsī: The Pantegni and Related Texts* (Leiden: Brill, 1994)

Busby, Keith, *French in Medieval Ireland, Ireland in Medieval French: The Paradox of Two Worlds*, Medieval Texts and Cultures of Northern Europe, 27 (Turnhout: Brepols, 2017)

Byrne, Aisling, and Victoria Flood, eds, *Crossing Borders in the Insular Middle Ages*, Medieval Texts and Cultures of Northern Europe, 30 (Turnhout: Brepols, 2019)

——, 'Insular Connections and Comparisons in the Later Middle Ages', in *Crossing Borders in the Insular Middle Ages*, ed. by Aisling Byrne and Victoria Flood, Medieval Texts and Cultures of Northern Europe, 30 (Turnhout: Brepols, 2019), pp. 1–22

Crossgrove, William, 'The Vernacularization of Science, Medicine, and Technology in Late Medieval Europe: Broadening Our Perspectives', *Early Science and Medicine*, 5.1 (2000), 47–63

Davies, Wendy, 'The Place of Healing in Early Irish Society', in *Sages, Saints and Storytellers: Celtic Studies in Honour of Professor James Carney*, ed. by Donnchadh Ó Corráin, Liam Breatnach, and Kim McCone, Maynooth Monographs, 2 (Maynooth: An Sagart, 1989), pp. 43–55

de Vries, Ranke, 'Medieval Medicine and the Healing of Caílte in *Acallam na Senórach*', *North American Journal of Celtic Studies*, 5.1 (2021), 49–82

eDIL = eDIL 2019: *An Electronic Dictionary of the Irish Language*, based on the Contributions to a Dictionary of the Irish Language (Dublin: Royal Irish Academy, 1913–1976) <www.dil.ie 2019>

Edmonds, Fiona, *Gaelic Influence in the Northumbrian Kingdom. The Golden Age and the Viking Age*, Studies in Celtic History, 40 (Woodbridge: The Boydell Press, 2019)

Eriksen, Stefka G., ed., *Intellectual Culture in Medieval Scandinavia, c. 1100–1350*, Disputatio, 28 (Turnhout: Brepols, 2016)

Etchingham, Colmán, Jón Viðar Sigurðsson, Máire Ní Mhaonaigh, and Elizabeth Ashman Rowe, *Norse–Gaelic Contacts in a Viking World*, Medieval Texts and Cultures of Northern Europe, 29 (Turnhout: Brepols, 2019)

Etheridge, Christian, 'Medieval Scientific Book Fragments Held in Swedish and Finnish Archives: The Tantalizing Remains of a Greater Scientific Corpus', in *Medieval Science in the North: Travelling Wisdom, 1000–1500*, ed. by Christian Etheridge and Michele Campopiano, Knowledge, Scholarship, and Science in the Middle Ages, 2 (Turnhout: Brepols, 2021), pp. 111–40

——, 'The Transmission and Reception of Science in Medieval Scandinavia 1110–1525' (unpublished doctoral thesis, Odense, University of Southern Denmark, 2018)

Etheridge, Christian, and Michele Campopiano, eds, *Medieval Science in the North: Travelling Wisdom, 1000–1500*, Knowledge, Scholarship, and Science in the Middle Ages, 2 (Turnhout: Brepols, 2021)

Finnur Jónsson, *Lægekunsten i den nordiske oldtid*, Medicinsk-historiske Smaaskrifter, 1 (Copenhagen: Tryde, 1912)

Flint, Valerie J., 'The Early Medieval "Medicus", the Saint – and the Enchanter', *Social History of Medicine*, 2.2 (1989), 127–45

Green, Monica, 'Salerno on the Thames: The Genesis of Anglo-Norman Medical Literature', in *Language and Culture in Medieval Britain: The French of England, c. 1100–1500*, ed. by Jocelyn Wogan-Browne (Woodbridge: Boydell and Brewer, 2013), pp. 220–32

Griffin, Carrie, and Emer Purcell, eds, *Texts, Transmission and Transformation in the European Middle Ages, 1000–1500*, Cursor Mundi, 34 (Turnhout: Brepols, 2018)

Grøn, Fredrik, *Altnordische Heilkunde* (Harlem: Erven Bohn, 1908)

Jolly, Karen Louise, *Popular Religion in Late Saxon England: Elf Charms in Context* (Chapel Hill: The University of North Carolina Press, 1996)

Harris, Jason, 'Latin Learning and Irish Physicians, *c.* 1350 – *c.* 1610', in *Rosa Anglica: Reassessments*, ed. by Liam P. Ó Murchú, Irish Texts Society Subsidiary Series, 28 (London: Irish Texts Society, 2016), pp. 1–25

Hayden, Deborah, 'Attribution and Authority in a Medieval Irish Medical Compendium', *Studia Hibernica*, 45 (2019), 19–51

——, '*Auraicept na nÉces* and the *Art of Medicine*', in *Glossing Practice: Comparative Perspectives*, ed. by Franck Cinato, Aimée Lahaussois, and John Whitman (Lanham, MD: Lexington Books, 2023), pp. 113–35

——, 'Observations on the "Doors of Death" in a Medieval Irish Medical Catechism', in *Rosa Anglica: Reassessments*, ed. by Liam P. Ó Murchú, Irish Texts Society Subsidiary Series, 28 (London: Irish Texts Society, 2016), pp. 26–56

——, 'Old English in the Irish Charms', *Speculum*, 97.2 (2022), 349–76

——, 'A Sixteenth-Century Irish Collection of Remedies for Ailments of the Male Reproductive Organs', *Celtica*, 33 (2021), 248–76

——, 'Textual Transfer, Irish Remedy Collections and the Vernacularization of Medical Learning in Late-medieval Europe', in *An Eoraip: Ireland in Medieval and Early Modern Europe*, ed. by Brendan Kane and Patrick Wadden (Leiden: Brill, forthcoming)

——, 'Three Versified Medical Recipes Invoking Dían Cécht', in *Fír Fesso: A Festschrift for Neil McLeod*, ed. by Anders Ahlqvist and Pamela O'Neill, Sydney Series in Celtic Studies, 17 (Sydney: Celtic Studies Foundation, University of Sydney, 2018), pp. 107–23

Hayes, Richard, 'Irish Medical Links with the Continent', in *What's Past is Prologue: A Retrospect of Irish Medicine*, ed. by William Doolin and Oliver Fitzgerald (Dublin: Monument Press, 1952), pp. 23–28

Heizmann, Wilhelm, *Wörterbuch der Pflanzennamen im Altwestnordischen*, Ergänzungsbände zum Reallexikon der Germanischen Altertumskunde, 7 (Berlin: Walter de Gruyter, 1993)

Hindley, Katherine Storm, *Textual Magic. Charms and Written Amulets in Medieval England* (Chicago and London: University of Chicago Press, 2023)

Holck, Jakob Povl, 'Middelalderens danske lægebog. Et kontaktfænomen' (unpublished doctoral thesis, University of Copenhagen, 2001)

Horden, Peregrine, 'What's Wrong with Early Medieval Medicine?', *Social History of Medicine*, 24 (2011), 5–25

Hunt, Tony, *The Medieval Surgery* (Woodbridge: Boydell Press, 1992)

——, *Plant Names of Medieval England* (Cambridge: D. S. Brewer, 1989)

ISOS = *Irish Script on Screen – Meamrám Páipéar Ríomhaire* (School of Celtic Studies, Dublin Institute for Advanced Studies) <www.isos.dias.ie> [accessed 3 August 2022]

Jón Viðar Sigurðsson and Timothy Bolton, eds, *Celtic-Norse Relationships in the Irish Sea in the Middle Ages 800–1200* (Leiden: Brill, 2013)

Kaiser, Charlotte, *Krankheit und Krankheitsbewältigung in den Isländersagas. Medizinhistorischer Aspekt und erzähltechnische Funktion* (Cologne: Seltman & Hein Verlag, 1998)

Kesling, Emily, *Medical Texts in Anglo-Saxon Literary Culture* (Cambridge: D. S. Brewer, 2020)

Kwakkel, Erik, and Francis Newton, *Medicine at Monte Cassino: Constantine the African and the Oldest Manuscript of his 'Pantegni'* (Turnhout: Brepols, 2019)

Langum, Virginia, *Medicine and the Seven Deadly Sins in Late Medieval Literature and Culture* (New York: Palgrave Macmillan, 2016)

Ledderose, Hannelore, *Heilkundige Männer und Frauen und ihre medizinischen Behandlungsmethoden in der altnordischen Überlieferung* (Munich: Utzverlag, 2020)

Leja, Meg, *Embodying the Soul. Medicine and Religion in Carolingian Europe* (Philadelphia: University of Pennsylvania Press, 2022)

MacKinney, Loren C., 'Medical Ethics and Etiquette in the Early Middle Ages: The Persistence of Hippocratic Ideals', *Bulletin of the History of Medicine*, 26.1 (1952), 1–31

Maraschi, Andrea, *Similia similibus curantur. Cannibalismo, grafofagia e 'magia' simpatetica nel Medioevo (500–1500)* (Spoleto: Cisam, 2020)

———, 'Sympathetic Graphophagy in Late Medieval Scandinavian Leechbooks and Collections of Charms', in *Civilizations of the Supernatural: Witchcraft, Ritual, and Religious Experience in Late Antique, Medieval, and Renaissance Traditions*, ed. by Fabrizio Conti (Budapest: Trivent Publishing, 2020), pp. 247–64

McCleery, Iona, 'Introduction: The Cultural History of Health', in *A Cultural History of Medicine in the Middle Ages*, ed. by Iona McCleery, A Cultural History of Medicine, 2 (London: Bloomsbury Academic, 2021), pp. 1–19

McDougall, Ian, 'The Third Instrument of Medicine. Some Accounts of Surgery in Medieval Iceland', in *Health, Disease and Healing in Medieval Culture*, ed. by Sheila Campbell, Bert Hall, and David Klausner (London: MacMillan, 1992), pp. 57–83

McNeill, John T., 'Medicine for Sin as Prescribed in the Penitentials', *Church History*, 1.1 (1932), 14–26

McVaugh, Michael, *Medicine before the Plague. Practitioners and their Patients in the Crown of Aragon, 1285–1345* (Cambridge: Cambridge University Press, 2002)

Metzler, Irina, *Disability in Medieval Europe. Thinking about Physical Impairment during the High Middle Ages, c. 1100–1400* (Abingdon and New York: Routledge, 2006)

Mitchell, Stephen A., 'Faith and Knowledge in Nordic Charm Magic', in *Faith and Knowledge in Late Medieval Scandinavia*, ed. by Karoline Kjesrud and Mikael Males, Knowledge, Scholarship, and Science in the Middle Ages, 1 (Turnhout: Brepols, 2020), pp. 193–211

———, 'Leechbooks, Manuals, and Grimoires. On the Early History of Magical Texts in Scandinavia', *ARV. Nordic Yearbook of Folklore*, 70 (2014), 57–74

———, *Witchcraft and Magic in the Nordic Middle Ages* (Philadelphia: University of Pennsylvania Press, 2011)

Murray Jones, Peter, and Lea T. Olsan, 'Medicine and Magic', in *The Routledge History of Medieval Magic*, ed. by Sophie Page and Catherine Rider (London: Routledge, 2019), pp. 299–311

Nic Dhonnchadha, Aoibheann, 'The Irish *Rosa Anglica*: Manuscripts and Structure', in *Rosa Anglica: Reassessments*, ed. by L. P. Ó Murchú, Irish Texts Society Subsidiary Series, 28 (London: Irish Texts Society, 2016), pp. 114–97

———, 'Medical Writing in Irish', *Irish Journal of Medical Science*, 169.3 (2000), 217–20 (repr. from J. B. Lyons, ed., *2000 Years of Irish Medicine* [Dublin: Eireann Healthcare Publications, 1999], pp. 21–26)

———, 'Tráchtas leighis ón 14ú haois: lámhscríbhinn, téacs agus foinsí', in *Léann na Sionainne*, ed. by Aengus Ó Fionnagáin and Gordon Ó Riain, Aistí Léannta, 3 (Dublin: Cló Léann na Gaeilge, 2022), pp. 1–60

Oliver, Lisi, *The Body Legal in Barbarian Law* (Toronto: University of Toronto Press, 2011)

Olsan, Lea T., 'Charms and Prayers in Medieval Medical Theory and Practice', *Social History of Medicine*, 16.3 (2003), 343–66

Ó Máille, Tomás, 'The Authorship of the *Culmen*', *Ériu*, 9 (1921–1923), 71–76

Ó Muraíle, Nollaig, 'The Hereditary Medical Families of Gaelic Ireland', in *Rosa Anglica: Reassessments*, ed. by L. P. Ó Murchú, Irish Texts Society Subsidiary Series, 28 (London: Irish Texts Society), pp. 85–113

Owen, Morfydd E., 'The Doctor in the Laws of Hywel', *Transactions of the Physicians of Myddfai Society* (2018), 69–80

——, 'Meddygon Myddfai: A Preliminary Survey of Some Medieval Medical Writing in Welsh', *Studia Celtica*, 10–11 (1975–1976), 210–33

——, 'The Medical Books of Medieval Wales and the Physicians of Myddfai', *The Carmarthenshire Antiquary*, 31 (1995), 34–83

——, 'Medics and Medicine', in *The Welsh King and his Court*, ed. by T. M. Charles-Edwards, Morfydd E. Owen, and Paul Russell (Cardiff: University of Wales Press, 2000), pp. 116–41

——, 'Names for Sicknesses and Disease in Medieval Welsh', in *Kelten am Rhein: Akten des dreizehnten Internationalen Keltologiekongresses, 23. Bis 27. Juli 2007 in Bonn*, 2 vols, vol. 2: *Philologie: Sprachen und Literaturen*, ed. by Stefan Zimmer (Mainz: Philipp von Zabern, 2009), pp. 205–16

Pahta, Päivi, and Irma Taavitsainen, 'Vernacularisation of Scientific and Medical Writing in its Sociohistorical Context', in *Medical and Scientific Writing in Late Medieval English*, ed. by Irma Taavitsainen and Päivi Pahta (Cambridge: Cambridge University Press, 2004), pp. 1–22

Parina, Elena, 'Medical Texts in Welsh Translation: *Y Pedwar Gwlybwr* and *Rhinweddau Bwydydd*', in *Crossing Borders in the Insular Middle Ages*, ed. by Aisling Byrne and Victoria Flood, Medieval Texts and Cultures of Northern Europe, 30 (Turnhout: Brepols, 2019), pp. 47–63

Poppe, Erich, Simon Rodway, and Jenny Rowland, eds, *Celts, Gaels, and Britons. Studies in Language and Literature from Antiquity to the Middle Ages in Honour of Patrick Sims-Williams*, Medieval Texts and Cultures of Northern Europe, 35 (Turnhout: Brepols, 2022)

Sif Rikharðsdóttir, *Medieval Translations and Cultural Discourse: The Movement of Texts in England, France and Scandinavia* (Cambridge: D. S. Brewer, 2012)

Robbins, Rossell Hope, 'Medical Manuscripts in Middle English', *Speculum*, 45.3 (1970), 393–415

Schwabe, Fabian, 'Den norrøne legemiddelboktradisjonen', in *Translation – Adaptation, Interpretation, Transformation. Proceedings from the 28th Study Conference of IASS, Lund 3–7 August 2010*, ed. by Claes-Göran Holmberg and Per Erik Ljung (Lund: Lunds Universitet, 2010), pp. 1–13

Sheehan, Áine, 'Locating the Gaelic Medical Families in Elizabethan Ireland', in *Early Modern Ireland and the World of Medicine: Practitioners, Collectors and Contexts*, ed. by John Cunningham (Manchester: Manchester University Press, 2019), pp. 20–38

Sims-Williams, Patrick, *Irish Influence on Medieval Welsh Literature* (Oxford: Oxford University Press, 2011)

Siraisi, Nancy, *Medieval and Early Renaissance Medicine: An Introduction to Knowledge and Practice* (Chicago: University of Chicago Press, 2009)

Skemer, Don C., *Binding Words. Textual Amulets in the Middle Ages* (University Park, PA: The Pennsylvania State University Press, 2006)

Smyth, Marina, 'Isidorian Texts in Seventh-Century Ireland', in *Isidore of Seville and his Reception in the Early Middle Ages: Transmitting and Transforming Knowledge*, ed. by Andy Fear and Jamie Wood (Amsterdam: Amsterdam University Press, 2016), pp. 111–30

Tarsi, Matteo, 'Loanwords and Native Words in Old and Middle Icelandic (12th c. – 1550)' (unpublished doctoral thesis, University of Iceland, 2020)

Temkin, Owsei, *Hippocrates in a World of Pagans and Christians* (Baltimore and London: Johns Hopkins University Press, 1991)

Tuomi, Ilona, John Carey, Barbara Hillers, and Ciarán Ó Gealbháin, eds, *Charms, Charmers and Charming in Ireland. From the Medieval to the Modern* (Cardiff: University of Wales Press, 2019)

Turner, Wendy J., 'Mind/Brain: Medieval Concepts', in *A Cultural History of Medicine in the Middle Ages*, ed. by Iona McCleery (London: Bloomsbury, 2021), pp. 155–75

Voigts, Linda Ehrsam, 'Multitudes of Middle English Medical Manuscripts, or the Englishing of Science and Medicine', in *Manuscript Sources of Medieval Medicine: A Book of Essays*, ed. by Margaret R. Schleissner (London and New York: Routledge, 1995), pp. 183–95

Whaley, D. C., 'Miracles in the *Biskupa sögur*. Icelandic Variations on an International Theme', in *Preprints of the 9th International Saga Conference* (Rekjavík: Stofnun Árna Magnússonar, 1994), pp. 847–62

Whaley, D. C. and D. Elliot, 'Dupuytren's Disease: A Legacy of the North?', *Journal of Hand Surgery* (European Volume), 18.3 (1993), 363–67

Wormald, Patrick, 'The *Leges Barbarorum*: Law and Ethnicity in the Post-Roman West', in *Regna and Gentes. The Relationship between Late Antique and Early Medieval Peoples and Kingdoms in the Transformation of the Roman World*, ed. by Hans-Werner Goetz, Jörg Jarnut, and Walter Pohl (Leiden: Brill, 2003), pp. 21–53

Part I

Materia Medica and Medical Knowledge

CONAN T. DOYLE

2. Humoral and Elemental Theory in Early Medieval English Medicine

Reviewing the unprecedented volume of medical material from early medieval England that survives primarily in Anglo-Norman translations of the twelfth century and Latin manuscripts of English origin, Monica Green remarks that 'were it not for certain key elements suggesting southern Italian origin (e.g. unique elements of *materia medica* with Arabic names and preparations such as syrups), it would be nearly impossible to tell, on the basis of the manuscript evidence, that "Salerno" was not on the Thames!'[1] Green's article is primarily concerned with the survival of Latin texts belonging to the early Salernitan corpus of the long twelfth century and their reception in Anglo-Norman England, as documented by Tony Hunt and Ruth Dean, but does not fail to mention the older vernacular corpus of Old English medical compilations, which she describes as 'a truly unique phenomenon'.[2]

This study is primarily concerned with the textual evidence in Latin and Old English for the understanding of human physiology in early medieval England from the period before Monica Green's long twelfth century. While the pre-Norman period is often held to end in the year 1066, the year 1100 serves more globally as an approximate milestone in the history of medicine. The eleventh century saw the production and dissemination of a new textual tradition of medicine translated from Arabic by Constantinus Africanus, heavily associated with the famed medical school at Salerno. This watershed gave rise to the terms 'Pre-Salernitan' and 'Salernitan', respectively, to refer to early medieval medicine before and after 1100. Two useful points of contrast exist between the pre-Salernitan and Salernitan periods. The first is that the majority of those physicians engaging with scholarly medical texts in the earlier period were monastically educated: with the exception of Salerno, the university as an institution did not exist until the late eleventh century, and

1 Green, 'Salerno on the Thames', p. 222.
2 Green, 'Salerno on the Thames', p. 220.

Conan T. Doyle • Charles University in Prague; conan.doyle@fhs.cuni.cz

Medicine in the Medieval North Atlantic World: Vernacular Texts and Traditions, ed. by Deborah Hayden and Sarah Baccianti, KSS, 5 (Turnhout, 2025), pp. 55-74
BREPOLS PUBLISHERS DOI 10.1484/M.KSS-EB.5.143980

did not serve as a locus of medical education until the thirteenth century.[3] The practising physician from early medieval England is very hard to locate, but the most famous example was an abbot as well as a court physician to both Harold and William, namely Baldwin of Bury St Edmunds.[4] The second point of contrast is that the Latin medical corpus we are dealing with predates the production of Latin translations of Arabic authors, although scholarly opinion on what texts actually comprised the pre-Salernitan corpus is changing rapidly thanks to better engagement with manuscript witnesses.[5] The absence of work translated from Arabic in the intellectual climate of the period means that the scholastic influence of Aristotle was yet to leave its mark on medical theory in the Latin West, but that does not mean that this medicine was atheoretical.

This study will thus explore the ways in which the Neoplatonic philosophy of early Christianity was influential in shaping the theory and practice of medicine in late antiquity and the early Middle Ages.[6] Another aspect of this early medieval Latin corpus is its epistemological heterogeneity. Latin medical texts of antiquity and the Middle Ages were not composed with monolithic conformity to a single sect or philosophy of medicine. While the first-century AD encyclopaedist Celsus drew extensively on elite Greek medical theory and practice, Pliny the Elder scorned the theoretical approach to medicine and the practice of regimen and dietetics, and presented the cures he collected in a pragmatic utilitarian form devoid of the learned sophistication and reliance on Greek vocabulary that marked Celsus. It is ironic then that nine centuries later, Pliny is described as 'se micla læce' (the great physician) in Old English, and indeed is the only classical authority cited by name in Bald's *Leechbook* I.[7] Part of Pliny's fame as a great physician, despite his hostility to the learned medicine of his own lifetime, stems from the existence of two purely medical compilations based on his *Historia naturalis*, namely the *Physica Plinii* and *Medicina Plinii*, both of which were disseminated widely.[8] By contrast to

---

3 Rashdall, *The Universities of Europe*, I, pp. 75–86; Siraisi, 'The Faculty of Medicine' and Duranti, 'The Origins of the Studium of Medicine of Bologna'.

4 For a survey of known physicians in early medieval England, see Rubin, *Medieval English Medicine*, pp. 98–100.

5 Green, 'Rethinking the Manuscript Basis'.

6 Since this study is concerned with a vernacular corpus which was translated and compiled between the ninth and eleventh centuries, we find ourselves firmly within the pre-Salernitan period of medical history. The most important medical texts from the pre-Salernitan corpus are only slowly reaching the attention of competent editors, meaning that any research into them must by necessity engage directly with the manuscript sources which have been catalogued by Beccaria, *I codici di medicina*.

7 *Leechbook* I.87 in *Leechdoms*, ed. and trans. by Cockayne, II, pp. 154–55 (London, BL, MS Royal 12 D XVII. fol. 57ᵛ), ironically relating to a recipe in Alexander, not Pliny: see Cameron, *Anglo-Saxon Medicine*, p. 23 n. 11. Although Bald's *Leechbook* and *Leechbook* III are printed in the second of Cockayne's three-volume *Leechdoms*, all quotations from the text provided here are directly transcribed from the manuscript. All translations are my own unless stated otherwise.

8 For the use of these texts in Anglo-Saxon England, see Adams and Deegan, 'Bald's *Leechbook* and the *Physica Plinii*'. The *Medicina Plinii* is *Plinii secundi iunioris qui feruntur de medicina libri*

the popularity of these compilations based on Pliny, Celsus' *De medicina* survives in only two complete manuscript witnesses and a third witness to extracts of the text from our time period.[9] Late antique compilations such as *Marcelli de medicamentis liber* freely mixed invocations of pagan gods such as Helios, or magical formulae such as the *SATOR* square with therapies from sources such as Vindicianus, Celsus, Pliny, and Scribonius Largus, alongside pseudo-Hippocratic explications of humoral theory.[10]

While the early English, and indeed the early medieval Latin West in general, may not have frequently read Celsus, there was no shortage of texts which preserved and transmitted the core canon of what Owsei Temkin calls 'Galenic Hippocratism' in Latin.[11] Most of these texts seem to have been translated and compiled from Greek sources either in Roman North Africa before the Vandal invasion, or during the Byzantine Exarchate of Ravenna in the sixth and seventh centuries.[12] The volume of texts is too large to list here, but for our present purposes, the most important works with vernacular fortunes in pre-Conquest England are the Latin translations of Alexander Trallianus and Oribasius, the *Tereoperica*, and an ensemble of medical texts which were transmitted alongside the Galen's *Ad Glauconem*, later recompiled by Gariopontus as the *Passionarius Galieni*.[13] Where medical historians such

---

tres, ed. by Önnerfors. The text has been recently re-edited and translated into English by Hunt, *The Medicina Plinii*. The *Physica Plinii* exists in multiple recensions, of which only the *Physica Plinii Bambergensis* and *Physica Plinii Florentino-Pragensis* have been published.

9 Beccaria, *I codici di medicina*, items 29, 88 and 102 (= Paris, BnF, MS Lat 7028; Florence, Biblioteca Medicea Laurenziana, MS Plut. 73.1; and Rome, BAV, MS Lat. 5951).

10 On the *SATOR* square, see also the chapter by Deborah Hayden in this volume. The sources of *De medicamentis liber* are demonstrated by the inclusion of dedicatory epistles transmitted with it, including an epistle on weights and measures, the pseudo-Hippocratic letters to Antiochus and Maecenates, the preface to the *Medicina Plinii*, Celsus' letter to Pullius Natalis and Vindicianus's letter to Velentinian: see Marcellus, *De medicamentis liber*, ed. by Liechtenhan and Niedermann, pp. 2–52.

11 When saying that 'Galenic Hippocratism was formally installed' by Oribasius, Temkin was referring to his Greek-language medical works, as edited by J. Raeder for the *Corpus medicorum Graecorum*. See Temkin, *Hippocrates*, p. 214; for the printed Latin texts, see *Oeuvres d'Oribase*, ed. by Bussemaker and Daremberg, vols v–vi. For more modern editions, see Oribasius, *Synopsis I–II*, ed. by Mørland; *Euporista* i in 'Oribasius Latinus', ed. by E. W. Goos; and *Synopsis VII*, ed. by Gomez Costoya.

12 For the date and origin of the Oribasius Latinus, see Mørland, *Die Lateinischen Oribasiusübersetzungen*, pp. 187–94. For the date and place of origin of the Latin Alexander, see Alexander of Tralles, *The Latin Alexander*, ed. and trans. by Langslow, pp. 35–36. The only complete print edition is the early modern *Practica Alexandri yatros greci*, ed. by Fradin. Glaze discusses the use of Agnellus of Ravenna in the compilation of the *Tereoperica* in 'Master–Student Medical Dialogues'. On the African authors see Cilliers, *Roman North Africa*.

13 On the *Tereoperica*, the *Liber tertius*, and the related *Passionalis*, see Fischer, 'Two Latin Pre-Salernitan Medical Manuals', 'Der Pseudogalenische *Liber tertius*' and 'Dr Monk's Medical Digest'. On the reception of the *Tereoperica* see Maion, 'The Fortune of the So-Called *Practica Petrocelli Salernitani* in England'.

as Talbot noted parallels between Bald's *Leechbook* and the *Passionarius*, this indicates that the sources can most likely be found in the original ensemble, rather than the later recompilation.[14] These compilations, together with older herbal literature transmitted alongside the *Herbarius Apulei*, the *Physica Plinii*, and the *Medicina Plinii*, provide the bulk of cures so far identified in Old English translation.[15] These texts exhibit the same kinds of epistemological pluralism which I noted above contrasting Pliny and Celsus, insofar as they mix simple herbal cures with more complex philosophical medicine, but they also supplement these cures with Christian prayers, as used by Alexander Trallianus or copied into the last book of Oribasius' *Synopsis*.[16] This juxtaposition of Galenic humoralism with petitions to divine intercession has made many historians of medicine squeamish about the medicine of the pre-Salernitan period, creating a problematic dichotomy between those elements of the medical textual tradition — described as rational insofar as they conform to classical notions of physiology — and those elements of the tradition which are derided as superstitious, or, in the words of Charles Singer, 'the final pathological disintegration of that great system of Greek Medical thought'.[17]

I attempt to make no distinction between 'rational' and 'irrational' elements in these texts. A quotation from the *Carmen Paschale* or Revelations is just as important a literary reference in these texts as an allusion to the Hippocratic *Aphorisms*,[18] and just as rational when we consider that these texts were compiled by and for the use of Christian monks at a time when any form of education, including medical education, could be obtained only in the cloister or in the cathedral school.

---

14 Talbot, 'Some Notes on Anglo-Saxon Medicine', noted many parallels between Bald's *Leechbook* and the *Passionarius*, but as the Passionarius did not exist when Bald's *Leechbook* was copied, these texts must have come from the original ensemble. See Glaze, 'Galen Refashioned' and 'Gariopontus and the Salernitans'.

15 The *Herbarius Apulei* and related texts are found in *Antonii Musae De herba uettonica liber*, ed. by Howald and Sigerist; for the Old English translation, see *The Old English Herbarium*, ed. by de Vriend. For the sources of Bald's *Leechbook*, see Talbot, 'Some Notes on Anglo-Saxon Medicine'; Cameron, 'Bald's *Leechbook*', 'The Sources of Medical Knowledge' and *Anglo-Saxon Medicine*; Meaney, 'Variant Versions'; Adams and Deegan, 'Bald's *Leechbook* and the *Physica Plinii*'; D'Aronco, 'How "English" is Anglo-Saxon Medicine?', Doyle, 'Anglo-Saxon Medicine and Disease', and Kesling, *Medical Texts in Anglo-Saxon Literary Culture*.

16 See August Molinier's edition of the additional chapters of the *Synopsis* printed in *Oeuvres d'Oribase*, ed. by Bussemaker and Daremberg, VI, pp. 397–402. The manuscript of the New Latin translation in question is Laon, Bib. mun., MS 424, while similar recipes follow the Old Latin translation of the *Synopsis* in Paris, BnF, MS NAL 1619, fols 184va–206rb; on 'magical' recipes in Alexander, see Alexander of Tralles, *The Latin Alexander*, ed. and trans. by Langslow, pp. 8 and 29–36.

17 Grattan and Singer, *Anglo-Saxon Magic and Medicine*, p. 94. For a discussion of the problem, see Horden 'What's Wrong with Early Medieval Medicine?'.

18 Sedulius, *Carmen Paschale* III, ll. 23–25 is quoted in *Leechbook* I.62, in *Leechdoms*, ed. and trans. by Cockayne, II, pp. 136–37 (London, BL, MS Royal 12 D XVII, fol. 51^{v}).

Natural Philosophy in the Monastic Curriculum

The monastic curriculum of seven liberal arts is the essential precursor to the medieval university curriculum. The seven arts were divided into the essential preliminary arts of the *Trivium* and the higher arts of the *Quadrivium*. Although not officially part of the *Quadrivium*, the art of medicine seems to have taken its place alongside them as one of the higher faculties fit for study in either monastic institutions or, later, universities. Those aspects of philosophy which concern the natural and physical world, such as natural history and astronomy, were useful in the exegesis of scripture and in the execution of the pastoral duties of a bishop. Thus, Bede informs us, in his *Historia ecclesiastica*, that his mentor Theodore was knowledgeable about lunar prognostics for phlebotomy.[19] Bede's concern with timekeeping significantly intersects with the more learned aspects of classical medical theory and he draws upon two different medical authorities in his *De temporum ratione*. He quotes directly from the last two paragraphs of the pseudo-Hippocratic *Epistola ad Antiochum regem* in his chapter on solstices and equinoxes, while M. L. Cameron and Faith Wallis suggest that he paraphrased his description of the four humours from the *Epistola Vindiciani ad Pentadium*, a pithy digest of humoral theory written by an African medical professor to his nephew.[20] Bede's Neoplatonism comes to the fore in his explicit association of the qualities of the four Platonic elements and the four humours of the human body, the four seasons, the four ages of man and the four cardinal points of the compass.[21] He also enshrines the notion of man as a microcosm of the universe in stating: 'Sed et homo ipse, qui a sapientibus microcosmos, id est, minor mundus appellatur, hisdem per omnia qualitatibus habet temperatum corpus.' (But man himself, who is called a microcosm by the wise, that is a smaller world, through all things has a body tempered in every respect by the very same qualities).[22]

Bede's association of the four humours with four stages of life does not exactly match Vindicianus, but more closely matches the *Epistola Ippocratis et Galieni contemplantes quattuor esse humores in corpore humano*, which circulated

19 Bede, *Historia ecclesiastica* v.3, ed. and trans. by Colgrave and Mynors, p. 460.

20 For the *Epistola ad Pentadium*, see *Theodori Prisciani*, ed. by Rose, pp. 484–92. See Cameron, 'The Sources of Medical Knowledge', p. 150 and Wallis, 'Medicine in Medieval Calendar Manuscripts', p. 122. On the career of Vindicianus, see Cilliers, 'The Contribution of the 4th Century North African Physician'.

21 Here, Bede was possibly following Isidore, *Etymologiae*, IV.5, as these correspondences are rarely explicated in medical texts unless we count such epistolary fragments as the *Interrogationes medicinali* in Paris, BnF, MS lat. 11219, fol. 39ra, a part of the collection known as the *Liber epistolarum*. It contains the sentence 'Sanguis similat aerem, flegma similat aqua, colera rubea similat igni, colera nigri similat terra' (Blood resembles air, phlegm resembles water, red bile resembles fire, black bile resembles earth), bizarrely in answer to the question *quante ydropicie sunt?* ('how many species of dropsy are there?').

22 Bede, *Opera de temporibus*, ed. by Jones, p. 247.

as part of the *Tereoperica*.[23] Very similar accounts circulated in collections of epistles, such as the *Epistola Ippocratis de quattuor humoribus*, which circulated as part of a collection of pseudo-Hippocratic epistolary texts known as the *Liber epistolarum*. Vindicianus states that both childhood and old age are ruled by phlegm, youth is ruled by red bile mixed with blood and adulthood is ruled by black bile mixed with blood. In the further development of the Neoplatonic scheme of the pseudo-Hippocratic *epistolae*, these four ages of man are realigned to correspond to the elemental qualities of the four seasons, giving us the scheme followed in the *Liber epistolarum*: 'Singulos istos scito per diuersas aetates regnare. maxime infantibus sanguinem. iuuenibus fel rufum. maturis fel nigrum. flegma in senibus' (Know that these each rule through different ages, blood especially in infants, red bile in youths, black bile in adults, phlegm in the old).[24] Infancy is ruled by blood in the rearranged system because it is the springtime of life, and therefore hot and moist, and blood must rule it because blood is the hot moist humour. This is a logical rearrangement of what had originally been an observation that infants and old people tend to get more runny noses, and must therefore be ruled by phlegm. The clinical observation, crude as it is, has been replaced by a theoretical desire for the microcosm (man) and macrocosm (universe) to harmonize.

It is quite possible that this rearrangement of the humoral properties of the four ages of man originated with Bede, and that texts such as the *Epistola Ippocratis et Galieni contemplantes quattuor esse humores in corpore humano* were rearrangements of the original letter of Vindicianus in an attempt to bring medical theory into line with the Neoplatonism of patristic authority. The scheme which comes to prominence fully extends the analogous relationship between the four humours of man and the four elements, the four seasons with the four ages of man, and the four cardinal directions, but in so doing seems to discard whatever kernels of clinical observation had existed in Vindicianus' description of the temperaments of people in the stages of life. The full Neoplatonic schema following Bede is expounded in both Old English and Latin by Byrhtferth of Ramsay in his *Enchyridion*,[25] while Byrhtferth's source, Bede, also mentioned the associated psychological characteristics of the four humours in his *De temporum ratione* xxxv.5:

> Item sanguis eos in quibus maxime pollet facit hilares, laetos, misericordes, multum ridentes et loquentes; cholera vero rubea facit macilentos, multum tamen comedentes, veloces, audaces, iracundos, agiles; nigra

23 The text is printed as chapter 151 of the *Tereoperica*, ed. by de Renzi in *Collectio Salernitana* iv, pp. 285–86 but omitted in *Tereoperica*, ed. by Lopéz Figueroa.

24 Paris, BnF, MS lat. 11219 fol. 19ra. The version of the *Epistola* printed in Rose from a much later manuscript contains a different schema. The version on fol. 103va, i.e. following the *Tereoperica*, contains scribal corrections, bringing it into agreement with the text quoted above.

25 Byrhtferth, *Enchiridion*, ed. by Baker and Lapidge, pp. 10–12.

bilis, stabiles, graves, compositos moribus, dolososque facit. Phlegmata, tardos, somnolentos, obliviosos generant.

> (Likewise those in whom blood is especially strong, it makes them cheerful, happy, merciful, laughing greatly and talkative; red bile, however, makes them thin though they eat much, swift, rash, hot tempered and alert; black bile makes them steadfast, heavy, sedate in habits, and sorrowful; phlegmatic humours generate slowness, drowsiness and forgetfulness.)[26]

This description seems closer to a paraphrase of Vindicianus' *Epistola ad Pentadium* than to the pseudo-Hippocratic *Epistola de quattuor humoribus*, insofar as the latter text specifically separates the natural states of the four ages of man based on their dominant humours from the pathological effects of overabundant humours *cum alienatione mentis* (with disturbance of the mind). This concept of man as a microcosm had an enduring legacy in monastic education, as attested by the lavish diagrams of the relationship between microcosmic man and macrocosmic universe not only in such Insular witnesses associated with Byrhtferth of Ramsey, such as Oxford, St John's College, MS 17 fol. 7v or London, BL, MS Harley 3667 fol. 8r, to name just two examples.[27] While Plato's *Timaeus* was almost certainly not among the Greek works brought to England by Theodore and Hadrian, the most basic elements of Plato's atomic theory of four elements and the related physiological theory of four humours seem to have been an essential part of the monastic curriculum in England from the period of the conversion onwards.[28] While Anne Van Arsdall rightly argues that there was a fundamental difference between the philosophical and practical study of medicine, it remains true that medical theory rooted in Galenic Hippocratism was considered appropriate for advanced study in early English monasteries.[29]

More practical, but still quite theoretical, medical texts were also useful to Bede in his scriptural exegesis. He names Hippocrates in his *Retractio in actus apostolorum* as part of a direct quotation from Cassius Felix.[30] The purpose of the quotation is to explain the nature of a disease term which occurs in Acts 28. 8. Bede's exegesis in his *retractio* is highly philological and demonstrates that he was engaging directly with a Greek text of Acts.[31] This

26 Bede, *Opera de temporibus*, ed. by Jones, p. 247.

27 For continental examples, see Munich, BSB, MSS Clm 13002, fol. 7v and Clm 2655, fol. 105v.

28 For an overview of the relationship between humoralism and Plato's *Timaeus*, see De Lacy, 'Galen's Platonism'. For a more philosophical discussion of Neoplatonism in early Christianity, see Kurdziałek, 'Medieval Doctrines' and Otisk, 'The Four Elements and their Characteristics'.

29 Van Arsdall, 'Medical Training in Anglo-Saxon England', p. 406.

30 *Retractio in actu* 28.8, PL 92, col. 1032 directly quotes Cassius Felix 48, including a quotation of the Hippocratic *Aphorisms*: see Love, 'The Library of the Venerable Bede', p. 624.

31 Love, 'The Library of the Venerable Bede'.

use of a medical text in scriptural exegesis demonstrates the double function of the study of medicine in the monastic curriculum both as a practical discipline for the healing of the sick, as suggested in the sixth-century *Institutiones* of Cassiodorus, and as extension of the liberal arts, which could be studied for better comprehension of the world and of scripture.[32]

Humoral Theory in Medical Practice

The reception of humoral theory as part and parcel of Neoplatonic atomism in early medieval Christianity by itself would be thoroughly unsurprising. The true test of the reception of classical and late antique physiology is whether it has any bearing in the specifically medical literature of the Insular world, and in the case of this article, early medieval England. Searching for evidence of the theoretical basis of medical texts can prove useless unless there is first some understanding of how humoral theory affected medical practice in classical and late antique medicine. The elite medical practice of Galenic Hippocratism, scorned by Pliny the Elder[33] but transmitted to late antiquity by such authors as Oribasius, did not tend to reiterate the theory of the four humours in such trivial detail as the pseudo-Hippocratic *epistolae* or Vindicianus' didactic address to his nephew. Rather, the system of nosology, differential diagnosis, and therapeutics relied upon a thorough internalization of the Neoplatonic microcosm. There is a strong emphasis on regimen in these elite texts, that is, the maintenance of health by the precise control of food, drink, exercise, sexual intercourse, bathing and, where possible, the climate enjoyed, essentially the six *res non naturales* of later scholastic Galenism.[34] Therapeutics often focuses on the removal of overabundant humours, or the correction of temperament by the theory of opposites. This is succinctly described by Vindicianus to his nephew: 'nam si sit causa sanguinis, qui est dulcis umidus et calidus, occurrendum est sic ut adhibeatur e contrario quod sit frigidum amarum et siccum' (for instance, if the disease is of blood, which is sweet, moist and hot, it is to be opposed thus, to invite from the opposite, which is cold, bitter and dry).[35] Humours are thus purged through vomiting, stimulation of nasal discharge, diuretics and laxatives as well as phlebotomy (the cutting of veins), scarification (the drawing of blood through shallow scratches with a cupping glass), and very occasionally, with hirudotherapy (the application of live leeches).[36]

32 Cassiodorus, *Institutiones*, ed. by Baskerville Mynors, I, pp. 31–32.

33 See Nutton, 'The Perils of Patriotism' and Fagan, 'Bathing for Health with Celsus and Pliny'.

34 See Doyle, 'Foods for Body and Soul'.

35 Vindicianus, *Epistola ad Pentadium* in *Theodori Prisciani*, ed. by Rose, p. 491.

36 Hirudotherapy is completely absent from the Old English vernacular corpus but is attested in the *Tereoperica* at 72.3 and 102.1 in Lopez Figueroa's edition. See also London, BL, MS Sloane 2839 on fols 79^{r}, 94^{r,} 95^{v}, 99^{v}, 102^{r} and 105^{v}, where the application of *sansugia* (for

Most texts prescribe phlebotomy with caveats that it should only be done if the patient has sufficient strength and if the astrological conditions are correct. It was expressly forbidden during the *dies caniculares* (dog days of summer) and during certain days of the lunar month, known as *dies aegyptianes*.[37] Dog days are explained in Old English in *Leechbook* I.72: 'Blodlæs is to forganne | fiftyne nihtum ær hlafmæsse 7 æfter fif 7 þritig nihtum for þon þonne ealle æterno þing fleogaþ 7 mannum swiðe deriað' (bloodletting must be foregone for fifteen nights before the first of August and afterwards for thirty-five nights because at that time all poisonous things fly and do much harm to men).[38] Later in the same chapter, bloodletting is prohibited on every fifth day of the calendar month, i.e. the fifth, tenth, fifteenth, twentieth, twenty-fifth, and thirtieth days of the moon.[39] Ultimately, this seems to be a conflation of the *dies aegyptianes*, being a small number of certain inauspicious days in each calendar month as described, for example, in London, BL, MS Harley 3271, fol. 122^{r-v}, with the predictable occurrence of crises on numbered days after the accession of a fever as described in Galen's *Ad Glauconem*, sometimes circulating separately under the title *De diebus criticis*.[40]

Phlebotomy was not only prescribed to draw off pathological humours, but also as a form of prophylaxis against the accumulation of harmful humours, especially phlegm, which was associated with the constriction of the natural flow of bodily fluids resulting ultimately in apoplexy and death. In Bald's *Leechbook*, for example, it is stated that:

> 7 nis nan blodlæs tid swa god swa on foreweardne lencten þon*ne* þa yfelan wætan beoþ gegaderode | þe on wintra gedruncene beoð 7 on kalendas aprilis ealra selest þonne treow 7 wyrta ærest up spryttað þon*ne* weaxeð sio yfele gillestre 7 þæt yfele blod on þam holcum þæs lichoman.
>
> > (and there is no better time for phlebotomy than at the beginning of spring when the harmful humours are gathered that are absorbed in winter, and on the first day of April, when trees and herbs may first sprout up, then the harmful phlegm and evil blood increases in the cavities of the body.)[41]

---

sanguisugia) is mentioned. Oribasius suggests the use of *sanguisugas* at least three times in *Synopsis*, VIII, chs 40, 50 and 58 for application to the head and face.

37 In addition to these instances in purely medical texts, medical and non-medical prognostics circulated widely and have been the subject of relatively recent monographs: see Liuzza, 'Anglo-Saxon Prognostics in Context' and *Anglo-Saxon Prognostics*, as well as Chardonnens, *Anglo-Saxon Prognostics*.

38 London, BL, MS Royal 12 D XVII, fol. 55^{r-v}.

39 Læcas lærað eac þæt nan man on þone fif nihta ealdne monan 7 eft x nihta 7 fiftyne 7 twentiges 7 fif 7 twentiges 7 þritiges nihta eadlne monan ne læte blod ac betweox þara sex fifa ælcum (Doctors teach that no one should let blood on the five nights old moon, and again the ten, and fifteen and twenty and twenty-five and thirty nights old moon, but between each of the six fives).

40 See, for example St Gall, Stiftsbibliothek, MS 761, pp. 11–18.

41 Bald's *Leechbook* I.72, in *Leechdoms*, ed. and trans. by Cockayne, II, pp. 146–49 (London, BL, MS Royal 12 D XVII, fol. 55^{rv}).

While a specific Latin source for this Old English passage has not yet been located, there is a general agreement of detail between the advice given in the chapter overall and those epistolary fragments on phlebotomy which circulate alongside the *Tereoperica*.[42]

Phlebotomy was certainly not the only means of expelling those humours which abound at certain times of year. The *Physica Plinii*, for example, prescribes a mouthwash of honey and mustard boiled in water and strained through a linen cloth to purge the head of phlegm in winter (*Item purgatorium capitis hyeme*). A direct translation of this into Old English survives in *Leechbook* I.29,[43] although there it occurs in the context of treating chronic headaches. For gentler seasonal prophylaxis, Oribasius suggests such pharmaceuticals as aloe vera and terebinth in his *Euporista* I.9. This is faithfully translated in an excerpt in Bald's *Leechbook* that contains a long list of laxatives and purgatives, where it is noted that all these expurgations should be carried out 'on forweardne lencten ær þon sio yfele wæte se þe on wintra gesomnad bið hie togeote geond oþera lima' (at the beginning of spring before the harmful humours which are gathered in winter overflow throughout the other organs).[44]

Explicit statements of humoral pathology do not necessarily refer to one of the four bodily fluids by name, but an implicit suggestion of hot, boiling humours or cold turgid humours, etc., is more typical of late antique humoralism. Consider, for example, the following description of the cause of migraine from Bald's *Leechbook* I.1:

> Tacnu þære adle, sio adl cymð of yfelre wætan ufan flowendre oþþe of æþme oþþe of bam. Þonne sceal mon ærest on ða adle foreweardre blod lætan of ædre, æfter þon sceal man wyrt drenc sellan 7 lacnian siþþan þa saran stowa. Gif seo adl sie cumen of micelre hæto þonne sceal mon mid cealdum læcedomum lacnian. Gif hio of cealdum intingan cymð, þonne sceal mon mid hatum læcedomum lacnian, gehwæþeres sceal mon nyttian 7 miscian þæt þone lichoman hæle 7 afer mægen hæbbe.
>
> (Signs of the disease: the disease comes from a harmful upward flowing humour or from steam or from both. Then one should first let blood from a vein at the beginning of the disease, after that one

42 A text on phlebotomy occurs in London, BL, MS Sloane 2839, fols 110^{rv}, 109^{rv}, 108^{rv}, 107^{r}. The folios have been bound out of order. The *dies eqyptiani* are described somewhat differently in this text than in Old English. The *Liber epistolarum* in Paris, BNF, Lat 11219 fols 32ra–35vb also contains a series of tracts on phlebotomy.

43 London, BL, MS Royal 12 D XVII, fol. 9^{v}. It is closest to the *Physica Plinii Florentino Pragensis* I, 1. 27 (ed. by Winkler, pp. 60–61), while the *Physica Plinii Bambergensis* 1. 27 (ed. by Önnerfors, p. 24) does not mention the season; see Adams and Deegan, 'Bald's *Leechbook* and the *Physica Plinii*'.

44 *Leechbook* II.30, in *Leechdoms*, ed. and trans. by Cockayne, II, pp. 228–29 (London, BL, MS Royal 12 D XVII, fol. 85^{rv}) is directly translated from *Euporista* I. 9, specifically the New Latin translation, not the Old.

should give herbal drinks and then treat the sore place. If the disease comes from great heat, then one should treat with cold medicines. If it comes from a cold cause then one should treat with hot remedies, one should mix and choose from either so that the body becomes healthy, and always has strength.)[45]

Here, the humours other than blood are not specifically named, but the humoralism is explicit insofar as excesses are to be purged with cathartic medicines (*catartico* in the Latin Alexander), the cold is to be heated and the hot is to be cooled. Following such advice requires a knowledge of the natural properties of *materia medica,* and for that purpose the early English medic may have had recourse to Oribasius *Synopsis* II, which defines *materia medica* and foodstuffs by their principal properties, or *Euporista* IV, which is more concerned with dietetics. While there is no direct manuscript evidence that *Synopsis* II existed in pre-Conquest England, Oribasius' pharmacological writings were consulted by the compiler of Bald's *Leechbook,* who interpolated Oribasian lists of foods into therapies from the Latin Alexander for a patient suffering from *bulismus* or vomiting with syncope from travel sickness.[46]

Humoral Terminology in Medical Texts

As discussed above, medical application of humoral theory does not rely on a consistent lexis to define the four humours themselves. While the terms *phlegma, sanguis,* and *humor* are relatively universal across the Latin medical corpus, terms for the biles are not consistent in the colours they represent. *Χολη ξανθή* (yellow bile) may be rendered as a loanword, though the colour is normally altered to *rufum* or *rubeum* (red), as in Vindicianus' *Epistola ad Pentadium,* while the bile itself may be called *fel, choler,* or even *bilis.* More than naming the humours, the *sine qua non* of humoral theory in medical literature is the consistent use of concepts of heat and cold, superfluity and purgation, and the general conception of the whole body as a hydraulic system, disrupted by such pathological processes as *emphraxis* (*ἔμφραξις*) — meaning stoppage or constriction — which could give rise to such deadly conditions as *hemiplegia, apoplexia* or *paralysis* (what we might call a stroke or paralysis).[47]

45 The Latin source here is Alexander of Tralles, I.45–46, ed. by Fradin, fol. 7v. The chapter numbers differ in Paris, BnF, MS Lat. 9332; see Alexander von Tralles, *Original-Text,* ed. by Puschmann, I, pp. 499–501 for the Greek.

46 *Leechbook* II.16, in *Leechdoms,* ed. and trans. by Cockayne, II, pp. 192–97 (London, BL, MS Royal 12 D XVII, fol. 73r–v) translates Alexander, II.23 and Oribasius, *Synopsis,* IV.16–17; see Doyle, 'Foods for Body and Soul'. *Synopsis* II is essentially an abridgement of Galen *De simplicium medicamentorum temperamentis et facultatibus.*

47 The last recipe in the 'Leechbook Fragment' in London, BL, MS Harley 55, fol. 1v, 'wið þære healfdeadan adle' (for paralysis), translates Oribasius, *Synopsis,* VIII.14, which includes *enfraxin* as one of the aetiologies of *paralysis.*

In the same way, Old English does not have a single set of terms for the four humours. The generic term for fluid was *wæta* or *wæte*, a weak masculine or feminine substantive denoting moisture which could translate *humor* or *liquor*. Lois Ayoub noted that 'the Old English word *wæta* in Anglo-Saxon medical texts is consistently chosen to render references in Latin sources to the doctrine of the humours'.[48] Having analysed all instances of the term in Old English medical texts, I have noted that it translates Latin *humor* in about half of instances where a Latin source lemma can be identified. The Old English term also translates a range of other Latin terms, including *rheuma*, *flegma*, *pituitas*, or even *potio*, suggesting that it has a wider semantic range than *humor* alone: the fact that these usages occur in the Old English medical corpus breaks Langslow's criterion of absolute synonymy and total translatability in translated technical prose.[49] In medical contexts, the adjectives used to describe fluids are often more important than the words meaning fluid themselves. When referring to drinks, the use of temperature adjectives or adjectives of quality is common, while adjectives qualifying bodily fluids are of the utmost importance in understanding how medical authors and translators understood disease aetiology. I identified sixteen adjectives denoting humoral pathology that are used in agreement with *wæta* in the medical corpus: *æterno* (poisonous), *æterberend* (poisoning), *bitend* (biting), *biter* (bitter), *ceald* (cold), *fæt* (fat or moist), *hat* (hot), *horheht* (phlegmatic) *lið* (synovial) *ofset* (oppressive) *omig* (erysipelatic), *slipig* (slippery), *slitend* (cutting), *þicc* (thick), *ungemet* (immoderate) and, most commonly, *yfel* (harmful).

While blood (*sanguis*) is normally *blod* (unless vomited or in a seeping wound, in which case it is *wyrms*, translating *sanies*), terms for phlegm are many and varied. Byrhtferth of Ramsey invokes the action of coughing and sneezing (*hraca oððe geposu*) to denote this humour and in strictly medical texts it is much more often denoted by the use of *wæta* with one or more of the attributives listed above, while elsewhere the terms *horh*, *horheht*, and possibly even *bræc* can denote phlegm.[50] Indeed, the fact that the Old English translators of Oribasius, Alexander and other late antique elite medical texts chose to avoid excessive use of jargon and loanwords means that pathological concepts are often explicated with great clarity, if greater verbosity and at the cost of the stylistic concision that normally characterizes technical texts.[51] For example, six Greek pathology terms recur in the late antique medical corpus that derive from Galen's *Ad Glauconem* and the pseudo-Galenic *Liber tertius*:

apostema (*ἀπό-στημα*), meaning collection of humours into a swelling
syrrexis (*σύρρηξις*), meaning the rupture of an *apostema*

48 Ayoub, 'Old English *wæta*', p. 341.

49 Doyle, 'Anglo-Saxon Medicine and Disease', I, pp. 151–52; Langslow, *Medical Latin*, pp. 21–22.

50 On the association of *bræcseoc* with phlegm, see Lockett, 'The Limited Role of the Brain', pp. 46–51.

51 On the stylistic features of medical Latin, see Langslow, *Medical Latin*.

helcosis (ἕλκωσις) meaning an ulceration
phlegmone (φλεγμονή) meaning an inflammation
scleria (σκληρία) meaning a sensitive induration
and *scirrosis* (σκίρρωσις) meaning an insensitive induration

These six terms are never borrowed into Old English, but are explained quite well in Bald's *Leechbook*, as they pertain to hepatic pathology:

> II.17: Be sex þingum þe þone liferwærc wyrceað ærest geswel *þæt* is aþundenes þære lifer. Oþer is þæs geswelles toberstung. Þridde is wund þære lifre. Feorþe is welmes hæto mid gefelnesse 7 mid sare geswelle. Fifte is aheardung þæs magan mid gefelnesse 7 mid sare. Sexte is aheardung þære lifre butan gefelnesse 7 butan sare.[52]
>
> > (Concerning the six things that cause liver disease. First is swelling, that is inflammation of the liver, the second is rupture of the swelling, the third is a wound of the liver, the fourth is boiling heat with sensitivity and with painful swelling, the fifth is hardening of the stomach [understand liver] with sensitivity and with pain, the sixth is hardening of the liver without sensitivity and without pain.)

The Latin source here is obviously the pseudo-Galenic *Liber tertius*:

> *LT* 36.1. Incipiunt causae epaticae. Epar una res est, id est iecur, quae ex nomine causam designat periculosam, sed habet causas sex. Quae causae diuersis signis suis agnoscuntur uel demonstratur, id est: Apostema in iecore, syrrexis id est ruptio apostematis, helcosis id est uulneratio, phlegmone hoc est feruor uel tumor, scleria hoc est duritia cum sensu et dolore, scirrosis id est nimia duritia sine dolore et sine sensu, qui[a] in iecore habetur.[53]
>
> > (Here begin the causes of hepatitis. *Epar* is one thing, that is the liver, which designates a most perilous disease, but has six pathologies, which are recognized and revealed by diverse signs, that is: apostema in the liver; syrrexis, that is rupture of the apostema; helcosis, that is wound; phlegmone, that is heat or swelling, scleria, that is hardness with feeling and pain, scirrhosis, that is excessive hardness without pain and without feeling, which is held in the liver.)

These definitions of the possible fate of the initial *apostema* recur throughout the section of Bald's *Leechbook* which concerns the liver (II.17–22), using the extended definitions of the pathologies in each instance rather than making

52 Talbot, 'Some Notes on Anglo-Saxon Medicine', p. 161 notes some parallels with other medical compilations, namely the *Tereoperica* and *Passionarius*, but the *Liber tertius* provides a more convincing source.

53 Pseudo-Galen, *Liber tertius*, ed. by Fischer, p. 311.

recourse to loan-translation or borrowing. Of course, these pathologies are not limited to the liver, but it is in the chapters of the *Leechbook* concerning the liver that they are treated most consistently by the vernacular compiler.

The ability to synthesize a coherent and internally consistent medical compilation from multiple Latin sources including Alexander, pseudo-Galen and Oribasius, which use differing vocabulary to define the same conditions, is perhaps the strongest evidence that early English medics undertook a scholarly approach to medicine with a good understanding of the physiological system of Galenic Hippocratism transmitted in Latin through the Ravenna school.

Conclusion

Humoral theory is not only relevant to disease aetiology in Bald's *Leechbook*: it also informs the very structure of that text and the pre-Norman English understanding of human anatomy and physiology. Without direct access to Galen's Greek, the textual study of anatomy and physiology in the early medieval Latin West was limited to the short compilations attributed to Helvius Vindicianus, namely the *Gynaecia*, the *Epitome altera*, and *De natura generis humani*.[54] These texts provide the most cursory information about human anatomy, but also inform us about the humoral and even spiritual and cognitive functions of specific organs that are described in more detail, such as the brain, heart, stomach, liver, and spleen. While these texts, which may or may not have developed from authentic works of Vindicianus, were sparingly used in the compilation of Bald's *Leechbook*, two of the longer chapters of the *Epitome altera* are deployed to open the very long sections of *Leechbook* II on the liver and spleen respectively, explaining their functions before their pathologies are discussed over many chapters.[55] These sources, together with the Latin Alexander, are used to create a coherent narrative of human physiology. This centred on the role of the stomach, where food is first received and decocted and then sent on to the intestines where the five-lobed liver refines the chyle into blood, which is in turn sent out by the heart. The spleen (which is the seat of black bile) and the intestines (where decocted food undergoes decay before excretion) are also of great importance due to their capacity to influence the humoral temperament of the whole body. This is structurally represented in the arrangement of *Leechbook* II: chapters 1–16 concern the stomach, 17–24 concern the liver, 25–35 concern the small intestines, 36–45 concern the spleen,

54 *Epitome altera* and *Gynaecia* in *Theodori Prisciani Euporiston*, ed. by Rose, pp. 427–83; *De natura generis humani* in Vazques Buján, 'Vindiciano y el tratado *De natura generis humani*'. For a translation of one recension of the *Gynaecia*, see Cilliers, 'Vindicianus Gynaecia: Text and Translation'.

55 *Leechbook*, II.17 (ed. and trans. by Cockayne, II, pp. 196–99) opens with *Epitome Altera* 19 on the liver, while II.36 (ed. and trans. by Cockayne, II, pp. 242–43) contains a paraphrase of *Epitome altera* 20 on the spleen. See Cameron, *Anglo-Saxon Medicine*, pp. 93–94.

46–51 concern the lungs, and 55–58 concern the large intestines and bladder, with a significant lacuna after II.56. The compilation of the book must then have required a thorough internalization of humoral theory and physiology, not just at the level of faithfully preserving individual recipes, therapies and disease descriptions, but creatively combining multiple Latin sources into a coherent and consistent outline of the most important organs of the body within the humoral physiology of Late Antiquity and the early Middle Ages. The very structural arrangement of Book II is not just a convenient ordering of chapters from diverse sources, but a synthesis and distillation of a system of health that combined preventative medicine with therapeutics up to and including abdominal surgery. It was set out in a way which gave primacy to the anatomical seats of the four humours and explained the necessary steps to keep those humours in balance for the health of the whole body and mind.

Works Cited

Manuscripts

Florence, Biblioteca Medicea Laurenziana, MS Plut. 73.1
Laon, Bibliothèque municipale, MS 424
London, British Library, MS Harley 55
London, British Library, MS Harley 3271
London, British Library, MS Harley 3667
London, British Library, MS Royal 12 D XVII
London, British Library, MS Sloane 2839
Munich, Bayerische Staatsbibliothek, MS Latinus monacensis 2655
Munich, Bayerische Staatsbibliothek, MS Latinus monacensis 13002
Paris, Bibliothèque nationale de France, MS fonds latin 7028
Paris, Bibliothèque nationale de France, MS fonds latin 9332
Paris, Bibliothèque nationale de France, MS fonds latin 11219
Paris, Bibliothèque nationale de France, MS Nouvelle acquisition latine 1619
Oxford, St John's College, MS 17
Rome, Biblioteca Apostolica Vaticana, MS Latin 5951
St Gall, Stiftbibliothek, MS 761

Primary Sources

Alexander of Tralles, *The Latin Alexander: The Text and Transmission of a Late Latin Medical Book*, ed. and trans. by David Langslow, Journal of Roman Studies Monographs, 10 (London: Society for the Promotion of Roman Studies, 2006)

——, *Original-Text und Übersetzung nebst einer einleitenden Abhandlung: ein Beitrag zur Geschichte der Medicin*, ed. by Theodor Puschmann (Vienna: Braumüller, 1878)

——, *Practica Alexandri yatros greci cum expositione glose interliniaris Jacobi de partibus*, ed. by François Fradin (Lyon: F. Fradin, 1504)

Antonii Musae De herba uettonica liber, Pseudo-Apulei Herbarius. Anonymi De taxone liber, Sexti Placiti Liber medicinae ex animalibus, ed. by Ernst Howald and Henry Ernest Sigerist, Corpus medicorum latinorum, 4 (Leipzig: Teubner, 1927)

Anglo-Saxon Prognostics: An Edition and Translation of Texts from London, British Library, MS Cotton Tiberius A.iii, ed. and trans. by Roy M. Liuzza, Anglo-Saxon Texts, 8 (Cambridge: Brewer, 2011)

Bede, *Historia ecclesiastica*, ed. and trans. by Bertram Colgrave and Roger Aubrey Baskerville Mynors (Oxford: Clarendon Press, 1969)

Bede, *Opera de temporibus*, ed. by C. W. Jones (Cambridge, MA: Medieval Academy of America, 1943)

Byrhtferth, *Enchiridion*, ed. by Peter Baker and Michael Lapidge, Early English Text Society Supplemental Series, 15 (Oxford: Oxford University Press, 1995)

Cassiodorus, *Institutiones*, ed. by Roger Aubrey Baskerville Mynors, digitized by Raffaella Tabacco and Maurizio Lana, Biblioteca digitale di testi latini tardoantichi <https://digiliblt.uniupo.it/opera.php?id=DLT000078> [accessed 8 March 2022]

Isidore of Seville, *Etymologiae siue origiones*, ed. by Wallace Martin Lindsay, digitized by Bill Thayer <penelope.uchicago.edu/Thayer/e/roman/texts/isidore/home.html> [accessed 8 March 2022]

Leechdoms, Wortcunning and Starcraft of Early England, ed. by Thomas Oswald Cockayne, Rerum Brittanicarum medii aevi scriptores, 35, 3 vols (London: Longman, 1864–1866)

Marcellus, *De medicamentis liber*, ed. by Eduard Liechtenhan and Max Niedermann, trans. by Jutta Kollesch and Diethard Nickel, Corpus medicorum latinorum, 5 (Berlin: Verlag, 1968)

The Medicina Plinii: Latin text, Translation and Commentary, ed. by Yvette Hunt (Abingdon: Routledge 2021)

Oeuvres d'Oribase, ed. by A. C. Bussemaker and C. Daremberg, 6 vols (Paris: L'Imprimier Nationale, 1850–1876)

The Old English Herbarium and Medicina de quadrupedibus, ed. by Hubert Jan de Vriend, Early English Texts Society, o.s. 286 (London: Oxford University Press, 1984)

Oribasius, 'Oribasius Latinus ad Eunapium Eporiste liber primus: editie van de beide overleveringen van het eerste boek van de Euporista met commentaar', ed. by E. W. Goos (unpublished doctoral thesis, Rijksuniversiteit te Utrecht, 1989)

——, *Synopsis I–II*, ed. by Henning Mørland, *Oribasius Latinus (Erster Teil)*, Symbolae Osloenses Fasciculi suppletorii, 10 (Oslo: Brøger, 1940)

——, *Synopsis VII*, ed. by Gomez Costoya, in 'Estudio y edición critica de la traducción latina del libro VII de la Synopsis de Oribasio' (unpublished doctoral thesis, University of Santiago de Compostela, 2015)

——, *Synopsis* and *Euporista*, ed. by Joseph Raeder, Corpus Medicorum Graecorum, 6.3 (Leipzig: Teubner, 1926)

Pliny, *Physica Plinii Bambergensis*, ed. by Alf Önnerfors (Hildesheim: Georg Olms Verlag, 1975)

Pliny, *Physicae que fertur Plinii Florentino-Pragensis liber primus*, ed. by Joachim Winkler, Lateinische Sprache und Literatur des Mittelalters, 17 (Frankfurt: Peter Lang, 1984)

Pliny, *Plinii Secundi Iunoris qui feruntur de medicina libri tres*, ed. by Alf Önnerfors, Corpus Medicorum Latinorum, 3 (Berlin: Akademie Verlag, 1964)

Pseudo-Galen, *Liber tertius*, ed. by Klaus-Dietrich Fischer, in 'Galeni qui fertur ad Glauconem liber tertius ad fidem codicis Vindocinensis 109', in *Galenismo e Medicina tardoantica. Fonti greche, latine e arabe Atti del seminario internacionale di Siena*, ed. by Ivan Garofalo and Amneris Roselli, Analli Del'istituto Universitario Orientale di Napoli, 7 (Naples, 2003), pp. 283–346

Tereoperica, ed. by Laura Lopéz Figueroa, in 'Estudio y edición críticia de la compilación médica latina denominada *Tereoperica*' (unpublished doctoral thesis, University of Santiago de Compostela, 2011)

Tereoperica, ed. by Salvatore de Renzi, as 'Practica Petrocelli Salernitani', in *Collectio Salernitana*, 5 vols (Naples: Filiatro Sebezio, 1852–1859),IV.185–286

Theodori Prisciani Euporiston Libri III, ed. by Valentino Rose (Leipzig: Teubner, 1894)

Vindicianus, *Gynaecia*, in Louise Cilliers, 'Vindicianus Gynaecia: Text and Translation of the Codex Monacensis (Clm 4622)', *Journal of Medieval Latin*, 15 (2005), 153–236

Secondary Studies

Adams, James Noel, and Marilyn Deegan, 'Bald's Leechbook and the *Physica Plinii*', *Anglo-Saxon England*, 21 (1992), 87–114

Ayoub, Lois, 'Old English *wæta* and the Medical Theory of the Humours', *Journal of English and Germanic Philology*, 94 (1995), 332–46

Beccaria, Augusto, *I codici di medicina del periodo Presalernitano: secoli ix, x e xi* (Rome: Edizioni di storia e letteratura, 1956)

Cameron, Malcolm Laurence, *Anglo-Saxon Medicine*, Cambridge Studies in Anglo-Saxon England, 7 (Cambridge: Cambridge University Press, 1993)

——, 'Bald's *Leechbook*: Its Sources and their Use in its Compilation', *Anglo-Saxon England*, 12 (1983), 153–82

——, 'The Sources of Medical Knowledge in Anglo-Saxon England', *Anglo-Saxon England*, 11 (1982), 135–55

Chardonnens, Sándor, *Anglo-Saxon Prognostics, 900–1100*, Texts and Sources in Intellectual History, 155 (Leiden: Brill, 2007)

Cilliers, Louise, 'The Contribution of the 4th Century North African Physician, Helvius Vindicianus', in *Medicine and Healing in the Ancient Mediterranean*, ed. by Demetrios Michaelides (Oxford: Oxbow, 2014), pp. 123–29

——, *Roman North Africa: Environment, Society and Medical Contribution* (Amsterdam: Amsterdam University Press, 2019)

D'Aronco, Maria A., 'How "English" is Anglo-Saxon Medicine? The Latin Sources for Anglo-Saxon Medical Texts', in *Britannia Latina: Latin in the Culture of Great Britain from the Middle Ages to the Twentieth Century*, ed. by Charles Burnett and Nicholas Mann, Warburg Institute Colloquia, 8 (London: Warburg Institute, 2005), pp. 27–41

De Lacy, Phillip, 'Galen's Platonism', *The American Journal of Philology*, 93.1 (1972), 27–39

Doyle, Conan T., 'Anglo-Saxon Medicine and Disease, A Semantic Approach', 2 vols (unpublished doctoral thesis, University of Cambridge, 2017) <https://doi.org/10.17863/CAM.14430>

——, 'Foods for Body and Soul: The Application of Late Antique Regimen in Anglo-Saxon Medical Texts', in *Cultivating the Earth, Nurturing the Body and Soul: Daily Life in Early Medieval England*, ed. by Christine Voth (Turnhout: Brepols, 2025), pp. 267–93

Duranti, Tommaso, 'The Origins of the Studium of Medicine of Bologna: A Status quaestionis', *CIAN: Revisita de Historia de las Universidades*, 21 (2018), 121–49 DOI:10.20318/cian.2018.4193

Fagan, Garret, 'Bathing for Health with Celsus and Pliny the Elder', *The Classical Quarterly*, 56 (2006), 190–207

Fischer, Klaus-Dietrich, 'Dr Monk's Medical Digest', *Social History of Medicine*, 13 (2000), 139–251

——, 'Der Pseudogalenische "Liber tertius"', in *Galenismo e medicina tardoantica fonte greche, latine e arabe: Atti del seminario internazionale di Siena*, ed. by Ivan Garofalo and Amneris Roselli, Annali dell'Istituto universitario orientale di Napoli, 7 (Naples: Istituto Universitario Orientale, 2003), pp. 101–32

——, 'Two Latin Pre-Salernitan Medical Manuals, the *Liber passionalis* and the *Tereoperica* (Ps. Petroncellus)', in *Medical Books in the Byzantine World*, ed. by Barbara Zipser, Eikasmos Online, 2 (Bologna: Eikasmos 2013) pp. 35–56 <www2.classics.unibo.it/eikasmos/doc_pdf/studi_online/02_zipser_medical_books.pdf> [accessed 11 March 2022]

Glaze, Florence Eliza, 'Galen Refashioned: Gariopontus in the Later Middle Ages and Renaissance', in *Textual Healing: Essays on Medieval and Early Modern Medicine*, ed. by Elizabeth Lane Furdell, Studies in Medieval and Reformation Traditions: History, Culture, Religion, Ideas, 110 (Leiden: Brill, 2005), pp. 53–75

——, 'Gariopontus and the Salernitans: Textual Traditions in the Eleventh and Twelfth Centuries', in *La Collectio Salernitana di Salvatore De Renzi*, ed. by Danielle Jacquart and Paravicini Bagliani, Edizione Nazionale La Scuola Medica Salernitana, 3 (Florence: SISMEL, 2008), pp. 149–90

——, 'Master–Student Medical Dialogues: The Evidence of London, British Library, Sloane 2839', in *Form & Content of Instruction in Anglo-Saxon England in Light of Contemporary Manuscript Evidence*, ed. by Patrizia Lendinara, Loredana Lazzari, and Maria Amalia D'Aronco, Textes et Études du Moyen Âge, 39 (Turnhout: Brepols, 2007), pp. 467–94

Gratton, John Henry Grafton, and Charles Singer, *Anglo-Saxon Magic and Medicine Illustrated Specially from the Semi-Pagan Text 'Lacnunga'*, Publications of the Wellcome Historical Medical Museum, n.s. 3 (London: Oxford University Press, 1952)

Green, Monica, 'Rethinking the Manuscript Basis of Salvatore de Renzi's *Collectio Salernitana*: The Corpus of Medical Writings in the Long Twelfth Century', in *La Collectio Salernitana di Salvatore de Renzi: Convegno internazionale, Università degli Studi di Salerno, 18–19 giugno 2007*, ed. by Danielle Jacquart and Agostino Paravicini Bagliani (Florence: SISMEL, 2008), pp. 15–60

——, 'Salerno on the Thames: The Genesis of Anglo-Norman Medical Literature', in *Language and Culture in Medieval Britain: The French of England, c. 1100 – c. 1500*, ed. by Jocelyn Wogan-Browne, with Carolyn Collette, Maryanne Kowaleski, Linne Mooney, Ad Putter, and David Trotter (York: York Medieval Press, 2009), pp. 220–31

Horden, Peregrine, 'What's Wrong with Early Medieval Medicine?', *Social History of Medicine*, 24 (2011), 5–25

Kesling, Emily, *Medical Texts in Anglo-Saxon Literary Culture*, Anglo-Saxon Studies, 38 (Cambridge: D. S. Brewer, 2020)

Kurdziałek, Marian, 'Medieval Doctrines on Man as Image of the World', *Roczniki Filozoficzne*, 62.4 (2014), 205–46

Langslow, David, *Medical Latin in the Roman Empire* (Oxford: Oxford University Press, 2000)

Liuzza, Roy Michael, 'Anglo-Saxon Prognostics in Context: A Survey and Handlist of Manuscripts', *Anglo-Saxon England*, 30 (2001), 181–230

Lockett, Leslie, 'The Limited Role of the Brain in Mental and Emotional Activity According to Anglo-Saxon Medical Learning', in *Anglo-Saxon Emotions: Reading the Heart in Old English Language, Literature and Culture*, ed. by Alice Jorgensen, Frances McCormack, and Jonathan Wilcox, Studies in Early Medieval Britain and Ireland (Abingdon: Routledge, 2015), pp. 35–51

Love, Rosamund, 'The Library of the Venerable Bede', in *The Cambridge History of the Book in Britain*, ed. by Richard Gameson (Cambridge: Cambridge University Press, 2011), pp. 606–32

Maion, Danielle, 'The Fortune of the So-Called *Practica Petrocelli Salernitani* in England: New Evidence and some Considerations', in *Form and Content of Instruction in Anglo-Saxon England in the Light of Contemporary Manuscript Evidence: Papers Presented at the International Conference, Udine, 6–8 April, 2006*, ed. by Patricia Lendinaria, Loredana Lazzari, and Maria Amalia D'Aronco, Textes et Études du Moyen Âge, 39 (Turnhout: Brepols, 2007), pp. 495–512

Meaney, Audrey L., 'Variant Versions of Old English Medical Remedies and the Compilation of Bald's Leechbook', *Anglo-Saxon England*, 13 (1984), 235–64

Mørland, Henning, *Die Lateinischen Oribasiusübersetzungen*, Symolae Osloenses Fasciculi suppletorii, 5 (Oslo: Brøgger, 1932)

Nutton, Vivian, 'The Perils of Patriotism: Pliny and Roman Medicine', in *Science in the Early Roman Empire: Pliny the Elder, his Sources and Influence*, ed. by Roger French and Frank Greenway (London: Croom Helm, 1986), pp. 30–58

Otisk, Marek, 'The Four Elements and their Characteristics according to the Schema in the Early Medieval Anonymous Fragment *De quattuor elementis*', *Cosmos and History: The Journal of Natural and Social Philosophy*, 17.3 (2021), 462–500

Rashdall, Hastings, *The Universities of Europe in the Middle Ages*, ed. by Frederick Maurice Powicke and Alfred Brotherston Emden, 3 vols, rev. edn (Oxford: Oxford University Press, 1936)

Rubin, Stanley, *Medieval English Medicine* (Newton Abbot: David & Charles, 1974)

Siraisi, Nancy, 'The Faculty of Medicine', in *A History of the University in Europe I: The Universities in the Middle Ages*, ed. by Hilde de Ridder-Symoens (Cambridge: Cambridge University Press, 1991), pp. 360–87

Talbot, Charles, 'Some Notes on Anglo-Saxon Medicine', *Medical History*, 9 (1965), 156–69

Temkin, Owsei, *Hippocrates in a World of Pagans and Christians* (Baltimore: Johns Hopkins University Press, 1991)

Van Arsdall, Anne, 'Medical Training in Anglo-Saxon England: An Evaluation of the Evidence', in *Form and Content of Instruction in Anglo-Saxon England in the Light of Contemporary Manuscript Evidence: Papers Presented at the International Conference, Udine, 6–8 April, 2006*, ed. by Patricia Lendinaria, Loredana Lazzari, and Maria Amalia D'Aronco, Textes et Études du Moyen Âge, 39 (Turnhout: Brepols, 2007), pp. 415–34

Vazques Buján, Manuel Enrique, 'Vindiciano y el tratado *De natura generis humani*', *Dynamis*, 2 (1983), 25–56

Wallis, Faith, 'Medicine in Medieval Calendar Manuscripts', in *Manuscript Sources of Medieval Medicine: A Book of Essays*, ed. by Margaret Rose Schleissner (Abingdon: Routledge, 1995), pp. 105–44

ELISA RAMAZZINA

3. Therapeutic Baths in Medieval English Medicine*

Introduction

This study challenges some of the most widespread misconceptions related to medieval medicine, according to which balneotherapy was absent either for the entire duration of the medieval period or for at least part of it, being oftentimes forbidden due to epidemics and religious morals.[1] According to these theories, after the fall of the Roman Empire, where baths were medical and social hubs, the use of therapeutic baths declined and eventually disappeared. Some scholars even claim that only in the nineteenth century did the rise in popularity of leisure activities such as casinos, theatre, opera, and music concerts lead to a resurgence in public bathing practices.[2] Other scholars, instead, argue that the abandonment of Roman thermal baths corresponded to a lack of interest in the therapeutic functions of water, which is reflected in the lack of medical and scientific literature on water in the early Middle Ages.[3] This interest would undergo a revival only in the late Middle Ages, giving rise to the social practice of public baths on the one hand, and to the

* This publication is part of the results of a research project entitled 'Cleansing Water: Water and Baptism in Old English Poetry' that has received funding from the European Union's Horizon 2020 research and innovation programme under the Marie Skłodowska-Curie grant agreement No. 744615.

1 See for example Quintela, 'Contribution of Health', p. 76; Kosso and Scott, 'Preliminary Material', pp. i–viii; Rawcliffe, *Urban Bodies*, especially pp. 4–7 and 30–32; and Howes, *Transformative Waters*.

2 See for instance Cătănescu and Racolța, 'The Use of Decorative Elements', p. 2, and Nora, 'Turismo de Saúde', p. 1457.

3 See for example Bradley, *Health, Hedonism and Hypochondria*, pp. 3 and 65; Danzi, 'Le terme in Europa', p. 43; Silişteanu and others, 'Balneoclimatology', p. 58; and Zuccolin, 'Ruolo ed evoluzione della balneoterapia', p. 98.

Elisa Ramazzina • Queen's University Belfast; e.ramazzina@qub.ac.uk

Medicine in the Medieval North Atlantic World: Vernacular Texts and Traditions, ed. by Deborah Hayden and Sarah Baccianti, KSS, 5 (Turnhout, 2025), pp. 75-102
BREPOLS PUBLISHERS DOI 10.1484/M.KSS-EB.5.143981

production of medical-scientific texts on water and its therapeutic functions on the other.

The purpose of this contribution is to analyse the development of bathing practices in the English Middle Ages through examination of a selection of medical texts from the Old and Middle English corpora, with a view to demonstrating that medicinal baths have played a pivotal role in English medical practices since the early Middle Ages. It will be argued that, similar to what has been shown to be the case in medieval European medicine,[4] we can distinguish two phases regarding the therapeutic use of baths in English medical practices. In the first phase, corresponding to the early Middle Ages, water plays an important role in patient care, despite references to baths being scattered and bathing always being part of a more complex remedy that included the drinking of potions and the application of ointments. During this phase, the instructions for the preparation of baths and their use are very brief and general. In the second phase, which coincides with the late Middle Ages, balneotherapy started playing an increasingly vital role in healing practices. This is reflected in the medical literature of the time, with either sections of treatises or specific tracts entirely devoted to bathing, thermal waters, and their therapeutic virtues.

In this chapter, the curative and scientific properties of baths and their role in achieving the patient's psycho-physical wellbeing are examined in relation to other remedies, including potions and diets, to establish that the increasing relevance of bathing in medical practice throughout these two phases is directly related to the elemental and humoral theories that dominated natural philosophy and views of medicine and healing throughout the medieval period.[5]

It should be noted that in medieval England, there was a distinction between therapeutic bathing in private settings and public baths serving various functions beyond therapeutic purposes. Jaglarz emphasizes the importance of public bathing dating back to ancient Greece and Rome.[6] In these ancient civilizations, practices related to cleanliness, hygiene, and health took place in public areas, also symbolizing the status of free citizens. Public baths in Ancient Rome served as significant social hubs, comparable to modern venues like restaurants, urban squares, and recreational centres, where cultural and social activities flourished. These communal spaces played a crucial role in promoting both physical and mental well-being by enabling discussions, relaxation, games, artistic pursuits, and intellectual endeavours. In contrast, Jaglarz notes how the Middle Ages are known for their public bath houses,

4 For the evolution of therapeutic baths in medieval Europe, see Ramazzina, 'Bathing in Medieval Europe'.

5 On humoral theory in Old English sources, see also the chapter by Conan Doyle in this volume.

6 Jarglaz, 'The Evolution of Public Hygiene', p. 193.

which were popular primarily for entertainment rather than hygiene.[7] These medieval bathing establishments served as centres of pleasure and amusement, where activities like swimming and bathing were more focused on enjoyment than cleanliness. Erotic experiences often took precedence over the practical aspect of bathing, with water becoming a medium for physical delights and sensual pleasures. Elements such as wine, food, music, and secluded alcoves with curtains were essential in enhancing the overall experience of medieval baths. Despite this focus on entertainment, medieval European hydrotherapy and thermal treatises demonstrate that the public nature of some balneological resorts did not exclude their use for therapeutic purposes. An illustrative example is *De balneis Puteolanis*, a Latin poem by Peter of Eboli from the late twelfth century. This literary work provides a detailed description of the baths of Pozzuoli and Baiae near Naples, outlining their names, therapeutic properties, and successful treatments through the consistent use of medical terminology.[8]

Bathing in Early Medieval England

The earliest written records for medical practice in medieval England, which date to around the tenth century,[9] indicate that water was considered a fundamental element for patient care and was used both as an ingredient in potions and concoctions and in the preparation of baths. As noted by Smith, 'inner (and outer) bodily "cleansing" is ultimately connected to the more profound principle of "wholesomeness" within the general system of homeostasis that balances and sustains all bodily functions'.[10] Hippocrates was the first to claim that all diseases were due to an imbalance of bodily humours and, in order to restore that balance, he recommended remedies involving changes in habits, diet, and environment, as well as bathing, perspiration, and exercise.[11] This view was shared by medieval physicians, who, as I discuss below, prescribed medicinal baths as a way to contrast and heal such an imbalance.

Isidore of Seville (*c.* AD 560–636), whose works were very influential throughout the Middle Ages, associates thermal baths with psychological wellbeing in his *Etymologies*, relating the etymology for 'bath' to the curative properties of this practice, which was thought to be beneficial for sorrow and anxiety:

---

7 Jarglaz, 'The Evolution of Public Hygiene', p. 193.

8 On this topic see Ramazzina, 'Bathing in Medieval Europe', pp. 112–19.

9 London, BL, MS Royal 12 D XVII is the first manuscript entirely dedicated to medicine. It contains *Bald's Leechbook* (*Leechbooks I* and *II*), *Leechbook III*, and a prognostic text on 'Dog Days'.

10 Smith, *Clean*, p. 9.

11 See Galen, *On Hippocrates' On the Nature of Man*, ed. and trans. by Lewis and Beach, especially Part One.

Thermas appellatas quod caleant; Graeci enim θερμόν calorem vocant. Balneis vero nomen inditum a levatione maeroris; nam Graeci βαλανεῖον dixerunt, quod anxietatem animi tollat. Haec et gymnasia dicuntur, quia ibi athletae uncto corpore et perfricato manibus exercitantur; nam γυμνάσιον Graece, Latine exercitium dicitur. [...] Propina Graecus sermo est, quae apud nos corrupte popina dicitur: est autem locus iuxta balnea publica, ubi post lavacrum a fame et siti reficiuntur. Unde et propina et propinare dicitur. Πείνα enim Graece famem significat, eo quod hic locus famem tollat.

> (Hot baths [*thermae*] are so called because they are warm, for the Greeks call heat *θερμόν*. Baths [*balneum*] are assigned their name from the idea of the lifting of sorrow, because the Greeks called it *βαλανεῖον* [cf. *βάλλειν*, 'cast away'; *ἀνία*, 'grief'], since it takes away one's anxiety of spirit. Gymnasiums [*gymnasium*] are so called because there athletes are trained, with their bodies anointed and massaged, for γυμνασιον in Greek means 'training' in Latin. [...] *Propina* is a Greek word, which now among us has been corrupted to *popina*. It is a place next to a public bath where after bathing one may be refreshed of one's hunger and thirst. From this are named both *propina* and *propinare* ['to drink a toast'], for *πεῖνα* in Greek means 'hunger' — because this place relieves hunger.)[12]

As is evident from Isidore's discussion of the different rooms that make up a bathhouse, bathing is related not only to exercise, but also to food and drinks in a process of restoring psycho-physical wellbeing that also includes massaging the body with ointments. Interestingly, all these elements are instructions that can be found in many remedies that involve the use of balneotherapy and which are examined in this chapter.

Although some medieval Christians condemned bathing because they considered nudity to be a potentially dangerous temptation for the senses,[13] others considered balneotherapy to be a useful medical practice to help the poor and sick. The *Benedictine Rule* even prescribed bathing as a healing procedure for the sick, who should be allowed to benefit from baths as often as may be beneficial:

Quibus fratribus infirmis sit cella super se deputata et servitor timens Deum et diligens ac sollicitus. Balnearum usus infirmis quotiens expedit

12 Isidore of Seville, *The Etymologies*, XV.ii.39–42 (ed. by Lindsay, I, p. 164; trans. by Barney and others, pp. 307–08).

13 For instance, before the Council of Nicaea, the Church Fathers disapproved of bathing as they saw it as immoral, promiscuous, and unhealthy. Thus Clement of Alexandria, in the *Pedagogus* (*c.* AD 198), denounces public baths as places where the aristocracy indulge in excessive drinking, greed, as well as meaningless displays of wealth. In his *De habitu virginum* (*c.* AD 249), Cyprianus harshly criticizes the practice of displaying nudity in public baths. Addressing Christian women who go to mixed public baths, he accuses them of prostituting their bodies to appease the eyes of the libidinous and the curious rather than devoting themselves to modesty and chastity.

offeratur — sanis autem et maxime iuvenibus tardius concedatur. Sed et carnium esus infirmis omnino debilibus pro reparatione concedatur; at, ubi meliorati fuerunt, a carnibus more solito omnes abstineant.

> (For these sick let there be assigned a special room and an attendant who is God-fearing, diligent and solicitous.
> Let the use of baths be afforded the sick as often as may be expedient; but to the healthy, and especially to the young, let them be granted more rarely.
> Moreover, let the use of meat be granted to the sick who are very weak, for the restoration of their strength; but when they are convalescent, let all abstain from meat as usual.)[14]

According to Benedict, bathing is more effective when accompanied by a specific diet, as the consumption of meat helps the restoration of the patients' strength. The fact that the *Rule* explicitly prescribes bathing for the sick, while reminding healthy and convalescent monks to abstain from meat and bathe more rarely, is related to the humble and austere monastic lifestyle, which prescribed bathing only a few times a year, for example at Easter, when hygiene became part of a ritual to achieve spiritual cleansing. On the other hand, this also testifies to the fact that bathing was considered a particularly successful medical remedy, so much so that the sick could be treated with baths as often as was necessary for their healing.[15]

In line with the Benedictine *Rule*, the tenth-century English *Regularis concordia*[16] contains references to the care of the sick. Chapter XII is devoted to the care of sick brethren, who should be assisted by a carer, who will provide them with all they need; if required, a responsible brother should

14 St Benedict, *The Rule of St Benedict*, ed. by Venarde, ch. 36, p. 131.

15 For the monastic orders in the English Middle Ages, bathing was immensely important. Howes claims that most abbeys and monasteries possessed *lavatoria* with exceptional, innovative water systems. Baths were vital for both physical and spiritual purification, with baptism, churching (i.e., the purification of women after childbirth), and foot washing as the three principal rituals. See Howes, *Transformative Waters*, pp. 90 and 143. An anonymous rule from the early thirteenth century titled *Ancrene Wisse*, addressed specifically to female anchoresses, serves as an example of this. Here, religious meditation is compared to medicine for the spirit; in fact, the anchoress's cell, a focal point of meditation, is described as a medical procedure, and associated with curative postpartum bloodbaths and bloodletting particularly for their curative properties. See also Perk, '"Idleness Breeds Disgust for the Cell"', p. 17.

16 Attributed to Bishop Æthelwold of Winchester, who lived in the tenth century, the *Regularis concordia* entailed detailed instructions for daily monastic life, conduct, and rituals. The text is preserved in two extant versions dating to the eleventh century, the first of which is contained in London, BL, MS Cotton Tiberius A III (in Latin, with interlinear glosses in Old English; fols 3–27). The second text, in Old English and Latin, was dismembered by Sir Robert Cotton and its first part is preserved at fols 174–77 of MS Cotton Tiberius A III, whereas the second part is now contained in London, BL, MS Cotton Faustina B III (fols 159^r–198^r).

enlist the assistance of servants. The sick should also be visited often, until their health has improved and visiting can be discontinued.[17] Among the instructions regarding monastic life, the *Regularis concordia* contains some references to hygiene, especially in relation to ritual cleansing before Easter. Here, the ablution of (part of) the body relates to the purifying aspects of baptismal water, symbolically cleansing the monks from their sins and healing their souls. The brethren's Maundy is described in Chapter IV, and it is interesting to observe how various ritualistic gestures remind readers of analogous steps in some of the medical prescriptions examined in this chapter. Both the doctor and the abbot must wash the attendees in a basin; after being cleansed, both the patients and the ritualists must dress and dry; and during both processes, drinking liquids is required (potions or syrups in medical recipes and Eucharistic wine in the religious ritual).[18] Subsequently, on Holy Saturday, the monks should prepare for Easter by dedicating themselves to bodily and facial cleansing and, if Saturday is not sufficient, the monastic community must shave and bathe themselves after the veneration of the Cross.[19]

Similarly to what we find in continental sources during the early Middle Ages, English medical texts of this period contain scattered references to baths in relation to other remedies, such as potions and diets. Baths were considered as constituents of leechdoms that included a series of healing practices to cure a variety of diseases and in which bathing water was often mixed with different ingredients (mostly herbs) that varied depending on the symptoms of the patient. For example, in the first book of the so-called *Bald's Leechbook*, bathing is mentioned numerous times and for a variety

17 *Regularis concordia*, ed. and trans. by Symons, p. 64.

18 'fratrum agant post quam tempore congruo eorundem agatur Mandatum; qui tamen fratres prius pedes suos diligenter emundet; [...] quos subsequitur abbas in concha sua singulorum pedes lauans, ministrantibus sibi quos uoluerit ad hoc obsequium, [...] Quo peracto resideat abbas in sede sua ueniantque priores et ei eadem exhibeant; deinde surgens det aquam in manibus singulorum rursumque ei eadem seruitus exhibeatur. Interim uero dum manus lauantur diaconus hebdomadarius et reliqui ministri eant et induant se, [...]. Interim abbas propinando circumeat fratres cum singulis potibus singulorum osculans manus, [...] tunc a priore propinetur abbati et reliquis ministris qui assistebant. Euangelio finito potibusque haustis, praecedat processio' (the brethren shall then have their meal and thereafter, at the proper time, their Maundy shall take place; but they must wash their feet carefully beforehand. [...] the abbot shall wash the feet of all in his own basin, drying and kissing them, [...]. When he has done this, the abbot shall sit in his own place and the seniors shall minister to him in like manner, then, rising, he shall offer water for the hands of the brethren and again the like service shall be rendered to him. During the washing of the hands, the deacon and other ministers of the week shall vest; [...]. Meanwhile the abbot shall go round among the brethren drinking the health and kissing the hand of each. [...] Then the prior shall drink to the abbot and to the ministers who assisted him. When the gospel has been read and the healths have been drunk, the procession shall move on) (*Regularis concordia*, ed. and trans. by Symons, pp. 40–41).

19 *Regularis concordia*, ed. and trans. by Symons, pp. 45–46.

of conditions in relation to other remedies that are organized according to the Hippocratic head-to-foot order. Here, bathing involves both individual bodily parts as well as the whole body. The prescriptions of medicinal baths are usually brief and simple: they indicate the kind of water that should be used, sometimes referencing its temperature or the liquids that need to be used as an alternative to water, in addition to other ingredients. For example, for mist in the eyes, sea water must be mixed with the juice of celandine; the mixture then has to be smeared on the eyes, which are subsequently washed therewith: 'Eft ƿið þon ilcan celeþonian seap 7 sæƿæter smire mid þa eagan 7 beðe' (Again for the same [mist in the eyes], juice of celandine and sea water; smear and bathe the eyes therewith).[20] Similarly, for pain in the eyes, herbs have to be boiled in beer or ale and the solution has to be used to wash the eyes. The prescription suggests that the more often one does this, the better: 'Ƿið eagna ece genim þa readan hofan aƿyl on surum sƿatum oþþe on surúm ealað 7 beþe þa eagan on þam baþe betere swa óftor' (For ache of eyes, take the red hove, boil it in sour beer or in sour ale, and bathe the eyes in the bath, the oftener the better).[21] Moreover, in order to cure certain heart diseases, the invigorating and curative properties of full-body warm baths are combined with dietary prescriptions:

> Ƿiþ heort ece gif hím ón Innan hearð heort ƿærc sie þonne hím ƿyxþ ƿind on þære heortan 7 hine þegeð þurst 7 biþ unmehtiglic.
> Ƿyrc hím þonne stan bæð 7 ón þam ete suþerne rædic mid sealte þy mæg wesan sio wund gehæled.
>
> > (For heart ache, if there be to him within, a hard heart wark, then wind waxeth in the heart for him, and thirst vexes him and he is languid. Work him then a stone bath, and in that let him eat southern radish with salt, by that the wound may be healed.)[22]

In the second book of *Bald's Leechbook*, treatments involving bathing appear to have been arranged in a more coherent and organized way. Although therapeutic baths are mentioned in relation to a variety of diseases, prescriptions involving this practice have been grouped together in Chapters 32 and 36, where they are prescribed in addition or as an alternative to bloodletting and salves for disorders of the digestive system and for pain in the spleen:

> Læcedomas hu mon sƿa gesadne mán lacnian scule. ge mid blodlæse 7 sealfe 7 baðo 7 lácnúng on ꝥ hrif to Sendanne. 7 þas læcedomas magon ƿið lendenece. 7 gif món fonde mige. ƿiþ ut ƿærce. ƿið magan adlum 7 claƿunga 7 ƿifa dedternessum. 7 be þære coðe hu man lyfte utgan 7 ne mæg. 7 gif se utgang sie ƿindig 7 ƿæterig 7 blodig .xii. ƿifan. [...]

20 *Leechdoms*, ed. and trans. by Cockayne, II, pp. 28–29 (§ 3).
21 *Leechdoms*, ed. and trans. by Cockayne, II, pp. 34–35 (§ 19).
22 *Leechdoms*, ed. and trans. by Cockayne, II, pp. 60–61 (§ 17.1–2).

> Læcedomas be milte pærce 7 þ he bið on þa pinstran sidan 7 tacn ðære adle hu higeleafe hi beoð 7 hu lang se milte sie 7 be þæs miltes filmene on þa pinstran healfe be hleahtre þe óf milte cymð. hu se milte æghpæt þropað þæs þe oþer limo ge hát ge ceald. 7 be bæðe 7 hæmed þinge 7 hpanan sio hæto cume 7 cele þæs miltes eahta cræftas.
>
> > (Leechdoms how a man shall cure one so afflicted, whether with bloodletting, and salve, and baths, and *how* to send curatives into the belly. And these leechdoms are efficacious against loin ache, if a man mie [urinate] sand, for dysentery, for diseases of the maw, and gripings, and women's tendernesses, and of the disease where a man would evacuate and is not able (*tenesmus*), and if the discharge be windy, and watery, and bloody. Twelve methods. [...] Leechdoms of pain in the milt [spleen], and that the milt is on the left side, and tokens of the disease, how reckless the sick are, and how long the milt is, and of the film or membrane of the milt on the left side, and of splenetic laughter, which cometh of the milt, how the milt suffereth everything of that which other limbs suffer either hot or cold; and of the bath, and of sexual [intercourse], and whence the heat cometh and the cold of the milt: eight receipts.)[23]

In this book, balneotherapy is mostly recommended for disorders of the gastrointestinal tract and the spleen. As regards this organ, it can be noted that the cause of the disease is related to humoral theory, with heat or cold being the main reasons for the ailment.

Information on how the bath should be prepared and on its duration and frequency is also more detailed, as stated in a remedy for the sensitive hardness of the liver:

> Þiþ þære gefelan heardnesse þære lifre ðonne is sio to beðianne mid hatan pætre ón þám sien gesodene pyrta. Þermod. 7 pildre magþan pyrttruman. fenogrecum hatte pyrt. 7 eorð gealla. þonne þa sien ealle gesodene beþe þonne mid miclum spryngum þa saran stope lange. forlæt spa .iii. dagas. Þyrc þonne sealfe óf hpætenum gryttum geporht oððe óf bripe óf permode. 7 óf pine. 7 óf aprotanean 7 cymene. 7 of laures croppan do huniges to þ þu þyrfe sele him þ þry dagas. oþre þrie sete him horn ón oþþe glæs teoh ut. Sel þu lácnast gif þu seoþest rudan ón ele 7 grenne permod oððe drigne. 7 hpit cpudu þy ealle beþe lege on ufan. læt beón ealne dæg 7 eác fela daga þas þing sint to donne 7 þám monnum synd to sellanne migole drincan.

23 *Leechdoms*, ed. and trans. by Cockayne, II, pp. 164–67 (§§32 and 36). It should be noted that Cockayne originally translated *hǽmed-þing* as 'sexual commerce', perhaps because bathhouses were also associated with prostitution from Roman times. However, the term simply means 'sexual intercourse' without any commercial connotation, of which the text is also devoid. Hence the decision to amend the translation in this instance.

(For the sensitive hardness of the liver; it is to be bathed with hot water, on which worts have been sodden, wormwood and roots of wild maythe, a wort that hight fenugreek, and earth gall; when they are all sodden, then bathe the sore places for a long time with copious water fomentations; leave it so for three days; then work a salve wrought of wheaten groats or of a brewit [poultice] of wormwood, and of wine, and of abrotanum, and of cumin, and of bunches of laurel berries; add thereto as much honey as thou needest; give the man that for three days; on the other three set on him a cupping horn or glass, draw out by that, what comes out. Thou shalt treat the sick better if thou settest rue in oil, and green or dry wormwood, and gum mastic, with all that bathe him, also lay it upon him, let it be for a whole day, and also for many days these things are to be done, and to the men must be given diuretic drinks.)[24]

Here, the patient must bathe for a long time (*lange*) in hot water where herbs have been soaked, and the sore parts must be washed with copious water fomentations. To be effective, this treatment must be repeated for many days (*fela daga*) and accompanied by a salve. A better option for a more effective bath for this ailment is also offered, but since it employs oil — a more expensive ingredient — it was probably accessible to fewer people. According to this version, the patient should bathe for the whole day (*ealne dæg*), and this must be repeated many times.

Prescriptions recommending food, drinks, and exercise are more often combined with instructions to bathe. For example, for a deadened stomach, the patient must drink a syrup in the morning after a night's fast, have sharp[25] drinks and meats, and rub himself with mustard while bathing: 'Þis sceal pið adeadodum magan. gením huniges 7 eced togædere gemenged 7 gebeatenne pipor sele ón morgenne cucler fulne neahtnestigum nyttige scearpera drincena. 7 metta. 7 æt baþe mid sinope gnide 7 smerpe' (This shall apply for a deadened maw; take some honey and vinegar mingled together, and pepper beaten up, give in the morning a spoon full of it to the man after his night's fast, let him employ sharp drinks and meats; and at the bath let him rub and smear himself with mustard).[26] The therapeutic function of bathing — tempering the humours, re-establishing their balance — is then hinted at in a remedy for the hot and excessively inflamed stomach:

Þis sint tacn þæs hatan magan omihtan ungemet fæstlican. 7 þæs ofercealdan. þæs hatan magan ungemetfæstan tacn sindon þonne he bið mid omum

24 *Leechdoms*, ed. and trans. by Cockayne, II, pp. 206–07 (§ 22).

25 The adjective *scearp* ('sharp') is widely used in Old English medical texts to describe a bitter but also acid and pungent taste. Synaesthetically, it can refer either to food or to drinks, such as vinegar, wine, and herbal decoctions. See also Williams, 'Synaesthetic Adjectives', pp. 461–78.

26 *Leechdoms*, ed. and trans. by Cockayne, II, pp. 186–87 (§ 7).

gespenced þam men bið þurst getenge 7 nearones 7 gespogunga 7 modes tpeonung 7 unluft 7 plætta. him is nyt þ he hlaf þicgen on cealdum pætre oððe on ecede 7 spiðe fæste gesoden ægra offe gebrædde to undernes 7 pyrta. 7 lactucas þ is leahtric 7 mealpan 7 hænne flæsc næs spiþe gesoden. 7 gose þa ytmestan limo. 7 fixas þa þe heard flæsc habban. 7 pine pinclan. 7 ostran 7 oþru pysena cyn 7 mylsce æppla 7 bæþ of spetum ferscum pæterum sceal beon geporht hat bæþ him ne deah.

> (These are tokens of the hot flegmatic maw, irretentive, and of the overcold [excessive cold]. Of the hot or irretentive maw are tokens, when it is vexed with inflammations, thirst is incident to the man, and oppression, and swoonings, and vacillation of mind, and loss of appetite, and nausea. It is beneficial for him that he should eat bread in cold water or in vinegar, and eggs very hard boiled or roasted (at nine o'clock in the morning), and worts, and lactucas, that is lettuces, and mallow, and hen's flesh not much sodden, and the extremest parts of the limbs of goose, that is giblets, and fishes which have hard flesh, and periwinkles, and oysters, and others; various sorts of peas, and mild apples, and a bath of sweet fresh waters shall be wrought; a hot bath will not suit him.)[27]

In this case, the inflammation is caused by hot temperature, which, as Cockayne adds in his translation, can be referred to an excess of phlegm. The dietary advice to re-establish the body's humoral balance is very detailed and precise, noting when the patient should eat, that is *to undernes* (at nine in the morning), and how the food should be cooked — eggs should be hard boiled or roasted and poultry should be 'næs spiþe gesoden' (not much sodden). The temperature of the food is also extremely important, so much so that bread should be soaked in a cold liquid — either water or vinegar — to contrast the heat of the inflammation. Similarly, the temperature of the bath is also crucial: to counterbalance the stomach's temperature, hot water should be avoided, but the use of fresh sweet water is recommended instead. It should be noted that bathing is not recommended in a number of other remedies, when the patient is affected by certain symptoms. For example, in the case of liver diseases, it is recommended that the patient should avoid certain foods but also baths,[28] while elsewhere it is stated that baths are even harmful after the consumption of food and after sexual intercourse.[29]

Since herbal decoctions were one of the main ingredients of medicinal baths, the *Old English Herbarium*[30] contains a number of references to therapeutic

---

27 *Leechdoms*, ed. and trans. by Cockayne, II, pp. 192–95 (§ 16.1).

28 *Leechdoms*, ed. and trans. by Cockayne, II, pp. 191–93 (§ 16).

29 *Leechdoms*, ed. and trans. by Cockayne, II, pp. 244–45 (§ 36).

30 The *Old English Herbarium* is preserved in four manuscripts dating from the tenth to the twelfth centuries, one of which (London, BL, MS Cotton Vitellius C III) is beautifully illustrated. The other non-illustrated manuscripts are London, BL, MS Harley 585 (late

baths. In this text, each entry contains the name of an ingredient (plant or animal), followed by descriptions of the ailments it can treat and instructions on how to find and use it. Most of the remedies referencing baths prescribe that individual bodily parts rather than the full body are cleansed with the mixture of water and herbs. Information about how the affected part must be washed is brief and general, whereas the preparation of the medicine is usually precise and detailed. The instructions explain how the plant must be used, whether it must be pounded, mixed with other ingredients and boiled to prepare either a potion, a medicinal bath, a compress, or a salve. The quantities of the ingredients are often listed; for example, to cure swollen feet one should wash in a bath of waybread, i.e., plantain pounded in vinegar: 'Gif mannes fet on syþe tydrien: genim þonne wegbrædan ða wyrt; gnid on ecede; beþe ða fet þærmid, ond smyre. Ðonne þwineþ hy sona' (If a person gets footsore on a journey, then take the plant plantain; crush it in vinegar; bathe the feet with it and rub it in. They will quickly become less swollen.)[31] Similarly, to relieve sore legs, the same quantities of pennyroyal and pepper should be pounded together to make a salve that must be smeared wherever the patient is sore while bathing: 'Wiþ lendena ece ond wið þara þeona sare: genim þas ylcan wyrte *polleium* ond pipor, ægþres gelice mycel be gewihte; cnuca tosomne. Ond þonne þu on bæþe sy, smyre þærmid þær hyt swiþost derige' (For pain in the loins and for sore thighs: take this same plant pennyroyal plus pepper, the same amount of each by weight; pound them together. And when you are bathing, smear it on where it hurts the most.)[32]

An Intermediate Phase in Medieval English Balneotherapy

An intermediate phase in medieval English medicine, at the crossroads between the Old English and the Middle English periods, is represented by the *Peri didaxeon*, a translation of the Latin *Epistola peri hereseon*, contained in London, British Library, MS Harley 6258B, a codex of the twelfth century that also contains one of the four copies of the *Old English Herbarium*. The *Peri didaxeon* is a collection of remedies that is incomplete in the final part; it is preceded by a brief epistle illustrating humoral theory as the basis of medical doctrine and explaining health as the qualitative and quantitative balance of the four bodily humours. The fact that the text is preceded by a

tenth–early eleventh centuries), Oxford, Bodleian Library, MS Hatton 76 (eleventh century), and London, BL, MS Harley 6258B (late twelfth century). It has been edited and translated by Oswald Cockayne in *Leechdoms*, I, pp. 70–325, and more recently translated by Anne Van Arsdall in *Medieval Herbal Remedies* and edited and translated by John D. Niles and Maria A. D'Aronco in *Medical Writings from Early Medieval England*.

31 *Medical Writings*, ed. and trans. by Niles and D'Aronco, pp. 68–69 (§ 2.17).

32 *Medical Writings*, ed. and trans. by Niles and D'Aronco, pp. 220–21 (§ 94.13).

prefatory letter stressing the importance of the harmony between the four humours for a healthy body marks a clear difference with the early Middle Ages, during which, as discussed above, humoral theory was often implied in the remedies, but not explicitly mentioned. The recipes of *Peri didaxeon* demonstrate greater awareness of and attention to the elemental qualities[33] of the ingredients used for medical preparations, with hot constituents being used to contrast diseases caused by an excess of cold humours and cold ingredients counterbalancing an excess of hot humours. Dietary advice is also prescribed accordingly, with cold food counteracting hot humours and hot foodstuffs compensating for cold ones. The remedies are arranged according to different types of disease and follow the traditional order *de capite ad pedem*, but in this case, the final part of the treatise got lost and the text ends with recipes for stomach ailments.[34] If compared to the medical treatises analysed so far, this text is more precise in the description of the processes to prepare the remedies, including the quantities of the ingredients to be used and how they have to be processed to be effective. As the prefatory epistle suggests, the treatment of different diseases varies according to circumstances and conditions related to humoral and elemental theories. This is also reflected in the few prescriptions featuring therapeutic baths. For example, for loss of appetite caused by cold humours, the patient must bathe and, subsequently, drink a potion, the preparation of which is thoroughly described:

> Þis hys god ta þan mann þe hura metes ne lyst. Þæt Greccas hataþ *blaffesis*. And Ypocras seggeþ þæt seo untrumnyss cymþ of þrim þingum: oþþer of cyle, oþþer of miclum æte and drince oþþer of lytte æte and drince, oþþer of miclum wernesse.
>
> Gif hyt cumeþ of þam cyle, þanne scealt þu him helpan mid baþe. Gif hyt cymet of mycele drence, þanne scel he habba forhæfdnysse. [...] Gif þa untrumnysse cumþ of þan cyle, þanne nim þu beferes herþan and barne to duste, and grind piper and meng piper and þæt dust togader, and nim sticcan fulne þas gemengdede dustes and do in ane cuppefulle wynes, and wlece þanne þæt win mid þæt duste, and sile him drinca.

33 In Chapter 9 of his *De natura rerum*, Isidore of Seville explains, drawing on Hippocrates and Galen, that 'mundus conpetenter homo significatur, quia sicut ille ex quattuor concretus est elementis, ita et iste ex quattuor constat humoribus uno temperamento conmixtis' (the world properly signifies the human being, because just as the former is compounded out of four elements, so also the latter is made up out of four humours mixed together in one temperament): see Isidore of Seville, *De natura rerum* (*On the Nature of Things*), ed. by Tombeur, trans. by Kendall and Wallis, p. 127. In the *Etymologies* (VI.iv.1–3), Isidore links the four elements to each bodily humour and to the four seasons, clarifying that they share the same primary qualities: thus, phlegm is associated with water, yellow bile with fire, black bile with earth, and blood with air. Health is the result of the balance of the four humours, and all diseases are caused by their imbalance, and more specifically, by a fluid excessively accumulating in one bodily organ.

34 On the *Peri didaxeon*, see also Maion, 'Il trattato medico antico inglese "Peri Didaxeon"', pp. 1–29.

> (This is good for a person who has no appetite for food. The Greeks call this condition *blaffesis*. And Hippocrates states that this infirmity arises from three things: either from chills, or from too much food and drink or too little food and drink, or from extreme fatigue.
> If it comes from chills, then you should help him by making a bath. If it comes from overdrinking, then he should maintain abstinence. [...] If the ailment comets from chills, then take castoreum and burn it to a powder, and grind some pepper, and mix the pepper and the powder together, and take a spoonful of this composite powder and add a cupful of wine, and then warm the wine with the powder, and give him that to drink.)[35]

The procedure for preparing the potion, the quantities of its ingredients, and the temperature of the drink the patient should ingest are precisely described. First, a mixture of powders should be obtained by grinding peppercorns and burning beavers' testicles, as it was believed that they contained castoreum, a substance capable of healing various diseases.[36] Then a spoonful of this mixture had to be added to a cup of wine, which had to be heated until the liquid was lukewarm. This concoction was thought to contrast the excess of cold humours.

The remedy for asthma is another good example of the relevance of the elemental qualities of the prescribed remedies for their effectiveness. The ailment is explained as caused by an excess of humours coming from the stomach and oppressing the chest. After a long description of symptoms and of the processes to cure the ailment, the text prescribes the consumption of food with opposite qualities to those of the excessive humours, such as dry (*drige*) bread and cheese and a warm (*wearm*) loaf. The patient should also avoid cold (*cyle*) places, dwell in a warm house, and as soon as he gets better, take a warm bath:

> Þes læcedom sceal to þan mann þe byð yfele on þan breostam. Þur þa breost fela freccenysse synden þe on þe manne becumeþ. And soþ hys þæt ælc wætt cymd ærest ut of þan magan, and þur þane wæten þa breorst beoþ geheafugede and þa heorte ge sydu byð gefullede mid yfele blode. [...] Þanne sceal he etan drigne half and cyse. And ne cume he on nane cyle þe he hwile þe he seoc beo, ac beo hym on wermum huse, and hæte hym man bæþ swa hraþa swa hys wisa godige. [...] Nim þanne wulle þe ne com næfre awaxen and wyrc cliþan þærof. Lege þæruppa þa sealfe, wel þicce. Wryð þanne to þan breostan, swa hæt swa he hattest forberan mæge. Þanne þeo beo acoled, lege oþerne wearme þarto, and do þus ðe hwyle hym þearf sy.

35 *Medical Writings*, ed. and trans. by Niles and D'Aronco, pp. 562–65 (§ 50).

36 Castoreum is an exudate contained in the beavers' anal glands. It contains high concentrations of salicylic acid, an antiseptic, bactericide, and anti-inflammatory substance. In the Middle Ages, castoreum was erroneously believed to be contained in beavers' testicles: see Gow, *Bringing Back the Beaver*, pp. 46–47 and Walker-Meikle, 'Animals', p. 101.

Wyrce hym drenc gode, þe ægþer clænsige ge þa breost ge þane innoþ. And bace hym man þanne wearmen hlaf be heorþe, and ete þane manige dæges þane hlaf þe wyrm. Nim eft cicenemete and wermod and lauberigan, and do hwyt cudu oþer gerusodne ele to, and gnid eall togadere mid ele mid eall. Wyrme þane þa breost to heorþan, 7 smyre hy þanne mid þare scealfe.

(This medicine is for someone suffering from a chest ailment. There are many infirmities which come to a person through the chest. And it is the case that each humour originates first of all in the stomach, and it is through that humour that the chest is weighed down and the heart and sides are filled with noxious blood. [...]. Then he should eat dry bread and cheese. And he should not be allowed to suffer any chills as long as his illness persists, but have him stay in a warm house, and have a bath heated for him as soon as his condition improves. [...] Then take some wool that has never been washed and fashion a poultice from it. Spread the salve on it, a thick amount. Then tie this to the chest, as hot as he can stand. When this one has cooled, then apply another warm one, and do this as long as he requires.
Then make up a good drink for him, one that will purge both the chest and the inner organs. And bake him a warm loaf at the hearth, and for many days afterward have him eat the bread you have warmed. Then take chickweed and wormwood and laurel berries, and add gum mastic to it or extract of roses, and knead it all thoroughly together with the oil. Then warm the person's chest at the fireside, and then rub the salve into it.)[37]

The text clearly mentions *wætan* (humours), and in particular *yfel blod* (evil blood), as the cause of the disease. The preparation of a salve and a compress is also an important part of the remedy: for it to be effective, the objects used, such as the container and the woollen cloth on which the compress is going be spread, must be clean and new (*niwe*), as it is stated that the fabric should be *næfre awaxen* (never have been washed). Temperature is a key factor for the effectiveness of the remedy as it serves to counterbalance the excess of blood. Therefore, not only must the water for the bath be heated (*hæte*), but also the salve that is to be applied onto the patient's chest has to be 'swa hæt swa he hattest forberan mæge' (as hot as he can bear). In addition, the remedy prescribes the constant replacement of the cooled compress with a warm one, so that its active ingredients can be better absorbed. Moreover, to make the patient's chest more responsive to the active ingredients of the salve and of the compress, the chest must be also warmed up before smearing.

37 *Medical Writings*, ed. and trans. by Niles and D'Aronco, pp. 566–71 (§ 52).

Bathing in Late Medieval England

The second phase in the development of balneotherapy corresponds to the late Middle Ages, when bathing started playing a vital role in medical practice, so that entire sections of medical treatises were devoted to remedies involving baths and specific treatises on their therapeutic virtues were produced. Bathing practices were also related to elemental and humoral theories more explicitly than in the early Middle Ages, thus marking a further development of the notions contained in the *Peri didaxeon*. This European revolution in the treatment of bathing practices was brought about by two main cultural factors that deeply influenced medieval science and medicine. The first one — a turning point not only in the history of medicine, but also in the use of baths as a treatment within medical practice — was the development of the Salernitan School, the most important centre for the introduction and the spread of Greek and Arabic medicine into western Europe.[38] Here Greek texts, including those by Hippocrates, Galen, and Dioscorides were translated into Latin, and Arabic medical lore (coming from Sicily and North Africa) was integrated into medical practice. The influence of the Salernitan School on European medicine is universally recognized, being considered as 'the forerunner of modern university medical schools'.[39] Throughout European universities, the teaching of medicine was based on the collection of texts called the *Articella*, developed by the masters of Salerno.

The second important scientific turn involving water and hygiene, deeply related to Aristotelianism and Scholasticism, is the revival of thermalism. The

38 The Salernitan School was a medical institution founded in the southern Italian city of Salerno that gathered local and foreign students and physicians. Its foundation date has been debated for a long time. Some scholars date it back to the ninth century (see for example Bifulco and others, 'Dental Care', p. 87 and Stelmaschuk, 'The School at Salerno', p. 65). Sudhoff ('Salerno', p. 44) considers the account of the historian Richer of Reims, reporting the dispute between two doctors at the French court, as evidence that at the end of the ninth century there was a 'place dedicated to medical training in Salerno' ('Wir sehen daraus, daß schon im 9. Jahrhundert in Salerno eine ärztliche Lehrstelle bestand.') Hunt points out how there are no records of the Salernitan School before *c.* 950. This would not necessarily mean that the institution did not exist before that date, but simply that 'its origins remain shrouded in obscurity' and that 'it is only the emergence of a curriculum of prescribed texts which encourages us to speak of a school at all' (Hunt, *Popular Medicine*, p. 12). Kristeller, instead, traces its origins back to the late tenth century (Kristeller, 'The School of Salerno', p. 193). Other scholars (see for example Garcia-Ballester and others, *Practical Medicine*, p. 27, and Green, *The Trotula*, pp. 9–10) even claim that there is no evidence of any physical or legal entity in Salerno before the thirteenth century. It thus appears that, starting from the ninth century, there gathered in Salerno what Green has defined as 'an informal community of masters and pupils who [...] developed more or less formal methods of instruction and investigation' (Green, *The Trotula*, p. 9). This community flourished between the eleventh and thirteenth centuries. On the influence of the Salernitan School on medieval European balneotherapy, see Ramazzina, 'Bathing in Medieval Europe'.

39 de Divitiis and others, 'The "Schola Medica Salernitana"', p. 739.

development of thermal tourism gave rise to a specific scientific literature on waters and their beneficial effects.[40] Moreover, the tendency to systematize balneology as related to diet, exercise, and psycho-physical wellbeing within medical practice started in Salerno and benefited from the development and expansion of university medical schools.[41] England was not immune to all this. Indeed, as observed by Black, due to shared language and culture, 'medical texts [travelled] quickly from Monte Cassino and Salerno in Italy to Normandy and Anglo-Norman England around the turn of the twelfth century'.[42] As a result, many of the earliest copies of the translations of Constantinus Africanus, who was probably the most famous Salernitan master, and the works of other southern Italian authors, were copied there. In particular, Hunt has identified the Latin medical texts contained in Oxford, St John's College, MS 17,[43] dating to the first decade of the twelfth century, as the collection 'which represents the moment when Anglo-Saxon medicine gave way to the doctrines and practices of Salerno'.[44] Additionally, Green points out how England and northern France played a pivotal role in the dissemination of the medical texts produced in Salerno, with up to 25 per cent of the codices being produced there.[45] Furthermore, Gilbertus Anglicus (*c.* AD 1180 – *c.* 1250), one of the most famous medieval English physicians, had been a student of the Salernitan School and helped to disseminate its teaching throughout France and England.[46] This is well exemplified by the *System of Physic*, a re-writing of Gilbertus Anglicus's *Compendium medicinae* in Middle English, contained in the fourteenth-century codex Glasgow, University Library, MS Hunter 307.[47] After a definition of the four humours and their properties, their correspondence with the elements and their qualities, the four ages of man, the seasons of the year, and an explanation of uroscopy, the text provides an extensive description of disorders of the human body ordered according to the usual head-to-toe method. The nature and symptoms of each disease, the excess of humours causing it, and the cures, including advice on nutrition, recipes for potions, ointments, plasters, and other therapies, such as fumigations and baths, are carefully explained. The number of mentions of therapeutic baths — about once every four manuscript pages — demonstrates the relevance of bathing practices at that time. For example, we can find dozens of remedies for curing ophthalmic diseases that entail washing the eyes with solutions of water

40 On thermalism in medieval Europe see Nicoud, 'Le thermalisme'.

41 See Ramazzina, 'Bathing in Medieval Europe', and Jacquart, 'Medical Scholasticism'.

42 Black, 'A Star is Born'.

43 According to Wallis ('The Calendar and the Cloister'), this manuscript was copied at Thorney Abbey, Cambridgeshire, *c.* 1110.

44 Hunt, *Popular Medicine*, pp. 24–25.

45 Green, 'Salerno on the Thames', p. 221.

46 de Divitiis and others, 'The "Schola Medica Salernitana"', p. 738.

47 For an edition of the text see Gilbertus Anglicus, *Healing and Society in Medieval England*, ed. by Getz, and *System of Physic*, ed. by Esteban Segura.

and/or wine and herbs. Steam baths, often including fumigations, are also frequently prescribed. For example, to cure diseases of the spleen caused by cold humours, a steam bath using herbs with hot qualities, such as oregano, thyme, and rosemary, among others is prescribed on the third day of the treatment, together with bloodletting:

> if it be of cold humours ȝiue him oxymel to defie þe humours aftirward ȝiue him iera pigra to purge þe humours or sich an oþere medecyn aftir þe • iij • day make him a stufe of hote erbis as of origane calamynte hore howne tyme rose maryn and siche oþere and þe next day aftir let him blood vndir þe ancle in þe hyndir side of þe lift foot • and siþe mak him hoot plastris þat ben duryng and consumyng þe humours and leie to þe splene as of rewe celedoyne nettlis and of comyn sode and of siche oþere and let anoynte him bifore þe splene wiþ warm hony.
>
> > (if it is caused by cold humours give him oxymel [a preparation of vinegar and honey] to fight the humours, afterwards give him hiera picra to purge the humours or a similar other medicine. After the third day make him a stove of hot herbs such as oregano, storax tree resin, horehound, thyme, rosemary and other similar ones, and the next day let him bleed under the ankle under the side of the left foot. Subsequently, make him a durable hot plaster to consume the humours, made of raw celandine, nettle and cumin seed, and other similar ones and apply to the spleen. Smear him in front of the spleen with warm honey.)[48]

As is evident from this remedy, the medical procedures the patient undergoes and the ingredients used in the preparations are explicitly aimed at contrasting the excess of cold humours that are causing the disease, as the verbs *defie*, *purge* and *consumyng* clearly suggest. Moreover, the temperature of the plaster to be applied onto the patient's spleen is again a key factor for the recovery of the patient. To counterbalance cold humours, the paste must be *hoot* (hot) and *duryng* (durable), i.e., it must be kept constantly warm.

In comparison with to the other medical treatises that have been analysed in this study, prescriptions of baths in the *System of Physic* are more detailed, not only as regards the herbs that must be used and their qualities, but also as regards what bodily parts need to be soaked and the appropriate time for the bath. For instance, for kidney diseases caused by cold, the patient must drink a decoction of diuretic herbs and then bathe in another solution with their body immersed up to the navel. Moreover, if the patient has stones in his kidneys, he must bathe in the same solution often and in the third or fourth parts of the month:

48 Glasgow, Univ. Lib., MS Hunter 307, fol. 120^{r}; the translations from the *System of Physic* are my own.

> But if it come of cold let him vse oxymel duretik or oxymel squillitik and aftir mak abaþ of þe rotis of fenel of persily of march of carawey dauk saxifrage and milium solis sode in water and let him sitte in þe baþ vp to þe nauel • and siþe ȝiue him triacle with wyn þat saxifrage and milium solis ben sode inne and amorwe opene þe veyne þat is vndir þe ancle. And if þe stoon be in þe reynes let him ofte vse þis baþ in þe • iij • or þe • iiij • age of þe moneþe and let him vse þis sirip •.
>
> > (But if it comes from cold let him use diuretic oxymel or oxymel containing squill, and after, make a bath with the root of fennel, parsley, celery, caraway, wild carrot, saxifrage, and millet; boil in water and let him sit in the bath up to the navel. Subsequently, give him a medicine with wine that has been boiled with saxifrage and millet, and in the morning open the vein that is under the ankle. And if there are stones in the kidneys, let him often use the bath in the third or fourth part of the month and let him use this syrup.)[49]

The remedy for strangury, on the other hand, is representative of how baths combine with other therapies to rebalance the four humours. Different treatments are provided according to the cause of the disease. Thus, if the affection comes from hot humours, after bloodletting, the patient must drink a syrup and bathe in decoctions made with cold herbs, whereas if the sickness derives from an excess of cold humours, a steam bath of hot herbs has to be prepared. This must be accompanied by a series of treatments that include drinking a potion, bloodletting, and the internal administration of the medicine through a urinary catheter:

> Jf strangurie come of hete let hym blede vndir þe ancle •and ȝiue him þe electuarie of þe iuys of roses • and siþe baþe him in a baþ of colde erbis • and ȝiue him euery day at morwe and at euene sugre violet or diapenydion or diagragantum þat is cold and let him drinke water þat hertistonge or endyue is sode [...] but if þis greuaunce come of cold ȝiue him oxymel duretik and siþe make him a stufe of hote erbis •& and whan he comeþ out of þe baþ ȝiue him triacle with þe iuys of mynte or wyn þat castorie is sode in • and þe nexte day after let him blod vndir þe ancle and distempre triacle þoruȝ þe iuys of mynte and let hym resseyue it þoruȝ an enargale.
>
> > (If strangury comes from heat, let him bleed under the ankle and give him an electuary made with the juice of roses and then bathe him in a bath of cold herbs and give him every day in the mornings and in the evenings sugar violet or diapenidion or gum tragacanth that is cold; and let him drink water in which hart's-tongue fern or endive have been boiled [...]. But if this ailment comes from cold give him diuretic oxymel, and then make him a stove with hot herbs. And when

49 Glasgow, Univ. Lib., MS Hunter 307, fol. 128^r–v^.

he comes out of the bath give him a medicine with mint juice or wine in which castoreum has been boiled. And the day after, let him bleed under the ankle and mix the medicine with mint juice and administer it through a urethral catheter.)[50]

The reason why the patient has to ingest oxymel and sugar violet in the morning and evening is expressly stated: these ingredients have been chosen 'þat is cold' (because they are cold), therefore, they can effectively contrast hot humours.

Finally, the *Secreta secretorum*, one of the late medieval 'bestsellers' *par excellence*,[51] demonstrates how the elemental and humoral theories dominated the worldview of the time, and how this reflected also on balneology. The *Secreta secretorum*, an encyclopaedic treatise dealing with a wide range of topics, including government, cosmology, astrology, medicine, alchemy, and magic, was probably composed in Arabic during the tenth century and translated into Latin in the mid-twelfth century, and was subsequently translated into several vernacular languages. Among the topics covered by the text is a variety of suggestions regarding therapies, exercise, diet, and hygiene according to elemental theory. The foods that are recommended, as well as the medicinal herbs prescribed in the remedies, thus have certain qualities that make them compatible with the seasons. For instance, the chapter on winter, contained in the Middle English translation from French,[52] recommends the consumption of hot food and hot meats, such as chicken and mutton, as this season is cold and moist. Additionally, bloodletting should be avoided, whereas bathing is beneficial in this time of the year, as it helps gather all the natural heat of the body:

> Of wyntir tyme, and what it is
> Wintir bigynneth whan the sonne entrith into the first degre of þe signe that men callen Motoun [...] wyntir is cold and moyste, and therfore it nedith to ete hoote metis, as chekenys, hennes, motoun, and othir hoot metes, and fatte ffiges, notes, and reed wyne, and be ware that thou be not laxatijf, and lete no blood, but it were the gretter nede, and enfebille not þi stomak with excesse of mete ne of drynke. No companye thou nought moche with women, but it be attemperatly. And bathis are goode to be vsid in tyme of colde. þe hete naturalle gederith togidre in the body, and there good digestioun is bettir in wyntir, and in ver than in hervest or in somer, ffor in hervest and in somer the wombe is colde, and þat tyme be the pores open, for hete of that tyme and nature spredith it through alle parties of the body, and therfore the stomak hath litille part of þe hete, and þat lettith the digestioun and the humoures gaderen.

50 Glasgow, Univ. Lib., MS Hunter 307, fol. 130^{r-v}.

51 The number of extant witnesses of the *Secreta secretorum* is about 600, of which nine are Middle English translations produced in the fifteenth century. See also Gaullier-Bougassas and others, *Les trajectoires européennes du Secretum Secretorum*, especially pp. 5–25.

52 Preserved in London, BL, MS Royal 18 A VII.

> (Of winter, and what it is:
> Winter begins when the sun enters in the first degree of the sign that men call Aries […]. Winter is cold and moist, and therefore you need to eat hot meat such as chicken, hen, mutton, and other hot food, and figs of good quality, nuts, and red wine; and beware from having freely moving bowels and avoid bloodletting except in case of great necessity; and do not fill your stomach with excessive food or drink. Do not have much intercourse with women but do it moderately. And baths are good in cold times. The natural heat gathers together in the body and good digestion is better in winter and in spring than in autumn and summer, as in autumn and in summer the womb is cold and in that time the pores are open, and therefore the stomach has a small part of the heat, and that lets the digestion, and the humours gather.)[53]

In addition to a list of beneficial foods according to their elementary qualities, the text advises against excesses and prescribes eating, drinking and having sexual intercourse moderately. It also elucidates how, according to humoral theory, the digestive system works better in winter and spring as in the other seasons cold prevails, which favours an accumulation of humours in the stomach.

Some versions of the *Secreta secretorum*, such as the one preserved in London, Lambeth Palace Library, MS 501, contain a chapter (no. 63) that is entirely devoted to baths, which are even considered 'one of the marvels of the world'. This chapter describes bathhouses as arranged according to the four seasons and hosting four chambers that reflect the qualities of the four seasons and of the four elements: one is cold, one is lukewarm, one is hot, and the last one is dry. To bathe properly, one should spend a little time in each of the rooms. The patient's body must not undergo sudden changes in temperature, but the passage from one room to another must be as harmonious as the transition of the four seasons and the four elements into each other. The chapter also suggests the proper place to build a bath, as well as what herbs should be used for the preparation of the waters, along with dietary advice according to the time of the year. It is presented as a series of 'teachings' on 'how to heal and nourish the body':

> Of ordinance of stuynge
> Bathes er on of þe merueylles of þys werld, ffor yt ys housyd after pe ffoure tymes of pe ȝeer, ffor cold accordes to wynter, leuk-warme to Veer, hoot to somer, drye to heruest. Greet wyt ys it to make ffoure dwellynges by ordre yn bathes. Þe firste be cold, þe seconde leuk-warme. þe þrydde hoot, þe ferthe drye; And whenne a man entrys first yn-to þe bathes, he sholde be a lytyl while yn þe firste: and after yn þe seconde. And þere dwelle a lytill; And after yn-to þe pridde, & þere dwell a litill; And after in

53 *Three Prose Versions of the Secreta Secretorum*, ed. by Steele, ch. 46 (p. 29). The modern English translations from the *Secreta secretorum* are my own.

to þe forth entre, & so doo in þe selue manure. And whenne he wyl passe out, kepe he þe self manere, makynge a litill dwellynge yn ilke chambret so þat he passe noght fro oner greet hete to oner greet cold, no fro ouer greet cold to ouer greet hete; […]. And it ys to vse þare-ynne odoures couenables to þe tyme þanne beand, pat is to wete, to vse in Veer and in somer, treble or quatreblee, In heruest and yn wynter to vse double. After, him awe to sitte on setys wete with water of Roses, and do wype hym with a fair towaille of lyn, onys and eft; And wherme al þys ys doon, and he deliciously wasshyd, passe he sone to oþer houses, and vse þe techinges and oynementȝ folwand. If ne be ouercome with hete, kembe his heued, an vse þe oynement clensyd, couenable to þe tyme; ffor yn Veer and in somer, he sholde vse oynement sesaryn, maad of sendałł and emlege. In heruest and wynter, he sholde vse oynement maad of myrre, […] And after he sholde wasshe his body, and rubbe it with waters, to he be wel wasshyd and clene. After, enoynt his body of oynementȝ couenables to þe tyme […]. If he haue þrist, drynke he a syrupe of roses, and etc electuary with musk. […].Þys is þe ordre of hele & norsshyng of be body; And he þat ys olde, or cold and moyst, dwelle noght loncre in be bathe. Noþeles he shałł sytte þare-yn, to his body be moyst of þe bathe, and water be cast on hym ofte sithes attemperly, and aft so sone as he wille. Hit ys noght couenable for a ffleumatyk man to entre yn Bathes but fastynge, and bat he enoynt hym with hote oynemeritȝ. And he þat ys of hote kynde, kepe þe techynge byfore taght.

(On the arrangement of bathhouses.
Baths are one of the marvels of this world, for they are arranged after the four seasons of the year; for cold corresponds to winter, lukewarm to spring, hot to summer, dry to autumn. It is very wise to devote four rooms in baths accordingly. The first is cold, the second lukewarm. The third hot, the fourth dry. And when a man first enters the bath, he should spend a little time in the first, and after [enter] the second. And there, dwell a little. And then [enter] the third one, and there, dwell a little. And then enter the fourth and do in the same manner. And when he wants to leave, he should keep [doing this] in the same manner, dwelling a little in each room, so that he does not go from a great heat to a great cold, or from overly great cold to overly great heat […]. And therein he should use appropriate fragrances according to the time [of the year], a paste must be mixed with in three or four parts in spring and summer, and in two parts in autumn and winter. Subsequently, let him sit, let him soak in water of roses and wipe him with a clean towel of linen once and a second time. And when all this has been done and he is deliciously washed, let him go to the other rooms, and use the following teachings and ointments. If he is not overcome by heat, comb his head, using the cleansing ointment appropriate to the time [of the year]; for in spring and in summer

> he should use an ointment made of myrrh, […]. And after this, he should wash his body and rub it with water, until he is well-washed and clean. After, anoint his body with ointments appropriate to the time […]. If he is thirsty, he should drink rose syrup and an electuary with musk […]. This is the order to heal and nourish the body. And he that is old, or cold and moist should not dwell in the bath for a long time. Nonetheless, he shall sit therein, until his body is moist from the bath; the phlegmatic man should enter the bath fasting and be anointed with ointments. And he that is of the hot kind should keep in mind these teachings.)[54]

As can be seen, the importance of humoral theory in balneology is explained, listing the qualities of the four elements and their correspondence with the four seasons, hence the use of specific ingredients only in particular times of the year. Their quantities also vary according to the seasons: for example, to make a paste to be used during the bath, a lower dosage will be employed in autumn and winter. For the same reasons, even the ointments to be spread on the body before and after the bath must follow a precise seasonal pattern. The instructions for the bath, then, are very accurate, prescribing, for example, the position of the patient, the substances to be used for bathing, and the materials for drying. The patient must *sitte on setys wete* (be seated while immersed) in rose water and, similarly to the *Peri didaxeon*, which suggested the use of a new woollen fabric, only a clean linen cloth must be used. Finally, advice is given according to the dominant temperaments so that everyone bathing should follow some fundamental precautions to avoid the bath being harmful: people with a phlegmatic nature will have to fast and use an additional ointment, while the elderly and people with a cold and moist nature will have to soak for a shorter period.

Conclusion

This study has identified two phases in medieval English balneotherapy: the early Middle Ages, when references to baths were scattered, and the second phase, when baths were part of more complex remedies involving ointments, decoctions, and the ingestion of foodstuffs. In the first period, the instructions for the preparation of baths were simple, schematic, and succinct, listing ingredients, temperature, and processes to prepare the remedy. Furthermore, humoral theory was usually not explicitly mentioned, but the remedies, including balneotherapic ones, tended to allude to it by referring to the elementary qualities of some of the ingredients. Bathing was seen to be more effective when accompanied by a specific diet, as in the case of the

54 *Three Prose Versions of the Secreta Secretorum*, ed. by Steele, ch. 63 (pp. 82–83).

Benedictine Rule, while in *Leechbook II*, it was considered particularly effective as a treatment for gastro-intestinal ailments. The *Old English Herbarium* included single-ingredient treatments and typically advised washing specific parts of the body. Therefore, when compared to the other texts examined in this chapter, the quantities of and the methods for transforming the herbs were more precise.

The *Peri didaxeon*, which dates to the twelfth century, represents an intermediate phase in balneotherapy, focusing on the rebalancing of the four humours as a means to obtain recovery. This is reflected in a greater precision in the instructions to prepare the ingredients for bathing waters. Here, humours were also explicitly mentioned as the cause of disease. If compared to earlier treaties, this translated into considerable attention to the elemental qualities of the ingredients, bathing waters and ointments.

The second stage of balneology began in the late Middle Ages, when chapters on bathing started appearing in medical treatises and bathing became increasingly important in patient care. This development in balneology has been attributed to two key sociocultural factors. Firstly, with its production of medical treatises, which were quickly transmitted from the nearby scriptorium of Monte Cassino into Normandy and Anglo-Norman England, the Salernitan School of medicine had a significant influence on medical education. Additionally, it contributed to propagating the study of medicine across medieval universities in Europe. Secondly, bathing practices were clearly linked to elemental and humoral theories as a result of the resurgence of thermalism, which also gave rise to a tendency to systematize balneotherapy. The *System of Physic*, for instance, represents an advance over the ideas presented in the *Peri didaxeon* in that it links the four seasons to the four humours, the elements, and their attributes as the foundation of medical practice. The lexicon employed in some of the remedies under study provides further evidence that the relationship between healing and the rebalancing of the humours was a key tenet in medical treatises. English physicians in the late medieval period began to prescribe more treatments including baths as they grew more aware of the critical function that water played in patient healing. Water, as one of the four elements, through bathing, is fundamental in restoring humoral balance. Medical procedures thus become more unequivocally aimed at contrasting humoral excess through the use of ingredients with elemental qualities opposite to the humours they have to counterbalance: for example, if the ailment is caused by cold humours, the physician will use hot ingredients and vice versa. The prescriptions become more detailed in terms of ingredients, quantities, processes for their preparation, and elemental qualities. This culminates in treatises like the *Secreta secretorum*, where the complexity of balneotherapic advice reaches its peak, with bathhouses having to be designed and built according to the four seasons and different ingredients, fragrances, and ointments being prescribed before, during and after the bath according to time of the year and the patient's temperament, age, and health condition.

Works Cited

Manuscripts

Glasgow, University Library, MS Hunter 307. Digitized version available at <https://hunter.uma.es/> [accessed 20 April 2021]
London, British Library, MS Cotton Faustina B III
London, British Library, MS Cotton Tiberius A III
London, British Library, MS Cotton Vitellius C III
London, British Library, MS Harley 585
London, British Library, MS Harley 6258B
London, British Library, MS Royal 12 D XVII
London, British Library, MS Royal 18 A VII
Oxford, Bodleian Library, MS Hatton 76
Oxford, St John's College, MS 17. Digitized and annotated version available at <http://digital.library.mcgill.ca/ms-17> [accessed 17 July 2022]

Primary Sources

Galen, *On Hippocrates' On The Nature of Man*, ed. and trans. by W. J. Lewis and J. A. Beach, *Medicina Antiqua* <https://www.ucl.ac.uk/~ucgajpd/medicina%20antiqua/tr_GNatHom.html> [accessed 21 March 2022]

Gilbertus Anglicus, *Healing and Society in Medieval England: A Middle English Translation of the Pharmaceutical Writings of Gilbertus Anglicus*, ed. by Faye M. Getz (Madison: University of Wisconsin Press, 1991)

——, *System of Physic (GUL, MS Hunter 509, ff. 1r–67v): A Compendium of Medicine including the Middle English Gilbertus Anglicus*, ed. by Laura Esteban Segura, Middle and Early Modern English Texts, 3 (Pieterlen: Peter Lang, 2012)

Isidore of Seville, *De natura rerum*, Library of Latin Texts, Brepolis, ed. by Paul Tombeur (Turnhout: Brepols, 2023) <https://clt-brepolis-net.may.idm.oclc.org/llta/pages/QuickResults.aspx?qry=351f94e9-c036-4f54-81bd-b842c40b11de> [accessed 22 April 2022]

——, *The Etymologies of Isidore of Seville*, trans. by Stephen A. Barney, W. J. Lewis, J. A. Beach, and Oliver Berghof (Cambridge: Cambridge University Press, 2010)

——, *Isidori Hispalensis Episcopi: Etymologiarum sive originum*, ed. by W. M. Lindsay (Oxford: Oxford University Press, 1911). Available online <https://penelope.uchicago.edu/Thayer/E/Roman/Texts/Isidore/home.html> [accessed 8 July 2022]

——, *On the Nature of Things*, ed. and trans. by Calvin B. Kendall and Faith Wallis (Liverpool: Liverpool University Press, 2016)

Leechdoms, Wortcunning, and Starcraft of Early England, ed. and trans. by Thomas O. Cockayne, 3 vols (Cambridge: Cambridge University Press, 1865; repr. 2012)

Medical Writings from Early Medieval England Volume 1: The Old English Herbal, Lacnunga, and Other Texts, ed. and trans by John D. Niles and Maria A. D'Aronco (Cambridge, MA: Harvard University Press, 2023)

Medieval Herbal Remedies. The Old-English Herbarium and Early Medieval Medicine, trans. by Anne Van Arsdall, 2nd edn (London: Routledge, 2023)

Regularis concordia Anglicae nationis monachorum sanctimonialiumque. The Monastic Agreement of the Monks and Nuns of the English Nation, ed. and trans. by Thomas Symons (London: Thomas Nelson and Sons Ltd, 1953)

St Benedict, *The Rule of St Benedict*, ed. and trans. by Bruce L. Venarde (Cambridge, MA: Harvard University Press, 2011)

Three Prose Versions of the Secreta Secretorum, ed. by Robert Steele, 2nd edn (Oxford: Oxford University Press, 1996)

Secondary Studies

Bifulco M., M. Amato, G. Gangemi, M. Marasco, M. Caggiano, A. Amato, and S. Pisanti, 'Dental Care and Dentistry Practice in the Medieval Medical School of Salerno', *British Dental Journal*, 221.2 (2016), 87–89

Black, Winston, 'A Star is Born: Reading Constantine the African in Medieval England', *Constantinus Africanus*, 22 August 2018 <https://constantinusafricanus.com/2018/08/22/a-star-is-born-reading-constantine-the-african-in-medieval-england/> [accessed 20 March 2022]

Bradley, Ian, *Health, Hedonism and Hypochondria: The Hidden History of Spas* (London: Bloomsbury Publishing, 2021)

Cătănescu, Alina, and Andrei Racolța, 'The Use of Decorative Elements in the Interior Design of the Nineteenth-century Spa Buildings', *Journal of Architecture, Urbanism and Heritage*, 2.1 (2019) <http://www.jauh.upt.ro/index.php/JAUH/issue/view/1> [accessed 7 July 2022]

Danzi, Massimo, 'Le terme in Europa tra letteratura e medicina', *Quaderns d'Italià*, 22 (2017), 43–56

de Divitiis, Enrico, Paolo Cappabianca, and Oreste de Divitiis, 'The "Schola Medica Salernitana": The Forerunner of the Modern University Medical Schools', *Neurosurgery*, 55.4 (Oct 2004), 722–44

Garcia-Ballester, Luis, Roger French, Jon Arrizabalaga, and Andrew Cunningham, *Practical Medicine from Salerno to the Black Death* (Cambridge: Cambridge University Press, 2004)

Gaullier-Bougassas, Catherine, Margaret Bridges, and Jean-Yves Tilliette, eds, *Les trajectoires européennes du Secretum Secretorum du Pseudo-Aristote (xiiie-xvie siècle)* (Turnhout: Brepols, 2015)

Gow, Derek, *Bringing Back the Beaver: The Story of One Man's Quest to Rewild Britain's Waterways* (White River Junction, VT: Chelsea Green Publishing, 2020)

Green, Monica H., 'Salerno on the Thames: The Genesis of Anglo-Norman Medical Literature', in *Language and Culture in Medieval Britain: The French of England c. 1100 – c. 1500*, ed. by Jocelyn Wogan-Browne (Woodbridge: Boydell & Brewer, 2009), pp. 220–32

——, *The Trotula: A Medieval Compendium of Women's Medicine* (Philadelphia: University of Pennsylvania Press, 2001)

Howes, Hetta E., *Transformative Waters in Late Medieval Literature* (Woodbridge: Boydell, 2021)

Hunt, Tony, *Popular Medicine in Thirteenth-century England: Introduction and Texts* (Cambridge: D. S. Brewer, 1990)

Jacquart, Danielle, 'Medical Scholasticism', in *Western Medical Thought from Antiquity to the Middle Ages*, ed. by Bernardino Fantini (Cambridge, MA: Harvard University Press, 1998), pp. 197–239

Jaglarz, Anna, 'The Evolution of Public Hygiene and Sanitary Facilities in the Context of Urbanization Processes and Social Conditions', in *Universal Access in Human-Computer Interaction: Design for All and Accessibility Practice. 8th International Conference, UAHCI 2014, Held as Part of HCI International 2014, Heraklion, Crete, Greece, June 22–27, 2014, Proceedings, Part IV*, ed. by Constantine Stephanidis and Margherita Antona (Berlin: Springer, 2014), pp. 192–203

Kosso, Cynthia, and Anne Scott, 'Preliminary Material', in *The Nature and Function of Water, Baths, Bathing and Hygiene from Antiquity through the Renaissance*, Technology and Change in History, 11, ed. by Cynthia Kosso and Anne Scott (Leiden: Brill, 2009), pp. i–viii

Kristeller, Paul O., 'The School of Salerno: Its Development and its Contribution to the History of Learning', *Bulletin of the History of Medicine*, 17.2 (1945), 138–94

Maion, Danielle, 'Il trattato medico antico inglese "Peri Didaxeon": problemi di traduzione', *Traduzione, società e cultura*, 10.4 (2002), 1–29

Nicoud, Marilyn, 'Le thermalisme médiéval et le gouvernement des corps: d'une *recreatio corporis* à une *regula balnei*?', in *Le thermalisme: Approches historiques et archéologiques d'un phénomène culturel et médical*, ed. by John Scheid, Marilyn Nicoud, Didier Boisseuil, and Joël Coste (Paris: CNRS Éditions, 2015), 79–104 <http://books.openedition.org/editionscnrs/26379> [accessed 16 July 2022]

Nora, Paula, 'Turismo de Saúde: um estudo comparativo', *Revista Turismo & Desenvolvimento*, 17–18 (2012), 1453–68

Perk, Godelinde G., '"Idleness Breeds Disgust for the Cell": Circumscribing Sloth, Acedia and Health in Anchoritic Literature', *Nordic Journal of English Studies*, 21.2 (2022), pp. 8–31

Quintela, Joana Alegria Ferreira Da Silva, 'Contribution of Health and Wellness Tourism to Happiness and Quality of Life: A Comparative Study between Portugal and Hungary' (unpublished doctoral thesis, Universidade de Aveiro, 2021)

Ramazzina, Elisa, 'Bathing in Medieval Europe', in *The Four Elements in the Medieval World: Interdisciplinary Perspectives, 'WATER'*, ed. by Marilina Cesario, Hugh Magennis, and Elisa Ramazzina (Leiden: Brill, 2024), pp. 99–139

Rawcliffe, Carole, *Urban Bodies: Communal Health in Late Medieval English Towns and Cities* (Woodbridge: Boydell, 2013)

Silișteanu, Sînziana Călina, Dumitru Mihăilă, Gabriela Dogaru, and Petruț-Ionel Bistricean, 'Balneoclimatology – Where To?', *Georeview*, 30 (2020), 42–64

Smith, Veronica, *Clean. A History of Personal Hygiene and Purity* (Oxford: Oxford University Press, 2008)

Stelmaschuk, Amber, 'The School at Salerno: Origin of the European Medical University', in *The Proceedings of the 10th Annual History of Medicine Days. Faculty of Medicine, The University of Calgary, March 23rd and 24th, 2001*, ed. by William A. Whitelaw (Calgary: Faculty of Medicine, University of Calgary, 2001) <https://prism.ucalgary.ca/handle/1880/51835> [accessed 9 July 2022]

Sudhoff, Karl, 'Salerno, eine mittelalterliche Heil- und Lehrstelle am Tyrrhenischen Meere', in *Sudhoffs Archiv für Geschichte der Medizin*, 21.1, ed. by Karl Sudhoff (Wiesbaden: Franz Steiner Verlag 1929), pp. 43–62

Walker-Meikle, Kathleen, 'Animals: Their Use and Meaning in Medieval Medicine', in *A Cultural History of Medicine: Middle Ages (800–1450), vol. 2*, ed. by Iona McCleery (London: Bloomsbury Academic, 2021), pp. 87–106

Wallis, Faith, 'The Calendar and the Cloister: Oxford – St John's College MS 17', McGill University Library Digital Collections Program, 2007 <http://digital.library.mcgill.ca/ms-17> [accessed 3 July 2023]

Williams, Joseph M., 'Synaesthetic Adjectives: A Possible Law of Semantic Change', *Language*, 52.2 (1976), 461–78

Zuccolin, Gabriella, 'Ruolo ed evoluzione della balneoterapia nel pensiero scientifico-medico in Italia dal XII al XVI secolo', in *Il Calore della Terra: Contributo alla Storia della Geotermia in Italia*, ed. by Marco Ciardi and Raffaele Cataldi (Pisa: Edizioni ETS, 2005), pp. 98–115

ANNE IRENE RIISØY

4. Body, *baugr*, and Sick-Maintenance

The Germanic Context of Early Medieval Norwegian Law on Wounds

In a seminal article of 2003 on the *Leges Barbarorum*, Patrick Wormald argued that the rules on bodily harm and their corresponding injury tariffs were fundamentally Germanic.[1] Whereas the Germanic laws (*c.* AD 500–900) consider bodily harm a personal affront, and therefore allocate the primary payment for such injury to the victim, according to Roman law, bodily harm was punished by the state. In addition to compensation, some Germanic laws accord the victim sick-maintenance, which 'is the responsibility of a person who has grievously injured another to provide for the victim until he is able to return to work'.[2] Following in the wake of Wormald came important works by Lisi Oliver, Przemyslaw Tyszka, and Han Nijdam.[3] In addition to the Germanic laws, Old Irish law-tracts on compensation for injuries and sick-maintenance have survived; above all, D. A. Binchy has edited, translated, and studied these sources.[4]

In recent years, the Nordic material has received renewed interest.[5] Of some relevance for this contribution are studies by Christine Ekholst and Jenny Benham. Ekholst explored how the Swedish medieval laws regulated injuries, typically wounds that followed from assault, and she found that in addition to compensation for the wound, some rules decree that the perpetrator also had to cover the expenses for bandages and the doctor's fee.[6] Benham compared rules of wounding from England and Scandinavia,

1 Wormald, '*Leges Barbarorum*', pp. 47–53.
2 Oliver, 'Sick-Maintenance in Anglo-Saxon Law', p. 304.
3 Oliver, 'Sick-Maintenance in Anglo-Saxon Law'; Oliver, *The Body Legal in Barbarian Law*; Tyszka, *The Human Body in Barbarian Laws*; Nijdam, 'Indigenous or Universal?'.
4 'Bretha Crólige', ed. and trans. by Binchy; Binchy, 'Sick-Maintenance in Irish Law'; 'Bretha Déin Chécht', ed. and trans. by Binchy.
5 For earlier scholarship, see Phillpotts, *Kindred and Clan*, pp. 1–101. In 2021 two studies of relevance to the wider topic of manslaughter, *wergild*, and wounds were published: see Vogt, 'The Kin's Collective Responsibility' and Lawing, 'Victims of Maiming in Sturlunga Saga'.
6 Ekholst, 'The Value of a Thumb', p. 46.

Anne Irene Riisøy • University of South-Eastern Norway; anne.irene.risoy@usn.no

Medicine in the Medieval North Atlantic World: Vernacular Texts and Traditions, ed. by Deborah Hayden and Sarah Baccianti, KSS, 5 (Turnhout, 2025), pp. 103-122
BREPOLS PUBLISHERS DOI 10.1484/M.KSS-EB.5.143982

and she included Norwegian legal material in the form of four paragraphs from the *Gulathing Law* (§§169, 179, 184, and 185), which are discussed in a twelfth- and thirteenth-century context.[7] My approach somewhat differs from Ekholst's and Benham's. I will focus exclusively upon the early Norwegian rules of wounding, which also contain clauses on sick-maintenance, namely a few paragraphs in the *Frostathing Law* and the *Gulathing Law*.[8] I agree with Benham that the rules on bodily harm also had relevance for High Medieval Norway; however, I work from the assumption that they were also relevant for a society that is considerably older. It should be noted that Benham too agreed with the position that the *Gulathing Law* contains older oral law.[9] The earliest Norwegian laws, the *Frostathing Law* and the *Gulathing Law*, contain elaborate regulations on bodily harm, and they stipulate compensation as well as the occasional fine to the king, calculated in terms of a *baugr* (ring) or fractions thereof.[10] The term *baugr* appears in all Germanic languages except Gothic, and it was used in various contexts. Rings were prestigious gifts, jewellery, and mediums of payment, typically of compensation; fines, dowries and rings were also applied in oath-swearing procedures.[11] Some paragraphs on bodily harm in the *Frostathing Law* stipulate compensation in rings made of gold, and archaeologist Dagfinn Skre saw this as a possible trace of migration-period law (*c.* 400–550), since it was the only gold-rich period in western Scandinavia.[12] However, other rules specify 'rings' in silver, which chronologically fits the Viking Age (*c.* 750–1050) when rings of silver were common and gold rings were quite rare.[13] The Norwegian rules on bodily harm are therefore chronological palimpsests that present themselves as suitable *comparanda* for similar provisions in the Germanic laws, and, as D. A. Binchy stated in his study on sick-maintenance in Irish law, 'the rules governing compensation for personal injuries offer perhaps the most fruitful field for the work of drawing parallels between ancient legal systems'.[14]

Oliver hypothesized that Germanic peoples had a common institution of sick-maintenance that was made up of two components, compensation

---

7 Benham, 'Wounding in the High Middle Ages', pp. 151–72.

8 The *Gulathing Law* and the *Frostathing Law* are abbreviated as G and F in the footnotes.

9 Benham, 'Wounding in the High Middle Ages', pp. 153–54.

10 Ebbe Hertzberg, who edited the glossary for the medieval laws of Norway, *Norges Gamle Love* (henceforth abbreviated to NgL; the glossary appeared in volume v), pp. 191 and 459, and Gerhard Hafström, 'Böter och baugar', pp. 1–7, who studied the system of fines in the earliest Norwegian laws, noted that a *baugr* never designated a fine to the bishop, only to the king. They, therefore concluded (correctly, in my opinion), that these fines had a pre-Christian origin.

11 Engeler, *Altnordische Geldwörter*, p. 86; Green, *Language and History*, pp. 67–68; Zimmermann and Capelle, 'Ring und Ringschmuck', pp. 3–12; Steuer and Beck, 'Ringgeld', pp. 16–19. See also 'baugr' in Cleasby and Vigfusson, *An Icelandic–English Dictionary*, pp. 53–54, and Fritzner, *Ordbog over Det gamle norske Sprog*, I, p. 118.

12 Skre 'Monetary Practices', pp. 292–93.

13 Skre 'Monetary Practices', pp. 292–93.

14 Binchy, 'Sick-Maintenance in Irish Law', p. 78.

and medical fees payable to the victim.[15] Sick-maintenance only occurred when the injury was unlawful, and not in cases of self-defence or in the case of slight corporal injury, which would heal quickly. Oliver's starting point can be found in a rule in the earliest Anglo-Saxon law of Æthelberht of Kent of *c.* AD 600, which is preserved in *Textus Roffensis* from the early 1120s. The section on personal injury in Æthelberht contains archaic syntax, which suggests that it had been preserved from an oral transmission predating AD 600.[16] Æthelberht § 63 stipulates:

> Gif man gegemed weorðeþ, XXX scill gebete.
> Gif man cearwund sie, XXX scill gebete.
>
>> (If a person becomes cured [after having been wounded] let him [i.e., the person who caused the wound] pay [with] 30 shillings.
>> If a person should be grievously wounded, let him pay [with] 30 shillings.)[17]

Oliver adduced two Germanic connections, one Old Norse and one Frankish. The Old Norse *kǫr* (sickbed), reflecting a wound that requires the victim to stay in bed, is cognate with *cear*, the first element in the hapax compound term *cearwund* in Æthelberht.[18] The laws of Æthelberht and the Salian Franks (481–507) have the same placement, grouping, and relative amounts of compensation, and Oliver suggested therefore that these similarities 'imply West-Germanic echoes of an orally transmitted ancestor which was fairly stable in a predecessor to at least the Salic and Anglo-Saxon laws'.[19] The second clause in the Frankish paragraph stipulates a fee for the doctoring (*de mendicatura*), presumably a parallel to the fine for the victim's having to be *gegemod* (cured) in Æthelberht § 63.[20]

---

15 Oliver, 'Sick-Maintenance in Anglo-Saxon Law', pp. 310–11.

16 Oliver, 'Sick-Maintenance in Anglo-Saxon Law', pp. 303–05; Oliver, *The Beginnings of English Law*, pp. 14–15; Wormald, *The Making of English Law*, pp. 29–30 and 93–101. Lambert, *Law and Order*, pp. 33–37 noted that almost every clause in Æthelberht's code prescribes compensation appropriate to a specific affront to honour, and that they were written down because they were the most prestigious rules in pre-Christian Kentish society.

17 § 63 in Oliver, *The Beginnings of English Law*, pp. 74–75.

18 Oliver, 'Sick-Maintenance in Anglo-Saxon Law', p. 308 noted that a literal translation of *cearwund* is 'bedriddening-wound' or, more intelligibly, 'wound causing a person to be bedridden'. Jurasinski, *The Old English Penitentials*, pp. 151–56 argued that although a term such as *cearwund* implies 'some faint awareness of sick maintenance in Anglo-Saxon law', the biblical influence of Exodus was the most likely source of inspiration. Against this, I would like to take heed of Oliver's statement that, although *cearwund* occurs in Æthelberht § 63 only, absence of evidence should not be taken as evidence of absence, because Æthelberht's law also contains other archaic terms that soon disappear from the language: see Oliver, 'Sick-Maintenance in Anglo-Saxon Law', p. 308 and Oliver, *The Beginnings of English Law*, pp. 29–30.

19 Oliver, 'Sick-Maintenance in Anglo-Saxon Law', pp. 308–09.

20 Oliver, 'Sick-Maintenance in Anglo-Saxon Law', p. 309. Oliver (p. 314) also pointed out that the Old English *læcefeoh* 'leech-fee' only has one pre-Conquest attestation.

As Oliver pointed out, the earliest Icelandic law *Grágás* does not contain personal injury tariffs, which typically were fractions of *wergild*.[21] Injury tariffs are found in other Scandinavian laws, such as the *Gulathing Law* and the *Frostathing Law*; however, it is necessary to reassess Oliver's statement that these laws do not contain clauses dealing with sick-maintenance.[22] Oliver found that Old Norse *kǫr* (f. gen. *karar*, a bed in which one lies bedridden, i.e. sickbed) and *kararmaðr* (a bedridden person) only appear in literary sources, not laws.[23] The *Gulathing Law* and the *Frostathing Law* have rules on sick-maintenance, although expressed in different terminology, where the victim is entitled to compensation, a doctoring 'leech fee' and refection, normally a fixed fee rendered in flour and butter. Moreover, the laws take into account that the wounded may need time to recuperate in a sick-bed, for example a person who wounded a slave had to provide victuals 'meðan hann liggr i sarom' (as long as he [i.e. the slave] lies wounded).[24] Henceforth, the main focus of this chapter will be on the *Gulathing Law* and the *Frostathing Law*. Oliver placed these laws in the mid-twelfth to the early thirteenth century. However, similarly to the earliest Anglo-Saxon and Irish laws, the *Gulathing Law* and the *Frostathing Law* may contain material which is considerably older than the earliest manuscripts and manuscript fragments.

Material and Method

Before the *Landslaw* was codified in 1274, there were four large legal provinces within the area that approximately corresponds to present day Norway: Gulathing, Frostathing, Eidsivathing, and Borgarthing, each of which codified legislation for ecclesiastical as well as secular affairs. From the Borgarthing and the Eidsivathing law provinces of south-east Norway, only the Christian law section has been preserved. The most pertinent paragraphs on bodily harm

21 Oliver, 'Sick-Maintenance in Anglo-Saxon Law', p. 308. It should be noted that *Grágás* has rules on *wergild*: see Phillpotts, *Kindred and Clan*, pp. 11–46. William Ian Miller discussed legal practice in Iceland, where compensation for injuries was often subject to the social standing and power of the victim and his kin. In a typical settlement in cases with multiple claims, corpse was balanced against corpse, and insult against injury, 'And in the formalized balancing of man against man or of man against property, we see one of the few explicit indicators of rank in a society virtually without formal ranking' (Miller, *Bloodtaking and Peacemaking*, p. 277).

22 Oliver, 'Sick-Maintenance in Anglo-Saxon Law', pp. 305–08.

23 Oliver, 'Sick-Maintenance in Anglo-Saxon Law', pp. 307–09. Similar terms with the same meaning are found in Norwegian diplomas, legal documents that concern witness statements. See Fritzner, *Ordbog over Det gamle norske Sprog*, II, p. 390: *kǫr* (sickbed), *kǫrlægr* (bedridden), which informs that a man Þormóðr had been bedridden for four years (*Diplomatarium Norwegicum* III 165, s.a. 1332), and *kǫrlægimaðr* (bedridden person) (*Diplomatarium Norwegicum* VII 102, s.a. 1324). The Norwegian medieval diplomas are accessible via <https://www.dokpro.uio.no/>.

24 G 215; NgL I, p. 73 (*Earliest Norwegian Laws*, trans. by Larson, p. 149).

are therefore in the section on 'Personal Rights' in the *Frostathing Law* and the *Gulathing Law*.[25] The oldest manuscript fragments date from *c.* 1200; however, these laws were written down earlier, probably in the eleventh century, and the secular law sections contain material that predates the eleventh century.[26] Rune Røsstad found that stylistic variation in medieval Norwegian legal language correlates somewhat with chronology, implying that the secular law sections in the *Gulathing Law* and the *Frostathing Law* contain Viking-Age law (*c.* 750–1050).[27] Moreover, as Skre's interdisciplinary study suggested, the term *baugr* in these laws appears to have its origin in the Migration Period.[28]

The Norwegian rules on manslaughter and *wergild* (a term designating 'remuneration for a man [person]'), have received more attention than those concerning wounds followed by compensation and sick-maintenance.[29] There is, however, an obvious connection between the two, as a case of wounding may turn into a case of manslaughter. Initially, though, it may have been undecided whether a case would eventually become one or the other. The Norwegian laws contain several different systems of *wergild* and several chronological layers, a mixture of old and new elements that have not been sufficiently sorted out. As Bertha S. Phillpotts noted, it is as if the compilers had heaped together all the *weregeld* clauses or fragments of *weregeld* regulations known to them.[30] Similarly, the rules on bodily harm and sick-maintenance may also contain material from different time periods.

---

25 These two laws applied to the coastal areas all along the western seashore of Norway.

26 In addition to the secular law (which regulates areas such as 'personal rights', property, and inheritance) there are the Christian laws, which contain paragraphs that go back to the first half of the eleventh century when Christianity was politically accepted. In NgL IV, pp. xiv–xv, Gustav Storm gave a short description of the surviving legal manuscripts, and seventeen are older than *c.* 1300, mostly fragments. The debate regarding when the laws were first written down has primarily focused upon the Christian laws, which may have been put on parchment before the secular law sections. Magnus Rindal, 'Dei eldste norske kristenrettane', argued for an early date in the 1020s, whereas for example Knut Helle, *Gulatinget*, p. 22, was sceptical of such an early date, but would not rule it out completely.

27 Røsstad, *A tveim tungum*.

28 Skre, 'Monetary Practices', pp. 289–94.

29 Haubrichs, 'Wergeld', pp. 94–96 and 107, discusses the west-Germanic term **wira-gelda*, which is earliest attested in Merovingian legal texts. The first element means man, person and the second (**geld-a-*) means retaliation, remuneration. *Wergild* was the central measure in the composition of various wrongs and affronts, and injury tariffs were often fractions of *wergild*: see Siems, 'Observations', p. 54.

30 Phillpotts, *Kindred and Clan*, p. 68. Phillpotts and Knut Robberstad, who edited and translated the *Gulathing Law*, were in agreement neither regarding the number of different systems of *wergild*, nor how the different systems should be ranked chronologically. Robberstad, *Gulatingslovi*, pp. 370–75, found five different systems of wergild in the *Gulathing Law*, in the main older than the revision undertaken in the 1160s, whereas Phillpotts, *Kindred and Clan*, pp. 56–63, operated with three complete sets of *wergild* regulations. Regarding chronology, Phillpotts and Robberstad agreed that G 316 is the youngest. I would like to point out that this paragraph too contains archaic traces, as the *baugr* is stipulated in gold.

Results: Bodily Harm, Compensation, and Sick-Maintenance

The point of departure for my enquiries is all the rules on bodily harm which entailed compensation, and which also include clauses on sick-maintenance embedded in the *Gulathing Law* and the *Frostathing Law*. Before compensation and sick-maintenance were due, it was imperative to assess the injury. A wound had to be publicly declared and examined in order to determine whether compensation should be awarded for wounding or for killing.[31] For example, if an injured man is still living 'en ruva se a sare' (after a scab has been formed on the wound), the offender shall 'bæte hanom sarbotom' (pay him the wound fine) and a *baugr* to the king.[32] Benham noted that the *Gulathing Law* prescribes immediate response, because if he can, the injured man should go on the same day with his wound unbound and show it to the first man he meets. The witness should name the offender on the same day, and consequently, the offender should be summoned to the assembly.[33] A wound may also be inspected after a scab has formed.

> En þegar er rúfa er á sáre. Þá scal sá er særði láta menn .ij. siá. En ef hinn sáre vill eigi sýna sár sín. þá er af hins ábyrgð er særði. oc svá þó at hinn verði dauðr. En ef hann sýnir. Þá sculo þeir bera vitni um er sá. en hann scal kenna þing oc bióða konungi lǫgbauga oc sárbœtr hinom sára oc sárbætr hinom sára oc læcnisfé [...][34]
>
> > (As soon as a scab has formed on the wound, the one who caused the wound shall have two men inspect it; but if the wounded man refuses to show his wound, the one who wounded him is no longer liable, even though the other man shall die. But if he does show it, they who view it shall bear witness concerning it. And he [the offender] shall summon a thing and offer to pay the fines to the king and the wound fine and the leech money to the wounded man [...])[35]

A rather elaborate rule 'Um beingiölld' (Concerning bone money) in the *Frostathing Law* prescribes compensation in every case where 'bein leysir or sári manns' (a bone has to be removed from a man's wound). Compensation is stipulated in a number of *eyrir* that is calculated on the basis of how many bones have to be removed from the wound as well as the size of those bones.[36] This rule also contains an archaic legal ritual involving a shield, or alternatively a bowl. In situations when a tiny bone was broken off a wounded person,

31 Benham, 'Wounding in the High Middle Ages', p. 155.

32 G 183, NgL I, p. 67 (*Earliest Norwegian Laws*, trans. by Larson, p. 138).

33 Benham, 'Wounding in the High Middle Ages', pp. 155–56; G 184, NgL I, p. 67 (*Earliest Norwegian Laws*, trans. by Larson, pp. 138–39).

34 F IV 12, NgL I, pp. 162–63.

35 *Earliest Norwegian Laws*, trans. by Larson, pp. 263–64.

36 F IV 49, NgL I, p. 172 (*Earliest Norwegian Laws*, trans. by Larson, pp. 277–78).

if the bone was making a rattling sound on the shield ('skellr á skialldi') a compensation of one *eyrir* was due. A comparable legal ritual was applied also in the Gulathing area, although here an alternative phrase of bones 'skellr i skalom' (rattling in a bowl) appears.[37] Strikingly similar rules are evidenced in several of the Germanic laws.[38]

According to the clauses above, the *Frostathing Law* stipulates that the person who caused the wound shall pay one *eyrir* and leech money every month and two months' supply of flour and butter.[39] The only comparable paragraph in the *Gulathing Law* prescribes sick-maintenance in cases where 'Nu særer maðr annan' (a man wounds another) and therefore has to 'sárbotom bœta' (pay the wound fine) as compensation.[40] Additionally, the culprit 'scal kaupa læcningar kaupi sa er særði oc fá þeim fœzlo manaðar mat hvárs a manaðe' (shall pay for the leech and the remedies and provide the injured man with victuals, a month's food of both kinds).[41]

The reference to food of both kinds is most likely flour and butter, and the expression *manaðarmatr* (a month's food) includes these two victuals also in other contexts. The *manaðarmatr* was used as a unit of value designating the food supply for the representatives sent to the Gulathing assembly as well as the men serving in the *leiðangr*-fleet, the seaborne defence system.[42] We do not know how far back in time the *manaðarmatr* goes, but regional assemblies and a seaborne military system presumably existed long before the Viking Age, and people who participated in them would have to be fed. Archaeological traces of so-called court-sites all along the western coast of Norway point to the existence of regional assemblies going back to Roman times, and a system of a sea-based military organization may have existed for an equally long time.[43] During the High Middle Ages, sick-maintenance, including the month's food, faded away. It is not stipulated in the *Landslaw* (1274), but presumably it was a legal reality until that time.[44] Likewise, also

37 G 185, NgL I, pp. 67–68 (*Earliest Norwegian Laws*, trans. by Larson, p. 139). The translation in Larson versus Robberstad presents a slightly different meaning, and here I follow Robberstad, *Gulatingslovi*, p. 190.

38 Hüpper-Dröge, 'Schutz- und Agriffswaffen', pp. 120–21; *Frostatingslovi*, ed. and trans. by Hagland and Sandnes, p. 221 n. 24.

39 F IV 11, F IV 49, NgL I, pp. 162 and 172.

40 G 185, NgL I, pp. 67–68 (*Earliest Norwegian Laws*, trans. by Larson, p. 139).

41 G 185, NgL I, pp. 67–68 (*Earliest Norwegian Laws*, trans. by Larson, p. 139).

42 *Frostatingslova*, ed. and trans. by Hagland and Sandnes, pp. 236–37, Helle, *Gulatinget*, p. 69; for example, attendees at the Gulathing assembly, G 3, NgL I, p. 5; men serving in the *leiðangr*-fleet, G 300, NgL I, p. 98.

43 Iversen, 'Houses of Representatives?'; Malmros, *Vikingernes syn på militær og samfund*, pp. 122–23, discussed the *leiðangr* in tenth-century skaldic poetry. See also Helle, *Gulatinget*, p. 32 and Stylegar, '"… An Ornament in Peace and a Defence in War"', pp. 243–63.

44 Sick-maintenance (with terms such as the *læknir* 'leech/doctor' and *læknisfé*) also appears in the oldest preserved town-law of Norway, the *biarkeyiarréttr*, which applied to Niðarós (present-day Trondheim). Most of the material is taken from the *Frostathing Law*, as Niðarós was situated within the Frostathing legal province. The *biarkeyiarréttr* was probably

in the context of attendance at assemblies and the *leiðangr*-fleet, references to a month's food disappeared during the High Middle Ages.[45]

Compared to the *Frostathing Law*, the *Gulathing Law* is less concerned with bones removed from a wound, but focuses on other aspects, each entailing one *eyrir* in compensation from the perpetrator, who shall 'sárbotom bœta þeim er hann særðe' (pay the wound fine to the one whom he injured), such as if the weapon touched him or cut the flesh.[46] Higher compensation was prescribed for a wound in the chest or abdomen, a wound that enters the marrow, if the flesh drops to the ground or if rough scars form on the head (6 *aurar*). Finally, wounds on the back shall be twice as dear as those on the breast.[47]

The other paragraphs in the *Frostathing Law* dealing with sick-maintenance are rather brief. They all prescribe 'wound fine and the leech money', compensation, and in addition 'the customary fines shall be owing to the king'. The rules in question, which have all the above criteria, concern pushing someone into a fire resulting in an injury so serious that it needs to be bandaged; pushing someone into the sea; kicking or jerking away a man from his oar bench; or hitting someone with a missile or an axe-head.[48] When any kind of weapon was hurled against someone, the question of whether blood was shed or not decided the size of the compensation.[49] Moreover, mutilation or wounding in several places and severing of limbs were covered by similar rules.[50]

---

codified in the eleventh century and it may have been first written down in the mid-twelfth century. The manuscript evidence is late; except for one thirteenth-century fragment, all the manuscripts are post-medieval. The manuscripts seem to stem from a mid-thirteenth-century redaction, which suggests that at least by that time the rules on sick-maintenance were still applied (see *Bjarkøyretten*, ed. and trans. by Hagland and Sandnes, pp. ix–xv).

45 According to the *Landslaw*, § 2 (NgL II, pp. 11–12), in the section on 'Travelling to the thing', representatives to the regional assemblies were reimbursed, not in flour and butter, but in *aurar* (silver), the amount depending on the travel distance. The *leiðangr* was a system in which people presented not only victuals but also ships and crew to the king. From the second half of the twelfth century, the royal power gained greater control over the *leiðangr*, and in addition, the benefits, victuals, crew, and ships were converted into a tax in peacetime.

46 G 185, NgL I, pp. 67–68 (*Earliest Norwegian Laws*, trans. by Larson, p. 139).

47 Only one more paragraph in the *Gulathing Law* mentions leech money and the procuring of victuals: G 215 *Um sarbætr*, NgL I, p. 73 (*Earliest Norwegian Laws*, trans. by Larson, p. 149). This paragraph does not represent the institution of sick-maintenance, because it concerns slaves who were treated as their master's property with regard to bodily harm. Here the owner of the slave was also entitled to compensation. This principle is similar to a clause in the Lombard *Edicts of Lothari* (*c.* 643). Here too, the restitution was paid to the owner when a working slave had been damaged (see Oliver, 'Sick-Maintenance in Anglo-Saxon Law', pp. 319–20).

48 F IV 16, F IV 17, F IV 19, NgL I, pp. 163–64 (*Earliest Norwegian Laws*, trans. by Larson, pp. 265–66).

49 F IV 21, NgL I, pp. 164–65 (*Earliest Norwegian Laws*, trans. by Larson, p. 267).

50 F IV 42, NgL I, pp. 170–71 (*Earliest Norwegian Laws*, trans. by Larson, pp. 274–75).

The Body, Honour, and Social Stratification

The compensation tariffs in the Germanic laws show great variation, however one consistent factor appears. The compensation for the principal limbs was normally reckoned in fractions of the total *wergild*, usually half for the loss of a hand, foot or an eye.[51] The same principle is also evidenced in Norway, where the *Gulathing Law* prescribes half *wergild* if a person's hand or foot is hewn off, and the same if an eye is put out. Moreover, 'En ef allt er af einum manne hoggvit hond oc fotr. Þa er sa verri livandi en dauðr. scal giallda sem dauðr se' (if both hands and feet are hewn away, the man is worse off living than dead, and the payment shall be as if he were dead).[52]

In addition to compensation for physical harm to the body, early medieval people expected compensation for intangible offences more akin to insults where the harm upsets the victim's social standing, reputation, and honour. This principle applied in Germanic and Celtic societies alike.[53] Honour affected not only a person's self-respect but also reflected their standing in society, as honour was publicly valuated and bestowed upon that person by those who knew them.[54] Both Lambert and Oliver observed that in many cases, a wounded honour could be more important than bodily injury.[55] For a compensation settlement to be effective, both parties had to come out of it with their honour intact. According to the social logic of honour, if too little was paid this would dishonour the victim, and if too much was paid, this would dishonour the offender.[56] Moreover, as Lambert pointed out, in the context of honour the existence of an authoritative compensation tariff covering a wide variety of affronts was crucial, and, in order to be effective, compensation tariffs needed to be prestigious.[57] Presumably, the tariffs were applied in practice but not rigidly adhered to. They provided a common ground and served as a starting point for the commencing negotiations, and multifaceted factors such as the wealth, prestige, and reputation of the parties involved were considered. Detailed descriptions of injuries with corresponding tariffs may also have saved time in court, and at the same time, also minimized the risk of conflict.

According to the Germanic laws, visible damage to honour may take precedence over physical harm, and, as Patricia Skinner noted, due to their visibility, wounds to the head and face were the most serious of injuries in

51 Oliver, *The Body Legal in Barbarian Law*, pp. 137–40.

52 G 179, NgL I, p. 66 (*Earliest Norwegian Laws*, trans. by Larson, p. 137).

53 Oliver, *The Body Legal in Barbarian Law*, pp. 165–71; Lambert, *Law and Order*, pp. 35–38. As Liam Breatnach has argued, satire was a powerful weapon to be feared because it could damage honour (Breatnach, 'Satire, Praise and the Early Irish Poet', p. 63).

54 Lambert, *Law and Order*, p. 35; Charles-Edwards, 'Honour and Status', p. 123.

55 Oliver, *The Body Legal in Barbarian Law*, pp. 165–71; Lambert, *Law and Order*, pp. 35–38.

56 Lambert, *Law and Order*, pp. 35–38.

57 Lambert, *Law and Order*, p. 38.

early medieval society.[58] The same principle is traceable in the Norwegian laws. The nose has a prominent place in the face, and according to the *Frostathing Law* injuries to the nose shall be compensated for visible blemish, 'oc scal svá hvervitna er eigi hyll háre eða klæðom' (and it shall be thus wherever a blemish is not concealed by hair or by clothes).[59] Moreover, if 'kamstaðr verðr i hofðe manne' (rough scars form on the head), this entailed higher payment, presumably because such scars would be very noticeable.[60] Wounds that could not be covered by hair or clothing also demanded higher compensation in the Germanic laws.[61] Even teeth had an honourable place. Molars, which are of vital importance for chewing and processing food, are often valued less than front teeth, whose cutting function can be replaced by a knife.[62] Here too, the Norwegian system of evaluation focused on looks rather than on functionality, stipulating one *eyrir* for a molar compared to four times that amount for knocking out one of the front teeth.[63]

Compensation for wounds is one of the two cornerstones of the Germanic system of sick-maintenance.[64] Moreover, compensation tariffs that correlate with social status indicate a context of honour.[65] Although many rules on wounds stipulate compensation according to physical damage, not rank, some rules take rank into account. The following formulation bears this out: 'er hinn sáre er burðum til' ([paying] according to the wounded man's rank).[66] The final part in the paragraph on the so-called *beingiölld* (bone-money), in the *Frostathing Law*, addresses cases where it is necessary to turn the injured man on his face, and the compensation is accentuated according to rank:

> Þá scal bœta ǫfundarbót. haulldi aurum .vj. þaðan scal vaxa hvers manns réttr þriðiungi uppfrá haulldi. oc svá þverra. árbornum manne .iiij. aura. recs þegni .iij. aura. en leysingia .ij. aura. En þat scal vera allt silfrmetit.[67]
>
> > (there shall be a fine for evil intent: six oras to a hauld, and as his rank rises above the hauld's rank, every man's compensation increases by one-third. And it shrinks in the same ratio: a free-born man's compensation is four oras; that of a reksthegn, three oras; and that of a freedman, two oras. All this shall be measured in burned silver.)[68]

58 Skinner, 'Visible Prowess?', p. 81.
59 F IV 45, NgL I, pp. 171–72 (*Earliest Norwegian Laws*, trans. by Larson, p. 276).
60 G 185, NgL I, p. 68 (*Earliest Norwegian Laws*, trans. by Larson, pp. 139–40).
61 Nijdam, 'Compensating Body and Honor', p. 34.
62 Oliver, *The Body Legal in Barbarian Law*, p. 168.
63 F IV 45, NgL I, pp. 171–72 (*Earliest Norwegian Laws*, trans. by Larson, p. 276).
64 Oliver, 'Sick-Maintenance in Anglo-Saxon Law', pp. 310–11.
65 Lambert, *Law and Order*, pp. 35–39.
66 F IV 12, NgL I, pp. 162–63 (*Earliest Norwegian Laws*, trans. by Larson, pp. 263–64.
67 F IV 49, NgL I, p. 172.
68 *Earliest Norwegian Laws*, trans. by Larson, pp. 277–78.

Compensation for evil intent (*ǫfundarbót*) occurred only when the wounded man had to be turned on his face. Presumably, the victim had been attacked from behind, which was perceived as a cowardly way of assaulting someone. The act was therefore clearly linked to notions of honour, and punished accordingly.

A paragraph in the *Gulathing Law* 'Um sara virðing' (Concerning the valuation of wounds) correlates the compensation to the offender's rank: if a *leysingi* (freedman) wounds a man, he shall pay one *baugr*, [that is] twelve *aurar*, a freedman's son two rings, for a *bóndi* (freeman) three rings, and from then on the compensation doubles for each step up the social ladder (six rings for a man born to odal right, twelve rings for a *lendrmaðr* (landed-man) or *stallari* (king's marshall), twenty-four rings for an earl), all the way to the top of the social pyramid, where the king had to pay forty-eight rings.[69] This rule may have been revised in the Viking Age, as indicated by the compensation reckoned in burned silver. It is perhaps possible to narrow down the redaction of this rule even further, to the Late Viking Age. The *stallari* is mentioned for the first time during the time of King Óláfr Tryggvason (r. 995–1000).[70] The *lendrmaðr*, who had received land and authority from the king, appears in tenth-century sources. In skaldic poetry *lendrmaðr* and *hersir*, a title for a chieftain who probably had an independent and hereditary position of power, were often used synonymously. The *hersir* disappears from the sources from around the year 1000, and it therefore makes sense that he is not included in the tariff where the new men of power, the *lendrmaðr* and *stallari*, appear.[71]

Wormald pointed out that although the Germanic compensation tariffs are 'broadly similar' they are also 'invariably divergent', implying that they served as markers of identity and ethnicity.[72] A comparison between the laws of the Gulathing and the Frostathing fits Wormald's description: similar, yet divergent. The greater focus upon bone-wounds in the Frostathing compared to the Gulathing may be due to the chance survival of the manuscripts. Regarding social stratification, real differences between these two neighbourly legal provinces are more easily discernible.

As quoted above, the *Frostathing Law* accords compensation to a wounded man who had to be turned on his face, which was specified according to rank, and the *hǫldr* (that may include anyone from higher yeoman to a nobleman) served as the point of departure. Every man's compensation increases by one-third from the *hǫldr*, and likewise, the compensation for social ranks

---

69 G 185, NgL I, pp. 67–68 (*Earliest Norwegian Laws*, trans. by Larson, p. 139). The pre-medieval term *oðal*, which even predates the Viking Age, refers to allodium, inherited land that was closely attached to the homestead and elevated above other kinds of property. *Oðal* was particularly protected by law from falling into the wrong hands when transferred (Ruthström, *Land och Fæ*, pp. 22–24 and 122–23).

70 Hamre, 'Stallar', p. 34.

71 Iversen, *Eiendom, makt og statsdannelse*, p. 27.

72 Wormald, '*Leges Barbarorum*', p. 41.

below the *hǫlðr* shrinks in the same ratio.[73] This one-third principle applied to wounds as well as wergild. In the Gulathing area, as we have seen, the conversion principle is different. In cases where an offender had wounded another, a *bóndi* (freeman) had to pay three rings, and from then on, the payment doubled for each step up the social ladder. Similarly, according to the *Gulathing Law*, *wergild* doubled for each step up from the *hǫlðr*.[74] The *hǫlðr*, who was the pivotal point in *wergild* in both the Frostathing and the Gulathing, was occasionally interpreted as 'farmer or peasant'; however, as Jo Rune Ugulen recently concluded, the *hǫlðr*, who had twice as high a *wergild* as the *bóndi*, must be regarded as a nobleman.[75] There are also some minor differences between the Frostathing and the Gulathing legal provinces regarding the number and names of the various social ranks. The *reksþegn*, for example, appears in the *Frostathing Law* only, and exclusively in the compensation tariffs. The etymology of this term has been debated, and the *reksþegn* had place between a *leysingi* (freedman) and an *árborinn maðr* (fully free person).[76]

An important part of the Frostathing and the Gulathing laws were rules or customs connected to affronts and their corresponding compensation tariffs. Within the Frostathing and the Gulathing legal province, people were concerned about their *lǫg* (law), with the set expressions 'innan laga várra' and 'utan laga várra', meaning inside (*innan*) or outside (*utan*) legal area/jurisdiction.[77] Comprehensive rules on affronts and compensation, which in these two areas were rather similar, yet in some respects clearly diverged, may therefore have been important markers of identity and served to separate 'our' law from 'their' law. In order to keep track of the detailed rules and customs connected to affronts, legal experts (*lǫgmenn*, sg. *lǫgmaðr*) may have learned

73 F X 34, NgL I, p. 225 (*Earliest Norwegian Laws*, trans. by Larson, p. 356): 'Haullðr scal taca at fullrétti sínu mercr .iij. Nú scal þriðiungi vaxa upp frá haullði réttr hvers manns. oc svá þverra annan veg frá haullði oc þriðiungi' (The hauld shall receive three marks as his full atonement. Now the amount of the atonement money shall be increased by one-third from the hauld upward and decreased by one-third the other way).

74 G 200, NgL I, p. 71 (*Earliest Norwegian Laws*, trans. by Larson, pp. 144–45): A freeman (*leysingi*), six aurar, his son one mark, freeman (*bóndi*) twelve aurar, *haullðmaðr* 3 marks, *lendrmaðr* or *stallari*, six marks, earl or bishop 12 marks. This version is presumably late Viking Age. Bishops are incorporated, and the first bishop, from England, may have appeared during the early years of the reign of King Hákon góði, 'the Good' (ruled *c.* 933–961). G 200 takes bishops' and priests' sons for granted, and accord them the same rights as their fathers, which indicates a date before the mid-twelfth century, when the Archbishopric of Niðarós was established. See also G 218, NgL I, p. 74 (*Earliest Norwegian Laws*, trans. by Larson, p. 150), stating that the man-fines increase or decrease in amount from the *oðalborenn*, that is the *höldr*, just as the other atonements do.

75 Ugulen, 'The *hauldr*', showed that tenth-century English sources describe the *hǫlðr* as an important warlord, worthy to be mentioned by name when he fell against the English. The *hǫlðr* was also a powerful man on a national level, and, presumably, his position was similar across the North Sea in contemporary Norway.

76 *Frostatingslova*, ed. and trans. by Hagland and Sandnes, p. 238; NgL V, p. 514.

77 In Norway, *lǫg* also had a second meaning as it denoted a geographical-judicial area where this law applied: see Riisøy, 'Outlawry', p. 113.

them by heart so they could be recited formally when needed in a public setting such as the assembly. Being a *lǫgmaðr* was prestigious; the written sources imply that individuals who held this office were rich and powerful, and that the position may have been inherited through certain families.[78]

The *baugr* and Fractions Thereof

The Norwegian rules on bodily harm, including sick-maintenance, operate with the following units of payment: *baugr*, *eyrir*, and *mǫrk* (pl. *merkr*), where one *baugr* equals twelve *aurar* and eight *aurar* equals one *mǫrk*. Whereas the *baugr* is anchored in the Migration Period, both etymologically and archaeologically, the etymological evidence for a Migration Period date of the *eyrir*/*aurar* is less secure.[79] As Skre has pointed out, migration period gold rings from western Scandinavia tend to correspond to multiple or fractions of a common weight unit, which is reflected in pre-AD 550 grave finds of scales and weights. Furthermore, many rings from the migration period were adjusted to three, six, nine, or twelve *aurar*, the weight unit that appears in the *Frostathing Law*. This corroborates the existence of the *eyrir*/*aurar* weight unit in the Migration Period.[80] Because *wergild* represents deeply rooted cultural practices, such a long judicial continuity is plausible.[81] As the rules on sick-maintenance demonstrate, the *baugr* was also an early word for punishment, as the king was entitled to a fine in regard to various sorts of bodily harm.[82] Whether this practice also goes back to the Migration Period is hard to say; however, there were larger political units and rulers in Norway, as elsewhere in Scandinavia during that time.[83] Otherwise, the earliest attestation of 'a ring to the king' appears in Æthelberht's law. Here the king was entitled to fifty shillings as *drihtinbeage*, a compound of 'lord' and 'ring', if a freeman was killed.[84] Daniela Fruscione suggested that the *drihtinbeage* emerged in the Migration Period when the size of a lord's retinue was of great importance, and where the interests of *drihtin* (a military lordship) were relevant to a larger community.[85] Hence, *drihtinbeage* in Æthelberht may have been part of the

78 Brink, 'Law and Legal Customs', pp. 87–89.

79 Skre, 'Monetary Practices', p. 284, shows how the *eyrir*/*aurar* appears in Viking Age sources, such as a runic inscription on the Swedish Forsaringen of the ninth or early tenth century and in tenth-century Anglo-Saxon documents.

80 Skre, 'Monetary Practices', pp. 283–86.

81 Skre, 'Monetary Practices', p. 289.

82 Kilger, 'Wholeness and Holiness', p. 320. For examples, see NgL v, p. 92; Engeler, *Altnordische Geldwörter*, p. 88; and Brink, 'The Hälsinge Law', pp. 44–47. In cases of manslaughter, the *baugr* denoted a compensation payment and a fine to the king in the *Hälsinge Law*.

83 Andersen, *Dansk etnicitet og identitet til ca. år 1000*; Iversen, 'Between Tribe and Kingdom'; Skre, 'Rulership and Ruler's Sites'.

84 Æthelberht § 12, in Oliver, *The Beginnings of English Law*, pp. 62–63.

85 Fruscione, 'Beginnings and Legitimation'.

orally transmitted legal heritage the settlers brought from their homelands, which also included Scandinavia.[86]

Doctoring, Victuals, and Even Traces of a Substitute Worker?

As shown above, medical fees, the second cornerstone in Oliver's exposition of the Germanic sick-maintenance, are prescribed in Norwegian law, and healers or doctors are mentioned in the sagas. For example, after a great battle in Norway in the early eleventh century, many severely wounded men were placed inside a building, and a healer woman was there, boiling water for cleansing wounds and bandaging these men. The healer women obviously knew how to inspect wounds and made a concoction where leeks and various herbs were boiled together. After the men had eaten, she could smell the leek through a wound which went into the body cavity. From one of her patients, the healer received a gold ring.[87] Additionally, the Norwegian laws require the procuring of victuals as part of the sick-maintenance. This component is not specified in the laws Oliver draws upon, but Early Irish law, which has the most elaborate and archaic rules on sick-maintenance, do proscribe victuals to the victim.[88] The Irish law on sick-maintenance developed over time. In the earliest stage the injured person was removed from his home to be nursed back to health under the direction of a leech. The basic fare for everyone was two loaves of bread every day, and if corn was unavailable, the equivalent of 'summer-food' was given, i.e. butter and milk products. Additionally, the patient was fed according to social rank.[89] The injurer also had a duty of provide a substitute worker for the injured person, and to feed the substitute.[90] In the second stage, the patient remained in their own home, and the defendant procured food and a physician.[91] This system was cumbersome and inconvenient, and already around the eighth century the separate obligations such as food and drink, leech, and substitute worker were amalgamated by a single all-inclusive fee. The payment varied according to the victim's rank, and it included physician's fee, food, and drink, and compensation for 'blemish, hurt or loss of limb'.[92] The standard

86 Oliver, *The Beginnings of English Law*, p. 6, suggested that the people of Kent spoke a Jutish-influenced dialect.

87 *Heimskringla, Saint Oláf's saga*, chap. 234, trans. by Hollander, pp. 519–20. Nicknames such as 'wooden-foot' show that healers also knew how to make protheses (Oliver, *The Body Legal in Barbarian Law*, p. 120).

88 Binchy, 'Sick-Maintenance in Irish Law', p. 78.

89 Binchy, 'Sick-Maintenance in Irish Law', p. 125.

90 Binchy, 'Sick-Maintenance in Irish Law', pp. 115–16.

91 Binchy, 'Sick-Maintenance in Irish Law', pp. 127–29.

92 Kelly, *A Guide*, p. 133; Oliver, 'Sick-Maintenance in Anglo-Saxon Law', pp. 315–16, Binchy, 'Sick-Maintenance in Irish Law', pp. 90–91.

provisions are rather similar in Irish and Norwegian law, e.g. loaves of bread for the Irish and flour for the Norwegians and butter (an excellent way to preserve milk products) for both. These similarities may have nothing to do with a common inheritance regarding sick-maintenance but may reflect the basic products from an agricultural economy, which was rather similar in North-Western Europe. The Germanic laws on sick-maintenance cannot be linked to an Indo-European past as they lack the third component in the institution of sick-maintenance, which occurs in early Irish and Hittite law: namely, that the wrongdoer provide a substitute worker for the wounded man or compensate the work.[93]

I would like to draw attention to one paragraph in the *Frostathing Law* which may suggest a substitute worker. This law has two paragraphs that concern blinding. One rather brief paragraph, which is otherwise similar to many other rules on bodily harm, simply stats that 'Ef en maðr höggr augu or höfði manni. Þá sculu uppi mercer .iij. oc læcnisfé oc lǫgbaugar konunge' (if a man puts out another man's eye, there shall be due three marks and the leech fee and the customary fines [reckoned in rings] to the king).[94] The previous paragraph concerns exactly the same case, although it does not resemble any other paragraphs on bodily harm. Neither leech fee nor victuals are specified, but the victim was granted a farm with livestock:

> Ef maðr stingr augu or höfði manne. Þá verða menn iij útlager um þat verc einn er sá er or stacc en ij er á helldu […] þá sculo þeir aller gera honum xij kúa bú oc ij rossa oc iij mansmanna.
>
> > (If a man puts out another man's eye, the deed shall send three men into outlawry, the one who put out (the eye) and the two who held (the man). […] they shall stock a farm for him with twelve cows, two horses and three tralls.)[95]

The very specific details concerning how two men who held the victim and one man poked out the eyes indicates that this passage reflects an actual case. The paragraph has been drawn into a discussion of the size of a freeman's farm, or perhaps even the typical farm of *hǫlðr*, as the *hǫlðr* after all was the pivotal point in compensation tariffs.[96] Of interest here is a suggestion by Tore Iversen that one of the three slaves may be a substitute worker for the blinded man.[97] The suggestion is plausible, but yet again it should be stressed that this paragraph is unique.

---

93 Oliver, 'Sick-Maintenance in Anglo-Saxon Law', p. 307.

94 F IV 45, NgL I, p. 171 (*Earliest Norwegian Laws*, trans. by Larson, pp. 275–76).

95 F IV 44, NgL I, p. 171 (*Earliest Norwegian Laws*, trans. by Larson, p. 275).

96 Sandnes, '"Tolv kyr, to hester og tre træler"'.

97 Iversen, *Trelldommen*, pp. 115–16.

Concluding Remarks

I have argued that early Norwegian law also contains traces of sick-maintenance, which entailed compensation, leech fee and in addition victuals (flour and butter). Far more such rules are preserved in the *Frostathing Law* than the *Gulathing Law*. This may be coincidental as very few manuscripts and manuscript fragments from these laws have been preserved, and, therefore, absence of evidence should not be taken as evidence of absence. Other 'Germanic traits', such as honour taking precedence over actual bodily harm as well as compensation graded according to social rank, is evidenced in both laws. A comparison between these two laws shows that they fit into Wormald's generalization of the Germanic compensation tariffs: they are similar yet divergent, and the rules on affronts and compensation may have served as identity markers for the people living within the two separate legal provinces.

A system of sick-maintenance including compensation, leech fee, and victuals was in place during the Viking Age, and perhaps even earlier. Chronologically, this study therefore places itself between Skre's (Viking Age, perhaps even Migration Period) and Benham's (twelfth and thirteenth centuries). During the High Middle Ages, a legal transformation occurred in Norway. The *Landslaw* (1274), which applied to the whole country, played down the principle of social stratification and other aspects relating to honour, such as revenge killings and compensation to a wide network of kin, which were curtailed.[98] Important facets relating to sick-maintenance, including the leech fee and the unit *manaðarmatr*, disappeared from the *Landslaw*. The *Landslaw* was codified during a period known as the heyday of Medieval Norway, characterized by a relatively strong central kingdom, and the fact that one law for the whole realm was codified attests to this political situation. A comparison with medieval Frisia is interesting, because there the situation was different. Central government was weak, honour was of high importance, and elaborate compensation tariffs were still written down in the lawbooks.[99]

In Norway, sick-maintenance was presumably a valid legal principle up to the time of the codification of the *Landslaw*, whereas in legal practice, it may have existed far longer. However, legal practice is hard to assess. Diplomas detailing crimes start to appear from *c.* 1300, but cases that concern lesser crimes (wounds on the body were after all less serious than manslaughter and murder) may not have been written down to the same extent as more serious cases.

---

98 Riisøy, *Sexuality, Law and Legal Practice*, pp. 63–67. Mundal, 'The View of Blood Vengeance', pp. 148–51, showed how in legal practice this principle gradually faded away during the Late Middle Ages.

99 Nijdam, 'Indigenous or Universal?', p. 11.

Works Cited

Primary Sources

Bjarkøyretten, ed. and trans. with introduction and notes by Jan Ragnar Hagland and Jørn Sandnes (Oslo: Det Norske Samlaget, 1997)
'Bretha Crólige', ed. and trans. by D. A. Binchy, *Ériu*, 12 (1938), 1–77
'Bretha Déin Chécht', ed. and trans. by D. A. Binchy, *Ériu*, 20 (1966), 1–66
Diplomatarium Norwegicum, ed. by Christian Christoph Andreas Lange, Carl Richard Unger, Henrik Jørgen Huitfeldt-Kaas, and Gustav Storm, 22 vols (Christiana/Oslo: Riksarkivet, 1847–1997
The Earliest Norwegian Laws: Being the Gulathing Law and the Frostathing Law, trans. by Laurence M. Larson (New York: Columbia University Press, 1935)
Frostatingslova, ed. and trans. with introduction and notes by Jan Ragnar Hagland and Jørn Sandnes (Oslo: Det Norske Samlaget, 1994)
Gulatingslovi, ed. and trans. with introduction and notes by Knut Robberstad, 4th edn (Oslo: Det Norske Samlaget, 1981)
Heimskringla. History of the Kings of Norway, trans. by Lee M. Hollander (Austin: University of Texas Press, 1964)
NgL I = *Norges Gamle Love indtil 1387. Förste Bind*, ed. by Rudolph Keyser and P. A. Munch (Christiania: Grøndahl & Søn, 1846)
NgL II = *Norges Gamle Love indtil 1387. Andet Bind*, ed. by Rudolph Keyser and P. A. Munch (Christiania: Grøndahl & Søn, 1848)
NgL V = *Norges Gamle Love indtil 1387. Femte Bind*, ed. by Gustav Storm and Ebbe Hertzberg (Christiania: Grøndahl & Søn, 1895)

Secondary Studies

Andersen, Kasper H., *Dansk etnicitet og identitet til ca. år 1000* (Aarhus: Aarhus Universitet, 2017)
Benham, Jenny, 'Wounding in the High Middle Ages: Law and Practice', in *Wounds in the Middle Ages*, ed. by Anne Kirkham and Cordelia Warr (London: Routledge, 2016), pp. 151–72
Binchy, D. A., 'Sick-Maintenance in Irish Law', *Ériu*, 12 (1938), 78–134
Breatnach, Liam, 'Satire, Praise and the Early Irish Poet', *Ériu*, 56 (2006), 63–84
Brink, Stefan, 'The Hälsinge Law between South and West, King and Church, and Local Customs', in *New Approaches to Early Law in Scandinavia*, ed. by Stefan Brink and Lisa Collinson (Turnhout: Brepols, 2014), pp. 37–56
——, 'Law and Legal Customs in Viking Age Scandinavia', in *The Scandinavians. From the Vendel Period to the Tenth Century*, ed. by Judith Jesch (Woodbridge: Boydell, 2002), pp. 87–127
Charles-Edwards, Thomas, 'Honour and Status in Some Irish and Welsh Prose Tales', *Ériu*, 29 (1978), 123–41

Cleasby, Richard, and Gudbrand Vigfusson, *An Icelandic-English Dictionary*, 2nd edn with a supplement by Sir William A. Craigie (Oxford: The Clarendon Press, 1957)

Ekholst, Christine, 'The Value of a Thumb: Injuries and Disability in Swedish Medieval Law', *Mirator*, 2.20 (2021), 38–53

Engeler, Sigrid, *Altnordische Geldwörter* (Frankfurt am Main: Peter Lang, 1991)

Fritzner, Johan, *Ordbog over Det gamle norske Sprog*, revised edn (Oslo: Universitetsforlaget, 1973)

Fruscione, Daniela, 'Beginnings and Legitimation of Punishment in Early Anglo-Saxon Legislation from the Seventh to the Ninth Century', in *Capital and Corporal Punishment in Anglo-Saxon England*, ed. by Jay Paul Gates and Nicole Marafioti (Woodbridge: Boydell, 2014), pp. 34–47

Green, David H., *Language and History in the Early Germanic World* (Cambridge: Cambridge University Press, 1998)

Hafström, Gerhard, 'Böter och baugar', in *Rättshistoriska studier*, II (Stockholm: Nordiska Bokhandeln, 1957), pp. 1–7

Hamre, Lars, 'Stallar', in *Kulturhistoriskt Lexikon för nordisk medeltid*, XVII (Malmö: Allhems förlag, 1972), pp. 34–36

Haubrichs, Wolfgang, 'Wergeld: The Germanic Terminology of *Compositio* and its Implementation in the Early Middle Ages', in *Wergild, Compensation and Penance. The Monetary Logic of Early Medieval Conflict Resolution*, ed. by Lukas Bothe, Stefan Esders, and Han Nijdam (Leiden: Brill, 2021), pp. 92–112

Helle, Knut, *Gulatinget og Gulatingslova* (Leikanger: Skald, 2001)

Hüpper-Dröge, Dagmar, 'Schutz- und Agriffswaffen nach den Leges und verwandten fränkischen Rechtsquellen', in *Wörter und Sachen im Lichte der Bezichnungsforschung. Arbeiten zur Frühmittelalterforschung*, ed. by Ruth Schmidt-Wiegand, Schriftenreihe des Instituts für Frühmittelalterforschung der Universität Münster, 1 (Berlin: de Gruyter, 1981), pp. 107–27

Iversen, Frode, 'Between Tribe and Kingdom – People, Land, and Law in Scandza AD 500–1350', in *Rulership and Ruler's Sites in 1st–10th-century Scandinavia. Royal Graves and Sites in Avaldsnes and Beyond*, ed. by Dagfinn Skre (Berlin: de Gruyter, 2020), pp. 245–304

——, *Eiendom, makt og statsdannelse. Kongsgårder og gods i Hordaland i yngre jernalder og middelalder* (Bergen: Universitetet i Bergen Arkeologiske Skrifter, 2008)

——, 'Houses of Representatives? Courtyard Sites North of the Polar Circle: Reflections on Communal Organisation from the Late Roman Period to the Viking Age', in *Power and Place in Europe in the Early Middle Ages*, ed. by Jayne Carroll, Andrew Reynolds, and Barbara Yorke (Oxford: Oxford University Press), pp. 174–202

Iversen, Tore, *Trelldommen: Norsk slaveri i Middelalderen* (Bergen: Historisk institutt Universitetet i Bergen, 1997)

Jurasinski, Stefan, *The Old English Penitentials and Anglo-Saxon Law* (Cambridge: Cambridge University Press, 2015)

Kelly, Fergus, *A Guide to Early Irish Law* (Dublin: Dublin Institute for Advanced Studies, 1998)

Kilger, Christoph, 'Wholeness and Holiness: Counting, Weighing and Valuing Silver in the Early Viking Period', in *Means of Exchange. Dealing with Silver in the Viking Age*, ed. by Dagfinn Skre (Århus: Aarhus University Press, 2008), pp. 253–325

Lambert, Tom, *Law and Order in Anglo-Saxon England* (Oxford: Oxford University Press, 2017)

Lawing, Sean, 'Victims of Maiming in Sturlunga Saga: Worse off Living than Dead', *Mirator*, 2.20 (2021), 54–72

Malmros, Rikke, *Vikingernes syn på militær og samfund. Belyst gjennom skjaldernes fyrstedigtning* (Aarhus: Aarhus Universitetsforlag, 2010)

Miller, William Ian, *Bloodtaking and Peacemaking: Feud, Law, and Society in Saga Iceland* (Chicago: University of Chicago Press, 1997)

Mundal, Else, 'The View of Blood Vengeance in Medieval Norwegian Sources', in *Approaching the Viking Age*, ed. by Erika Sausverde and Ieva Steponaviciute (Vilnius: Vilnius University Publishing House, 2009), pp. 139–52

Nijdam, Han, 'Compensating Body and Honor: The Old Frisian Compensation Tariffs', in *Medicine and the Law in the Middle Ages*, ed. by Wendy Butler and Sara Turner (Leiden: Brill, 2014), pp. 25–57

——, 'Indigenous or Universal? A Comparative Perspective on Medieval (Frisian) Compensation Law', in *How Nordic are the Nordic Laws? Ten Years After. Proceedings of the Tenth Carlsberg Conference on Medieval Legal History 2013*, ed. by Per Andersen, Kirsi Salonen, Helle Møller Sigh, and Helle Vogt (Copenhagen: DJØF Publishing, 2014), pp. 161–81

Oliver, Lisi, *The Beginnings of English Law* (Toronto: Toronto University Press, 2002)

——, *The Body Legal in Barbarian Law* (Toronto: University of Toronto Press, 2011)

——, 'Sick-Maintenance in Anglo-Saxon Law', *Journal of English and Germanic Philology*, 107.3 (2008), 303–26

Phillpotts, Bertha S., *Kindred and Clan in the Middle Ages and After* (Cambridge: Cambridge University Press, 1913)

Riisøy, Anne Irene, 'Outlawry: From Western Norway to England', in *New Approaches to Early Law in Scandinavia*, ed. by Stefan Brink and Lisa Collinson (Turnhout: Brepols, 2014), pp. 101–22

——, *Sexuality, Law and Legal Practice and the Reformation in Norway* (Leiden: Brill, 2009)

Rindal, Magnus, 'Dei eldste norske kristenrettane', in *Religionsskiftet i Norden. Brytinger mellom nordisk og europeisk kultur 800–1200 e.Kr.*, ed. by Jón Viðar Sigurðsson, Marit Myking, and Magnus Rindal (Oslo: Unipub Forlag, 2004), pp. 108–10

Røsstad, Rune, *A tveim tungum: om stil og stilvariasjon i norrønt lovmål* (Oslo: Noregs forskingsråd, 1997)

Ruthström, Bo, *Land och Fæ. Strukturellt-rättsfilologiska studier i fornnordiskt lagspråk* (Lund: Bloms, 2003)

Sandnes, Jørn, '"Tolv kyr, to hester og tre træler". Litt om omfanget av trælholdet i Norge i vikingtid og tidlig kristen tid', *Norsk Historisk Tidsskrift*, 62 (1983), 79–82

Siems, Harald, 'Observations Concerning the "Wergild System"': Explanatory Approaches, Effectiveness and Structural Deficits', in *Wergild, Compensation and Penance. The Monetary Logic of Early Medieval Conflict Resolution*, ed. by Lukas Bothe, Stefan Esders, and Han Nijdam (Leiden: Brill, 2021), pp. 38–64

Skinner, Patricia, 'Visible Prowess?: Reading Men's Head and Face Wounds in Early Medieval Europe to 1000 CE', in *Wounds and Wound Repair in Medieval Culture*, ed. by Larissa Tracy and Kelly DeVries (Leiden: Brill, 2015), pp. 81–101

Skre, Dagfinn, 'Monetary Practices in Early Medieval Western Scandinavia', *Medieval Archaeology*, 62 (2017), 277–99

——, 'Rulership and Ruler's Sites in 1st–10th-century Scandinavia', in *Rulership and Ruler's Sites in 1st–10th-century Scandinavia. Royal Graves and Sites in Avaldsnes and Beyond*, ed. by Dagfinn Skre (Berlin: de Gruyter, 2020), pp. 193–244

Steuer, Heiko, and Heinrich Beck, 'Ringgeld', in *Reallexikon der Germanischen Altertumskunde*, ed. by Heinrich Beck, Dieter Geuenich, and Heiko Steuer (Berlin: Walter de Gruyter, 2003), pp. 16–19

Stylegar, Frans-Arne, '… An Ornament in Peace and a Defence in War': Late Roman Weapon Graves and Military Organisation in Eastern Norway', in *Facets of Archeology: Essays in Honour of Lotte Hedeager on her 60th birthday*, ed. by Konstantinos Chilidis, Julie Lund, and Christopher Prescott (Oslo: Unipub forlag, 2009), pp. 243–62

Tyszka, Przemyslaw, *The Human Body in Barbarian Laws c. 500 – c. 800. 'Corpus Hominis' as a Cultural Category* (Frankfurt am Mein: Peter Lang, 2014)

Ugulen, Jo Rune, 'The *hauldr*: Peasant or Nobleman?', in *Law and Power in the Middle Ages: Proceedings of the Fourth Carlsberg Academy Conference on Medieval Legal History 2007*, ed. by Per Andersen, Mia Münster-Swendsen, and Helle Vogt (Copenhagen: DJØF Publishing, 2012 [2008]), pp. 139–45

Vogt, Helle, 'The Kin's Collective Responsibility for the Payment of Man's Compensation in Medieval Denmark', in *Wergild, Compensation and Penance. The Monetary Logic of Early Medieval Conflict Resolution*, ed. by Lukas Bothe, Stefan Esders, and Han Nijdam (Leiden: Brill, 2021), pp. 277–92

Wormald, Patrick, 'The *Leges Barbarorum*: Law and Ethnicity in the Post-Roman West', in *Regna and Gentes. The Relationship between Late Antique and Early Medieval Peoples and Kingdoms in the Transformation of the Roman World*, ed. by Hans-Werner Goetz, Jörg Jarnut, and Walter Pohl (Leiden: Brill, 2003), pp. 21–53

——, *The Making of English Law: King Alfred to the Twelfth Century*, I. *Legislation and its Limits* (Oxford: Wiley-Blackwell, 1999)

Zimmermann, Christiane and Torsten Capelle, 'Ring und Ringschmuck', in *Reallexikon der Germanischen Altertumskunde*, ed. by Heinrich Beck, Dieter Geuenich, and Heiko Steuer (Berlin: Walter de Gruyter, 2003), pp. 3–12

RANKE DE VRIES

5. Three 'Exotic' Brain Injuries in Medieval Irish Literature*

Medieval Irish saga texts frequently contain references to fantastical injuries and unusual treatments. Scholars typically interpret these injuries and treatments from a linguistic perspective (e.g. Irish medical term X is cognate with Welsh medical term Y); a literary perspective (e.g. what does the injury of X in text Y symbolize; injury X is connected with biblical reference Y) or a legal perspective (e.g. who is culpable for inflicting injury X on patient Y?). While nobody would contest that these are valid and important approaches, scholars rarely employ a medical approach when looking at saga texts. However, examining literary episodes that involve injury or medical treatment from a medieval medical perspective is at least as important as other theoretical approaches, as medieval medical theory often provides a logical explanation for the (at first glance) unusual nature of the injuries and/or medical treatments. This chapter will illustrate this point by examining three examples of brain injury and subsequent treatment from a medical perspective: the leaking brains of Cormac Cas from the thirteenth-century compilation *Acallam na Senórach* (The conversation of the old men); Conán's head worm, found in the same text; and Cenn Fáelad's loss of his brain of forgetfulness, as featured in the

* This chapter is a modified version of my presentation given at the *Medicine in the Medieval North Atlantic World* conference, which also included references to a number of other head conditions in *Acallam na Senórach*. I would like to thank all those present there for their comments and helpful suggestions, as well as the editors of this volume and the anonymous readers. I would also like to thank the following student research assistants for their work, analysing dozens of saga texts for the presence of medical references as part of the MMIST (Medicine in Medieval Irish Saga Texts) project, some of which has been included in the present article: Chelsey MacPherson, Rhiannon Walker, Abbie Benjamin, Adele Martel, Aidan Wallace, Caitlyn McEwing, Dustin King, Katie MacIntosh, Sarah Laffin, Ryan Washburn, and Ethan Sabatella. Finally, my thanks to St Francis Xavier University for a UCR grant to support this research.

Ranke de Vries • St Francis Xavier University, Nova Scotia, Canada; rdevries@stfx.ca

Medicine in the Medieval North Atlantic World: Vernacular Texts and Traditions, ed. by Deborah Hayden and Sarah Baccianti, KSS, 5 (Turnhout, 2025), pp. 123-142
BREPOLS PUBLISHERS DOI 10.1484/M.KSS-EB.5.143983

late Middle Irish or Early Modern Irish version of the text *Cath Maige Rath* (The battle of Mag Rath), dated to the thirteenth or fourteenth century.[1]

Medieval Irish authors appear to have been well aware of the danger of injuries to the head and brain. This is, for example, borne out by the fact that out of the twelve doors of the soul (a term for locations where injuries would be especially dangerous or difficult to heal), listed in the seventh-century legal text *Bretha Déin Chécht* (The judgements of Dían Cécht), the first four locations are related to the head.[2] These include the crown of the head or the suture (*mullach cinn*); the hollow of the occiput (*clais da chulad*); the hollow of the temple or temporal fossa (*toll arai*); and the Adam's apple (*huball braiget*).[3]

Injuries to the head and brain occur relatively frequently in medieval Irish saga texts.[4] Occasionally, such accounts provide intriguing insights into continental medical knowledge and theory known in Ireland. Thus, brain injury is the subject of what is undoubtedly the most famous passage in medieval Irish saga literature dealing with medicine. The passage in question occurs in *Cath Maige Tuired* (The [second] battle of Mag Tuired), an eleventh- or twelfth-century revision of a ninth-century text,[5] and involves the murder of Míach by his father Dían Cécht. Enraged at the superior healing skills of his son, Dían Cécht, healer of the Túatha Dé Danann, strikes Míach on the head four times, penetrating further and further into his head each time. Only with the final strike, when Dían Cécht actually removes Míach's brain, does he kill his own son.[6] As pointed out previously by Hayden, this description shows an understanding of the anatomy of the brain that conformed to medieval European and Arabic anatomical doctrine,[7] and the injuries listed reference

1 Dillon, 'A Note', p. 201. It is perhaps significant that both of these texts post-date the influx of learned literature from Europe as well as the appearance of Latin translations of a number of important Arabic medical works.

2 Breatnach places the date of composition of the *Senchas Már* tracts, to which *Bretha Déin Chécht* belongs, to between 660 and 680 based on both linguistic and non-linguistic evidence (Breatnach, *The Early Irish Law Text* Senchas Már, p. 42). Hayden has discussed two later instances of dangerous locations, so-called 'doors of death', from two sixteenth- and seventeenth-century manuscripts in 'Observations', pp. 42–44 and 49–50.

3 *Bretha Déin Chécht*, ed. and trans. by Binchy, pp. 24–25. It should be noted that the order of the various body parts in this list is not necessarily in order of importance, but essentially reflects the standard medieval medical practice of discussing body parts from head to toe.

4 This is not just the case in medieval Irish literature; head injury appears to have been one of the more commonly occurring types of injury, particularly in a martial setting — Skinner points out that once a medieval warrior had lost his helmet, his head would have been a prime target as it was least protected, and a blow to the head could incapacitate a person, leaving them defenseless (Skinner, 'Visible Prowess', p. 89; see also MacInnes, 'Heads, Shoulders, Knees and Toes', p. 119). Head wounds were also used in medieval literature to 'emphasize the strength and prowess of the warrior who delivers the blow and the gravity of the wound for the knight who receives it' (Tracy, 'Into the hede', p. 498).

5 *Cath Maige Tuired*, ed. and trans. by Gray, p. 11.

6 *Cath Maige Tuired*, ed. and trans. by Gray, pp. 33–34.

7 Hayden, 'Observations', pp. 39–40.

various layers of the head as discussed in later medical manuscripts, like the sixteenth-century surgical tract *Anathomia Gydo*, an Irish translation of part of Guy de Chauliac's *Chirurgia magna*.[8] This tract follows earlier tradition and cites the late tenth- and early eleventh-century Persian physician Avicenna when identifying the external and internal layers of the head.[9]

In addition to knowledge of the anatomy of the brain, saga literature provides evidence that at least some medieval Irish scholars followed Galenic medical tradition with regard to the function of the brain itself. In Galenic tradition, the brain, along with the liver and the heart (and in some cases, the testicles or ovaries), was seen as one of the so-called principal members of the body, which in turn governed other bodily parts and functions.[10] In other words, the brain was one of the most important organs, responsible for the so-called animal virtues, associated with the function of the soul.[11] This theory is reflected in medieval Irish saga literature. For this, we turn to a gruesome episode in the twelfth-century text *In Cath Catharda* (The Civil War), an adaptation of Lucan's *Bellum Civile*. During a fight at sea, Caesar's people throw a grappling hook onto a ship that accidentally catches hold of the torso of a hero, Lycidas, dragging him to the edge of the ship. When his shipmates try to pull him back to prevent him from going overboard, Lycidas is torn in two. His lower body stays on the ship; his entrails plunge into the sea; and his upper body remains stuck on the grappling hook. According to the text, while the lower body has no life left in it, it takes a long time for his upper body to die.[12] The reason for this, so the Irish text tells us, is that this part contains the principal members that govern life ('na baill beóthacha'), and the seats of the soul ('istudha na h-anma'), here identified as the liver, brain, heart and Adam's apple ('áe 7 inchinn 7 craidhe 7 ubhall braighet').[13]

This account differs from that in Lucan's original. There, Lycidas is also torn in two, but the description of the upper part of his body is as follows:

> At tumidus qua pulmo iacet, qua viscera fervent, Haeserunt ibi fata diu luctataque multum / Hac cum parte viri vix omnia membra tulerunt.

---

8 Hayden, 'Observations', p. 39; *Anathomia Gydo*, ed. and trans. by Ní Ghallchobhair, pp. 60–61.

9 *Anathomia Gydo*, ed. and trans. by Ní Ghallchobhair, pp. 60–61.

10 Siraisi, *Medieval and Early Renaissance Medicine*, p. 107.

11 Siraisi, *Medieval and Early Renaissance medicine*, p. 108. The term 'animal' here is connected with the Latin word *anima* (soul). The heart is connected with vital or spiritual powers, while the liver is connected with natural virtues. Galen was part of a group of scholars (including Ptolemy, Herophilus, Erasistratus, and Plato) who adhered to an encephalocentric stance (which considered the brain to be the controlling principle of the body), in opposition to cardiocentrist scholars who thought that the heart was the controlling principle (Rocca, *Galen on the Brain*, pp. xx and chapter 1, particularly pp. 18–21).

12 *In Cath Catharda*, ed. by Stokes, pp. 160–61, ll. 2092–93: 'in leth uachtarach immorro búi sein for anamthaigh fria ré cían' (The upper half, however, was for a long time at the last gasp).

13 *In Cath Catharda*, ed. by Stokes, pp. 160–61, ll. 2093–95.

> (but where the lungs were full of air and the heart of heat,[14] there death was long baffled and struggled hard with this part of the man, till with difficulty it mastered the whole body.)[15]

There is quite a difference between the organs mentioned in the two texts. The Irish text has clearly borrowed from Galenic medical tradition, but with a twist: the Irish text lists the principal members and the seats of the soul as the liver, brain, and heart, as expected, but it then also includes the Adam's apple, rather than the testicles. As far as I am aware, the Adam's apple does not feature elsewhere in medical tradition in this context. This should probably be seen as a necessary substitution by the author. Due to the incident, Lycidas's testicles are no longer with the other members, but rather are part of his now lifeless lower body. Based on the fact that four body parts are mentioned, it seems likely that the author of this part of the Irish text must have believed that there were four principal members: liver, heart, brain, and testicles (or ovaries). Since he had to list four organs, he had no choice but to replace the missing testicles with something else, and settled on the Adam's apple as the most suitable candidate (potentially due to its significance as one of the doors of the soul mentioned above).

The Lycidas episode, like the murder of Míach, shows quite clearly that Irish scholars of the eleventh and twelfth centuries were familiar with important concepts from continental European and Arabic medicine related to the brain.[16] Now that this has been established, we can turn to our three examples of brain injury and subsequent medical treatment. At the time of composition of these episodes (i.e. the early thirteenth century and after), a substantial number of continental European and Arabic medical tracts dedicated to the anatomy of the brain, or focused on brain injury and head afflictions would have been in circulation.[17]

Medieval medical literature of the time typically held that the brain was divided into three different main cells or ventricles.[18] The first cell or anterior

---

14 Literally, 'where the vitals seethe'. This could potentially be a reference to the heart as a vital member.

15 Lucan, *Bellum civile*, ed. by Duff, 3.644–45 (pp. 160–61).

16 For further evidence of familiarity of medieval Irish scholars with European and Arabic medical tradition, see for example De Vries, 'Medieval Medicine'; Mulligan, 'The Erasure', especially pp. 33–41, and Sharon Arbuthnot's contribution to this volume.

17 Of particular importance are the works by Galen cited below. Celsus' *De medicina* contains a discussion of head injuries, and later, important surgical texts such as those by Rhazes (in the *Liber Almansoris*, particularly the section on head wounds and fracture of the head bone), Albucasis (book thirty of the *Kitab al-Tasrif* on surgery and surgical instruments), translated into Latin in the twelfth century; and Roger Frugard's *Practica Chirurgiae* (probably composed in the late twelfth century) include discussions of brain surgery. No specific Irish medical tracts survive from the thirteenth and fourteenth centuries — those did not appear until the fifteenth century.

18 Demaitre, *Medieval Medicine*, p. 129. This differs from earlier Greek medical tradition, in which the brain typically had four cells. This is the case in for example the works of Erasistratus of Chios and Herophilus of Chalcedon, both connected with a school of

ventricle was located at the front of the head. This contained the *sensus communis*, which collected the information perceived by the five senses. This information was processed by the imaginative faculty (*vis imaginativa*), or by *fantasia*. In the second cell, located in the middle of the brain, this processed information was further formed into concepts (through the *vis cogitativa*), and judgements (by the *vis estimativa*). The third cell or posterior ventricle held the faculty of memory (*vis memorativa*) and, according to some physicians, had control over body movement.[19] Each of the episodes under discussion focuses on a different part of the brain — anterior, middle, and posterior, respectively.

The Leaking Brains of Cormac Cas

The first example of a brain injury with an unusual treatment plan occurs relatively early on in *Acallam na Senórach*. The text speaks of a battle that has taken place between the Munster king Cormac Cas and the Ulster king Eochaid Abratrúad. Eochaid is killed in the battle, and Cormac himself is seriously injured. It is Cormac's injury that is of relevance to us here:

> do buailed Cormac Cas ann, 7 ro bhái trí bliadna déc ica leighius 7 a inchinn (ac si)led [asa cin*n* A4, p. 16, column a, line 35/asa chinn A20 fol. 22^{v}9], 7 sé a ríghi Muman ris sin. Ocus dorónad dúnad (7 degbai)le aigi ac dún ar sléibh, 7 is amlaid ro bhái (in dúnad s)in, 7 lochtopar grin lainidi ar lár an (dúnaid), 7 dorónad ríghthech romhór aigi imon tiprait, 7 ro saidhit tri liagána [A4/A20 liaga] cloiche uimpe, 7 ro suidhiged leabaidh in ríg 7 a cenn siar idir na trí huaithnib cloiche sin, 7 óclach grádha da mhuintir ag tabairt uisce a cuach nó as sithal ima cenn. Ocus fuair[-sium] bas iarsin ann.[20]
>
> (Cormac Cas was struck there, and he was in recovery for 13 years, and his brain was dripping [from his head], and he was king of Munster during that time. And a fort and a fine dwelling were made by him at Dún ar Sléib 'The fort on the Mountain', and this is how that fort was: with a swift and full natural well [lit. 'lake-well'] in the foundation of

anatomy in Alexandria in the late fourth/early third century BC and in the works of Galen, second century AD (see Rocca, *Galen on the Brain*, especially pp. 41, 113 and 153). Galen's discussion of the ventricles can mainly be found in his works *De anatomicis administrationibus* and *De usu partium* (Rocca, *Galen on the Brain*, p. 166). It is not entirely clear where and when the localization of specific faculties within the brain developed; for one argument in this regard, see Green, 'Where'.

19 Demaitre, *Medieval Medicine*, p. 129. There were variations on this, of course; in Augustine's writings, for example, memory was located in the middle part of the brain: see Green, 'Where', pp. 139–40.

20 *Acallamh na Senórach*, ed. by Stokes, p. 33, ll. 1168–77.

> the fort, and a very big royal house was built by him around the well, and three stone pillars were placed around it [= the well], and the bed of the king was placed between those three stone pillars, with his head [tilted] backwards. A beloved/trusted young warrior of his retinue[21] kept bathing his head with water from a cup or basin. And he died there afterwards.)[22]

The salient facts of the injury are as follows: a blow to Cormac's head has resulted in continual leaking of a substance from the brain for a period of thirteen years, at which stage, Cormac dies. During this entire time, Cormac appears to be bedridden, and a trusted servant washes or bathes his head with water until Cormac's eventual demise.

The Irish term used for the loss of fluid is connected with the verb *silid* (drips). This verb mainly occurs in connection with (thin) liquids like water, tears, ink, urine, or blood (eDIL s.v. *silid*).[23] Use of this term then suggests that this is not a leak of actual brain matter (which a patient would be unlikely to survive for an extended period of time). Blood would indicate a skull fracture, in which case the patient required surgical intervention.[24] As there is no indication of any such intervention in the text, the substance is unlikely to be blood. Rather, this may have been considered a more regular

21 The reference to a beloved or perhaps trusted warrior may here refer to the fact that a king was supposed to be without blemish or he was no longer considered fit to rule (Kelly, *A Guide*, p. 19). A trusted warrior might not mention the blemish to anyone else, thus allowing Cormac to remain king. This type of loophole (the law only applies if it is acknowledged [publicly] as a problem) is found elsewhere in Irish literature. For example, in the eighth-century text *Echtra Fergusa maic Léiti* (The adventures of Fergus mac Léiti), the face of king Fergus becomes permanently distorted. Here the problem is solved by keeping the king himself unaware of his condition by obscuring all mirrors and not allowing him to see his own reflection. Alternatively, the use of a trusted servant might be intended to aid in recovery as his presence might comfort the patient. Irish law provides descriptions of the type of house in which an injured party would have been receiving treatment, which is low in stimuli and free from loud sounds and disturbances: see Kelly, *A Guide*, pp. 130–31. While this pertains specifically to the practice of *folog n-othrusa* (sick-maintenance), which deals with responsibilities of someone who has (deliberately) injured a person, it is probable that this applied also to sick and injured people in general.

22 My translation.

23 See <dil.ie/37522>.

24 See for example Celsus' *De medicina*, 8.4.1 (ed. and trans. by Spencer, III, pp. 502–05): 'Igitur ubi ea percussa, protinus requirendum est, num bilem homo is vomuerit, num oculi eius occaecati sint, num obmutuerit, num per nares auresve sanguis ei fluxerit … haec enim non nisi osse fracto eveniunt; atque ubi inciderunt, scire licet necessariam sed difficilem curationem esse' (Therefore after a blow on the head first we must enquire whether the patient has had bilious vomiting, whether there has been obscurity of vision, whether he has become speechless, whether he has had bleeding from the nose or ears … for such signs do not occur unless with fractured bone; and when they are present, we must recognize that [surgical] treatment is necessary but difficult).

(even if continual and inconvenient) draining of a non-descript watery fluid from the head.[25]

Medieval medical texts frequently used the term *rheuma* to describe this condition. This term was further subdivided into different types, although variation existed among medical authors.[26] Avicenna, for example, described two specific afflictions related to loss of fluid from the brain, *coryza* and *catarrh,* although he pointed out that some use the term *catarrh* for both:[27]

> He due egritudines co*mmun*ica*n*tes sunt in hoc q*uod* vnaq*ua*m ear*um* est cursus materiei ex cerebro. Uer*um* q*ui*dam ho*min*um sunt q*ui* appropria*n*t no*min*e catarri ill*ud* q*uo*d desce*n*dit at guttur 7 no*min*e corize q*uo*d desce*n*dit ex via nasi. Et q*ui*da*m* ho*min*es sunt q*ui* no*min*ant totu*m* ill*ud* catarru*m*.[28]
>
> (These two afflictions share commonalities in this, namely that each of them involves the flowing of material from the brain. Now there are some people who attach the name *catarrh* to that which flows down to the throat, and designate that which descends via the nose with the name *coryza*; and there are some people who call all of that *catarrh.*)[29]

Although the Irish text does not provide further details, it is most likely that Cormac suffers from rhinorrhea, the leaking of fluid from the nose. Cormac is bedridden, and has his head positioned *siar*. The word *siar* typically means westwards, but it can also be translated as backwards or back, which I suggest is the case here. The reason for Cormac's having to remain in this position is then that it will prevent the leaking of fluid.[30] Discharge of mucus or liquid

---

25 From a modern medical perspective, it is likely that this is actually an example of the leaking of cerebrospinal fluid (a CSF-leak) as a result of a traumatic head injury, which is an extremely serious condition that can last for a long time and can lead to headaches, coma, strokes, and death. I hope to publish on this elsewhere.

26 Demaitre, *Medieval Medicine*, p. 186.

27 The *Salernitan Regimen of Health*, for example, identified *catarrhus* as flux to the chest; *branchus* was liquid flowing to the throat, and *coryza* was a flux to the nostrils: see Demaitre, *Medieval Medicine*, p. 186. In the works of Paul of Aegina, *coryza* is a defluxion of a redundant humour to the nose, *catarrh* is used when this is present in the pharynx and roof of the mouth, and *branchus* or *morbus arteriacus* when it attacks the larynx and arteria trachea (Paul of Aegina, *Medical Compendium*, ed. by Adams, I, p. 469).

28 Arnaldus de Villa Nova, *Libellus Avicene*, ed. by Bertochus, p. 339.

29 My translation. Avicenna further points out that *catarrh* and *coryza* can be caused by internal and external factors. Those with hot complexions are more susceptible to external factors, while those with cold complexions are more likely to suffer from coryza produced by the body itself (Arnaldus de Villa Nova, *Libellus Avicene*, ed. by Bertochus, p. 339: 'Et habentes complexionem calidam vehementius sunt preparati ad recipiendum causas extrinsecas facientes corimiam quam habentes complexiones frigidas 7 humidas 7 habentes complexiones calidas in se ipsis plus sunt secure ne accidat eis ex causis corporeis quam habentes complexiones frigidas').

30 This is consistent with CSF leak—see Prosser and others, 'Traumatic Cerebrospinal Fluid Leaks', p. 860. Some of the more conservative modern treatments of CSF include strict bed rest, elevation of the head, and avoiding pressure on the head (Prosser and others,

from the nose was typically connected with the anterior ventricle of the brain in medical literature, as physicians like Galen assumed a direct connection between the brain and the nasal cavities.[31]

Cormac's long-term medical treatment (head-washing and lying in a bed positioned over a well) may seem unorthodox to a modern reader, but in fact, at its core, it both supports the idea that Cormac's affliction involves the leaking of clear fluid and conforms to medical doctrine. In humoral theory, the brain was associated with the element water. The watery environment (a bed located over a natural well), and the continual washing of the head may thus have been intended to replace any lost watery fluids. The idea that a substance similar in appearance to the one that is lost or absent can be effective in curing an affliction (so-called sympathetic cures) was quite common in medieval medicine, and is reminiscent of the concept *similia similibus curantur* (like is healed by like) found in for example Pliny the Elder's *Naturalis Historia*.[32] Alternatively, pouring water onto a patient's head, and frequent bathing, is indicated as a cure for *catarrh* and *coryza* in persons with a naturally hot temperament in the works of the seventh-century Greek physician Paul of Aegina.[33]

The stone pillars are likely significant from a medicinal perspective, but unfortunately, the text does not specify the type of stone used here. A potential candidate is limestone, as the Irish term *cloch* (stone), used in the episode, is sometimes qualified by the genitive *áeil* (of lime); this may thus be an instance of ellipsis. Limestone caves are present in Ireland, and the pillars in the text should perhaps be taken not as carved pillars, but rather as naturally formed ones, i.e. stalactites or stalagmites. Dioscorides describes one of the types of limestone as the solid form of moisture found in certain caves, and limestone could be used to purge the head if diluted with water and dropped into the nostrils through wool.[34] In other words, limestone would fit the type of watery medical treatment provided to Cormac.

'Traumatic Cerebrospinal Fluid Leaks', pp. 863–64).

31 Rocca, *Galen on the Brain*, p. 135.

32 Hayden, 'A Sixteenth-Century Irish Collection', p. 255. This often relates to, for example, the shape of plants or parts of plants (e.g. a walnut looks like a brain and is therefore helpful in curing afflictions of the brain), but see the use of plants that contain a milky sap or latex for afflictions related to lactation in Pliny (Stannard, 'Medicinal Plants', p. 15). This watery environment can be taken as an extrapolation of this idea.

33 Paul of Aegina, *Medical Compendium*, ed. by Adams, I, p. 470. This cure is then connected with the opposite medical concept that contraries are healed by contraries, found in the works of for example Galen. The Irish text provides no indication of Cormac's temperament, unfortunately, so it is not possible to determine which of these doctrines underlies the treatment plan.

34 Dioscorides, *De materia medica*, trans. by Osbaldeston, p. 801. Limestone was also thought to contain some heat and burn in water (Isidore, *Etymologiae*, XVI.iii.8: ed. Lindsay, II, p. 189; trans. Barney and others, p. 319). In a contraries healing contraries setting, it could counteract some of the water, or perhaps serve to heat up his body.

The 'Envenomed Head Worm' of Conán

The second example of an unusual brain affliction occurs about midway through *Acallam na Senórach*. In the episode in question, the ancient warriors Caílte and Oisín tell St Patrick about the death of a certain Conán:

> 'Crét aidhidh in Chonáin-sin?' ar Pátraic. 'An cethramad fer,' ar Cáilte, 'fuair bás re hadhart don Ḟéinn hé .i. cruimh neime do ghabh'na chinn, 7 fuair bás ón trath co araile.[35]
>
> ('How did that Conán die?'[36] said Patrick. 'He was one of four men of the *fían*,' said Caílte, 'who died in his bed.[37] A *cruimh neime* (envenomed/penetrating/putrid worm/maggot) assailed his head and he died in the space of a day.')[38]

Joseph Nagy has previously discussed this episode in his 2014 article 'Death by Pillow', in which he links the unheroic death of Conán with the secretive manner in which he has wormed himself into Finn's *fían*.[39] But a medical interpretation (or at least a medical origin for this episode) is also possible.

The episode within the *Acallam* itself is quite short on details — it just mentions a *cruimh neime* and a swift death. Fortunately, there is another text that provides more information. A mid-twelfth-century Fenian poem termed 'The abduction of Eargna', which was edited in the collection *Dúanaire Finn*,[40] links Conán's death with a blow to the head, inflicted in battle by Aodh Rinn. This poem, which slightly predates the *Acallam*, can be found in UCD OFM MS A20, 2[r], and Conán's injury and demise are recorded as follows:[41]

Mairc do rad in béim co prap	(Woe worth who gave the sudden blow
do Chonán issin chomhnart	to Conan in the equal fight:

35 *Acallamh na Senórach*, ed. by Stokes, p. 102, ll. 3589–92.

36 The term *aidhidh* here refers to a violent death or by extension a death from unnatural causes. This means that St Patrick assumes here that warriors did not typically die a natural death — something that is confirmed by Caílte in the next sentence.

37 The expression 'bás (écc) fri hadart' literally means 'death on a pillow', and can be used to indicate that someone did not die a violent death, but a natural one (eDIL s.v. *adart*, dil.ie/314).

38 My translation. The term *cruimh neime* will be discussed below as it can mean several different things.

39 Another example of a headworm, this one connected with Cían, can be found in *Toruigheacht Dhíarmada agus Ghráinne* — see Nagy, 'Vermin Gone Bad', but I am unable to discuss that episode here for reasons of length.

40 For the date, see *Dúanaire Finn*, ed. and trans. by Murphy, III, p. 3.

41 *Dúanaire Finn*, ed. and trans. by Murphy, III, pp. 3 and 98. I have added some corrections to the Irish text based on manuscript readings.

dar ledair in cenn co cnáimh	when he [= Aodh] cleft the head to the bone
tré c(h)ertlár c(h)athbharr Conáin	through the middle of Conan's helmet.
[...]	
Sechtmhoin is mí na luighe	A week and a month a-bed
do bhí Conán cathaighe	was battle-waging Conan:
leis na leghaiph do badh dóigh	the leeches had expected
ternamh a chnedh a ccedóir	him to come whole of his wounds at once.
Bliadhain do Chonan ar bith	A year was Conan in the world
gus in laithe rod buaidhredh	until the day when he became confused[42]
seachnóin Sligheadh[43] Dála duind	along the road of Dáil the brown
is in maighin ós Echdhruim	in the plain above Eachdhruim.
Cnuimh neime ro ghaph na chinn	An envenomed worm had entered his head
tre n[e]imh[44] chloidhimh Aodha Rinn	through the venom of Aodh Rinn's sword:
marph ar Moigh Dála na n-áth	he died on Magh Dála of the fords
do ghalar ceithre ccert-tráth	of an illness of four day-thirds)

In this poem, Conán's cause of death is ultimately a blow to the middle part of the head with Aodh Rinn's sword. This leads to a head wound that takes unexpectedly long to heal. A year or so later, Conán's health takes a turn and he dies about a day later as a result of the *cnuimh* (= *cruimh*) *neime* present in his head, which may appear rather unusual from a modern perspective.

There are several different ways in which to interpret this *cruim neime*. The word *cruim* typically means worm or maggot, although it is possible that it was used as a general term for worm-like objects and creatures, much like the Old English term *wyrm*.[45] It is used to gloss the Latin term *vermis* in the Yellow Book of Lecan version of Cormac's Glossary, connected with Cormac mac Cuilennáin (d. 908), under the entry *cruimther* (priest) (*ego sum* ***vermis*** = *conad* ***cruim*** *me*).[46] The word *neim* usually means poison, but when used in

42 The edition here has 'when he went mad', but the verb *búaidrid* (eDIL s.v. dil.ie/7230) means disturbs, troubles, harasses, confuses — which is rather an indication that Conán became confused or muddled than that he lost his mind.

43 MS Slighigh.

44 MS neimh.

45 Cf. Meaney, 'The Anglo-Saxon View', p.14. I am grateful to Deborah Hayden for referring me to this article.

46 The gloss can be found as part of the Early Irish Glossaries Database: <https://www.asnc.cam.ac.uk/irishglossaries/texts.php?versionID=9&readingID=17187#17187>.

combination with a term for sword, it may also mean 'virulence, keenness, penetrating force' (eDIL s.v. *neim*).[47] In a medical context, it may perhaps also be used to express putrid material or material that must be extracted from a wound as it can lead to infection.[48] This means that *cruim neime* has three potential base translations when it comes to the element *neime*:

Penetrating worm/maggot
Putrid worm/maggot
Envenomed worm/maggot

The Penetrating Worm/Maggot

Our first option is to read *neim* in the sense keenness, penetrating force, giving us worm of penetrating force, penetrating worm. This means that we can translate the lines 'Cnuimh neime ro ghaph na chinn | tre neimh chloidhimh Aodha Rinn' as 'A penetrating (= burrowing?) worm (or maggot) took hold in his head, | through the keenness of the sword of Aodh Rinn'. Penetrating worms occur in other medical literatures outside of Ireland, including the fourth-century Latin text *Medicina Plinii* and Old English medical texts; Bald's *Leechbook*, *Leechbook* III and *Lacnunga*, for example, all contain references to and remedies for penetrating worms (*smeoga wyrmum*).[49] Meaney has suggested that these may in fact be examples of fistulous ulceration, as fistulas, abnormal, tunnel-like passageways between two organs or between an organ and the exterior of the body, 'look like worms, spreading along channels under the skin'.[50]

The Putrid Worm/Maggot

This second option is also reasonably straightforward. Aodh Rinn has inflicted a head wound on Conán that is not healing, and for whatever reason (be it poison or putrid matter on the sword, for example) the wound becomes infected, and putrefies. This is exactly the environment that would produce maggots, according to medieval medical thought. As the seventh-century scholar Isidore of Seville, who was well-known in Ireland, put it, 'Proprie autem vermis in carne putre nascitur' (In particular, vermin [*vermis*, here specifically 'maggots'] are generated in putrid meat).[51] In this interpretation, the infected head wound produces (a) maggot(s), which then enter(s) his head and results in death for Conán.

47 dil.ie/33028.
48 See De Vries, 'Medieval Medicine', p. 64.
49 Meaney, 'The Anglo-Saxon View', p. 15.
50 Meaney, 'The Anglo-Saxon View', p. 15.
51 Isidore, *Etymologiae*, XII.v.18 (ed. by Lindsay, II, p. 60; trans. Barney and others, *Etymologies*, p. 259).

The Envenomed Worm/Maggot

This final option is, medically speaking, perhaps the most intriguing one. The poem from *Dúanaire Finn* clearly suggests that the *neim*, in this reading meaning poison, comes from the sword of Aodh Rinn, which must then have somehow transferred onto a worm or maggot. In the previous two options under discussion, the worms were external factors. And in this instance, that is of course also possible. An external worm could have come from a previous victim of Aodh Rinn's that was still present on his sword, which then entered Conán's head; or a maggot may have crawled into Conán's head, passing through an envenomed wound and carrying the poison into Conán's head. There is an alternative option, however, and that is that the worm was present in Conán's head all along.

Medical literature discusses the various types of worms that could form inside the human body. Of these, intestinal worms were probably the most common.[52] Medical compendia contain large numbers of recipes attempting to cure worms of various kinds. Theories as to where or how such worms originated varied, although they were often seen as the result of putrefied phlegmatic humour.[53] The expulsion of worms could take place in a variety of ways, including discharge by mouth or sometimes by the nose,[54] which might suggest a connection with the head.

Indeed, medical compendia discuss a number of different locations inside the head that could house or become infested with worms. These include ear worms, thought to cause itching or tingling in the head;[55] tooth worms;[56] and actual head worms, thought to be the underlying cause of a specific type of headache. In his *Canon of Medicine*, Avicenna mentions such a head worm in an overview of various types of headache (*soda*) that may originate near the membrane of the brain:

> Quidam vero medici indi [*sic* for inde] dixerunt quod quandoque est causa in soda vermes generati in partibus capitis motu suo ledentes. Et quidam remouerunt hoc; sed non est necessarium vt remoueantur. Nam vermes

52 Demaitre, *Medieval Medicine*, pp. 258–59. Paul of Aegina, a seventh-century Byzantine physician, for example, distinguished three different types of intestinal worm: round worms, broad worms, and ascarides. Round worms formed in the small intestines; broad worms were a conversion of the membrane which lines the inside of the intestine into a living body; and ascarides were earthworm-like and formed in the intestines as well (Paul of Aegina, *Medical Compendium*, ed. by Adams, II).

53 As early as the seventh century, Paul of Aegina posited that all worms were the 'offspring of crude and thick pituitous matters with a suitable putrefaction. [...] But they do not grow from hot, acrid, or melancholic humours' (Paul of Aegina, *Medical Compendium*, ed. by Adams, II, p. 139). Phlegmatic humour, of course, was connected with the brain in particular.

54 Paul of Aegina, *Medical Compendium*, ed. by Adams, II, p. 140.

55 Demaitre, *Medieval Medicine*, p. 180.

56 For a historical overview, see for instance Gerabek, 'The Tooth-Worm'.

multotiens nascuntur in anteriore capite super locum qui est in stricture narium; 7 possibile est vt nascantur apud velamina 7 si raro contingat.[57]

> (But some physicians have therefore said that sometimes the cause for the headache is worms that are produced in parts of the head, who cause pain through its [the head's] motion; And some [physicians] have removed these; but it is not necessary to do so. For oftentimes worms are created [lit. born] in the front of the head, above the place that is in the narrow part of the nose; and it is possible that they are born near the membrane of the brain and if so, it [the headache] rarely takes hold.)

In addition to these internal worms, there is one further option. The poem suggests that Conán's head wound was located in the middle of the head. This is also the location of a worm-shaped section of the brain termed *vermis* (worm). This was thought to be a worm-like passage that connected two sections of the brain, usually the anterior and the middle part.[58] It was rolled up like a worm ('sicut vermis reuolutus'),[59] and could contract and expand. As stated above, the Irish term *cruim* is used to translate Latin *vermis*; the idea expressed in the text might then be at its core that Aodh's sword injured this specific part of the brain.[60] All of these options are viable from a medieval medical perspective. The accounts in the *Acallam* and the poem differ, of course, which makes it difficult to determine what the medieval diagnosis might have been — the *Acallam* passage suggests that Conán was bedridden and died suddenly, while the poem suggests that he was bedridden for six weeks and then took a sudden turn for the worse a year later. Diagnosing Conán's head wound, however, is not the purpose of this article — that is merely to demonstrate that this episode can be explained from a medieval medical perspective.

Cenn Fáelad's Brain of Forgetfulness

The final example of a fantastical brain injury concerns the infamous head injury of Cenn Fáelad, a scholar connected with the monasteries of Túaim Drecan and Daire Luráin, whose death was recorded in the annals under the year 679.[61] The account of his injury is connected with the battle of Mag Rath, and can be found in three separate sources belonging to the Middle Irish

57 Arnaldus de Villa Nova, *Libellus Avicene*, ed. by Bertochus, p. 264.

58 Galen used the term 'worm-like outgrowth' (σκωληκοειδὴς ἐπίφυσις) for the cerebellar vermis, which he deemed responsible for the regulation of psychic pneuma from the third ventricle to the fourth ventricle, and which he thought was able to move (Rocca, *Galen on the Brain*, p. 150).

59 Arnaldus de Villa Nova, *Libellus Avicene*, ed. by Bertochus, p. 252.

60 It is perhaps also possible to combine options one and three, and see in this a wound that penetrated to the *vermis*.

61 Qiu, 'Law, Law-Books and Tradition', p. 138.

period (*c.* AD 900 – *c.* 1200): appended to the Old Irish legal text *Bretha Éitgid* (Judgements of Inadvertence), as part of *Auraicept na n-éces* (The Scholars' Primer), and in the thirteenth or fourteenth-century longer version of the narrative *Cath Maige Rath* (The Battle of Mag Rath).[62]

This last text contains the most detailed description of the injury. In the battle of Mag Rath, Congal Cláen encounters Cenn Fáelad. Congal hits Cenn Fáelad with his sword, cleaving his helmet and cutting his head so that part of his brain flows out ('co n-urrainn do'n indchinn ina fhoirleanmuin').[63] Cenn Fáelad survives, however, and is taken away for recuperation:

> Ocus ro íodhnaic Senach Ceannfaeladh iar sin go Bricin Tuama Dreaccan, ocus do bhi aicce go ceann m-bliadhna aga leigheas; ocus do shil a inchin chúil as ris an re sin, co nach bi ní da g-cluineadh gan a bheith do ghlain meabhrae aige; doig amh an t-aiceapt do nidh Bricin do tri scolaib do bhiodh sin do ghlain-mheabhra aige-sium, gur bo fear tri scol iaromh Ceannfaeladh, mac Oiliolla, gur ab é do athnuadaidh Uraiceapt na n-Eicces, i n.-Doire Lurain ierttain.
>
> (After this Senach conducted Cennfaeladh to Bricin of Tuaim Dreagan, with whom he remained for a year under cure, and in the course of this time, his back brain had flowed out,[64] which so much improved his memory that there was nothing which he heard repeated, that he had not distinctly by heart, and the instruction which Bricin had delivered to his three schools he [Cennfaeladh] had treasured up in his clear memory; so that Cennfaeladh, the son of Oilell, afterwards became a man [i.e. a teacher] of three schools, and it was he that afterwards renewed Uraicept na n-Eges, at Doire Lurain.)[65]

The loss of Cenn Fáelad's brain of forgetfulness has elicited a fair amount of scholarly discussion,[66] which has mainly focused on the topics of learning and intellectualism, and oral versus written tradition. Cenn Fáelad remembers everything taught at the three different schools of learning that cover *fénechas* (native Irish law), *filidecht* (poetry), and *léigind* (monastic/Latin learning).[67] This episode has a clear symbolic meaning, as these subjects represent the three main strands of learning in medieval Ireland. Cenn Fáelad thus ends up as 'a prototype for a learned person', and the outcome of the injury is undoubtedly an 'allegory to components of Irish intellectualism', as stated

62 Qiu, 'Law, Law-Books and Tradition', p. 138 and Dillon, 'A Note', p. 201. As Qiu points out on that same page, the material on Cenn Fáelad is probably the result of accretion over time.

63 *The Banquet of Dun na n-Ged*, ed. and trans. by O'Donovan, pp. 278–81.

64 Note that the verb is once again *silid* (drips). It is possible that this is another example of traumatic CSF leak, particularly as this dripping takes place over the course of a year.

65 *The Banquet of Dun na n-Ged*, ed. and trans. by O'Donovan, pp. 282–85.

66 For an overview and references, see Qiu, 'Law, Law-Books and Tradition', pp. 138–39.

67 Breatnach, *A Companion*, pp. 381–82.

by Qiu.[68] The significance of the episode, as pointed out by Mac Cana, was that Cenn Fáelad was the first to commit native learning to writing; at a later stage, when this significance was obscured or forgotten, Cenn Fáelad's 'prodigious powers of memory [...] were rendered appropriately fabulous by the legend of his wound and subsequent medical treatment'.[69] I would like to argue here that the injury does not elevate this episode to the realm of the fabulous. Rather, as is the case for the other examples under discussion, it is solid medical theory that underlies it.

At its most basic level, Cenn Fáelad's affliction is a brain injury that affects memory. There are two terms used to designate the specific section of Cenn Fáelad's brain that is affected. *Cath Maige Rath* mentions the back of the brain (*inchinn chúil*), while both the *Auraicept* and *Bretha Éitgid* refer to it as the *inchind dermait* (brain of forgetfulness). Assuming that these two sources are intended to refer to the same location, the injury is to the back of the brain, which in the text is clearly connected with memory. I would suggest that the term *inchinn* has been used here to signify not the entire brain, but rather a ventricle. Combined with the element *cúl* (back), the term *inchind chúil* would then refer to the posterior ventricle of the brain. The term *dermait* (of forgetting) could be taken as a qualifying genitive that indicated the result produced by injury to this part of the brain, i.e., memory loss; alternatively, this may be a deliberate play on words/medical concepts — an injury to the part of the brain which houses memory (the *vis memorativa*) leads to the opposite of remembering: loss of memory. By describing this section of the brain as the ventricle of forgetting, the injury might be thought to produce the opposite effect: loss of forgetting, i.e. remembering everything. Alternatively, the word *inchinn* can perhaps refer to the cerebellum (literally, small brain),[70] a structure located at the back of the brain that resembles a small brain in appearance, and that was linked with memory by for example the fourth-century author Nemesius: 'The organ of memory, too, is the posterior cavity of the brain, which they call the cerebellum and the enkranis, and the psychic pneuma within it.'[71]

The idea that injury to the back of the brain could affect memory occurs in medical literature as early as the fourth century AD. Poseidonius of Byzantium,

---

68 Qiu, 'Law, Law-books and Tradition', p. 138.

69 Mac Cana, 'The Three Languages', pp. 64–65.

70 This connection was also made by O'Donovan in his edition of the text: see *The Banquet of Dun na n-Ged*, ed. and trans. by O'Donovan, footnote on pp. 282–83.

71 Nemesius, *On the Nature of Man*, trans. by van der Eijk and Sharples, p. 121. Although in modern medical theory, the cerebellum is involved with the processes related to balance and movement, there is some recent literature that suggests that the cerebellum is also involved in certain cognitive processes; see for example Schmahmann, 'The Cerebellum and Cognition'. Note that Galen, who adhered to the idea that the brain consisted of four ventricles, considered the cerebellum the fourth ventricle, which was connected with the cerebrum via a canal or aqueduct (known since the seventeenth century as the Aqueduct of Silvius); see Rocca, *Galen on the Brain*, p. 151.

for example, described the effects of localized brain damage. Injury to the front of the brain could impair a person's imagination; injury to the middle of the brain could cause issues with rational thought; and issues to the back of the head could affect memory.[72] Similar references can be found in the work of Nemesius,[73] and in the work of Aetius of Amida in the sixth century.[74] It is hardly surprising, then, that an injury to the *inchind chúil* would impact memory in some form.

Some scholars have pointed out the unlikelihood of this type of injury, and mention that brain injury typically involves loss of memory, rather than an inability to forget.[75] This is also the case in most medieval discussions of memory. It is therefore possible that we here find a deliberate inversion of medical theory in service of the narrative. From a medical perspective, however, it should be mentioned that an injury such as this is not impossible. As O'Donovan has pointed out, there are modern examples of brain injury that lead to improvement of learning.[76] The condition of acquired savant syndrome is particularly relevant in this light, as it is a condition in which people acquire a specific skill as a result of injury, and some of these skills involve memory.[77]

Cenn Fáelad's brain injury is a clear example of medical theory used in service of a legal allegory: as Cenn Fáelad is eyewitness (or earwitness) to the teachings of the various schools, he can give reliable testimony, and his infallible memory allows for all this learning to be committed to writing without mistakes, and indicates the absolute reliability of everything produced by Cenn Fáelad. To attribute a text to Cenn Fáelad, then, means to have an authoritative text. Regardless of the allegorical meaning attached to the learning, however, this is at its core a perfectly straightforward medical condition.

Conclusion

As stated at the beginning of the article, head and brain injuries occur frequently in medieval Irish literature, as they do elsewhere in medieval Europe. While elements in the Irish tales that contain these injuries may have subsequently been embellished, exaggerated, reinterpreted, or used in an allegorical sense, all three examples discussed above have a solid foundation in European and Arabic medieval medical doctrine related to both the anatomy and the function of the brain.

Interpreting saga material such as the examples above from a medical perspective helps to place them in context and takes away some of the

72 Tascioglu and Tascioglu, 'Ventricular Anatomy', p. 58.
73 Nemesius, *On the Nature of Man*, trans. by van der Eijk and Sharples, pp. 118–23.
74 Poulakou-Rebelakou and others, 'Dementia on the Byzantine Throne', p. 407.
75 See for example Slotkin, 'Medieval Irish Scribes', p. 439.
76 *The Banquet of Dun na n-Gedh*, ed. and trans. by O'Donovan, pp. 282–83.
77 See Treffert, 'The Savant Syndrome', and Treffert and Ries, 'The Sudden Savant'.

perceived strangeness of the tales themselves: after all, head trauma to the back of the brain can certainly affect memory, as that was the area where memories were stored. Traumatic brain injury can cause the leaking of fluid from a patient's head, one of the cures for which was the application of water; and medieval physicians identified various different types of head worms, as well as a worm-like structure in the middle of the brain itself.

Medical interpretation of texts is rarely attempted when it comes to medieval Irish saga literature. This article has hopefully demonstrated that a medical approach should be an important part of textual interpretation, in addition to other, more frequently used approaches, like legal interpretations or literary comparisons with biblical, classical, and medieval sources. We need to employ all of these approaches (and others as well — one might for example think of areas such as philosophy) if we wish to understand medieval Irish texts in a manner that is as closely connected as possible to the world in which they were written. Our reactions to these injuries when we first read about them — which typically comprise a spectrum ranging from bafflement to derision — really have more to do with our own lack of knowledge of medieval medicine than with the overactive imagination of their authors. This needs to change, and scholars should be encouraged to adopt a holistic approach to medieval Irish literature that includes medicine.

Works Cited

Manuscripts

Dublin, University College Dublin, MS OFM A4

Dublin, University College Dublin, MS OFM A20

Primary Sources

Acallamh na Senórach, ed. by Whitley Stokes, in *Irische texte mit Wörterbuch*, 4.1, ed. by Ernst Windisch and Whitley Stokes (Leipzig: Hirzel, 1900)

Anathomia Gydo, ed. and trans. by Eithne Ní Ghallchobhair, Irish Texts Society, 66 (London: Irish Texts Society, 2014)

Arnaldus de Villa Nova, trans., *Libellus Avicene de viribus cordis*, ed. by Dionysius Bertochus (Venice, 1498–1490)

The Banquet of Dun na n-Ged and the Battle of Magh Rath: An Ancient and Historical Tale, ed. and trans. by John O'Donovan (Dublin: University Press, 1842)

Bretha Déin Chécht, ed. and trans. by D. A. Binchy, *Ériu*, 20 (1966), 1–66

In Cath Catharda: The Civil War of the Romans, ed. by Whitley Stokes, in *Irische Texte*, 4.2, ed. by Ernst Windisch and Whitley Stokes (Leipzig: Hirzel, 1909)

Cath Maige Tuired, ed. and trans. by Elizabeth Gray, Irish Texts Society, 52 (London: Irish Texts Society, 1982)

Celsus, *De medicina*, ed. and trans. by Walter George Spencer, 3 vols (Cambridge, MA: Harvard University Press, 1935–1938)

Dioscorides, Pedanius, *De materia medica*, trans. by Tess Anne Osbaldeston (Johannesburg: Ibidis, 2000)

Dúanaire Finn: The Book of the Lays of Fionn 3, ed. and trans. by Gerard Murphy, Irish Texts Society, 43 (London: Irish Texts Society, 1941 [1953])

Early Irish Glossaries Database, ed. by Paul Russell, Sharon Arbuthnot, and Pádraic Moran <https://www.asnc.cam.ac.uk/irishglossaries> [accessed 2 February 2022]

Isidore of Seville, *Etymologiae sive origines libri* xx, ed. by Wallace Martin Lindsay (Oxford: Clarendon Press, 1911)

——, *The Etymologies of Isidore of Seville*, trans. by Stephen Barney, W. J. Lewis, J. A. Beach, and Oliver Berghof (Cambridge: Cambridge University Press, 2006)

Lucan, *Bellum Civile*, ed. and trans. by J. D. Duff, Loeb Classical Library, 220 (Cambridge, MA: Harvard University Press, 1928)

Nemesius, *On the Nature of Man*, trans. by Philip van der Eijk and R. W. Sharples (Liverpool: Liverpool University Press 2008)

Paul of Aegina, *Medical Compendium in Seven Books*, ed. by Francis Adams, 3 vols (London: The Sydenham Society, 1844–1847)

Secondary Studies

Breatnach, Liam, *A Companion to the Corpus Iuris Hibernici*, Early Irish Law Series, 5 (Dublin: Dublin Institute for Advanced Studies, 2005)

——, *The Early Irish Law Text* Senchas Már *and the Question of its Date*, E. C. Quiggin Memorial Lectures, 13 (Cambridge: Department of Ango-Saxon, Norse and Celtic, 2011)

Demaitre, Luke, *Medieval Medicine. The Art of Healing from Head to Toe* (Santa Barbara, CA: Praeger, 2013)

de Vries, Ranke, 'Medieval Medicine and the Healing of Caílte in the *Acallam na Senórach*', *North American Journal of Celtic Studies*, 5.1 (2021), 49–82

Dillon, Myles, 'A Note on the Texts of "Cath Maige Rath" Preserved in the Yellow Book of Lecan', *Éigse*, 7 (1953), 199–201

eDIL 2019:= *An Electronic Dictionary of the Irish Language*, based on the Contributions to a Dictionary of the Irish Language (Dublin: Royal Irish Academy, 1913–1976) <www.dil.ie 2019> [accessed 7 July 2022]

Gerabek, W. E., 'The Tooth-Worm: Historical Aspects of a Popular Medical Belief', *Clinical Oral Investigations*, 3 (1999), 1–6

Green, Christopher D., 'Where Did the Ventricular Localization of Mental Faculties Come From?', *Journal for the History of Behavioral Sciences*, 39.2 (2003), 131–42

Hayden, Deborah, 'Observations on the "Doors of Death" in a Medieval Irish Medical Catechism', in *Rosa Anglica: Reassessments*, ed. by Liam P. Ó Murchú, Irish Texts Society Subsidiary Series, 28 (London: Irish Texts Society, 2016), pp. 26–58

——, 'A Sixteenth-century Irish Collection of Remedies for Ailments of the Male Reproductive Organs', *Celtica*, 33 (2021), 248–76

Kelly, Fergus, *A Guide to Early Irish Law*, Early Irish Law Series, 3 (Dublin: Dublin Institute for Advanced Studies, 1988)

Mac Cana, Proinsias, 'The Three Languages and the Three Laws', *Studia Celtica*, 5 (1970), 62–78

MacInnes, Iain, 'Heads, Shoulders, Knees and Toes: Injury and Death in Anglo-Scottish Combat, *c.* 1296 – *c.* 1403', in *Wounds and Wound Repair in Medieval Culture*, ed. by Larissa Tracy and Kelly DeVries (Leiden: Brill), pp. 102–27

Meaney, Audrey L., 'The Anglo-Saxon View of the Causes of Illness', in *Health, Disease and Healing in Medieval Culture*, ed. by Sheila Campbell, Bert Hall, and David Klausner (London: Palgrave Macmillan, 1992), pp. 12–33

Mulligan, Amy, 'The Erasure of a Warrior's Body: Cú Chulainn, Isidore of Seville, and Irish Independence', in *From Enlightenment to Rebellion: Essays in Honor of Christopher Fox*, ed. by James Buickerood (Lewisburg, PA: Bucknell University Press, 2018), pp. 33–47

Nagy, Joseph Falaky, 'Death by Pillow', in *Rhetoric and Reality in Medieval Celtic Literature: Studies in Honor of Daniel F. Melia*, ed. by Georgia Henley and Paul Russell, with Joseph F. Eska, CSANA Yearbook, 11–12 (Hamilton, NY: Colgate University Press, 2014), pp. 128–36

——, 'Vermin Gone Bad in Medieval Scandinavian, Persian, and Irish Traditions', in *Old Norse Mythology — Comparative Perspectives*, ed. by Pernille Hermann, Stephen A. Mitchell, and Jens Peter Schjødt, with Amber J. Rose, Milman Parry Collection of Oral Literature, 3 (Cambridge, MA: Milman Parry Collection of Oral Literature 2017): <http://nrs.harvard.edu/urn-3:hul.ebook:CHS_HermannP_etal_eds.Old_Norse_Mythology.2017> [accessed 2 February 2022]

Poulakou-Rebelakou, Effie, George Kalantzis, Costas Tsiamis, and Dimitris Ploumpidis, 'Dementia on the Byzantine Throne (AD 330–1453)', *Geriatrics & Gerontology International*, 12.3 (2012), 405–12

Prosser, John Drew, John R. Vender, and Clementine Arturo Solares, 'Traumatic Cerebrospinal Fluid Leaks', *Otolaryngologic Clinics of North America*, 44 (2011), 857–73

Qiu, Fangzhe, 'Law, Law-Books and Tradition in Early Medieval Ireland', in *Law/Book/Culture in the Middle Ages*, ed. by Thom Gobbitt, Explorations in Medieval Culture, 14 (Leiden: Brill, 2021), pp. 126–46

Rocca, Julius, *Galen on the Brain: Anatomical Knowledge and Physiological Speculation in the Second Century AD* (Leiden: Brill, 2003)

Schmahmann, Jeremy D., 'The Cerebellum and Cognition', *Neuroscience Letters*, 688.1 (2019), 62–75

Siraisi, Nancy, *Medieval & Early Renaissance Medicine. An Introduction to Knowledge and Practice* (Chicago: University of Chicago Press, 1990)

Skinner, Patricia, 'Visible Prowess?: Reading Men's Head and Face Wounds in Early Medieval Europe to 1000 CE', in *Wounds and Wound Repair in Medieval Culture*, ed. by Larissa Tracy and Kelly DeVries (Leiden: Brill), pp. 81–101

Slotkin, Edgar, 'Medieval Irish Scribes and Fixed Texts', *Éigse*, 17.4 (1978–1979), 437–50

Stannard, Jerry, 'Medicinal Plants and Folk Remedies in Pliny, "Historia Naturalis"', *History and Philosophy of the Life Sciences*, 4.1 (1982), 3–23

Tascioglu, Ali Oguz, and Ayse Beliz Tascioglu, 'Ventricular Anatomy: Illustrations and Concepts from Antiquity to Renaissance', *Neuroanatomy*, 4 (2005), 57–63

Tracy, Larissa, '"Into the hede, throw the helme and creste": Head Wounds and a Question of Kingship in the Stanzaic *Morte Arthur*', in *Wounds and Wound Repair in Medieval Culture*, ed. by Larissa Tracy and Kelly DeVries (Leiden: Brill), pp. 496–518

Treffert, Darold A., 'The Savant Syndrome: An Extraordinary Condition. A Synopsis: Past, Present, Future', *Philosophical Transactions of the Royal Society B*, 364 (2009), 1351–57

Treffert, Darold A., and Hunter Ries, 'The Sudden Savant: A New Form of Extraordinary Abilities', *Wisconsin Medical Journal*, 120.1 (2021), 69–73

VIKTORIIA KRIVOSHCHEKOVA

6. Early Irish Literature and the Embodied Mind*

Introduction: The Meaning of Embodiment

The easiest and most natural way for us to make sense of an abstract concept is to find a clear and tangible analogy for it: so, for instance, love is often described as a kind of illness.[1] More generally, our physical experiences in the world give structure to concepts which otherwise lack spatial and perceptual grounding. The mechanism that underlies such semantic mappings is that of metaphor.

In recent decades, metaphor or, more specifically, conceptual metaphor has become one of the foundational concepts of cognitive linguistics. Broadly understood, metaphors are 'general mappings across conceptual domains'.[2] Zoltán Kövecses further noted: 'The domain of experience that is used to comprehend another domain is typically more physical, more directly experienced, and better known than the domain we wish to comprehend, which is typically more abstract, less directly experienced, and less known.'[3] The domain of physical experience, which includes movement, sense-perception, and object interaction, can, through metaphorical transfer, help organize meaning at more abstract levels of cognition.[4]

One omnipresent but notoriously elusive entity that benefits from the mechanism of conceptual metaphor is the human mind. Many of the metaphorical mappings related to the mind fall under the umbrella of the

* I would like to thank Professor Liam Breatnach (Dublin Institute for Advanced Studies), Dr Elizabeth Boyle (Maynooth University), Dr Bernhard Bauer (University of Graz), and the editors of this volume for reading through different drafts of this article. All remaining errors are my own.

1 For medieval uses of this idea and on viewing love as an actual medical condition, see Wack, *Lovesickness in the Middle Ages*.

2 Lackoff, 'The Contemporary Theory of Metaphor', p. 203.

3 Kövecses, *Where Metaphors Come From*, p. 2.

4 Johnson, *The Body in the Mind*, pp. xix–xx.

Viktoriia Krivoshchekova • Dublin Institute for Advanced Studies, School of Celtic Studies; viktoriia@celt.dias.ie

Medicine in the Medieval North Atlantic World: Vernacular Texts and Traditions, ed. by Deborah Hayden and Sarah Baccianti, KSS, 5 (Turnhout, 2025), pp. 143-165
BREPOLS PUBLISHERS DOI 10.1484/M.KSS-EB.5.143984

'mind-as-body' metaphor which co-opts the language of bodily experience for describing mental states, including such metaphors as 'mind is a container', 'understanding is seeing', 'conscious is up/unconscious is down', etc.[5] This paradigm in cognitive linguistics received the name of 'embodied realism' or simply 'embodiment' and holds that 'many aspects of cognition are grounded in embodiment, especially in terms of the phenomenological experience of our bodies in action'.[6]

Exploring these ideas in medieval texts may be particularly fruitful since the strict separation between mind and body did not exist in pre-Cartesian thought. Consequently, as John E. Joseph noted, projecting 'the divide between medicine as the science of the body, and philosophy and linguistics as sciences of the mind' onto pre-modern thought is likewise incorrect.[7] Medieval theories of cognition do explore its underlying anatomical mechanisms, and, conversely, bodily functions are understood to depend on mental processes. The most prominent example of this is Galen's ventricular theory, or the theory of the inner senses, which became influential in the Middle Ages and according to which mental faculties, such as imagination, estimation, and memory, are located in the cerebral ventricles, i.e. are rooted in physiology.[8] At the same time, motor functions, most notably speech, were commonly understood to be the result of cognitive processes.[9] In addition, mental disorders were often explained by means of the humoral theory — one of the pillars of medieval medical thought.[10]

The connection between mind and body was not only the subject of scientific study. The insights of medicine and philosophy were also encoded in literary language. One of the most comprehensive explorations of embodied realism in a medieval context is Leslie Lockett's study of the so-called hydraulic model of the mind in Old English literature. The hydraulic model associates changes in a person's psychological states with 'dynamic changes of pressure and temperature in the chest cavity'.[11] Lockett posits a challenging question: should the hydraulic model be understood exclusively as conceptual metaphor (that is, an explanatory mechanism for the work of the mind, which is otherwise understood as incorporeal) or does it reflect actual views on human physiology and entails a corporeal view of the mind?[12] Lockett

---

5 Lackoff and Johnson, *Metaphors We Live By*; Sweetser, *From Etymology to Pragmatics*, pp. 28–32. See also Reddy, 'The Conduit Metaphor'.

6 Gibbs, *Embodiment and Cognitive Science*, p. 3; see also Lackoff and Johnson, *Philosophy in the Flesh*, p. 90.

7 Joseph, *Language, Mind and Body*, p. 21.

8 Green, 'Where Did the Ventricular Localization of Mental Faculties Come From?'; Kemp and Fletcher, 'The Medieval Theory of the Inner Senses'.

9 Wollock, *The Noblest Animate Motion*, p. xxxviii.

10 Demaitre, *Medieval Medicine*, pp. 133–40; Trenery and Horden, 'Madness in the Middle Ages', pp. 65–68. I thank the editors of this volume for drawing my attention to these references.

11 Lockett, *Anglo-Saxon Psychologies*, p. 5.

12 Lockett, *Anglo-Saxon Psychologies*, pp. 7–8.

herself suggested that it might have started as the latter but came to be seen predominantly as a metaphor, due to the increasing influence of the Latin learned tradition on early English scholars.[13] The existence and popularity of the hydraulic model in Old English prose and verse show that medical or general physiological observations played a major part in conceptualizing human experience in literary language.

A similar, though very brief, study of Irish literature was carried out by Liam Mac Mathúna, who analysed the uses of the word *cride* (heart) in connection with metaphorical expressions for various mental states.[14] Although his specific interest is in the concept of 'heartbreak', Mac Mathúna also showed that the heart could be viewed as the seat of religious belief, as in the mid-eighth-century Würzburg glosses on the Pauline epistles.[15]

The present study similarly builds on the paradigm of embodied cognition in order to explore some of the ways in which Irish intellectuals of the early Middle Ages conceptualized the work of the mind through the use of metaphor, both explicit and implicit. It shows how authors of non-medical texts were drawing on wider intellectual currents for their understanding of mental processes. The following discussion will focus on two items of Old Irish vocabulary which refer to properly incorporeal entities — *menma* (mind) and *imrádud* (thought). Using the embodiment thesis, I will explore the semantic and syntactic contexts in which they are used and what this can tell us about Irish views on the mind and its functioning.

This analysis comprises two sections. In the first section, I discuss two vernacular poems that focus specifically on the work of the mind. These will provide a frame of reference for the embodied understanding of the mind through poetic metaphor. The second section takes an entirely different approach to the problem by analysing metaphorical mappings across a number of Old Irish scholarly (non-poetic, non-narrative) texts which address the problems of mental activity by means of conventional language. This is done using the resources of network analysis as a small-scale case-study and is not intended to be a comprehensive exploration of the topic.

The Embodied Mind in Vernacular Poetry: An Exercise in Close Reading

The first text to be considered is one of the most famous early Irish poems, sometimes referred to as *Pangur bán* or *The Scholar and His Cat*. It is one of a number or vernacular poems in the manuscript produced by an Irishman in Leinster and/or Western Francia in the 840s, entitled the *Reichenauer*

13 Lockett, *Anglo-Saxon Psychologies*, pp. 9–14.
14 Mac Mathúna, 'Lexical and Literary Aspects'.
15 Mac Mathúna, 'Lexical and Literary Aspects', pp. 8–10.

Schulheft or the Reichenau Primer by Hildegard Tristram.[16] The poem itself is an extended analogy between the intellectual effort of a scholar and the feline activities of his pet cat.[17] Here, I present four out of its total of eight stanzas:

1 Messe ocus Pangur bán,
cechtar nathar fria ṡaindán:
bíth a menmasam fri seilgg,
mu menma céin im ṡaincheirdd. [...]
4 Gnáth, hūaraib, ar gressaib gal
glenaid luch inna línsam;
os mé, du-fuit im lín chéin
dliged ndoraid cu ndronchéill
5 Fūachidsem fri frega fál
a rosc, a nglése comlán;
fūachimm chēin fri fēgi fis
mu rosc rēil, cesu imdis. [...]
8 Hē fesin as choimsid dáu
in muid du-ngní cach ōenláu;
du thabairt doraid du glé
for mu mud cēin am messe.

1 (I and white Pangur practice each of us his special art:
his mind is set on hunting, my mind on my special craft. [...]
4 It is usual, at times, for a mouse to stick in his net, as a result of warlike battlings.
For my part, into my net falls some difficult rule of hard meaning.
5 He directs his bright perfect eye against an enclosing wall.
Though my clear eye is very weak I direct it against keenness of knowledge. [...]
8 He it is who is master for himself of the work which he does every day.
I can perform my own work directed at understanding clearly what is difficult.)[18]

---

16 The manuscript is now kept in Austria (Carinthia, St Paul im Lavanttal, Stiftsbibliothek, MS 86a/1). For a description, see Tristram, 'Die irischen Gedichte'; Oskamp, 'The Irish Material', pp. 386–87; Toner, '"Messe ocus Pangur Bán"', p. 2 n. 7. The connections to Leinster are evident in the choice of vernacular poems, one of which is a eulogy for Aed mac Diarmata of the Uí Muiredaig, a Leinster dynasty, and another is ascribed to St Mo Ling (d. 697) whose cult is firmly rooted in Leinster, with two foundations called Tech Moling, one in Co. Carlow (present-day St Mullins) and one in Co. Kildare (present-day Timolin). See Flower, *The Irish Tradition*, pp. 27–33; Ní Dhonnchadha, 'The Cult of St Moling', pp. 4–8, 19–21. According to Hildegard Tristram, some of the material in the codex could have been copied in Ireland while other portions (e.g. the Greek contents) would require access to continental libraries, as she considered the presence of such materials in Ireland less likely. Tristram, 'Die irischen Gedichte', pp. 516–17.

17 Toner, '"Messe ocus Pangur Bán"', pp. 5–10.

18 *Early Irish Lyrics*, ed. and trans. by Murphy, pp. 2–3.

Although the metaphorical resources of the poem have a clear artistic intent, they follow the utilitarian logic of embodied realism: the scholar's lofty and ephemeral intellectual exercise is constantly paralleled in the cat's simple instinctual habits. The scholar is hunting for meaning like the cat hunting for mice; he is contemplating philosophical problems just as the cat is intently observing its surroundings. The complexities of thought are creatively imagined as watching, moving and catching — all physical experiences helping to give structure to the otherwise amorphous concept of cognition.

The first stanza offers an opportunity for further scrutiny. The way in which lines 3–4 are structured is important: 'a menma fri seilgg' and 'mu menma im ṡaincheirdd', literally 'his mind towards hunting' and 'my mind in my special craft'. Both lines are construed as prepositional phrases that depict the mind itself and the concepts that it contemplates as physical objects in Euclidean space, either moving or stationary. In line 3, the preposition *fri* (towards) implies that the mind moves in a straight line, whereas in line 4 the mind is in a state of rest, as suggested by the preposition *i* (in). These details may not be coincidental: the mind moving towards something may represent acquiring an idea or an impulse to act and is more instantaneous in nature, like the cat is fully prepared to attack prey on sight. The mind being within the object of contemplation, on the other hand, refers to continuous consideration of a particular idea. The subtle semantic difference between the two constructions was previously pointed out by Anders Ahlqvist, who observed that the preposition *i* implies a 'somewhat firmer mental relationship than *fri*'.[19] Ahlqvist offered two further examples to support his position, taken from the Würzburg glosses on the Pauline epistles (*c.* 750):

> .i. bíith amenme frisso bad samlid pridchaid (i.e. let his mind be to this: let him preach thus.)[20]

> beith formenme and arnafoircnea forcrabud and .i. hibarpeccad cenaithirgi (i.e. let your mind be there [literally 'in it'], lest it should put an end to your piety therein, i.e. in your sin without repentance.)[21]

In the first example, the glossator comments on 1 Corinthians 14.37: 'si quis uidetur propheta esse aut spiritalis, cognoscat quae scribo uobis, quia Domini sunt mandata' (If any seem to be a prophet, or spiritual, let him know the things that I write to you, that they are the commandments of the Lord). The phrase 'bíith amenme frisso' (let your mind be to this) therefore echoes the apostle's request for people who consider themselves prophets to learn of God's commandments. The preposition *fri* here emphasizes a rapid change of mental focus to a new set of ideas. The second gloss is a comment on

---

19 Ahlqvist, '*Pangur Bán*', pp. 230–31.

20 *Thesaurus Palaeohibernicus*, ed. and trans. by Stokes and Strachan, I, p. 582 (Wb. 13a22). The *Thesaurus* is hereafter referred to as *Thes.*

21 *Thes.* I, p. 628 (Wb. 20b13).

Galatians 5.15: 'quod si inuicem mordetis et comeditis, uidete ne ab inuicem consumamini' (But if you bite and devour one another, take heed you be not consumed one of another). This verse is an iteration of the commandment to love one's neighbour, and the glossator reminds the audience to be mindful of it constantly without fail. For this purpose, the preposition *i* is used: 'beith formenme and' (let your mind be in it).

This pair of examples thus provides additional evidence for the difference between the metaphorical meaning of *fri* and *i* in the descriptions of mental activity. The case for this can be strengthened even further by considering another instance where the two constructions appear side-by-side, just as they do in *Pangur bán*. The following stanza closes the earliest recension of the tale *Reicne Fothaid Canainne* (The Death of Fothath Cananne), which appears to be contemporary with the Würzburg glosses:[22]

> A ben nacham·aic i-lle!
> ni frit ita mu meenma:
> Ata mo menma co lléic
> Isind imairec oc Féc.
>
> > (O woman, do not entreat me (to come) hither!
> > My mind is not upon you:
> > Still is my mind
> > Upon the encounter at Féc.)[23]

The agreement in the choice of prepositions between this stanza and *Pangur bán* is quite remarkable. Here too, *menma* is paired with *fri* first and with *i* immediately after. The quatrain is spoken by Fothath's severed head and is addressed to the woman whom he had won from his rival Oilill mac Eochain — the deed that cost him his life. Lamenting his own fate, Fothath says to the nameless woman that he is not thinking of her: 'ni frit ita mu meenma', literally 'not towards you is my mind'. Indeed, such thoughts would appear incongruent with the gravity of the situation and their fleeting nature is expressed with the help of *fri*. Instead, Fothath's mind is 'isind imairec oc Féc', literally 'in the encounter at Féc'. The use of *i* in this contrasting statement gives more weight to Fothath's continuous dwelling on the tragic circumstances of his death. Similarly to *Pangur bán* and the Würzburg glosses, this verse juxtaposes two different types of mental activity through the use of spatial metaphors: movement towards something represents a more immediate and transient kind of thinking or acquiring a new idea, while position in a place suggests a more carefully considered and contemplative thought.

---

22 'The Death of Fothath Cananne', ed. and trans. by Hull, p. 400. A longer, tenth-century version of the tale, where this verse serves as the opening of a longer poem (forty-nine stanzas), has been edited and translated in *Fianaigecht*, ed. and trans. by Meyer, pp. 4–21.

23 'The Death of Fothath Cananne', ed. and trans. by Hull, pp. 401 and 404.

These considerations bring to mind a study conducted by William Short on the spatial metaphors for cognition in Classical Latin. Short's findings are, indeed, very similar to what has been observed so far regarding Irish sources. He examined different aspects of the metaphor 'ideas are locations' and discovered that the vocabulary of 'moving towards' (prepositions *in* or *ad* + accusative) refers to acquiring new knowledge or focusing on an idea that was not previously at the forefront of one's attention, whereas phrases referring to 'being in' (*in* + ablative) express established beliefs or methodical consideration of ideas.[24] In light of this, it can be concluded that basic spatial metaphors are a fundamental element of the language of embodiment.

The texts discussed thus far certainly present the mind as a body capable of motion but not necessarily as an animated body. The anthropomorphic metaphor comes to prominence in the tenth-century anonymous Middle Irish poem known by its opening words 'Is mebul dom imrádud' (Shame on my thought), or, as Kuno Meyer christened it, 'On the Flightiness of Thought'.[25] Below are five out of the total twelve stanzas to appreciate the consistency of the metaphor:

1 Is mebul dom imrádud
a mét élas úaimm:
atágur a imgábud
i lló brátha búain.
2 Tresna salmu sétaigid
for conair nád cóir,
rethid, búaidrid, bétaigid
fiad roscaib Dé móir.
3 Tre airechtu athluma,
tre buidnib ban mbóeth,
tre cholltib, tre chathracha,
is lúaithiu ná in góeth. [...]
7 Ce trialltar a chuibrech-sum
nó gemel na chois,
ní cundail, ní cuimnech-sum
co ngabad feidm fois.
8 Fóebur nó fúaimm flescbuille
ní tráethat co tailc,
slemnithir eirr escuinge
oc dul as mo glaicc.

1 (Shame to my thought how it strays from me!
I dread great danger from it on the day of lasting Doom.

24 Short, 'Thinking Places, Placing Thoughts', pp. 106–18.

25 The poem survives in the fifteenth-century *Leabhar Breac* (Dublin, RIA, MS 23 P 16 [1230], p. 262), with an additional copy in an early-seventeenth-century manuscript Dublin, RIA, MS B iv 2 (1080), fol. 141. See *Early Irish Lyrics*, ed. and trans. by Murphy, pp. 189–90.

2 During the psalms it wanders on a path that is not right:
it runs, it disturbs, it misbehaves before the eyes of great God.
3 Through eager assemblies, through companies of wanton women,
through woods, through cities — swifter it is than the wind.
[...]
7 Though one should try to bind it or put shackles on its feet,
it is neither constant nor mindful to take a spell of rest.
8 Neither sword-edge nor swish of lash will keep it down strongly:
as slippery as an eel's tail it glides out of my grasp.)[26]

The object of the author's worry here is *imrádud* (thought). Interestingly, Kuno Meyer, whose translation, with modifications, is offered above, rendered it as plural 'thoughts' throughout the poem, seemingly for stylistic reasons, even though *imrádud* in the first stanza is singular and is accompanied by singular verbal forms in the second stanza: *sétaigid* ([it] wanders), *rethid* ([it] runs), *búaidrid* ([it] disturbs), *bétaigid* ([it] misbehaves). I suggest that this is an important detail which should not be left to artistic liberty as it constitutes the core of the poem's metaphorical schema. By making thought singular, the author emphasizes its agency as an individual and singular actor, the inner self. In this regard, the poem can be considered to belong to the long-standing intellectual tradition that conceptualizes various aspects of a person's mental life as a unified anthropomorphic entity, a sort of an 'inner man'. This idea can be traced back to Plato but it gained particular prominence in Christian thought via Paul the apostle, whose use of the 'inner man' metaphor (*ὁ ἔσω ἄνθρωπος* or *homo interior*) ensured its longevity in the patristic and medieval tradition.[27]

In the poem, too, the metaphor likens various activities of the mind with those of the body. *Imrádud* (thought) is understood as a distinctly animated and conscious entity capable of experiencing many exploits of the body and perhaps even more voracious in its activities due to the lack of physical limitations. The image of putting 'shackles on its feet' provides a definitive comparison to the human body. But alas, thought cannot be imprisoned because its body is paradoxically incorporeal.

The metaphorical language of *Is mebul* is well-defined and vivid. However, it may not be wholly original. The work that left an indelible impression on the

26 'A Religious Poem', ed. and trans. by Meyer, pp. 14–15 (translation modified). A more recent edition and translation can be found in *Early Irish Lyrics*, ed. and trans. by Murphy, pp. 38–43. I chose Meyer's edition as it contains fewer emendation and represents the *Leabhar Breac* text more closely.

27 The relevant Pauline passages are: II Corinthians 4. 16, Romans 7. 22, Ephesians 3. 16. For a discussion of the Platonic roots of the Pauline metaphor, see Hecht, 'The "Inner Man"'. He argues that, like Plato, St Paul understands the 'inner man' to be 'a continuous agent' 'within a permanent flux of interior phenomena of the soul' (p. 292). See also van Kooten, 'St Paul on Soul', pp. 35–43; Matthews, 'The Inner Man'.

author's imagination is John Cassian's *Conlationes* (Conferences) — a collection of conversations with ascetics in the Egyptian desert. This text was known in Ireland already in the sixth century and had a significant influence on Irish monastic practice.[28] Cassian's presence in *Is mebul* is unmistakeable. Apart from the fact that Cassian himself made great use of the 'inner man' metaphor, he also appears to be the originator of some of the poem's imagery. The seventh conference titled *De animae mobilitate et spiritalibus nequitiis* ('On the Inconstancy of the Soul and Spiritual Wickedness') often has recourse to the concept of *homo interior* to emphasize the necessity of maintaining purity of mind in order to prevent the body from transgression. So, for example, Serenus, Cassian's interlocutor, is said to practice strict fasts and pray zealously in order that the victory over the desires of his heart 'which had been bestowed on his inner man by a gift of God' ('quae interiori homini suo dono dei fuerat adtributa') might translate into external purity.[29] In the same conference some familiar imagery appears:

> siquidem per momenta singula lubricis discursibus animus euagatus cum ad [...] contemplationem reducitur spiritalem, priusquam firmetur in ea, rursum fugacius euanescit, cum que eum [...] deprehenderimus ab intentione proposita deuiasse [...] uoluerimus eum tenacissima cordis intentione uelut quibusdam *uinculis obligare*, in ipso conatu nostro *ocius quam anguilla* de recessibus mentis *elabitur*.
>
>> (When the mind that has gotten involved in silly distractions for a few moments returns [...] to spiritual contemplation, before it becomes fixed there, it disappears again still more quickly. When we [...] realize that it has wandered away from its proposed intent [...] we want to *bind it* by the most tenacious attentiveness of heart, *as if by chains*, but even as we are attempting this *it slips away* again, *speedier than an eel*, from the recesses of our mind.)[30]

The parallels to *Is mebul* are difficult to ignore. To start with a more trivial one, *animus* (mind), which in this passage acts as the subject, is indeed a singular agent. Moreover, the imagery of a chained mind and likening its escape from the chains to an eel slipping away seem too specific to have been used by the Irish poet coincidentally. Given the monastic setting of the poem — the author describes a struggle with concentration during the singing of the psalms — these motifs are likely to be a borrowing from Cassian. In both cases, the freedom that thought enjoys is viewed as a source of frustration.[31]

---

28 Follett, 'Cassian, Contemplation'; Lake, 'Knowledge of the Writings of John Cassian', pp. 38 and 41.

29 John Cassian, *Conlationes*, VII, II.1, ed. by Petschenig, p. 180, trans. by Ramsey, p. 247.

30 John Cassian, *Conlationes*, VII, III.4, ed. by Petschenig, p. 182, trans. by Ramsey, p. 249 (italics are mine).

31 On Cassian's preoccupation with the problem of wandering thoughts, see Powell, 'The Quest for "quies mentis"'.

Its vagrancy and various transgressions disrupt the pious intentions of the person to whom it belongs. This lack of control clearly caused much anxiety to those devoted to the monastic ideals.

The wandering mind is not an uncommon trope in Irish literature. An eleventh-century Latin poem composed by an Irishman and known as *Mentis in excessu* ('In Ecstasy of Mind') offers an expansive tableau of a mental journey envisaged as an allegory for studying Scripture.[32] Closer to the topic at hand, mental journeying as an undesirable experience is also acknowledged in the ninth-century text now bearing the name 'The Monastery of Tallaght'. It is a work relating the teachings of Máel Ruain (d. 792), the founder of Tallaght and advocate for ascetic ideals and rigorous devotional practices as means to create 'a more personal, spiritually committed relationship with the Deity'.[33] One section of the text is concerned with inconstancy of mind, which is described as *foíndel* (wandering): 'andand mbis a foindel inda menmain commór fri mimradud a timtasad for caúlae feib dorrontar 7 tuidecht légind nó a scrutain fris 7 menme isind aurnaigti' (when the thoughts are constantly straying towards ill meditations, they must be checked and recalled as far as possible; and he should resort to reading or to examining himself against it, and keep his mind fixed on prayer).[34] This passage makes use of both of our key terms — *menma* (mind) and *imrádud* (thought). *Menma* here acts as the agent while *imrádud* (appearing as the compound *míimrádud* 'wrong thought') is presented as the destination of the unruly mind. Note, too, how the mind wanders *towards* an ill thought. This type of phrase, construed with the preposition *fri*, has already been discussed in relation to *Pangur bán*, where it represents, as I suggested, an immediate intention to act or an impulsive thought rather than steady contemplation. This idea is evident here as well, with the mind directing itself at various undesirable considerations and momentary passions rather than staying fixed on God.

Embodied Cognition in Old Irish through the Lens of Semantic Network Analysis

There is thus no doubt that the language of embodiment constituted a crucial part of the way in which the work of the mind was conceptualized in early Irish literature. In the previous section I applied the method of close reading to analyse two examples of embodied cognition used as a literary trope

32 The author of the poem was considered to be Patrick, bishop of Dublin (d. 1084). However, this attribution has been called into question. For a discussion of *Mentis in excessu*, including authorship and textual parallels with *Is mebul*, see Boyle, 'Allegory, the *áes dána* and the Liberal Arts', pp. 24–30.

33 Follett, *'Céli Dé' in Ireland*, p. 214; on 'The Monastery of Tallaght', see pp. 101–02.

34 'The Monastery of Tallaght', ed. and trans. by Gwynn and Purton, p. 151 (§ 62).

in vernacular poetry. In the second section, I propose to take an opposite approach by asking the question: can similar linguistic patterns be observed on a larger scale and in texts which are not specifically dedicated to artistic representations of the mind?

Of course, it would be impossible to answer this question fully within this essay. However, in what follows, I will offer a case-study that begins to address it, with a more extensive project currently in the works. The methodological approach which can help us recognize implicit systematic patterns of language use, including metaphorical language, is semantic network analysis. Network analysis is a powerful heuristic tool for abstracting information from large datasets. Its theoretical foundations lie in complex networks theory, which seeks to represent and understand the relationships between elements of a complex system.[35] Examples of complex networks range from social relations to the Internet and neural networks, and, indeed, language.

Network analysis in linguistics can take on many different shapes. This study is concerned with the notion of conceptual metaphor, that is, with the mechanism of semantic transfer, and it can therefore be further informed by the resources of semantic network analysis, which is a tool for reconstructing implicit patterns of meaning on a systematic level.[36] Since language networks can be said to approximate the human cognitive system,[37] a study of the semantic associations between words and their underlying concepts also promises to provide insights into the conceptual mechanisms that govern certain semantic patterns.

In this study, I am interested in establishing a semantic network which would represent the concepts that connote or are connoted by the words *menma* and *imrádud* in Irish. Given that the network will be built around just two focal nodes, it can be classified as an ego-network, that is, a network which consists of all items, or nodes, connected to the focal node within a specified distance.[38] These connections are called links or edges. In order to test this methodology, I have been collecting attestations of mind-related vocabulary, including, among others, the terms *menma* and *imrádud,* in a variety of Old Irish texts. For the present case-study, I am using a small corpus comprised of just five texts from the Old Irish period. The texts in question are:

Apgitir Chrábaid ('The Alphabet of Piety') (*c.* 700–750): seven tokens;
The Würzburg Glosses (*c.* 750): twenty tokens;

35 For an overview of the field, see Strogatz, 'Exploring Complex Networks'; Newman, 'The Structure and Function'; Boccaletti and others, 'Complex Networks'.

36 For a valuable introduction to the aims and methods of semantic network analysis in the context of historical linguistics, with a case-study of the ancient Egyptian language corpus, see Elwert and Gerhards, 'Tracing Concepts'.

37 Beckage and Colunga, 'Language Networks as Models of Cognition', p. 4.

38 Elwert and Gerhards, 'Tracing Concepts', p. 318.

The Milan Glosses (*c.* 800): forty-two tokens;
The St Gall Glosses (*c.* 850): six tokens;
'The Monastery of Tallaght' (*c.* 815–840): twelve tokens.

In total, the corpus for the case-study contains eighty-seven tokens. It is important to define what constitutes a token. For an ego-network, it is a fragment of text that contains a target term (in this case, *menma* or *imrádud*). It has been argued that the optimal length of a textual unit for the accuracy of semantic analysis is a sentence.[39] I followed this principle for simple sentences containing the words *menma* and *imrádud*. However, for complex sentences, I only included the clause that contains a relevant key word in my corpus.

The processing for the corpus consisted of several procedures. The first step in preparing the data for visualization is syntactic parsing. Generally, two strategies are available for semantic analysis: a co-occurrence network and a dependency network. A co-occurrence network is undirected, that is, all relations between nodes are considered to be symmetrical. The inferences about the significance of different edges are based purely on the frequency of co-occurrence of two words. A dependency network, on the other hand, is directed and takes into account the semantic hierarchy of a phrase or a sentence and distinguishes between source and target in every pair of nodes. It has been shown that networks based on syntactically annotated corpora are 'more effective in capturing the properties of the mental lexicon than simple co-occurrence networks'.[40] For this case study, dependency trees were created for each of the eighty-seven tokens.[41]

As the next step, each individual surface form was lemmatized in order to avoid the difficulties of dealing with multiple inflected forms of a single lemma. After that, certain parts of speech that do not significantly affect semantic relations were excluded from the analysis (e.g. pronouns, conjunctions, the copula, the substantive verb), leaving only nouns, verbs, adjectives, and prepositions. These two steps resulted in a list of 138 lemmata.[42] Each lemma then was assigned to one of four broad semantic categories, to facilitate detection of metaphors. The categories are:

abstract concepts (e.g. *menma* [mind], *ainimm* [soul], *fírinne* [truth]);

39 Elwert and Gerhards, 'Tracing Concepts', p. 318.

40 De Deyne, Verheyen, and Storms, 'Structure and Organization of the Mental Lexicon', p. 51. In network analysis, the dependency approach, not the constituency approach, is the preferred method for syntactic mark-up. See Čech, Mačutek, and Liu, 'Syntactic Complex Networks', pp. 168–69. On syntactic dependency, see Mel'čuk, 'Levels of Dependency in Linguistic Description', pp. 197–211.

41 For the Milan and St Gall glosses, the existing parsed corpora were used. See respectively Griffith and Stifter, *A Dictionary of the Old-Irish Glosses*; Bauer, Hofman, and Moran, *St Gall Priscian Glosses*.

42 Spelling and translation of the lemmata are based on the *Electronic Dictionary of Irish Language* (eDIL).

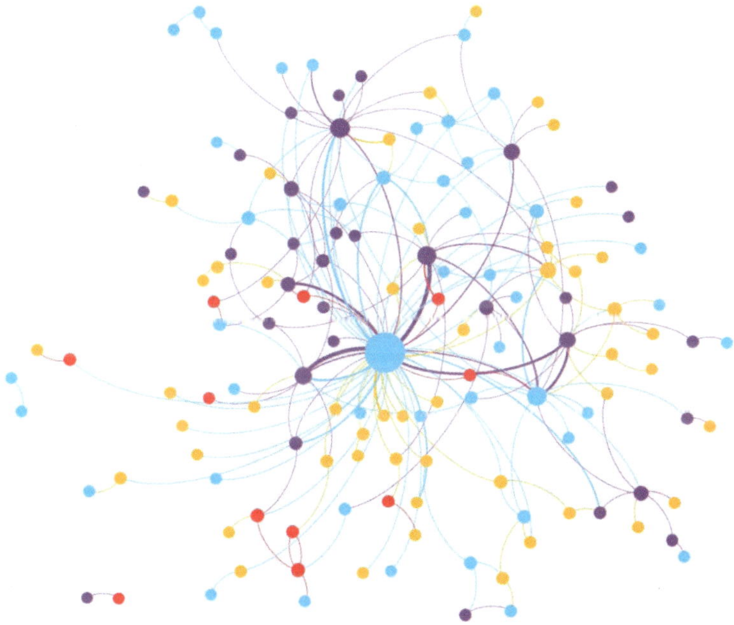

Figure 6.1. Network generated from eighty-seven tokens containing the words *menma* and *imrádud*. Image by the author.

space and motion (e.g. *téit* [goes], *cáel* [narrow], *fri* [towards]);
body and object interaction (e.g. *rét* [thing], *énirt* [weak], *fo-ben* [attacks]);
language (e.g. *as-beir* [says], *bríathar* [word], *labrad* [speech]).

One should, of course, bear in mind that this classification, though meant to be objective, is not immune to a certain degree of arbitrariness. Some words are particularly problematic to categorize. For instance, such concepts as *coibsenugud* (confession) or *mess* (judgement) can be seen as acts of the mind or as ritual actions grounded in the physical world, or even as linguistic events. Ultimately, I assigned them to the category 'body and object interaction' based on the pronounced performative nature of these concepts in early medieval societies. In the final step, this data was imported into the open-source software *Gephi*, and the spatial layout algorithm *Force Atlas* was used for the visualization of the network graphs. In what follows, I present a few exemplary graphs that can be generated in response to different queries. The bird's eye view of the whole network can be seen in Figure 6.1. It consists of 138 nodes and 207 edges. The size of nodes and thickness of edges are directly proportional to their weight, that is, the number of connections. As expected, the giant component in the middle of the network is *menma*. The four semantic categories are colour-coded as follows (edges are the colour of the source node):

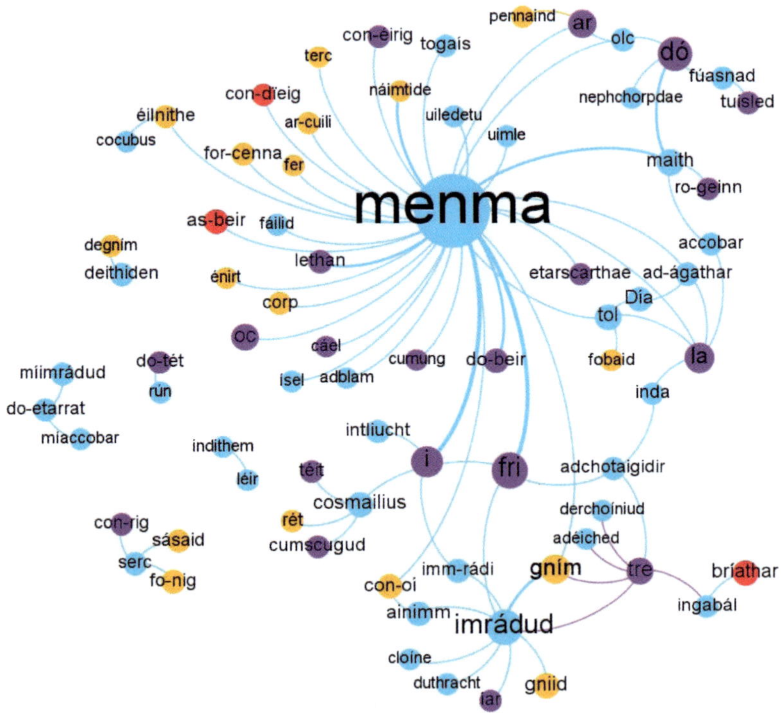

Figure 6.2. Sub-network displaying all links with abstract concepts as source. Image by the author.

blue: abstract concepts (forty-six nodes, eighty-two edges);
purple: space and motion (thirty-one nodes, sixty-seven edges);
yellow: body and object interaction (fifty nodes, forty-five edges);
red: language (eleven nodes, thirteen edges).

In order to draw some inferences from the network, specific queries need to be created. One can, for example, filter edges by source. Figure 6.2 is a graph that shows all occurrences where an abstract concept is the governing element. While they are not the most numerous group of concepts (there are more nodes in the category 'body and object interaction'), they generate the largest number of links. This is due to the fact that our two key terms, *menma* and *imrádud*, belong to this group. Each of them forms a conceptual community, dominating the top and the bottom of the graph respectively. Since *imrádud* is less frequently attested in the corpus, its community is smaller. However, both of them have a direct link to the preposition *fri* ('towards'), which has been discussed in the previous section. This further demonstrates that 'to have one's mind/thought directed towards something' was a common strategy

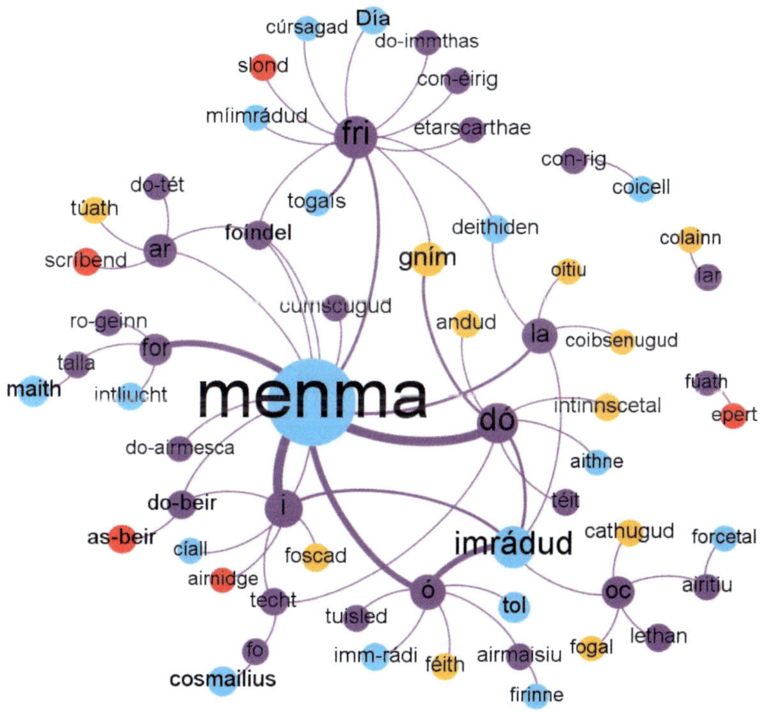

Figure 6.3. Sub-network displaying all links with 'space and motion' concepts as source. Image by the author.

for expressing the more fluent aspects of mental activity.[43] It is worth noting that the edge connecting *menma* and *fri* is one of the strongest in the graph, as the two words occur together three times in the corpus. The same can be said for the preposition *i*, which has been analysed in conjunction with *fri* earlier and is likewise paired with *menma* three times in the corpus. Again, the mind is depicted as being within another object, for instance, *isin cheil* ('in the meaning' of the psalms) or *isind aurnaigti* (in prayer).[44] This type of construction conveys the idea of mental concentration.

Applying the same filter to space and motion concepts yields a network of nodes governed by them. This is represented in Figure 6.3. Predictably, we see that prepositions play the most important role here: prepositions like *fri* (towards), *i* (in), *ó* (from) and *do* (for) are the strongest and best-connected

43 Examples of this construction are found in the Würzburg and Milan glosses: *Thes.* I, pp. 59 (Ml. 28c14), 528 (Wb. 5b37) and 582 (Wb. 13a22).

44 For these constructions, see 'The Monastery of Tallaght', ed. and trans. by Gwynn and Purton, §§39 and 62 (pp. 142 and 151).

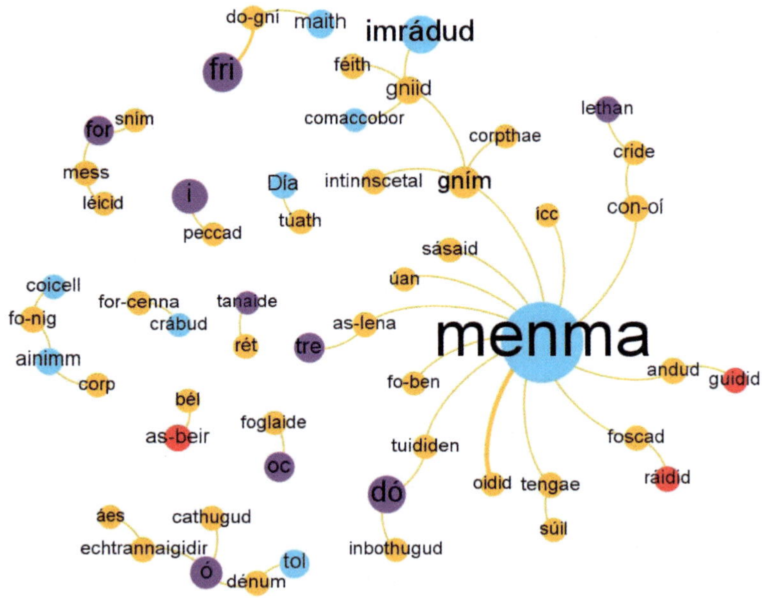

Figure 6.4. Sub-network displaying all links with 'body and object interaction' concepts as source. Image by the author.

nodes in the graph beside *menma* and *imrádud*. Indeed, they are crucial in creating the geometry of mental space at the most fundamental level of cognition. But at the same time, among the nodes that govern *menma* are such words as *foíndel* (wandering), *cumscugud* (motion) and *do-airmesca* (constrains), which reiterate the themes of the roaming mind and the act of thinking as a sort of mental traversal.[45] In the same graph we also find another facet of the 'mind-as-body' metaphor, namely the imagery of fighting undesired thoughts, represented by the words *cathugud* (battle) and *fogal* (attack), which occur in different texts and are therefore independent attestations of the same metaphor.[46]

---

45 *Foíndel* occurs in the already discussed passage from § 62 of the 'Monastery of Tallaght', ed. and trans. by Gwynn and Purton, p. 151 (see p. 152 above). *Do-airmesca* is found in the same text: *fobíthin fobenad 7 doairmescad menmain* ('because it might harass and constrain the mind'): 'The Monastery of Tallaght', ed. and trans. by Gwynn and Purton, § 2 (pp. 127–28, although Gwynn and Purton translate *doairmescad* as '[it might] disturb'). The phrase *innacumscaigthe inmenman* ('of the motions of the mind') is found in the Milan glosses. *Thes.*, I, p. 14 (Ml. 15a2).

46 *Cathugud* is attested in the Milan glosses in the phrase 'ó menmain naimtinech oc inchathugud' (fighting with hostile mind): *Thes.*, I, p. 220 (Ml. 65b10). *Fogal* occurs in 'The Monastery of Tallaght', ed. by Gwynn and Purton, § 39, p. 142 where the mind, along with the eye and the tongue, are the said to be the three adversaries of a pious person. For a discussion of combat imagery in hagiographic descriptions of monastic meditative practice, see Powell, 'Demonic Daydreams'.

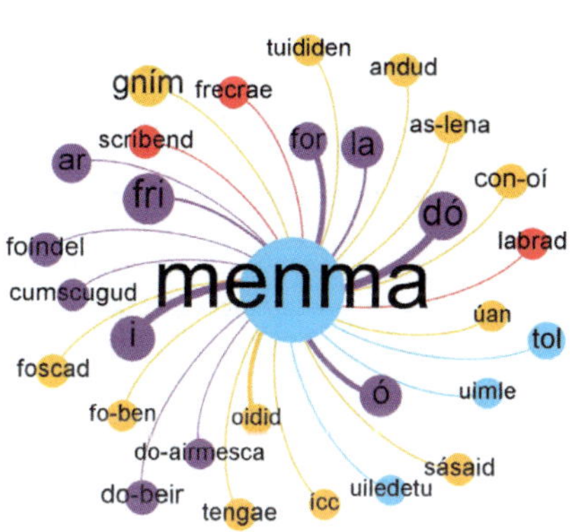

Figure 6.5.1. Ego-network of menma as target (path length = 1). Image by the author.

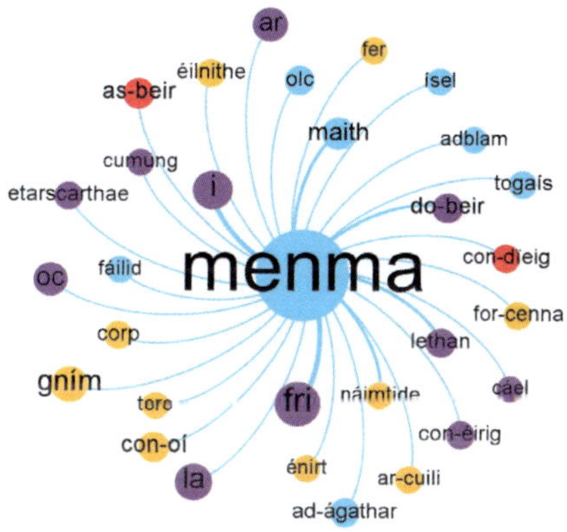

Figure 6.5.2. Ego-network of *menma* as source (path length = 1). Image by the author.

When the network is filtered to reflect links generated by the concepts from the category 'body and object interaction' (Fig. 6.4), we notice that they often control abstract concepts beyond *menma* and *imrádud*. So, for instance, the verb *fo-nig* (cleanses) governs the nouns *coicell* (thought) and *ainimm* (soul), conveying the idea that to be virtuous or pious is to be clean. On the contrary, one of the concepts connected to *menma* in this graph is *as-lena* (defiles), which suggests that deficient morality is imagined as a lack of purity. These examples, again, come from different texts but utilize the same metaphor.[47] This reaffirms the role of body-related vocabulary in the metaphorical representation of various aspects of mental life.

Another way to extract information from this network is to consider the immediate neighbourhood of *menma* (there is not enough data in the corpus at this stage to do the same for *imrádud*). The graphs in Figure 6.5.1 and 6.5.2 represent all nodes connected to *menma* by only one edge, that is, they govern or are governed by *menma* directly, without any intermediaries. In Figure 6.5.1 *menma* acts as the target and in Figure 6.5.2 as the source. When *menma* is the dependent element in a phrase (Fig. 6.5.1), it is almost exclusively governed by space (purple) and body (yellow) concepts. The latter include such words as *ícc* (medicine) and *sásaid* (soothes), invoking the metaphor of the mind as a sick person in need of treatment and care.[48]

---

47 Love of God is said to cleanse the soul and thoughts in 'Apgitir Chrábaid', ed. and trans. by Hull, § 6 (pp. 60–61). The phrase *aslentis amenma* ('they used to defile their mind') is found in the Milan glosses. *Thes.*, I, p. 253 (Ml. 74c3).

48 See respectively *Thes.*, I, p. 10 (Ml. 2d13); 'Apgitir Chrábaid', ed. and trans. by Hull, § 6 (pp. 60–61).

A handful of linguistic concepts can be seen in the category of 'language': *labrad* (speech), *scríbend* (writing) and *frecrae* (answer). They occur in genitival constructions: 'the speech of the mind', 'the writing of the mind', 'the answer of the mind', which hint towards another kind of metaphor, namely that thought functions like a language.[49]

With *menma* as the head of a phrase (Fig. 6.5.2), we can observe a group of spatial adjectives such as *cáel* (narrow), *cumung* (constrained), *lethan* (broad).[50] These are mappings that belong to the container metaphor. They imagine the mind as a more or less capacious storage space for ideas. In addition to this, the anthropomorphic metaphor makes another appearance with concepts from the language category: *as-beir* (says) and *con-dïeig* (demands).[51] Here the mind acts as a speaker.

Overall, this case-study helped detect various aspects of metaphorical language discussed in the first section within a larger and more varied group of texts. This includes the most fundamental spatial metaphors as well as more complex mappings that conceptualize the mind as a human-like agent. Although the present study is limited by the small size of the textual corpus, it shows definite potential of applying the method of semantic network analysis to facilitate the tracing of stable linguistic patterns on a large scale.

Conclusion

The study has shown that the language of embodiment was a crucial part of Irish vocabulary for describing the work of the mind. On the most fundamental level, this language imagines the movement of ideas and the mind itself towards, from or into various locations within mental space, thus creating thoughts, feelings, memories, or other cognitive content. The next step on the embodiment scale is imagining the mind as an animated being, and more specifically a human being. As such, it can take on different roles: a wanderer, a fugitive and an outlaw, a patient, an interlocutor, an adversary to be fought. These mappings manifest themselves with equal strength in poetic metaphors and in conventional language not specifically concerned with the problems of cognition. Overall, the way in which Irish scholars understood

49 The phrases *frecrae menmman* ('mental answer' [literally 'the answer of the mind']) and *scríbend menmman* ('intended writing' [literally 'the writing of the mind']) are attested in the St Gall glosses: *Thes.*, II, pp. 79 (Sg. 28b15) and 174 (Sg. 178b3,4). The gloss from the Milan collection sums up the entire metaphor: *airis imradud álabradsidi in menman* (for the speech of the mind is thought): *Thes.*, I, p. 468 (Ml. 138a3).

50 The mind is described as 'narrow' (*cáel*) and 'constrained' (*cumung*) in 'Apgitir Chrábaid', ed. and trans. by Hull, § 33 (pp. 74–75). *Lethan* is attested in the Würzburg glosses in the phrase *badlethan formenme etforcride* ('let your mind and your heart be enlarged'). *Thes.*, I, p. 605 (Wb. 16a15).

51 Both lemmata are attested side-by-side in the Würzburg glosses: *Thes.*, I, p. 558 (Wb. 10a15: *con-dïeig*; Wb. 10a16: *as-beir*).

and conceptualized the work of the mind is rooted in the experience of the human body. This once again confirms that psychology and physiology are intertwined in medieval thought.

It is hoped that beside the exploration of the stated topic, this study will also draw some attention to the advantages of the two methodological paradigms used here. Indeed, cognitive linguistics has much to offer to the analysis of premodern material, as a number of successful examples in the field of early medieval English studies have demonstrated.[52] There is similar potential for such work in Celtic Studies. The same can be said about complex network theory and network analysis. Although computational methods have long been in the arsenal of historical linguists, there is also much value to be derived from this approach for the study of intellectual history.[53] Here, semantic network analysis offers many untapped opportunities to explore historical mentalities through language use.

Works Cited

Manuscripts

Carinthia, St Paul im Lavanttal, Stiftsbibliothek, MS 86a/1
Dublin, Royal Irish Academy, MS B iv 2 (1080)
Dublin, Royal Irish Academy, MS 23 P 16 (1230) 'The Leabhar Breac'

Primary Sources

'Apgitir Chrábaid: The Alphabet of Piety', ed. and trans. by Vernam Hull, *Celtica*, 8 (1968), 44–89

'The Death of Fothath Cananne', ed. and trans. by Vernam Hull, *Zeitschrift für celtische Philologie*, 20 (1936), 400–04

Early Irish Lyrics: Eighth to Twelfth Century, ed. and trans. by Gerard Murphy (Oxford: Clarendon Press, 1956) [reprinted Dublin: Four Courts Press, 1998]

Fianaigecht, Being a Collection of hitherto Inedited Irish Poems and Tales Relating to Finn and His Fiana, ed. and trans. by Kuno Meyer (Dublin: Hodges and Figgis, 1910)

John Cassian, *The Conferences*, trans. by Boniface Ramsey, Ancient Christian Writers, 57 (New York: Newman Press, 1997)

——, *Conlationes XXIIII*, ed. by Michael Petschenig, Corpus Scriptorum Ecclesiasticorum Latinorum, 13 (Vienna: Gerold, 1886)

52 In addition to Lockett, *Anglo-Saxon Psychologies*, a few other notable studies are: Harbus, *Cognitive Approaches to Old English Poetry*; Low, 'The Anglo-Saxon Mind'. For Medieval Studies in general, see Dresvina and Blud, eds, *Cognitive Sciences and Medieval Studies*.

53 Network analysis has gained particular prominence in the study of social and intellectual networks throughout history. For an exhaustive bibliography, see 'HNR Bibliography'.

'The Monastery of Tallaght', ed. and trans. by Edward J. Gwynn and W. J. Purton, *Proceedings of the Royal Irish Academy: Archaeology, Culture, History, Literature*, 29 (1911–1912), 115–79

'A Religious Poem', ed. and trans. by Kuno Meyer, *Ériu*, 3 (1907), 13–15

Thes. = *Thesaurus Palaeohibernicus. A Collection of Old-Irish Glosses Scholia Prose and Verse*, ed. and trans. by Whitley Stokes and John Strachan, 2 vols (Cambridge: Cambridge University Press, 1901–1903)

Secondary Studies

Ahlqvist, Anders, '*Pangur Bán*', in *Ollam: Studies in Gaelic and Related Traditions in Honor of Tomás Ó Cathasaigh*, ed. by Matthieu Boyd (Madison, NJ: Fairleigh Dickinson University Press, 2016), pp. 227–36

Bauer, Bernhard, Rijcklof Hofman, and Pádraic Moran, *St Gall Priscian Glosses*, version 2.0 (2017) <http://www.stgallpriscian.ie/> [accessed 9 May 2022]

Beckage, Nicole M., and Eliana Colunga, 'Language Networks as Models of Cognition: Understanding Cognition through Language', in *Towards a Theoretical Framework for Analyzing Complex Linguistic Networks*, ed. by Alexander Mehler, Andy Lücking, Sven Banisch, Philippe Blanchard, and Barbara Frank-Job (Berlin: Springer, 2016), pp. 3–28

Boccaletti, S., V. Latora, Y. Moreno, M. Chavez, and D.-U. Hwang, 'Complex Networks: Structure and Dynamics', *Physics Reports*, 424 (2006), 175–308. DOI: <https://doi.org/10.1016/j.physrep.2005.10.009>

Boyle, Elizabeth, 'Allegory, the *áes dána* and the Liberal Arts in Medieval Irish Literature', in *Grammatica, Gramadach and Gramadeg: Vernacular Grammar and Grammarians in Medieval Ireland and Wales*, ed. by Deborah Hayden and Paul Russell (Amsterdam: John Benjamins, 2016), pp. 11–34

Čech, Radek, Ján Mačutek, and Haitao Liu, 'Syntactic Complex Networks and Their Application', in *Towards a Theoretical Framework for Analysing Complex Linguistic Networks*, ed. by Alexander Mehler, Andy Lücking, Sven Banisch, Philippe Blanchard, and Barbara Frank-Job (Berlin: Springer, 2016), pp. 167–86

De Deyne, Simon, Steven Verheyen, and Gert Storms, 'Structure and Organization of the Mental Lexicon: A Network Approach Derived from Syntactic Dependency Relations and Word Associations', in *Towards a Theoretical Framework for Analysing Complex Linguistic Networks*, ed. by Alexander Mehler, Andy Lücking, Sven Banisch, Philippe Blanchard, and Barbara Frank-Job (Berlin: Springer, 2016), pp. 47–79

Demaitre, Luke, *Medieval Medicine: The Art of Healing, from Head to Toe* (Santa Barbara: Praeger, 2013)

Dresvina, Juliana, and Victoria Blud, eds, *Cognitive Sciences and Medieval Studies: An Introduction* (Cardiff: University of Wales Press, 2020)

eDIL = eDIL 2019: *An Electronic Dictionary of the Irish Language, Based on the Contributions to a Dictionary of the Irish Language* (Dublin: Royal Irish Academy, 1913–1976) <www.dil.ie> [accessed 11 May 2022]

Elwert, Frederik, and Simone Gerhards, 'Tracing Concepts – Semantic Network Analysis as a Heuristic Device for Classification', in *Classification from Antiquity to Modern Times: Sources, Methods, and Theories from an Interdisciplinary Perspective*, ed. by Tanja Pommerening and Walter Bisang (Berlin: De Gruyter, 2017), pp. 311–38. DOI: <https://doi.org/10.1515/9783110538779-012>

Flower, Robin, *The Irish Tradition* (Oxford: Clarendon Press, 1947)

Follett, Westley, 'Cassian, Contemplation, and Medieval Irish Hagiography', in *'Insignis sophiae arcator': Essays in Honour of Michael W. Herren on His 65th Birthday*, ed. by Gernot R. Wieland, Carin Ruff, and Ross G. Arthur (Turnhout: Brepols, 2006), pp. 87–105

——, *'Céli Dé' in Ireland: Monastic Writing and Identity in the Early Middle Ages* (Woodbridge: Boydell Press, 2006)

Gibbs, Raymond W., Jr., *Embodiment and Cognitive Science* (Cambridge: Cambridge University Press, 2005)

Green, Christopher D., 'Where Did the Ventricular Localization of Mental Faculties Come From?', *Journal of History of the Behavioral Sciences*, 39.2 (2003), 131–42

Griffith, Aaron, and David Stifter, *A Dictionary of the Old-Irish Glosses in the Milan Codex Ambrosianus C 301 inf.* (Institut für Sprachwissenschaft, Universität Wien, 2007–2013) <http://www.univie.ac.at/indogermanistik/milan glosses.htm> [accessed 9 May 2022]

Harbus, Antonina, *Cognitive Approaches to Old English Poetry*, Anglo-Saxon Studies, 18 (Woodbridge: Brewer, 2012)

Hecht, Stephan, 'The "Inner Man" – Fundamental Concept of Pauline Anthropology?', *The Biblical Annals*, 12.2 (2022), 279–94

Historical Research Network Community (HNR), 'HNR Bibliography: Network Analysis in the Historical Sciences' <https://historicalnetworkresearch.org/bibliography/> [accessed 12 May 2022]

Johnson, Mark, *The Body in the Mind: The Bodily Basis of Meaning, Imagination, and Reason* (Chicago: The University of Chicago Press, 1990)

Joseph, John E., *Language, Mind and Body: A Conceptual History* (Cambridge: Cambridge University Press, 2018)

Kemp, Simon, and Garth J. O. Fletcher, 'The Medieval Theory of the Inner Senses', *The American Journal of Psychology*, 106.4 (1993), 559–76

Kövecses, Zoltán, *Where Metaphors Come From: Reconsidering Context in Metaphor* (Oxford: Oxford University Press, 2015)

Lackoff, George, 'The Contemporary Theory of Metaphor', in *Metaphor and Thought*, ed. by Andrew Ortony, 2nd edn (Cambridge: Cambridge University Press, 1993), pp. 202–51

Lackoff, George, and Mark Johnson, *Metaphors We Live By* (Chicago: The University of Chicago Press, 1980)

——, *Philosophy in the Flesh: The Embodied Mind and Its Challenge to Western Thought* (New York: Basic Books, 1999)

Lake, Stephen, 'Knowledge of the Writings of John Cassian in Early Anglo-Saxon England', *Anglo-Saxon England*, 32 (2003), 27–41

Lockett, Leslie, *Anglo-Saxon Psychologies in the Vernacular and Latin Traditions* (Toronto: University of Toronto Press, 2011)

Low, Soon Ai, 'The Anglo-Saxon Mind: Metaphor and Common Sense Psychology in Old English Literature' (unpublished doctoral thesis, University of Toronto, 1998)

Mac Mathúna, Liam, 'Lexical and Literary Aspects of "Heart" in Irish', *Ériu*, 53 (2003), 1–18

Matthews, Gareth B., 'The Inner Man', *American Philosophical Quarterly*, 4.2 (1967), 166–72

Mel'čuk, Igor, 'Levels of Dependency in Linguistic Description: Concepts and Problems', in *Dependenz und Valenz: Ein internationales Handbuch der zeitgenössischen Forschung. Dependency and Valency: An International Handbook of Contemporary Research*, ed. by Vilmos Ágel, Ludwig M. Eichinger, Hans-Werner Eroms, Peter Hellwig, Hans Jürgen Heringer, and Henning Lobin (Berlin: De Gruyter, 2003), pp. 188–229

Newman, M. E. J., 'The Structure and Function of Complex Networks', *SIAM Review*, 45.2 (2003), 167–256. DOI: <https://doi.org/10.1137/S003614450342480>

Ní Dhonnchadha, Máirín, 'The Cult of St Moling and the Making of *Buile Shuibne*', in *Buile Shuibne: Perspectives and Reassessments*, ed. by John Carey (London: Irish Texts Society, 2014), pp. 1–42

Oskamp, Hans, 'The Irish Material in the St Paul Irish Codex', *Éigse*, 17.3 (1978), 385–91

Powell, Hilary, 'Demonic Daydreams: Mind-Wandering and Mental Imagery in the Medieval Hagiography of St Dunstan', in *New Medieval Literatures 18*, ed. by Laura Ashe, Philip Knox, David Lawton, and Wendy Scase (Cambridge: Brewer, 2018), pp. 44–74

——, 'The Quest for "quies mentis"', in *The Restless Compendium: Interdisciplinary Investigations of Rest and Its Opposites*, ed. by Felicity Callard, Kimberley Staines, and James Wilkes (Basingstoke: Palgrave, 2016), pp. 19–26

Reddy, Micheal J., 'The Conduit Metaphor – A Case of Frame Conflict in our Language about Language', in *Metaphor and Thought*, ed. by Andrew Ortony, 2nd edn (Cambridge: Cambridge University Press, 1993), pp. 164–201

Short, William M., 'Thinking Places, Placing Thoughts: Spatial Metaphors of Mental Activity in Roman Culture', *Quaderni del Ramo d'Oro*, 1 (2008), 106–29

Strogatz, Steven H., 'Exploring Complex Networks', *Nature*, 410 (2001), 268–76

Sweetser, Eve, *From Etymology to Pragmatics: Metaphorical and Cultural Aspects of Semantic Structure* (Cambridge: Cambridge University Press, 1990)

Toner, Gregory, '"Messe ocus Pangur Bán": Structure and Cosmology', *Cambrian Medieval Celtic Studies*, 57 (2009), 1–22

Trenery, Claire, and Peregrine Horden, 'Madness in the Middle Ages', in *The Routledge History of Madness and Mental Health*, ed. by Greg Eghigian (London: Routledge, 2017), pp. 62–80

Tristram, Hildegard L. C., 'Die irischen Gedichte im Reichenauer Schulheft', in *Studia Celtica et Indogermanica: Festschrift für Wolfgang Meid zum 70. Geburts-*

tag, ed. by Peter Anreiter and Erzsébet Jerem (Budapest: Archaeolingua, 1999), pp. 503–29

Van Kooten, George H., 'St Paul on Soul, Spirit and the Inner Man', in *The Afterlife of the Platonic Soul: Reflections of Platonic Psychology in the Monotheistic Religions*, ed. by Maha El-Kaisy and John Dillon (Leiden: Brill, 2009), pp. 25–44

Wack, Mary Frances, *Lovesickness in the Middle Ages: The 'Viaticum' and Its Commentaries* (Philadelphia: University of Pennsylvania Press, 1990)

Wollock, Jeffrey, *The Noblest Animate Motion: Speech, Physiology and Medicine in Pre-Cartesian Linguistic Thought* (Amsterdam: John Benjamins, 1997)

ERIN CONNELLY and CHRISTINA LEE

7. Menace or Medicine

What to do with Nettles?*

Strabo's *Hortulus*, a ninth-century text on the cultivation of gardens, records the author's surprise and dismay at finding his garden overgrown with nettles, such that he exclaims: *Quid facerem?* (What should I do?).[1] He tears the tangled roots out of the soil with diligence but acknowledges that the stubborn plant will likely return to his garden. Apparently the author deals with his rapidly spreading nettles during spring; other medieval authors suggest that the season of wild growth is August, which is aptly named the *Weodmonað* (weed month) in sources from Bede's *De temporum ratione*[2] to the late tenth-century poem, *Menologium*.[3] A fifteenth-century Middle English version of *De viribus herbarum* states that August is the best time to gather abundant nettles for medicinal purposes.[4] In these select examples there are shades of meaning to *weod*, a mixture of malevolence and benevolence, of menace and medicine, which reflect the character of nettles.[5] On the one hand, they are weeds which grow almost everywhere in the world; on the other, they could be used as food (when boiled), animal feed, fertilizer (they are rich in potassium), and as fibres for textile production. The term *weod* in Old and Middle English did not necessarily refer to a 'weed' and thus a nuisance, in the modern sense; rather, it could merely be an uncultivated plant.[6] *Nettle*, though widely used in healing remedies, is synonymous with

* This work was supported by an APEX award (Academies Partnership in Supporting Excellence in cross-disciplinary research award), administered by the British Academy, the Royal Academy of Engineering, and the Royal Society ('the Academies') and with generous support from the Leverhulme Trust. APEX Grant reference: APX\R1\180053. EC was supported by a UKRI Future Leaders Fellowship, MR/T020652/1.

1 Strabo, *Hortulus*, trans. by Payne, pp. 82–85.

2 Bede, *The Reckoning of Time*, ed and trans. by Wallis, p. 53.

3 *The Old English Metrical Calendar*, ed. by Karasawa, p. 80; see also n. 111.

4 Glasgow, Univ. Lib., MS Hunter 497, fol. 9v; see also *The Middle English Version of De Viribus Herbarum*, ed. by Calle-Martin and Miranda-García, p. 76.

5 The first definition in Bosworth-Toller is 'A useless or injurious plant, weed': see the Bosworth-Toller Anglo-Saxon Dictionary online <https://bosworthtoller.com> [accessed 21 May 2024].

6 See entry for *wed(e)* in McSparran and others, eds, *Middle English Compendium.*

Erin Connelly • University of Warwick; erin.connelly@warwick.ac.uk
Christina Lee • University of Nottingham; christina.lee@nottingham.ac.uk

Medicine in the Medieval North Atlantic World: Vernacular Texts and Traditions, ed. by Deborah Hayden and Sarah Baccianti, KSS, 5 (Turnhout, 2025), pp. 167-190
BREPOLS PUBLISHERS DOI 10.1484/M.KSS-EB.5.143985

sin, annoyance, brutal foes, or bad character in figurative contexts.[7] Nettles are ubiquitous in medieval and modern settings and were part of the pharmaceutical kit used across the period. They are a nuisance to some authors, and a vital part of healing processes to others. So, Strabo's question arises again: what should we do with nettles?

This paper answers Strabo's question by discussing the worth of nettles in select research outcomes from a project which examined the potential medicinal qualities of nettles (restricted to *Urtica dioica*), inspired by early and late medieval medical recipes from a range of medical manuscripts.[8] Our previous research showed that the efficacy of the remedy lay in the combination of ingredients, but given the sheer number of different plants and potential combinations in medieval medical texts, we had to find common patterns.[9] The humanities-led exploration involved researchers from the disciplines of early and late medieval studies, microbiology, and data science. By combining skills in medieval cultural history, manuscript studies, lab sciences, and analysis of complex datasets, we aimed to detect and examine common patterns of combinations, which includes the processes of preparation and application of medieval nettle-based remedies. The project explored to what extent this long tradition demonstrates continuity with modern uses and how such uses may benefit present day research. While modern science possesses a vast array of information on the chemistry of single ingredients, such as garlic or copper, less is known about combinations of plants. However, the chemicals from different plants can affect each other and testing existing combinations may reduce guesswork in future research.[10]

Medieval Medicine: Plants and Prejudice

Before we look at a range of nettle remedies, it may be important to consider if there is any value in medieval remedies at all. After all, ideas of illness and health are different between then and now, medieval 'science' was not based in labs, nor was it science in our modern sense.[11] For a long time, medieval medicine has been regarded as backward. In his seminal article on early

7 See examples in the entry for *netle* in McSparran and others, eds, *Middle English Compendium*; see also an Irish remedy for boiling nettle seed with salt and pepper in whey in order to ward off desire 'from clerics and other people' in Hayden, 'A Sixteenth-century Irish Collection of Remedies', pp. 256–57 and 267 (§ 10).

8 The project was funded by the Royal Society through an APEX Award and was carried out through the partnership of the University of Nottingham and the University of Warwick.

9 Furner-Pardoe and others, 'Anti-biofilm Efficacy'; Harrison and others, 'A 1,000-Year-Old Antimicrobial Remedy'; Connelly and others, 'Data Mining a Medieval Medical Text'.

10 See, for example, Cooper and Deakin, *Botanical Miracles*.

11 For early medieval concepts see Jolly, 'Magic, Miracle and Popular Practice' and Paz, 'Magic that Works'.

medieval medicine, Peregrine Horden points out the complexities of working with this period that led to such negative attitudes:

> The most basic terms we want to deploy — 'text', 'use', even 'medicine' — are all problematic. In addition, what we read often raises in acute form such vexed categories as 'magic', 'science', 'religion' and their interrelations.
>
> The outcome of all this is a field in which, by comparison with classical antiquity or the later Middle Ages, few scholars work; a field (I shall suggest) detached from wider currents in the historiography of the period; above all, a field that has no master narrative, however provisional, except a negative one defined in such prejudicial terms as 'decline' or 'lack', and coloured by nostalgia.[12]

Horden wrote this statement in the early decades of the twenty-first century. Since then there has been a vibrant interest in medicine in the medieval West as a lens through which we may explore the extent of knowledge in the period and understand people's reaction to illness and impairment.[13] In the study of remedies, the main focus has been on the transmission and cultural context of such remedies, but less on the question of whether they worked.[14] The treatment of medieval medical texts as literary documents of long-extinct knowledge may have been the established narrative at one time; however, over the last few decades, medieval medical scholarship has benefited from widespread re-evaluation of these texts through a scientific lens, including collaboration with scientists, who possess the expertise to see evidence of the scientific method in the texts of their medieval colleagues. Along such lines, Anne Van Arsdall, in her evaluation of medieval herbals, writes: 'Only twenty-first century hubris would dismiss as totally useless and ineffectual a more than 2000-year-old healing tradition, and with it, its texts and remedies.'[15] The reason why many of the early transcribers or commentators of manuscripts took a dim view of this material is because many of the remedies contain extra-medicinal aspects, such as prayers or actions which seem to serve no purpose at all.[16]

12 Horden, 'What's Wrong with Early Medieval Medicine?', p. 6.

13 There is a long list of scholars who have examined illness and impairment in early medieval England, e.g. Audrey Meaney, Debby Banham, Christine Voth, Jacqueline Fay, Maria D'Aronco, Conan Doyle, Erin Sweany, Rebecca Brackmann, Anne Van Arsdall, Renée Trilling, Megan Cavell, László Sándor Chardonnens, and Penelope Scott, to name but a few.

14 For tests of efficacy, see the works of Olivia Corcoran; Frances Watkins; Brennessel and others; the discussion in Cameron, *Anglo-Saxon Medicine*; and the introduction in Connelly and others, 'A Case Study of the Ancientbiotics Collaboration'.

15 Van Arsdall, 'Evaluating the Content of Medieval Herbals', p. 48. see also Falk, *The Light Ages*, in which the popular conception of the medieval period as a time of darkness and stagnation (awaiting salvation by the Renaissance) is challenged by an exploration of specific scientific achievements across medieval disciplines.

16 Joseph Payne declares in the 1903 Fitzpatrick Lecture (Payne, *English Medicine*, p. 57): 'It must be confessed that the Anglo-Saxons with all their zeal for learning and respect for the ancients, were unfortunate in the time of which they began to form their medical literature,

There is a vast corpus of medical texts that have survived from the long medieval period. Most of them have survived from 1000 onwards, and scholars, such as James Palmer and Claire Burridge, and Carine van Rhijn (Merovingian and Frankish texts), Diana Luft (Welsh medical manuscripts), Deborah Hayden and Siobhán Barrett (Irish sources) are currently making many of these sources accessible.[17] The medical texts of early medieval England form a group apart because of a careful incorporation of largely unnamed sources. While the direct influence of classical medicine is rather minor, as suggested by Debby Banham,[18] the influence of classical traditions of Antiquity, such as the works of Galen and Hippocrates, shaped at least some of the performance of medicine in the early Middle Ages and remained a significant influence until the twelfth century, when new Arabic-influenced medicine became available to Western Europeans. There are five major medical collections that have survived from early medieval England: Bald's *Leechbook*, named after Bald, who tells us in the colophon that he owned the book, and *Leechbook* III in the same manuscript (London, BL, MS Royal 12 D XVII). Further there is *Lacnunga* (London, BL, MS Harley 585), as well as the *Old English Herbarium* and *Medicina de Quadrupedibus* (London, BL, MS Cotton Vitellius C III)[19] and the late Old English *Peri Didaxeon* (London, BL, MS Harley 6258b). While these are the main medical manuscripts, remedies also survive in other texts, occasionally even copied into the margins of different manuscripts.[20]

---

namely the period from the ninth to the eleventh century. It was the time when European medicine stood at its very lowest level …' Even the prominent editor of Old English remedies, Oswald Cockayne, although giving some credit to the people who produced the manuscripts, wrote in the preface to his second volume of *Leechdoms, Wortcunning, and Starcraft of Early England* (p. xix) that 'Here a leech calmly sits down to compose a not unlearned book, treating of many serious diseases, and assigning for them something he hopes will cure them.' The wording chosen by Cockayne for his translations, as shown by Anne Van Arsdall, did not help, since it creates the impression that 'medieval medicine was frivolous': see *Medieval Herbal Remedies*, trans. by Van Arsdall, p. 109. For a re-evaluation of Cockayne, see Van Arsdall, 'Medical Training in Anglo-Saxon England'.

17 See e.g. *Medieval Welsh Medical Texts*, ed. and trans. by Luft. Claire Burridge's recent project 'Crossroads' pursued an 'in-depth analysis of the surviving early medieval Latin medical recipes found outside of established classical and late antique recipe collections': Crossroads <https://www.earlymedievalmedicine.com/> [accessed 24 May 2024]; see also her paper 'Incense and Medicine'. Burridge is also a co-applicant with Carine van Rhijn and PI James Palmer the Corpus of Early Medieval Latin Medicine (CEMLM) project: <https://www.thebritishacademy.ac.uk/projects/corpus-of-early-medieval-latin-medicine-cemlm/>.

18 Banham, 'Dun, Oxa and Pliny the Great Physician', p. 62.

19 The text survives in four manuscripts: the others are London, BL, MS Harley 585; BL, MS Harley 6258b; Oxford, Bodleian, MS Hatton 76. The manuscripts were edited as a parallel edition: *The Old English Herbarium and Medicina De Quadrupedibus*, ed. by de Vriend.

20 The manuscripts and the connections between versions, as well as between the Old English texts and their sources have been studied by a range of scholars, among them D'Aronco, 'How "English" is Anglo-Saxon Medicine?'; Meaney, 'Variant Versions'; *Medieval Herbal Remedies*, trans. by Van Arsdall; *Medical Writings*, ed. and trans. by Niles and D'Aronco; Doyle,

Monastic lists show the extent of medical texts which once existed in Europe.[21] This wealth of sources is due to a renaissance of book production in the Carolingian empire. King Alfred of Wessex (848–899 CE), who emulated much of the cultural climate of the Carolingian court, encouraged the production of texts. The proximity of Bald's *Leechbook* to other texts from the time of Alfred has been pointed out by scholars such as Audrey Meaney and, most recently, Emily Kesling.[22] The use of a large range of medical texts from various traditions suggests that the text was compiled in an environment that provided access to many different sources, which may have been the Old Minster at Winchester, or Worcester.[23] The compilation of medicine in an Alfredian environment indicates that the art of healing was also considered among the 'ða ðe niedbeðearfosta sien eallum monnum to wiotonne' ([books] most necessary to know for everyone).[24]

Lacnunga is a collection of vernacular remedies dated to the late tenth to the mid-eleventh century. The text does not just include remedies for humans but also for their livestock. More than any other of the Old English medical texts, *Lacnunga* was tarred with the label of superstition. Talbot declares it to be a 'rambling collection of about two hundred prescriptions, remedies and charms, derived from many sources [...]; it is a whole world apart from the scientific work of Byrhtferth, the monk of Ramsey'. *Lacnunga*, he continues, is the 'final pathological disintegration of Greek medical thought'.[25] This negative assessment belies the complexities of the text, which is a compilation of vernacular herbal remedies (drinks, poultices, and ointments) with the addition of more esoteric elements, ranging from dung to amulets and chants.

The idea that medieval medicine, which is often more holistic in its approach, is using prayers and formulas which may involve more action than just the interchange between physician and patient, is also not that new.[26] The

---

'Anglo-Saxon Medicine and Disease'; Cameron, *Anglo-Saxon Medicine*, pp. 35–58; Banham, 'Dun, Oxa and Pliny the Great Physician'; and Meaney, 'The Practice of Medicine in England'.

21 D'Aronco, 'How "English" was Anglo-Saxon Medicine?', especially pp. 35–37.

22 Cameron, *Anglo-Saxon Medicine*, p. 30; Kesling, *Medical Texts*, pp. 47–48. Reasons for the association are the dialect, but also a direct textual reference to the king which describes a remedy sent from Elias, Patriarch of Jerusalem, to Alfred. While scholars, such as Christine Voth, have regarded this passage as an addition, Kesling (*Medical Texts*, p. 47) points out that it is nevertheless a purposeful adaptation.

23 Meaney, 'Variant Versions', has noted that 'Bald's Leechbook' contains a range of remedies which are also known from other sources; this means that the compiler worked from a bank of texts which were in circulation at this time. Nokes, 'The Several Compilers', has identified a number of different contributors. On the basis of stylistic differences, he assumes that the manuscript is the result of at least two different compilers.

24 King Alfred, *King Alfred's West-Saxon Version of Gregory's Pastoral Care*, ed. and trans. by Sweet, p. 6.

25 Talbot, *Medicine in Medieval England*, p. 23.

26 There has been a lively discussion about the nature of charms and some radical rethinking of their role and purpose. See, for example, Olsan, 'The Language of Charms' and 'Charms and Prayers'; Arthur, *'Charms', Liturgies, and Secret Rites*, and Batten, '"Lazarus, Come Forth"'.

Enlightenment already saw a shift in which earlier practices were regarded with suspicion. An example where we can observe a change in attitude towards what are considered extra-medical elements are the instructions for preparing a cold and cough remedy from a late-seventeenth-century medical text, which captures the tension between the pre-Reformation remedy and the current understanding:

> Let it seeth together by the space that one may say the Psalme of Miserere mei Deus, (that is, the one and fiftieth Psalme in English, called in those dayes one of the seven Penitential Psalms: but now penitency is out of fashion. The Psalm will not hurt you, if you think it not too much superstition to read it; neither will your Reading it do the Psalm any hurt at all; nor your letting it alone, will not alter its Religion.)[27]

By judging such medical methods as superstitious, the reader may miss an important aspect of the preparation, which is time. As reflected in the seventeenth-century explanation, in a period without standardized or reliable time-keeping methods, practitioners could use well-known conventions, such as the Penitential Psalms or prayers, to measure the time required for manufacturing processes or the application of certain plasters or ointment. While it is perfectly possible that prayers or psalms were regarded as adding a special layer of efficacy by including spiritual assistance,[28] such formulas also have a pragmatic aspect. Similarly, poetry, formulaic utterances, and symbols or mnemonic devices which are more akin to poetry may also serve important functions. For example, in a largely oral society, the use of known texts may be a mnemonic aid with which practitioners and their apprentices could store, teach, and learn knowledge.[29] Secondly, these methods may contain critical information about active ingredient concentration or extraction principles. Many bioactive plant compounds are only active in freshly-crushed material or vary depending on harvest time,[30] and extraction method and temperature play an important role in efficacy of the recipe, such as soaking in cold water (artemisinin from *Artemisia annua* is a high-profile example).[31] The new dialogue between various disciplines, which has looked at historical medical texts as potential sources of active ingredients, has led to novel investigations

27 Moulton, *The Compleat Bone-Setter*, p. 127.

28 See, for example, Brackmann, '"It Will Help Him Wonderfully"'; we are indebted to Dr Brackmann for sharing an early draft of her essay. See also Lisa Weston, 'Language of Magic', who has examined the structure of the *Wið færsticce* charm. She underlines that rhetorical elements underpin the image of the power of the healer and thus the potency of the charm.

29 Junqi Zhang has explored the various linguistic/stylistic devices which suggest different addressees for remedies in the *Lacnunga* for his MRes dissertation, 'A Real-life Picture of Medieval Healing'.

30 See, for example, the discussion of *H. perforatum* in Watkins and others, 'Anglo-Saxon Pharmacopoeia Revisited'.

31 Tu, 'The Discovery of Artemisinin (*Qinghaosu*)'; Su and Miller, 'The Discovery of Artemisinin'.

of the processes behind such recipe constructions.[32] Pivotal to this research is the understanding that there are shared traditions and a transmission of medical knowledge across culture and time. While the remedies are clearly the products of their time, a comparative approach may point us to practical applications of novel ingredient combinations, which in turn may be the inspiration for new treatments.

Grasping the Nettle

Medieval medicine was not stagnant. It was influenced by classical knowledge, and there was a steady influence of new medical thinking via a range of sources across time.[33] Currently, nettles appear in a range of preparations from many traditions for the treatment of skin diseases, urinary disorders, respiratory diseases, arthritis, cancer, blood pressure, anaemia, bleeding, circulatory problems, and in consumer products for cosmetic applications.[34] Nettles have a long history of use in food and drink (e.g., tea, bread, cheeses, beers) and topical cosmetic products (e.g., shampoo, ointments, soap), as well as garment production (fibres). Given the widespread medical and culinary use of nettles, and an existing body of scientific pilot studies, nettles seemed to be a good candidate to explore in more detail.

Nettles appear frequently in a variety of recipes over this long period. Stinging nettle species (*Urtica* spp.) have a broad geographical distribution. These include the common nettle (*U. dioica*) and other *Urtica* species (such as *U. urens, U. pilulifera, U. membranacea*). The medieval texts in our dataset also mention dead-nettles (white or red), which may be defined as *Lamium* spp. The ubiquity of nettles may be gathered from other forms of evidence, such as place-names with nettle elements. Ann Cole shows that nettle names occur especially on routeways, and that the examples with Old English word formation are often situated on old Roman roads.[35] She speculates that the place-names indicate stopping places and areas where animal stock were tethered, since their excretions provided an excellent base for 'a luxuriant patch of nettles'.[36] The fact that nettles grow very well in certain conditions

---

32 It should be noted that scientific investigations of the efficacy of plant-based traditional or historical medicine is well established outside a European context.

33 For an overview of influences in early medieval England, see Cameron, 'The Sources of Medical Knowledge', and also the forthcoming book by Conan Doyle, *The Reception of Latin Medicine*, which will give a comprehensive overview of sources.

34 See, for instance, Kılıç, Yıldız, and Kılıç, 'Traditional Uses of Medicinal Plants'; Kregiel, Pawlikowska, and Antolak, 'Urtica spp.'; Kazancı, Oruç, and Mosulishvili, 'Medicinal Ethnobotany'; Ghedira, Goetz, and Le Jeune, 'Urtica dioica L., Urtica urens et/ou hybrides (Urticaceae)'; Vidyarthi, Samant, and Sharma, 'Traditional and Indigenous Uses of Medicinal Plants'.

35 Cole, 'The Use of *Netel* in Place-names'; Cole, 'The Use of ON *nata* in Place-Names'.

36 Cole, 'The Use of *Netel* in Place-Names', p. 54.

cannot have escaped people in the Middle Ages, and there is some indication that plants were collected from particular places because they contain more effective ingredients. Soil conditions can influence aspects of plant chemistry. Certain places may have produced noticeable variation in plant characteristics, which is perhaps why we are occasionally given instructions of where to collect species. The training of the medieval leech therefore may have included cumulative learning based on existing knowledge of poems and prayers, botany and geography. It may have also included specialized suppliers, as well as practitioners. For example, a remedy against lung disease in cattle in *Lacnunga* combines plants, making crosses from *cassuc* (hard grass, sedge) and a whole range of religious texts, including litanies and the Paternoster. A plant must be collected from an open space within a settled area: 'þær wexeð blaco bergean' (where black berries grow).[37] Soil conditions can make a difference to the chemical components of plants. Such instructions are helpful for the person collecting the plant materials and show perhaps that the maker of such a remedy was not necessarily the person who gathered the ingredients. This also suggests that there was at least a basic knowledge of the chemical advantages or disadvantages of different soil conditions. After all, the majority of people who lived in early medieval England were in contact with farming. It seems that certain conditions required nettles from specific places.[38] For example, consider the Old English charm *Wið færsticce* (Against a sudden pain), in which we are asked to get red nettles which grow through a building ('seo ræde netele ðe þurh ærn inwyxð').[39] Such instructions, although not very frequent, may have been based on pragmatic considerations: they are easy to obtain, but may have also been seen as inheriting some qualities of the place where they came from. For example, one remedy against *þeor*, which appears to be a kind of skin condition, in the eleventh-century *Lacnunga* specifies that the mint needs to have grown 'be þære ea' (by the water).[40] The compilers of medical texts seem to be aware that the gathering of plants may be time-consuming; a set of remedies to aid digestion in Bald's *Leechbook* describes the plants as 'þas wyrta sindon eac besta to þon ond eac be geatna' (These plants are each best for that and [are able to] be obtained).[41] Among the plants suggested are nettles boiled in water and salted, which is a combination that occurs in

37 *Medical Writings*, ed. and trans. by Niles and D'Aronco, p. 498. Other instructions include 'ivy grown on a stone on the earth': see *Medical Writings*, ed. and trans. by Niles and D'Aronco, p. 466.

38 For the use of nettles as fertilizer among other things, see di Virglio and others, 'The Potential of Stinging Nettle (*Urtica dioica L.*)'.

39 *Medical Writings*, ed. and trans. by Niles and D'Aronco, p. 494. Niles and D'Aronco translate *þurh* as 'around', which is more sensical, but given that this is one of the more complex remedies which includes a charm, it may as well be an abandoned or ruined building.

40 *Medical Writings*, ed. and trans. by Niles and D'Aronco, p. 502; for *þeor*, see Cameron, 'On *þeor* and *þeoradl*'.

41 London, BL, MS Royal 12 D XVII, fol. 85^{r}; *Leechdoms*, ed. and trans. by Cockayne, II, p. 226.

a range of wound-healing remedies from the Old English translation of the *Herbarium* and later medieval medical texts.

Exploring Nettles Remedies

As a starting point, our study aimed to trace and explore a dataset of nettle-based remedies from early- and late-medieval sources.[42] This approach allowed for comparison of the combination of ingredients and structure of the recipes. Particularly in the early medieval English remedies, there are plant names whose identification is not clear. A good example is *cropleac,* which appears to be an *Allium* species,[43] but it is not clear which one. Dialect variation and available sources seem to have resulted in some variety of names being assigned to plants.[44] Despite rationale for confidence in identifying certain species, the source language was used in the dataset to acknowledge the ambiguity and possible pitfalls in translating medieval plant names to modern scientific classifications.[45] Unlike many other plants, nettles have not experienced a great deal of human interference by breeding and widespread cultivation. Many modern plants have been cultivated across time, and it is very possible that this process has altered their chemical signatures. In considering possible genetic diversity in historical plants in comparison to modern plants, it is unlikely that modern wild nettles differ greatly from their predecessors as they have

42 This dataset focused on early- and late-medieval English with some additional Latin- and Welsh-language sources.

43 We consulted the *DOE*: 'a plant, a member of the *Allium* family, perhaps crow garlic'; we dismissed a secondary gloss from the Cotton Cleopatra glosses, which renders *cropleac* as *serpyllum* (thyme, wild thyme), *Dictionary of Old English Plant Names*, ed. by Bierbäumer and others: *Allium porrum* L., leek, Winter-Lauch? *Allium vineale* L., crow garlic, Kochs Lauch? *Allium sativum* L, garlic, Knoblauch? *Allium ascalonicum* L., shallot, Schalotte <http://oldenglish-plantnames.org/> and more recently Sauer and Kubaschewski, *Planting the Seeds of Knowledge*. Pettit, in his glossary to the *Lacnunga* (see *Anglo-Saxon Remedies*) thinks it is *Allium porrum*, 'leek'.

44 We may consider the plant *elehtre*, which according to the *DOE* occurs in sixty-two instances, but which may be anything from lupins (in medical texts) to mandrakes (in glosses). One of the important aspects to remember is that some, but not all, medical texts were transmitted in different manuscripts. Some go back to sources which are lost, others are derived from different manuscripts. Early medieval manuscripts have been described as florilegia, in contrast to later medieval medical texts, which were the result of university-based medicine: see Wallis, 'The Experience of the Book', esp. pp. 105–07. Aside from the fact that the context was collated from different sources, it leaves the question of whether the scribe or compiler made efforts to regularize plant names. There is also the question of variant versions of manuscripts. For an excellent overview, see D'Aronco, 'The Botanical Lexicon', esp. pp. 27–28.

45 For a detailed discussion of the challenges in processing medieval datasets see Connelly and others 'A Case Study of the Ancientbiotics Collaboration' and Connelly and others 'Data Mining a Medieval Medical Text'; see also Olalla, 'A Plea for Middle English Botanical Synonyma' and Grund, 'Editing Alchemical Texts in Middle English'.

not been widely cultivated or bred like other crops. The main cultivation or breeding effort, a recent development, appears to be to identify clones for increased fibre content in the natural textile industry.[46]

The early medieval dataset includes seventy-three recipes in total from five Latin sources and seven Old English sources ranging from the ninth to the twelfth century. The later medieval dataset includes thirteen Welsh recipes from four manuscripts[47] and fifty-three Middle English recipes from fourteen sources ranging from the thirteenth to the fifteenth century. This gives a final dataset of 139 recipes from thirty sources with a date range over seven centuries of time.[48] Types of remedies across early- and late-medieval sources include poultices, plasters, suppositories, gargles, drinks, salves, ointments, and external cleansing washes for many disease conditions such as dog bites, inflammation, post-surgical swellings, pustules, restraining blood, healing and cleaning wounds, swellings and abscesses of the mouth and throat, aches and pains, gout, dropsy, fevers, colic, cough, respiratory disorders, urinary disorders, 'leprosy' and skin disorders, bruises, and broken bones. The remedies typically specify the part of the plant being used, such as juice, seeds, root, powder, leaves, flowers, or the whole plant.[49] For experimental investigations, we chose to focus on nettle-based applications for wound care in combination with vinegar, or fats and oils due to the frequent occurrence in this specific dataset.

Often the nettles are combined with just one ingredient, such as salt or oil, and applied to the treatment site. Nettle leaves and salt are prescribed for deep wounds in the twelfth-century *Anglicanus ortus* of Henry of Huntingdon.[50] It appears that the leaves were used for plasters. An example is found in the ninth-century Carolingian *Lorscher Arzneibuch* (Bamberg, Staatsbibliothek, MS Msc. Med. 1, fol. 34^{r}), where crushed nettles are laid on the affected area against chills. The *Arzneibuch* is the oldest extant medical manuscript in Germany and the 482 Latin remedies cover a multitude of differing ailments, as well as an extraordinary defence of medicine in folios 1^{r}–5^{r}. Nettles, salt, and

---

46 Many thanks to Dr Charlotte Allender for discussing plant genetic diversity and nettle cultivation with us (conclusions here are our own); see also Di Virgilio and others, 'The Potential of Stinging Nettle' and Vogl and Hartl, 'Production and Processing'.

47 With thanks to Diana Luft for sharing her translations of these recipes, now available in her *Medieval Welsh Medical Texts*.

48 Limitations of the dataset include all recipes and sources that were not included in this study. The datasets are necessarily limited to sources available for access during the timeframe of the study. The outcomes and directions for future research presented here represent the results from this specific study and expansion of the dataset may reveal additional information not captured by this study.

49 Types and form of remedies also cited in Harrison and others, 'An Assessment of the Evidence for Antibacterial Activity'.

50 Henry of Huntingdon, *Anglicanus ortus*, ed. and trans. by Black, p. 270. The same combination of salt and nettles is also prescribed for sprains, abscesses, dog bites, and tumours.

oil appear as a combination in the *Old English Herbarium*, but this remedy is a translation of a Latin source, the *Pseudo-Apuleius*.[51] In other wound remedies, nettle and woad tops are pounded with butter and strained, and then salt is added.[52] Nettles are used as suppositories to help with conditions which appear to be connected to menorrhagia. For example, the *Old English Herbarium* recommends that nettles pounded well in a mortar with added honey should be put on moist, well-teaselled wool and 'laid under her' on the day of her period.[53] A combination of nettles and myrrh is suggested as a suppository in Henry of Huntingdon's *Anglicanus ortus*.[54] Dead-nettles, boiled with butter, *merscmergyllan*, and figwort are recommended for a person suffering from skin eruptions in the *Lacnunga*.[55] The use of nettles as a plaster continues into the later medieval period. For instance, the Middle English translation of *De viribus herbarum* advises:

> Stampe nettle leues with salte & make þer of a plastre & yt wol clense foule woundes & do good to bocches[.] Thys plastre ys good ayenst houndes bytyngge & cancres & þe syknes þat men callen parodyda.[56]
>
> (Stamp nettle leaves with salt and make thereof a plaster and it will cleanse foul wounds and do good to bocches. This plaster is good against hound bites and cancres and the sickness that men call parotida.)

---

51 *The Old English Herbarium*, ed. by de Vriend, pp. 222–23. We should not think of the *Herbarium* as just one text, since it has been transmitted in thirteen different manuscripts, some only partial. De Vriend's edition is based on two Old English manuscripts (MS V: London, BL, Cotton MS Vitellius C III and O: London, BL, Harley MS 6258 B) with additional material from other versions, as well as one parallel Latin version which is a composite of four manuscripts.

52 *Leechdoms*, ed. and trans. by Cockayne, p. 94; Doyle, 'Anglo-Saxon Medicine and Disease', p. 102 (Recipe I.38.17).

53 *Herbarium*, ed. by de Vriend, pp. 224–25: 'Wið wifes flewsan genim þas ylcan wyrte (nettle) on mortere wel gepunude oðþæt heo wel liþi sy, geyc þonne þærto sumne dæl huniges, nim syþþan wæt wulle, ond þa wel getæsede, smyre ðonne þa geweald mid þam læcedome ond syþþan hyne þam wife gesyle, þæt heo hyne hyre under gelecge' (Against a woman's flow: take the same herb [nettles] and pound it well in a mortar until it is very soft. Add to it some honey, then take moist wool that is well teaselled, smear the genitals with the remedy and then give it to the woman that she lays it under her). The remedy does not occur in all versions, and it is not quite clear what 'lays under' means, but it concurs with *supponas* (lay under) in the Latin variants. Wool becomes softer by teaselling.

54 Henry of Huntingdon, *Anglicus ortus*, ed. and trans. by Black, p. 270. Not every remedy against menstrual problems is necessarily external. In the *Lorscher Arzneibuch*, fol. 42[r], a complex remedy that contains all kinds of different plants, from nettles to mugwort to rue, suggests that the preparation should be ingested with wine for three days while following a diet of only boiled meat and little seasoning.

55 *Medical Writings*, ed. and trans. by Niles and D'Aronco, p. 91: the salve is put on after the person has bathed the swelling in cold water and lanced it.

56 *The Middle English Version of De Viribus Herbarum*, ed. by Calle-Martin and Miranda-García, p. 75. Translation authors' own.

A series of recipes from the later medieval hunting text *Master of Game*, for the treatment of 'men or bestes þat be byt with wode houndes',[57] contains an intriguing combination of medicinal ingredients:

> Þer is anoþer helpe, for men may [make] sause of salt, and vinegre, and strong garlyk ypilled and ystaumpe[d], and neteles, togidere and also hoot as it may be suffered, to ley vpon þe bityng. And þis is a gode medicine and a trewe, for it hath be preued. And euery day sholde it be leide vpon þe bityng ii. tymes, also hoot as it may be soffered, into þe tyme þat it be hool, or elles bi ix. daies. And ʒit þer is anoþer medicine better þan al þe oþir. Take lekes, and strong garlek, and chibols, and rywe, and neteles, and hakke hem smal with a knyf. And þan mengle hem with oile d'olif and vinegre, and boile hem togider. And þan take al þe herbes, also hoot as þei may be suffered, and ley vpon þe wounde, euery day [ii.] tymes til þe wound be wel hool, or at þe lest bi ix. daies.[58]
>
> > (There is another help, for men may make sauce of salt, vinegar and strong garlic pulled and stamped, and nettles together and as hot as it may be suffered to lay upon the bite. And this is a good medicine and a true, for it hath been proved, and every day should it be laid upon the biting twice, as hot as it can be suffered, until the time when it be whole, or else by nine days. And yet there is another medicine better than all the other. Take leeks and strong garlic and chives and rue and nettles and hack them small with a knife, and then mingle them with olive oil and vinegar, and boil them together, and then take all the herbs, also as hot as they may be suffered, and lay them on the wound every day twice, till the wound be healed, or at least for nine days.)

Such combinations containing salt, vinegar, garlic, leeks, and medicinal plants, which are ground, chopped, or boiled together, and plastered on a wound (along with temperature and timing instructions) are immediately interesting from an antimicrobial perspective. The acetic acid in vinegar is very well known to have antimicrobial activity at low concentration.[59] The antimicrobial activity of oils or fats (butter, lard, etc.), which often appear in the early medieval examples, are not well studied, and may be functioning primarily as palliative and binding agents or to absorb or restrain blood.

In modern natural product development, nettles appear largely in items intended for blood, hair, or skin care, which is not too far removed from its medieval precedent. In our systematic review of the scientific literature on the antimicrobial activity of nettles, it is notable how few authors discuss how the

57 McNelis, 'The Uncollated Manuscripts', l. 1440.

58 McNelis, 'The Uncollated Manuscripts', ll. 1455–66. Translation from *The Master of Game*, pp. 89–90.

59 Bjarnsholt and others, 'Antibiofilm Properties of Acetic Acid'; see also Halstead and others, 'The Antibacterial Activity of Acetic Acid'.

plant is prepared in traditional or historical methods or if that informed their choices of plant parts and extraction methods.[60] This is important because the plant part, cold or hot extraction, and method of preparation (e.g., boiling plant matter in water or pounding plants with fats, oils, or solvents) will extract different agents and produce different effects. In previous studies of natural product potential, following the historical recipe instructions has proved critical in observing successful activity (artemisinin and Bald's eyesalve are examples).[61]

The Ankaferd Blood Stopper (ABS, Ankaferd Health Products Ltd, Turkey) is based on a traditional combination of *Thymus vulgaris* (dried extract), *Glycyrrhiza glabra* (dried leaf extract), *Vitis vinifera* (dried leaf extract), *Alpinia officinarum* (dried leaf extract), and *Urtica dioica* (dried root extract).[62] In Turkey, it has been approved as a medicinal product for the management of external haemorrhage and bleeding in dental surgery. It is also licensed as a haemostatic agent in Turkey and Bosnia-Herzegovina.[63] Similarly, the skin care and wellness product company Weleda (established 1921) sells a product made of stinging nettle, wild strawberry, and honey 'historically used to support normal blood formation'.[64] The Ankaferd product is used for the management of bleeding in medical contexts (and has received approval for patient use in some countries), whereas the Weleda dietary supplement is advertised to consumers as a 'fortifying' and 'strengthening' agent for the blood, but it is unclear which historical or traditional practice inspired this product, nor does it appear to be connected with any scientific analysis.[65]

There is a limited body of research investigating the plant fibres or leaves of stinging nettle for antimicrobial activity, wound healing, and anti-inflammatory

60 Harrison and others, 'An Assessment of the Evidence for Antibacterial Activity'; the summary of the study given here is intended to be relevant to a humanities audience and interested readers are encouraged to consult complementary publications for full details. For those unfamiliar with the methodology of systematic reviews, see e.g. Khan and others, 'Five Steps to Conducting a Systematic Review'; Page and others, 'Updating Guidance for Reporting Systematic Reviews'; and Cheung and Vijayakumar, 'A Guide to Conducting a Meta-Analysis'.

61 Harrison and others, 'A 1,000-Year-Old Antimicrobial Remedy'; Tu, 'The Discovery of Artemisinin (Qinghaosu)'; also Connelly and others, 'A Case Study of the Ancientbiotics Collaboration'; Abdallah and others, 'Past Mastering of Metal Transformation'; Pitchon and others, 'How History can Help Present Research'.

62 It should be noted that of the studies identified in the systematic review concerning Ankaferd, none of them evaluated *U. dioica* independently from the other medicinal plants. The role *U. dioica* may be playing in this combination is unclear.

63 Kurt and others, 'Ankaferd Blood Stopper'; Chopra and Sivaraman, 'Ankaferd Blood Stopper'; Balcik and others, 'A Placebo-Controlled, Randomized, Double-Blinded, Cross-Over Phase-I Clinical Study'.

64 Weleda, 'Fragaria Urtica Compound'.

65 While Weleda products remain popular, it should be pointed out that they are not based in scientific or clinical trials. For instance, Oliver Rautenberg, described it as 'Pseudomedizin' <https://anthroposophie.home.blog/weleda-2/> [accessed 28 October 2021].

properties.[66] One example is a PhD project at Maastricht University to develop a novel dressing from the fibres and bioactive compounds of *U. dioica* for the treatment of chronic wounds.[67] In modern natural products for consumers, nettles appear frequently in hair care products and anti-dandruff shampoo. Based on uses in traditional Iranian medicine, one study (2015) identified by the systematic review examined ethanolic extracts of dried *U. dioica* leaves against clinical isolates of dandruff-causing fungal species, *Malassezia globosa, Malassezia furfur, Malassezia slooffiae*.[68] The authors found the *U. dioica* extracts were not as successful as other herbal extracts against the fungi. Nettles also appear in early medieval hair and beauty care. For example, the *Leiden Leechbook*, a small ninth-century collection of remedies in a number of languages, contains a remedy against lice which combines the roots, bark, and seeds of many medicinal plants, including *lanith*, which has been identified as either linseed or nettle.[69] The *Anglicanus ortus* recommends nettle seed juice against hair loss.[70] In the later medieval dataset examined here, nettles appear most frequently with wound care, and where nettle is applied to the head, it is to remove hair.[71]

Summary of Results

As the select examples of modern products above suggest, there is a tempting continuity in the applications of nettles across time and cultures. However, this is an under-studied area and the examples given here are not evidential; therefore, a systematic review was performed to establish a better picture of the research landscape and to determine if any conclusions are evident in the literature.[72] The systematic review shows that extracts of nettle leaves, oils, and stems continue to be used in a variety of contexts for antibacterial activity against various Gram-positive and Gram-negative bacteria, including species that cause antibiotic-resistant infections today, and antifungal activity against a range of species, such as *Candida* spp. and *Malassezia* spp. The majority of papers reviewed present pilot data from traditional remedies.

---

66 Such as Sabir and Ünal, 'The Using of Nettle Fiber in Towel Production', and Bouassida and others, 'Exploring the Urtica dioica Leaves'.

67 The project is currently on hold: see 'Novel Wound Dressing Derived from Stinging Nettles', Maastricht University, accessed September 2021 <https://www.maastrichtuniversity.nl/novel-wound-dressing-derived-stinging-nettles>.

68 Nazeri and others, 'Antifungal Activity of Herbal Extracts'.

69 Leiden, Univ. of Leiden, MS Vossianus lat. fol. 96A; see *The Leiden Leechbook*, ed. and trans. by Falileyev and Owen, pp. 9–10. For early medieval hair and beauty care, see Lee, 'The Art of Looking Good'.

70 Henry of Huntingdon, *Anglicanus ortus*, ed. and trans. by Black, p. 270.

71 See for instance *Medieval Welsh Medical Texts*, ed. and trans. by Luft, p. 256 (Recipe 9/47).

72 This summary is intended to benefit a humanities audience; for full details see Harrison and others, 'An Assessment of the Evidence for Antibacterial Activity'.

In summary, the published studies considered by the review varied in quality and used a wide variety of *Urtica* species, pathogen species, preparation methods, techniques and assay methods. The review did not find strong evidence for antibacterial activity. All of the studies used dried plant materials and no studies prepared nettles in vinegar or weak acid or in fats or oils, which are common combinations in our remedy dataset. This gap in the literature was addressed by new antibacterial tests of extracts of fresh *U. dioica* leaves prepared in vinegar, butter, or olive oil against the common opportunistic pathogens *Pseudomonas aeruginosa* and *Staphylococcus aureus*. The results of these tests found no evidence of antibacterial activity. Our systematic review and additional experimental data led us to conclude that there is no strong evidence for nettles containing molecules with clinically useful antimicrobial activity. However, the possibility that nettles do contain effective antimicrobial molecules cannot be excluded by this study, and we did not address any immunomodulatory potential. There is some evidence suggesting nettles may be more effective as an anti-inflammatory or immunomodulatory agent over antimicrobial activity.[73] Certainly, the continuity between historical and modern applications in the areas of skin and wound care (infection prevention and bleeding control) and cosmetic/hair care invites comparison; however, conclusions prove evasive as the systematic review shows that there is limited capacity to make meaningful comparisons.

In considering the frequency of appearance in traditional medicine globally and the diversity in methods applied by modern researchers, the systematic review revealed a series of questions that could be informative for further research purposes. Coming out of this work are questions about extraction temperature, plant parts, fresh or dry plant material (all the papers in the systematic review used dry materials, usually in aqueous or ethanolic preparations), lipophilic extract potential, and the method of preparation. For example, specification of plant juice is a frequent occurrence in medieval nettles remedies, but what does this translate to in a laboratory context? In Middle English, juice in a medical sense can mean the actual plant juice derived from squeezing or pounding the plant matter, but also the 'juice' obtained by boiling the herb/plant in water or an infusion or a mixture of ground herbs and liquids.[74]

When preparing fresh nettles for the experimental work in this study, by pounding the plant material with water or vinegar using a mortar and pestle, the researchers observed that the nettle leaves were highly absorbent: water or vinegar very quickly soaked up into the leaves, leaving no visible liquid in the mortar. Only very tiny (sub-ml) amounts of liquid could be released by attempts to squeeze the material or by pounding with the pestle once the liquid had been absorbed. This is an interesting outcome in considering if nettle in

73 For example, Johnson and others, 'Lipophilic Stinging Nettle Extracts'.

74 See entry *jus* in McSparran and others, eds, *Middle English Compendium*.

itself has a direct medicinal purpose or rather if such a readily available (and perhaps otherwise undesirable) plant made a good binding agent or vehicle for conveying medicinal preparations in poultices. For dangerous wounds (infected or at risk of infection), some remedies specify constant attention with application of medicines multiple times a day for many days. The ability to absorb and deliver a large volume of medicinal liquids (such as vinegar) to an injury or infection site may make nettles an excellent wound dressing. After considering our initial experimental results, Frances Watkins, medical herbalist, performed further experiments to extract nettle juice based on her practical experience of plant preparations. Using tools that would have been available to a medieval practitioner, she was able to extract 12.5ml of juice from 50g of nettle tops (freshly harvested) which did not require straining. She suggests that medieval practitioners may have expressed the nettle juice, poured it into a glass container, and then added oil over the top as means of preservation.[75]

The fats and oils so frequently combined with nettles may be functioning primarily as palliative vehicles to facilitate medicines or to restrain bleeding in a wound. However, there is a small body of studies that show lipophilic extracts are suggestive of anti-inflammatory activity, and this may be worth exploring in more detail to determine if there are effects beyond ointment construction. For instance, results from a 2013 study by Johnson and others, 'suggest that using lipophilic extracts of stinging nettle may be more effective than traditional tinctures (water, methanol, ethanol) in clinical evaluations for the treatment of inflammatory disorders especially arthritis'.[76] Only the antimicrobial nature of nettles was considered for the systematic review and experimental investigations. It may be worth considering anti-inflammatory or immuno-enhancing capabilities or medicinal plant combinations in future work.

Dead-nettles occur with frequency throughout the medieval remedies assessed by the dataset, but they were beyond the scope of experimental work and the systematic review performed in this study. However, *Lamium* spp. could be the subject of a whole separate experimental study. A cursory investigation of the major databases shows there is almost no scientific research on dead-nettles. Finally, it may also be worth noting that, as in the medieval recipe examples above, there are known antimicrobial medicinal plants being combined with the nettles in our dataset of medieval remedies. It is possible that additional biological activity is achieved when nettles are combined with other natural products, due to additive or synergistic interactions, as has been demonstrated in other combinations of natural products.[77]

75 Personal communication, 24 March 2022.

76 Johnson and others, 'Lipophilic Stinging Nettle Extracts', p. 143; see also Riehemann and others, 'Plant Extracts from Stinging Nettle'.

77 Caesar and Cech, 'Synergy and Antagonism in Natural Product Extracts'; Harrison and others, 'A 1,000-Year-Old Antimicrobial Remedy', Harrison and others, 'An assessment of the Evidence for Antibacterial Activity'.

Concluding Thoughts

The experimental results from our study of nettle preparations with single ingredients (vinegar, butter, or olive oil) showed that these treatments did not extract anything antibacterial from the nettles. However, the nettles acted as a highly effective sponge and delivery agent for vinegar, a well-known bactericidal agent: 'The nettles had no effect on viable bacteria numbers themselves, but were able to carry sufficient vinegar with them to completely eradicate the bacterial populations (all replicates of nettle + vinegar and vinegar treatments for both species had viable cell numbers below the limit of detection by plating).'[78] As many of the remedies identified in the dataset of historical medicines are external preparations or poultices, it is possible that nettles were used for their absorbent qualities and ability to deliver large volumes of medicinal liquid topically to a wound. There is an open door for many other avenues of research to consider further historical and traditional preparation methods, e.g. lipophilic extracts and anti-inflammatory capabilities; *Lamium* spp. in both historical and modern contexts; nettle species in combination with other medicinal plants; and efficacy claims of current consumer nettle-based products for blood, hair, wound, and skin care.

Returning to Strabo's question: we may need to have a bit more patience with our nettles. The search for new antimicrobials in historical or traditional sources is a well-established endeavour, but, as shown by our results, the search often yields pilot data that requires more extensive replication and investigation. Ethnopharmacological research has shown that plant medicines have clinically significant bioactivity, and a recent systematic review found that 50 per cent of the US Food and Drug Administration-approved antibacterial agents over the last four decades are from or derived from natural products,[79] while other ingredients may have been favoured simply as a structural component of a remedy. This may also be the case for many of the medieval recipes. Medieval remedies may offer some 'shortcuts' in the search for potential ingredient combinations, but they are also products of another time. Not only may plants have evolved from their medieval ancestors, but it is also important to understand the linguistic and cultural differences in which they were compiled. Medieval science was a combination of different disciplines and may comprise worldviews which are alien to modern scientific approaches. Essentially though, both are based on a quest for how things work and a desire to heal. We would do medieval medicine a great disservice if we reduced it to questions of efficacy in the modern lab, but at the same time it should not be dismissed as a purely text-critical exercise.[80]

---

78 Harrison and others, 'An Assessment of the Evidence for Antibacterial Activity'.

79 Porras and others, 'Ethnobotany and the Role of Plant Natural Products'.

80 We extend special thanks to Dr Freya Harrison who organized and conducted the lab work. Dr Harrison also co-led the systematic review with Dr Erin Connelly along with the final publication of those results. Thank you to Dr Jessica Furner-Pardoe for experimental work and thank you to Dr Cassidy Croci for work in preparing the dataset for display on our

Works Cited

Manuscripts

Bamberg, Staatsbibliothek, MS Msc. Med.1
Glasgow, University Library, MS Hunter 497
Leiden, University Library, MS Vossianus lat. fol. 96A
London, British Library, MS Cotton Vitellius C III
London, British Library, MS Harley 585
London, British Library, MS Harley 6258b
London, British Library, MS Royal 12 D XVII

Primary Sources

Anglo-Saxon Remedies. Charms, and Prayers from British Library MS Harley 585: The Lacnunga, ed. and trans. by Edward Pettit, 2 vols (Lewiston: Edwin Mellen Press, 2001)

Bede, *The Reckoning of Time*, trans. by Faith Wallis (Liverpool: Liverpool University Press, 1999)

Henry of Huntingdon, *Anglicanus ortus: A Verse Herbal of the Twelfth Century*, ed. and trans. by Winston Black (Oxford/Toronto: Bodleian Library/Pontifical Institute, 2012)

King Alfred, *King Alfred's West Saxon Version of the Pastoral Care*, ed. and trans. by Henry Sweet, Early English Text Society, o.s., 45 (London: Trübner, 1871)

Leechdoms, Wortcunning, and Starcraft of early England: Being a Collection of Documents, for the Most Part Never before Printed, Illustrating the History of Science in this Country before the Norman Conquest, ed. and trans. by Thomas Oswald Cockayne, 3 vols (London: Her Majesty's Stationery Office, 1864)

The Leiden Leechbook: A Study of the Earliest Neo-Brittonic Medical Compilation, ed. and trans. by Alexander Falileyev and Morfydd E. Owen (Innsbruck: Institut für Sprachen und Literaturen der Universität Innsbruck, 2005)

The Master of Game by Edward, Second Duke of York: The Oldest English Book on Hunting, ed. by William and Florence Baillie-Grohman (New York: Duffield and Company, 1909)

Medical Writings from Early Medieval England, ed. and trans. by John D. Niles and Maria D'Aronco (Harvard: Dumbarton Oaks, 2023)

Medieval Herbal Remedies: The Old English Herbarium and Anglo-Saxon Medicine, trans. by Anne Van Arsdall (New York: Routledge, 2002)

---

website. We also extend thanks to Dr Diana Luft for sharing her translations of medieval Welsh recipes. Thank you to Dr Frances Watkins for sharing her experimental results. We thank Dr Deborah Hayden and Dr Sarah Baccianti for feedback and editorial comments on an early draft and the reviewers for their comments.

Medieval Welsh Medical Texts, Volume 1: The Recipes, ed. and trans. by Diana Luft (Cardiff: University of Wales Press, 2020)
The Middle English Version of De Viribus Herbarum, ed. by Javier Calle-Martin and Antonio Miranda-García (Bern: Peter Lang AG, 2012)
The Old English Herbarium and Medicina de Quadrupedibus, ed. by Hubert Jan De Vriend, Early English Texts Society o.s., 286 (London: Oxford University Press, 1984)
The Old English Metrical Calendar (Menologium), ed. by Kazutomo Karasawa (Cambridge: D. S. Brewer, 2015)
Strabo, Walahfrid, *Hortulus*, trans. by Raef Payne (Pittsburgh: The Hunt Botanical Library, 1966)

Secondary Studies

Abdallah, Basma, Cendrine Seguin, Elora Aubert, Hassan Ait BenHassou, Laila Sbabou, Laurence Choulier, Catherine Vonthron, Isabelle J. Schalk, Gaetan L. A. Mislin, Sylvie Fournel, Véronique Pitchon, and Pierre Fechter, 'Past Mastering of Metal Transformation Enabled Physicians to Increase their Therapeutic Potential', *J. Trace Elem. Med. Biol.*, 71 (2022) <10.1016/j.jtemb.2022.126926> [accessed 16 January 2023]
Arthur, Ciaran, *'Charms', Liturgies and Secret Rites in Early Medieval England* (Woodbridge: Boydell and Brewer, 2018)
Balcik, Ozlem S., Mustafa Koroglu, Handan Cipil, Osman Kaftan, Senem Maral, Ayse Gurel, Hakan Goker, Ibrahim C. Haznedaroglu, and Ali Kosar, 'A Placebo-Controlled, Randomized, Double-Blinded, Cross-Over Phase-I Clinical Study Indicating the Safety of Topical Ankaferd Hemostat in Healthy Volunteers', *International Journal of Hematology and Oncology*, 4.22 (2012), 267–74 <https://doi.org/10.4999/uhod.10124> [accessed 29 October 2021]
Banham, Debby, 'Dun, Oxa and Pliny the Great Physician: Attribution and Authority in Old English Medical Texts', *Social History of Medicine*, 24.1 (2011), 57–73
Batten, Caroline, '"Lazarus, Come Forth": Pregnancy and Childbirth in the Life Course of Early Medieval English Women', in *Early Medieval English Life Courses*, ed. by Theijs Porck and Harriet Soper (Leiden: Brill, 2022), pp. 140–58
Bjarnsholt, Thomas, Morten Alhede, Peter Østrup Jensen, Anne K. Nielsen, Helle Krogh Johansen, Preben Homøe, Neils Høiby, Michael Givskov, and Klaus Kirketerp-Møller, 'Antibiofilm Properties of Acetic Acid', *Advances in Wound Care*, 4.7 (June 2015), 363–72 <https://doi.org/10.1089/wound.2014.0554> [accessed 29 October 2021]
Bouassida, Karama Zouari, Sana Bardaa, Meriem Khimiri, Tarek Rebaii, Slim Tounsi, Lobna Jlaiel, and Mohamed Trigui, 'Exploring the Urtica dioica Leaves Hemostatic and Wound-Healing Potential', *BioMed Research International* (October 2017) <https://doi.org/10.1155/2017/1047523> [accessed 29 October 2021]
Brackmann, Rebecca, '"It Will Help Him Wonderfully": Placebo and Meaning Responses in Early Medieval English Medicine', *Speculum*, 97.4 (2022), 1012–39

Burridge, Claire, 'Incense and Medicine: an Early Medieval Perspective', *Early Medieval Europe*, 28.2 (2020), 219–55 <https://onlinelibrary.wiley.com/doi/full/10.1111/emed.12394> [accessed 13 May 2024]

Caesar, Lindsay K., and Nadja B. Cech, 'Synergy and Antagonism in Natural Product Extracts: When 1 + 1 Does Not Equal 2', *Natural Product Reports*, 36.6 (June 2019), 869–88 <https://doi.org/10.1039/c9np00011a> [accessed 29 October 2021]

Cameron, Malcolm Laurence, *Anglo-Saxon Medicine*, Cambridge Studies in Anglo-Saxon England, 7 (Cambridge: Cambridge University Press, 1993)

——, 'On *þeor* and *þeoradl*', *Anglia*, 106 (1988), 124–29

——, 'The Sources of Medical Knowledge in Anglo-Saxon England', *Anglo-Saxon England*, 11 (1982), 135–55

Cheung, Mike W. L., and Ranjith Vijayakumar, 'A Guide to Conducting a Meta-Analysis', *Neuropsychology Review*, 26 (May 2016), 121–28 <https://doi.org/10.1007/s11065-016-9319-z> [accessed 29 October 2021]

Chopra, Aditi and Karthik Sivaraman, 'Ankaferd Blood Stopper: A Novel Hemostatic Agent with Unique Antimicrobial, Antineoplastic and Regenerative Properties', *Journal of Research in Pharmacy*, 23.5 (June 2019), 777–84 <https://doi.org/10.35333/jrp.2019.24> [accessed 29 October 2021]

Cole, Ann, 'The Use of *Netel* in Place-names', *Journal of the English Place-Name Society*, 35 (2002–2003), 49–58

——, 'The Use of ON *nata* in Place-names', *Journal of the English Place-Name Society*, 36 (2003–2004), 51–53

Connelly, Erin, Charo I. del Genio, and Freya Harrison, 'Data Mining a Medieval Medical Text Reveals Patterns in Ingredient Choice that Reflect Biological Activity against Infectious Agents', *mBio*, 11 (February 2020) <10.1128/mBio.03136–19> [accessed 17 October 2022]

Connelly, Erin, Christina Lee, Jessica Furner-Pardoe, Charo del Genio, and Freya Harrison, 'A Case Study of the Ancientbiotics Collaboration', *Patterns*, 3.12 (December 2022) <https://doi.org/10.1016/j.patter.2022.100632> [accessed 16 January 2023]

Cooper, Raymond, and Jeffrey J. Deakin, *Botanical Miracles: Chemistry of Plants that Changed the World* (London: CRC Press, 2016)

D'Aronco, Maria Amalia, 'The Botanical Lexicon of the Old English *Herbarium*', *Anglo-Saxon England*, 17 (1988), 15–33

——, 'How "English" is Anglo-Saxon Medicine? The Latin Sources for Anglo-Saxon Medical Texts', in *Britannia Latina: Latin in the Culture of Great Britain from the Middle Ages to the Twentieth Century*, ed. by Charles Burnett and Nicholas Mann (London/Turin: Warburg Institute, 2003), pp. 27–41

Di Virgilio, Nicola, Eleni G. Papazoglou, Zofija Jankauskiene, Sara Di Lonardo, Marcin Praczyk, and Kataryna Wielgusz, 'The Potential of Stinging Nettle (Urtica dioica L.) as a Crop with Multiple Uses', *Industrial Crops and Products*, 68 (June 2015), 42–49 <https://doi.org/10.1016/j.indcrop.2014.08.012> [accessed 29 October 2021]

Doyle, Conan Turlough, 'Anglo-Saxon Medicine and Disease: A Semantic Approach' (unpublished doctoral thesis, Cambridge University, 2017) <https://doi.org/10.17863/CAM.14430> [accessed 29 October 2021]

——, *The Reception of Latin Medicine in Early Medieval England: The Evidence of Old English Texts* (York: York Medieval Press, forthcoming)

Falk, Seb, *The Light Ages: The Surprising Story of Medieval Science* (New York: W. W. Norton & Company, 2020)

Furner-Pardoe, Jessica, Blessing Anonye, Ricky Cain, John Moat, Catherine Ortori, Christina Lee, David Barrett, Christopher Corre, and Freya Harrison, 'Anti-biofilm Efficacy of a Medieval Treatment for Bacterial Infection Requires the Combination of Multiple Ingredients', *Scientific Reports*, 10.12687 (2020) <https://doi.org/10.1038/s41598-020-69273-8> [accessed 8 July 2022]

Ghedira, K, P. Goetz, and R. Le Jeune, 'Urtica dioica L., Urtica urens et/ou hybrides (Urticaceae)', *Phytothérapie*, 7.279 (November 2009) <https://doi.org/10.1007/s10298-009-0408-5> [accessed 29 October 2021]

Grund, Peter, 'Editing Alchemical Texts in Middle English: The Final Frontier?', in *Probable Truth: Editing Medieval Texts from Britain in the Twenty-First Century*, ed. by Anne Hudson and Vincent Gillespie (Turnhout: Brepols, 2013), pp. 427–42

Halstead, Fenella D., Maryam Rauf, Naiem S. Moiemen, Amy Bamford, Christopher M. Wearn, Adam P. Fraise, Peter A. Lund, Beryl A. Oppenheim, and Mark A. Webber, 'The Antibacterial Activity of Acetic Acid against Biofilm-Producing Pathogens of Relevance to Burns Patients', *PLOS ONE*, 10. 9 (September 2015) <https://doi.org/10.1371/journal.pone.0136190> [accessed 29 October 2021]

Harrison, Freya, Jess Furner-Pardoe, and Erin Connelly, 'An Assessment of the Evidence for Antibacterial Activity of Stinging Nettle (Urtica dioica) Extracts', *Access Microbiology*, 4.3 (March 2022) <https://doi.org/10.1099/acmi.0.000336> [accessed 6 June 2022]

Harrison, Freya, Aled E. L. Roberts, Rebecca Gabrilska, Kendra P. Rumbaugh, Christina Lee, and Stephen P. Diggle, 'A 1,000-Year-Old Antimicrobial Remedy with Antistaphylococcal Activity', *mBio*, 6.4 (August 2015) <https://doi.org/10.1128/mBio.01129-15> [accessed 29 October 2021]

Hayden, Deborah, 'A Sixteenth-century Irish Collection of Remedies for Ailments of the Male Reproductive Organs', *Celtica*, 33 (2021), 248–76

Horden, Peregrine, 'What's Wrong with Early Medieval Medicine?', *Social History of Medicine*, 24.1 (April 2011), 5–25 <https://doi.org/10.1093/shm/hkp052> [accessed 6 June 2022]

Johnson, Tyler A., Johann Sohn, Wayne D. Inman, Leonard F. Bjeldanes, and Keith Rayburn, 'Lipophilic Stinging Nettle Extracts Possess Potent Anti-inflammatory Activity, Are Not Cytotoxic and May Be Superior to Traditional Tinctures for Treating Inflammatory Disorders', *Phytomedicine*, 20.2 (January 2013), 143–47 <https://doi.org/10.1016/j.phymed.2012.09.016> [accessed 29 October 2021]

Jolly, Karen, 'Magic, Miracle and Popular Practice in the Early Medieval West', in *Religion, Science and Magic in Concert and Conflict*, ed. by Jacob Neusner (Oxford: OUP, 1981), pp. 166–82

Kazancı, Ceren, Soner Oruç, and Marine Mosulishvili, 'Medicinal Ethnobotany of Wild Plants: A Cross-cultural Comparison around Georgia-Turkey Border, the Western Lesser Caucasus', *Journal of Ethnobiology and Ethnomedicine*, 16.71 (November 2020) <https://doi.org/10.1186/s13002-020-00415-y> [accessed 29 October 2021]

Kesling, Emily, *Medical Texts in Anglo-Saxon Literary Culture* (Cambridge: D. S. Brewer, 2020)

Khan, Khalid S., Regina Kunz, Jos Kleijnen, and Gerd Antes, 'Five Steps to Conducting a Systematic Review', *Journal of the Royal Society of Medicine*, 96.3 (March 2003), 118–21 <https://doi.org/10.1258/jrsm.96.3.118> [accessed 29 October 2021]

Kılıç, Murat, Kemal Yıldız, and Fatma Mungan Kılıç, 'Traditional Uses of Medicinal Plants in Artuklu, Turkey', *Human Ecology*, 48 (September 2020), 619–32 <https://doi.org/10.1007/s10745-020-00180-2> [accessed 29 October 2021]

Kregiel, Dorota, Ewelina Pawlikowska, and Hubert Antolak, 'Urtica spp.: Ordinary Plants with Extraordinary Properties', *Molecules*, 23.7 (July 2018), 1664 <https://doi.org/10.3390/molecules23071664> [accessed 29 October 2021]

Kurt, Mevlut, Ibrahim Koral Onal, Meral Akdogan, Murat Kekilli, Mehmet Arhan, Abdurrahim Sayilir, Erkin Oztas, and Ibrahim Celalettin Haznedaroglu, 'Ankaferd Blood Stopper for Controlling Gastrointestinal Bleeding due to Distinct Benign Lesions Refractory to Conventional Antihemorrhagic Measures', *Canadian Journal of Gastroenterology and Hepatology*, 24.6 (June 2010), 380–84 <https://doi.org/10.1155/2010/896819> [accessed 29 October 2021]

Lee, Christina, 'The Art of Looking Good: Hair and Beauty Remedies in Early Medieval Texts and Contexts', in *Art and Worship in the Insular World: Papers in Honour of Elizabeth Coatsworth*, ed. by Gale Owen-Crocker and Maren Clegg Hyer (Leiden: Brill, 2021), pp. 45–67

McNelis III, James Ignatius, 'The Uncollated Manuscripts of "The Master of Game": Towards a New Edition' (unpublished doctoral thesis, University of Washington, 1996) <https://www.proquest.com/docview/304321065/A54505570994F32PQ/1?accountid=14888> [accessed September 2021]

McSparran, Frances and others, eds, *Middle English Compendium* (Ann Arbor: University of Michigan Library, 2000–2018) <http://quod.lib.umich.edu/m/middle-english-dictionary/> [accessed September 2021]

Meaney, Audrey, 'The Practice of Medicine in England about the Year 1000', *Social History of Medicine*, 13.2 (2000), 221–37

——, 'Variant Versions of Old English Medical Remedies and the Compilation of Bald's Leechbook', *Anglo-Saxon England*, 13 (1984), 235–68

Moulton, Thomas, *The Compleat Bone-setter*, ed. and trans. by Robert Turner (London: Tho. Rooks, 1665) <https://books.google.com/> [accessed 29 October 2021]

Nazeri, Mehdi, Roya Ata-Bakhshian, Mohsen Taghizadeh, Rezvan Talaee, and Mohaddese Mahboubi, 'Antifungal Activity of Herbal Extracts against Malassezia Species', *Iranian Journal of Dermatology*, 18 (January 2015), 10–15 <https://doi.org/10.1007/s10745-020-00180-2> [accessed 29 October 2021]

Nokes, Richard Scott, 'The Several Compilers of Bald's *Leechbook*', *Anglo-Saxon England*, 33 (2005), 51–76

Olalla, David Moreno, 'A Plea for Middle English Botanical Synonyma', in *Probable Truth: Editing Medieval Texts from Britain in the Twenty-First Century*, ed. by Anne Hudson and Vincent Gillespie (Turnhout: Brepols, 2013), pp. 387–404

Olsan, Lea, 'Charms and Prayers in Medieval Medical Theory and Practice', *Social History of Medicine*, 16.3 (2003), 343–66 <https://doi.org/10.1093/shm/16.3.343> [accessed 13 May 2024]

——, 'The Language of Charms in a Middle English Recipe Collection', *ANQ*, 18.3 (2005), 31–37 <https://doi.org/10.3200/ANQQ.18.3.31-37> [accessed 21 May 2024]

Page, Matthew J., Joanne E McKenzie, Patrick M Bossuyt, Isabelle Boutron, Tammy C Hoffmann, Cynthia D Mulrow, Larissa Shamseer, Jennifer M Tetzlaff, and David Moher, 'Updating Guidance for Reporting Systematic Reviews: Development of the PRISMA 2020 Statement', *Journal of Clinical Epidemiology*, 134 (June 2021), 103–12 <https://doi.org/10.1016/j.jclinepi.2021.02.003> [accessed 29 October 2021]

Payne, Joseph, *English Medicine in the Anglo-Saxon Times* (Oxford: Clarendon, 1904)

Paz, James, 'Magic that Works: Performing *Scientia* in the Old English Metrical Charms and Dialogues of Solomon and Saturn', *Journal of Medieval and Early Modern Studies*, 45 (2015), 219–43

Pitchon, Véronique, Elora Aubert, Catherine Vonthron, and Pierre Fechter, 'How History Can Help Present Research of New Antimicrobial Strategies: The Case of Cutaneous Infections' Remedies Containing Metals from the Middle Age Arabic Pharmacopeia', in *Medicinal Plants as Anti-Infectives: Current Knowledge and New Perspectives*, ed. by François Chassagne (London: Academic Press, 2022), pp. 459–78 <https://doi.org/10.1016/B978-0-323-90999-0.00016-1> [accessed 3 June 2024]

Porras, Gina, François Chassagne, James T. Lyles, Lewis Marquez, Micah Dettweiler, Akram M. Salam, Tharanga Samarakoon, Sarah Shabih, Darya Raschid Farrokhi, and Cassandra L. Quave, 'Ethnobotany and the Role of Plant Natural Products in Antibiotic Drug Discovery', *Chemical Reviews*, 121.6 (March 2021), 3495–560 <https://doi.org/10.1021/acs.chemrev.0c00922> [accessed 29 October 2021]

Riehemann, Kristina, Bert Behnke, and Klaus Schulze-Osthoff, 'Plant Extracts from Stinging Nettle (Urtica dioica), an Anti-rheumatic Remedy, Inhibit the Proinflammatory Transcription Factor NF-κB', *FEBS Letters*, 442.1 (January 1999), 89–94 <https://doi.org/10.1016/S0014-5793(98)01622-6> [accessed 29 October 2021]

Sabir, Emel Ceyhun, and Belkıs Zervent Ünal, 'The Using of Nettle Fiber in Towel Production and Investigation of the Performance Properties', *Journal of Natural*

Fibers, 14.6 (February 2017), 781–87 <https://doi.org/10.1080/15440478.2017.1279102> [accessed 29 October 2021]

Sauer, Hans, and Elisabeth Kubaschewski, *Planting the Seeds of Knowledge: An Inventory of Old English Plant Names* (Munich: Herbert Utz, 2018)

Su, Xin-Zhuan and Louis H. Miller, 'The Discovery of Artemisinin and the Nobel Prize in Physiology or Medicine', *Science China Life Sciences*, 58 (October 2015), 1175–79 <https://doi.org/10.1007/s11427-015-4948-7> [accessed 29 October 2021]

Talbot, Charles, *Medicine in Medieval England* (London: Oldbourne, 1967)

Tu, Youyou, 'The Discovery of Artemisinin (Qinghaosu) and Gifts from Chinese Medicine', *Nature Medicine*, 17 (October 2011), 1217–20 <https://doi.org/10.1038/nm.2471> [accessed 29 October 2021]

Van Arsdall, Anne, 'Evaluating the Content of Medieval Herbals', in *Critical Approaches to the History of Western Herbal Medicine: From Classical Antiquity to the Early Modern Period*, ed. by Susan Francia and Anne Stobart (London: Bloomsbury Publishing, 2015), pp. 47–66 <https://doi.org/10.5040/9781474210577.ch-003> [accessed 29 October 2021]

——, 'Medical Training in Anglo-Saxon England: An Evaluation of the Evidence', in *Form and Content of Instruction in Anglo-Saxon England in the Light of Contemporary Manuscript Evidence: Papers Presented at the International Conference, Udine, 6–8 April 2006*, ed. by Patrizia Lendinara, Loredana Lazzari and Maria Amalia D'Aronco (Turnhout: Brepols, 2007), pp. 415–34

Vidyarthi, Shalini, Sher S. Samant, and Pankaj Sharma, 'Traditional and Indigenous Uses of Medicinal Plants by Local Residents in Himachal Pradesh, North Western Himalaya, India', *International Journal of Biodiversity Science, Ecosystem Services & Management*, 9.3 (August 2013), 185–200 <https://doi.org/10.1080/21513732.2013.823113> [accessed 29 October 2021]

Vogl, C. R., and A. Hartl, 'Production and Processing of Organically Grown Fiber Nettle (Urtica dioica L.) and its Potential Use in the Natural Textile Industry: A Review', *American Journal of Alternative Agriculture*, 18.3 (September 2003), 119–28 <https://doi.org/10.1079/AJAA200242> [accessed 29 October 2021]

Wallis, Faith, 'The Experience of the Book: Manuscripts, Texts, and the Role of Epistemology in Early Medieval Medicine', in *Knowledge and the Scholarly Medical Traditions*, ed. by Donald G. Bates (Cambridge: Cambridge University Press, 1995), 101–26

Watkins, Frances, Barbara Pendry, Olivia Corcoran, and Alberto Sanchez-Medina, 'Anglo-Saxon Pharmacopoeia Revisited: A Potential Treasure in Drug Discovery', *Drug Discovery Today*, 16.23–24 (2011), 1069–75

Weleda, 'Fragaria Urtica Compound' <https://www.weleda.com/product/f/fragaria-urtica-compound> [accessed September 2021]

Weston, Lisa, 'The Language of Magic in Two Old English Metrical Charms', *Neuphilologische Mitteilungen*, 86.2 (1985), 176–86

Zhang, Junqi, 'A Real-life Picture of Medieval Healing: A Stylistic Study of Old English Medical Text *Lacnunga*' (unpublished MRes dissertation, University of Nottingham, 2023)

LAURA POGGESI

8. Medical Knowledge in Two Middle English Manuscripts

Their Use and Users

Introduction

The process of vernacularization of medical texts that began in the second half of the fourteenth century sparked a huge interest in the practical dimension of science, and by the end of the following century a great heritage of medical knowledge was preserved in vernacular texts and enjoyed by a vast community of people.[1] Medicine was conceived on the one hand as a learned university discipline, and on the other as a profession requiring technical skills,[2] which is the reason why it was performed by a heterogeneous group of practitioners of different levels of education and training, ranging from university-educated physicians to surgeons, barbers, apothecaries, rural empirics, and laywomen. Various factors stimulated the process of translation of scientific texts from Latin: in the first place the growing levels of literacy, which promoted the transmission of medical knowledge in the vernacular in written form rather than orally, but also the growth in the commercial book trade and importation of paper, which offered a choice and availability of materials for book-making — including cheaper alternatives to parchment — thus encouraging an increasing demand for vernacular medical manuscripts for a diversified audience. Latin remained the lingua franca of science throughout the Middle Ages and beyond and during the fifteenth century was still the language used to produce university textbooks. However, the appeal of vernacular medical texts was also strong among learned physicians, and manuscript evidence demonstrates that medical books in English were to be found on the bookshelves of elite practitioners as well as on those of the less educated ones.

1 For an investigation on the renewed interest in practically oriented medicine in fifteenth-century England, see Jones, 'Information and Science'.

2 On the dichotomy of medicine as a science and a craft, see Voigts, 'Medical Prose', p. 315; Crossgrove, 'Introduction', p. 82; and Taavitsainen, 'Discourse Forms and Vernacularisation', p. 95.

Laura Poggesi • University of Genoa; laura.poggesi@edu.unige.it

Medicine in the Medieval North Atlantic World: Vernacular Texts and Traditions, ed. by Deborah Hayden and Sarah Baccianti, KSS, 5 (Turnhout, 2025), pp. 191-209
BREPOLS PUBLISHERS DOI 10.1484/M.KSS-EB.5.143986

Scholarship traditionally distinguishes between two main traditions of Middle English medical writings: a learned tradition represented by academic treatises dealing with the founding principles of physiology and natural philosophy; and the more popular one of remedybooks comprising recipes, texts of prognostication, and charms. These traditions are not mutually exclusive, but rather denote two poles of a continuum, since both draw their material from Hippocratic and Galenic thought grounded in humoral theory, and both have Latin antecedents. Among the most broadly disseminated genres dealing with medicine were medical recipes: short texts providing instructions on how to prepare a medicine or cure a disease.[3] The ancient origin of these texts, their practical function, and their versatile and flexible form made them widely sought after in late medieval England both by trained physicians and lay practitioners, and they were not only collected in remedybooks but were often embedded in learned treatises as well.[4] Although medical recipes sometimes have been dismissed as the product of folk wisdom,[5] they constitute a fertile and fascinating field of study for two reasons: firstly, because they are a meeting-point between learned and popular tradition — as they frequently occur in collections along with healing charms and were informed both by older vernacular traditions and academic study conducted at universities — and secondly, because the instructional form of recipes bears close witness to the practical application of medical knowledge.[6]

This chapter presents a comparative analysis of the medical recipes transmitted in two fifteenth-century manuscripts whose history is little known: Cambridge, Trinity College Library, MS R.14.32 (hereafter TCC), a medical compendium probably produced for a trained practitioner; and Naples, National Library, MS XIII.B.29 (hereafter N), an anthology of texts of different genres, among which there is a collection of recipes, likely addressed to a laywoman.[7] A first examination of these *receptaria* has revealed that a number of recipes occur in both manuscripts, a quite remarkable fact considering the different functions they seem to have served. This study aims to interpret the analogies and discrepancies found among the shared recipes in light of the presumed target audiences, and to understand if, and to what extent, the level of medical expertise of their readership might have influenced the form of the texts. In this way it will be possible to gain further insight into these hitherto little-studied codices.

3 A definition of medical recipes has been provided by Taavitsainen, 'Middle English Recipes', p. 86.

4 The distinction between the structure and function of medical recipes collected in remedybooks and those embedded in theoretical treatises has been investigated by Taavitsainen, 'Middle English Recipes', and by Carroll, 'Middle English Recipes'.

5 On this issue see Taavitsainen and Pahta, 'Vernacularisation of Medical Writing', p. 158.

6 For a study on the function of recipes as vehicles of practical knowledge, see Leemans, *Contextualizing Practical Knowledge*.

7 Weldon, 'The Naples Manuscript'.

Description of the Manuscripts

Identifying the exact readership of a medieval medical manuscript is quite often a challenging task. As pointed out by Irma Taavitsainen, evidence gathered both from documentary records, such as wills or library catalogues, and elements internal to the manuscripts, such as marginal annotations, demonstrates that the dissemination of medical knowledge in the late Middle Ages spread through different layers of society and not always in a linear way.[8] Due to the lack of conclusive information about the history of TCC and N, their original owners, and the use made of them, the reliance on external and internal codicological features is essential for collecting as much detail as possible to formulate plausible hypotheses concerning their function. To better understand the recipe contents of these manuscripts, it is thus necessary to relate the material evidence of the manuscripts' production, inferred from codicological analysis, to their textual contents.

Cambridge, Trinity College Library, MS R.14.32

TCC is a portable manuscript measuring 195 × 140mm and consisting of 173 folia, partly of parchment and partly of paper. The exact date of production is unknown, but codicological, palaeographical, linguistic, and textual scrutiny suggests that it was assembled in the second half of the fifteenth century. Most of the texts were copied by a single scribe in a mixed handwriting with elements of Anglicana and Secretary scripts, typical of the fifteenth century, while other coeval hands contributed to the copying of some items or portions of them. The codex does not contain overt references to the place of production. The linguistic profile provided by the electronic *Linguistic Atlas of Late Mediaeval English* (*eLALME*) locates it in Essex; however, this evidence does not necessarily point to the place of production of TCC, but merely to the dialect of its texts.[9] Almost all the texts of TCC are in the vernacular except for three items in Latin: a list of remedies against pestilence (fol. 92^r), a collection of recipes (fols 140^r–44^r), and a version of the *Circa Instans* attributed to Matthaeus Platearius (fols 151^r–68^r).

The manuscript contains thirty-eight texts of different genres dealing with medical topics: four herbals, various theoretical treatises on different subjects, and 288 Middle English medical recipes gathered in collections or inserted as individual texts. Almost all the items are in prose, except for a herbal and a treatise on rosemary that are in verse. The texts in TCC are for the most part

8 Taavitsainen, 'Genres and the Appropriation of Science', pp. 181–82. Taavitsainen notices that while we may expect learned texts to be used exclusively by physicians and recipe collections by non-specialized readers, there is evidence that recipes were also copied in books meant for professional use, and that many learned treatises were also transmitted into the notebooks of laymen and women.

9 Benskin and others, *A Linguistic Atlas* (LP 6300).

translations of some well-known Latin originals which were vernacularized into English between the end of the fourteenth and the beginning of the fifteenth centuries. Various annotations in sixteenth-century hands testify to the continued use of the codex. The nature of these notes is heterogeneous: there are moralizing short poems, some scribbles, and additional medical recipes which suggest that TCC continued to be used for medical purposes during the early modern period. Among the later additions there are also two signatures: one by a John Cheke at the end of a rather moralizing poem (fol. 149^r),[10] and the other by a *magister* R. Arche placed at the end of a group of medical recipes (fol. 95^r).[11] Although in the manuscript there are neither elements unveiling the identity of its original owner, nor traces of actual use on the part of medieval readers, it is possible to infer some clues based on internal evidence. A first significant aspect of TCC is its consistency at both a codicological and thematic level. The paper portion of the manuscript is made of quires with the same watermark and from the same paper-stock.[12] Moreover, as already noted, the common thread of the entire compendium is medicine. All these features indicate that the codex was designed as a homogeneous product. A closer examination of the contents also reveals a careful choice of texts and a precise compilation scheme, beginning with an herbal (fols 1^v–65^r) and followed by a series of treatises on various medical topics such as the four humours, uroscopy, and the plague, whereas medical recipes are inserted only in the second half of the codex, from fol. 92^v onwards. This arrangement of material seems to provide a guide for reading especially useful to anyone directly involved in the practice of medicine, who might strengthen their theoretical knowledge with the texts at the beginning of the codex, and then turn their attention towards practical instructions for the pharmaceutical preparations prescribed in the recipes.

The items selected for the compilation of TCC reveal that it was not used as a textbook in universities.[13] Nonetheless, the presence of texts in Latin and the

10 It can hardly be affirmed that the signature was by the well-known John Cheke, Cambridge professor and statesman to King Henry VIII.

11 The signature is accompanied by the date '1548'. So far, I have not been able to find any correspondence with a sixteenth-century doctor named R. Arche, but the appellative *magister* suggests that he could have been a primary physician probably at the service of some members of the aristocracy. An overview on the terminology used to denote different kinds of medical practitioners is described in Siraisi, *Medieval and Early Renaissance Medicine*, pp. 20–21.

12 The paper portion of the manuscript comprises quires VII–XV (fols 67–173). The watermark of quires VII–XIII is a bull's head with a star, whereas that of quires XIV–XV is a deer's head. The different watermark along with the distinctive consistency of the paper of the last two quires suggest that, in origin, this part of the manuscript may have constituted a separate booklet. I would like to thank Professor Orietta Da Rold for helping me during the analysis of the material used for the production of TCC.

13 A survey on the medical texts used in the academic context during the Middle Ages and on the teaching methods in vogue is provided by Siraisi, *Medieval and Early Renaissance Medicine*, pp. 70–77.

coverage of all the fundamental topics for the medical profession suggest that the original owner of this manuscript could have been a skilled practitioner, such as a (barber-) surgeon or an apothecary with a good level of education. Alternatively, the original owner of TCC could have been a university-trained physician who may have used the manuscript for reference purposes during daily practice. Thus, this manuscript can be classified as a leechbook.[14] Despite its richness in contents, TCC has not raised much interest among scholars so far. The codex is often cited in studies dealing with the writings it contains, but the publication of a complete edition is still a desideratum.[15]

Naples, National Library, MS XIII.B.29

N is a paper manuscript of seventy-four folia measuring 240 × 290mm. The date of its production is indicated in a colophon placed on fol. 73^v^: 'Hic pennam fixi penitet me si male scripci qd mprfi (drawing of a hare) Anno domini 1457' (Here I leave the quill pen. I repent if I wrote badly. For this, More. A.D. 1457). This inscription also seems to indicate the name of the scribe, who might have been Harry More: the expression 'qd mprfi' may be interpreted as 'quod More' and the drawing of the hare could be a play on words for the name 'Harry'.[16] The codex contains a collection of 151 recipes (fols 1^v^–11^r^), the romance *Beuys of Hampton*, the hagiographic poem *Of Saint Alex of Rome*, the romances *Libeaus Desconus* and *Sir Isumbras* (only a fragment), and an acephalous version of Chaucer's *The Clerk's Tale*. All the texts are in Middle English, Dorset dialect,[17] with occasional use of Latin for formulaic expressions.

It is unclear whether all the texts of the manuscript were transcribed by Harry More alone or by several copyists. Manly and Rickert are certain about the identity of a single scribe,[18] whereas Mills distinguishes between two hands: one who copied the first half of the romance *Beuys of Hampton*,

14 For a definition of leechbook and its distinction from remedybooks, see Connolly, 'Evidence for Continued Use of Medieval Medical Prescriptions', pp. 137–38, and Keiser, *Manual of the Writings in Middle English*, p. 3653.

15 The only editions entirely based on a text of TCC are the ones published by Keiser, 'A Middle English Rosemary Treatise', and Poggesi, *Farmacopea inglese tardomedievale*, which provides a critical edition with Italian translation of the medical recipes. Other scholars relied on TCC for the apparatus of variants of their editions: see Braekman, *Studies on Alchemy* for an edition of a collection of recipes for the preparation of the so-called 'Alchemical Waters of Saint Gyle'; and Voigts and Hudson, 'A Drynke that Men Callen Dwale' for an edition and study of a medical recipe for the preparation of an anaesthetic.

16 Manly and Rickert, *The Texts of the Canterbury Tales*, p. 377.

17 Benskin and others, *An Electronic Version* (LP 9490). Manly and Rickert, *The Texts of the Canterbury Tales*, p. 377, based on the version of *The Clerk's Tale*, locate the dialect of the text in the East Midlands, while the study of the poem on Saint Alex carried out by Andreani (Andreani, 'Of Saint Alex of Rome') confirms the southern provenance proposed by the *LALME*.

18 Manly and Rickert, *The Texts of the Canterbury Tales*, p. 377.

and the other who started copying from the middle of *Beuys* till the end of the codex.[19] Notably, the palaeographical analysis of Mills does not take into consideration the collection of recipes at the beginning of the manuscript. Even though it may be difficult to determine if a change of hand occurred in the copying of the romance, I argue that a different hand wrote the *receptarium*.[20]

As for TCC, information about the history of the Naples manuscript is scant: there are neither dedications nor declarations of ownership, nor documents recording when and under what circumstances the manuscript reached Italy. The name 'Hampton Henry' is written on the first flyleaf in a handwriting that looks quite modern, and it is thus difficult to relate it to a medieval owner; moreover, the initials 'h c' inserted on fol. 11^{v} make it even more problematic to establish any connection to a specific person. However, the choice of the texts and their arrangement in the manuscript have led James Weldon to classify it as 'an anthology, a thematically designed and carefully prepared volume for a female readership'.[21] Notwithstanding the paucity of evidence on the medieval history of N, some drawings and annotations in Italian datable to the seventeenth century demonstrate the continued use of the codex by Italian owners in later years. In particular, the drawing of a hand pointing towards a bell on fol. 1^{r} suggests that for a period N could have been in the possession of the Italian philosopher Tommaso Campanella (1568–1639).[22]

Although some studies have highlighted that the versions of the texts transmitted in N are distinctive and unique in respect to their textual tradition, the codex has not received much scholarly attention. Apart from the work of Weldon, which presents a global analysis of the manuscript, there have been

19 *Lybeaus Desconus*, ed. by Mills, p. 7.

20 The main difference between the hand that copied the recipes and the one (or, if we accept Mill's hypothesis, the two hands) that wrote the other texts is the script: the recipes are written in a small and quite elegant Secretary, whereas the other texts are in a mixed handwriting displaying elements of Secretary and Anglicana. The two scripts also differ in the realization of some letters.

21 Weldon, 'The Naples Manuscript', p. 704. Weldon lays particular emphasis on the placement of the collection of recipes at the beginning of the manuscript, claiming that it might have served 'as a prologue or filtering device which draws attention to women, their bodies, and female agency' (p. 707).

22 The first to propose Tommaso Campanella as a possible owner of N was *La novella del chierico di Oxford*, ed. by Vallese, pp. 8–9. This assumption is based on the evidence that Campanella (also known by the pseudonym 'Squilla', meaning 'little bell') usually signed his name with the drawing of a bell. The drawing in N is accompanied by the inscription 'Questo manoscritto in lingua tedesca (then corrected with "inglese") l'ho hauuto da Diomede De Leonardis e fu primieramente…' (I have had this manuscript in the German language (then corrected with 'English') by Diomede De Leonardis, and it was previously…). The sentence is not completed by a name, but the series of dots leads exactly to the figure of the bell. It is thus possible that the manuscript was donated by the philosopher to his lawyer Giovan Battista De Leonardis, who in turn might have given it to a relative named Diomede.

no attempts to produce a complete edition of the codex.[23] Nonetheless, some scholars have used the Neapolitan versions of these contents as the base text for their editions, among which the facsimile edition of the medical recipes published by Vallese in 1940 is of particular relevance here.[24]

The Corpus of Medical Recipes

The first step in the analysis of the *receptaria* under investigation here involved examining their overall structure. TCC contains 288 medical recipes in Middle English, four of which are inserted in the manuscript as independent texts, while the others are gathered in eleven *receptaria*. Some of these collections are thematically organized, others are arranged — at least partly — according to the traditional head-to-foot order, others apparently do not observe any specific pattern. Moreover, a fair number of recipes are embedded in some of the theoretical treatises,[25] and thirteen are gathered in a Latin collection. Since N contains neither recipes incorporated into theoretical treatises nor Latin remedies, I have not analysed them in this study. Four main kinds of recipes can be identified among the 288 items taken into consideration: (1) eighty-three recipes for the preparation of medicines; (2) 201 medical recipes to heal sicknesses; (3) one healing charm; (4) three prognosticatory texts. The distinction between the first two categories is taken from a study by Ruth Carroll, who highlighted that recipes may tell either 'how to make things', providing instructions for the preparation of a medicine, or 'how to do things', which means how to use ingredients to cure a particular condition.[26] The medical subject behind all the texts is the first indication of the specialized nature of TCC.

By contrast, among the 151 recipes that comprise N there are 133 remedies to heal ailments, nine recipes for the preparation of medicaments, and two healing charms. No prognosticatory texts occur in the *receptarium*. What is

---

23 A project for the creation of a digital edition of N has been launched by Khalaf and Cioffi, 'Un progetto di trascrizione ed edizione digitale.'

24 *Un ignoto ricettario medico inglese*, ed. and trans. by Vallese. The edition presents a transcription of the recipes mirroring the images from the manuscript, and it is supplied by a poor apparatus of notes and a quite incomplete glossary. An updated edition is still desirable. The other editions dealing with the texts of N are *La novella del chierico di Oxford*, ed. by Vallese; *Sir Bevys of Hampton*, ed. by Vallese; Andreani, 'Of Saint Alex of Rome'; *Lybeaus Desconus*, ed. by Salisbury and Weldon.

25 Taavitsainen has noted that medical recipes were often inserted in theoretical treatises to validate the notions transmitted in the texts and to prove the practitioner's expertise (Taavitsainen, 'Middle English Recipes', pp. 106–07). Because of this function and due to the different writing context, embedded recipes assumed a less standardized form. On the contrary, medical recipes arranged in collections were meant for easy consultation during practice, and usually followed a more definite structure.

26 Carroll, 'Middle English Recipes', p. 188.

most worth noticing is that the recipes for the preparation of medicaments are quite generic, as in '*A medicine* for him that may not wel hire'[27] (fol. 10^{r}), where the title does not mention the type of medicament to be prepared, and thus whether it should be, for example, an ointment, a pill, or a potion. Moreover, the headings of all these recipes overtly state the sickness the medicaments aim to cure (for example, 'A drink to destroy the hed ache' on fol. 3^{r}); thus, greater attention is always given to the ailment rather than to the preparation itself. On the contrary, in TCC we have recipes entirely concerned with pharmaceutical preparations, where indications for treatment are given only at the end of the recipe but not in the title (for example, 'To make unguentum ryall' on fol. 107^{v}). It is reasonable to think that texts of this kind were addressed to specialists, such as herbalists or trained practitioners.

In addition to the medical prescriptions, N contains non-medical items as well. These recipes include a concoction to lure rabbits from their holes; a culinary recipe to prepare a quince preserve; a recipe for a dye and one to make sealing wax. The remaining recipes include three items, the relation of which to medical practice is more ambiguous as they appear to sit between medicine and popular belief and may have been of greater interest in a domestic environment rather than to a physician. The first is 'An oynement for vanitees in the hedde' (fol. 6^{r}). The concept of vanity and its medical meaning has been investigated by Isabel de la Cruz Cabanillas, who, after demonstrating the wide circulation of this recipe in various medieval *receptaria*, has highlighted the double connotation — spiritual and physical — this word had in Middle English. On the one hand, it carries the meaning of 'foolishness, arrogance, pride, or madness', on the other it denotes 'dizziness or light-headedness' and conveys a general sense of 'weakness'.[28] The last connotation seems the most suitable in a medical context, but given the contents of the following recipes, I think that here the spiritual meaning should not be fully dismissed: the second recipe, 'For to do awey frightens' (fol. 6^{r}), is a remedy against sudden fear, consisting of a sort of ointment made with the blood of an animal; while the third item, 'For to stop manis lust fro wymmen' (fol. 6^{v}), prescribes a potion to help cease men's desire towards women: something which can hardly be considered strictly medical.

Comparative Analysis

The general framework of the two manuscripts' collections of recipes presented in the previous paragraph has highlighted some elements of their diverse nature. TCC offers a more specialized configuration, and N is more likely a repository of domestic knowledge useful in everyday life. Before comparing the two collections, it may be convenient to identify the categories of ailments

27 My emphasis.

28 De la Cruz Cabanillas, 'A Medicine for the Vanity in the Head', p. 159.

in both codices. In order to do so, I rely on the classification proposed by Hunt and Benskin, based on eight macro-groups of recipes dealing with: (1) topical conditions, (2) non-localized conditions, (3) skin conditions, (4) gynaecology, (5) sores, ulcers, and tumours, (6) prognostics, (7) medicaments, to which I have added healing charms.[29] Such categories include, in turn, smaller groups of recipes dealing with specific disorders or pharmaceutical preparations. Tables 8.1.1 and 8.1.2 report the categories of recipes identified for each manuscript.

Table 8.1.1. Categories of medical recipes in TCC

TOPICAL COND.	**NON-LOCALIZED COND.**	**SKIN COND.**	**SORES, ULCERS, TUMOURS**	**PROG-NOSTICS**	**MEDICA-MENTS**	**HEALING CHARMS**
Head	Pestilence	Leprosy	Purgation	Death	Oils	*Longinus miles*
Eyes	Blood	Warts	Cancer		Ointments	
Ears	Urine	Scabs	Carbuncle		Medicinal waters	
Teeth	Worms	Sweat			Plasters	
Face	Wounds	Itching			Potions	
Mouth	Thorn extraction				Balms	
Abdomen stomach intestine	Cramp				Powders	
Chest	Dropsy				Laxatives	
Breasts	Somniloquy				*Mundificatives*	
Kidneys	Poison antidote				*Dwale*	
Joints	Fever				*Drynke of Antioch*	
Throat	Bites				*Dewte*	
Side	Burns				*Popilion*	
Back	Sinews				*Neruale*	
Veins	Palsy					

29 Hunt and Benskin, *Three Receptaria*, distinguish between 'preparations' — pointing to the kinds of medicaments, such as oils, ointments, potions and so on — and 'medicaments', referring to those medicines denoted by a proper name (for example, *dwale* or *nervale*). Since the difference between these categories is quite slight as they both concern the preparation of medicaments, I decided to consider them jointly: see *Three Receptaria*, ed. by Hunt and Benskin.

Table 8.1.2. Categories of medical recipes in N.

TOPICAL COND.	NON-LOCALIZED COND.	SKIN COND.	GYNAE-COLOGY	MEDICA-MENTS	HEALING CHARMS	AMBIGUOUS RECIPES
Head	Pestilence	Warts	Childbirth	Ointments	*Maria peperit* (for childbirth)	Vanity
Eyes	Blood		Menstruation	Plasters	*Bironix* (to stop bleeding)	Sudden fear
Ears	Urine			Potions		Lust
Teeth	Worms			Powders		
Face	Wounds					
Mouth	Thorn extraction					
Abdomen stomach intestine	Stone					
Chest	Jaundice					
Breasts	Complexion					
Joints	Evil in the body					
Back						
Feet						
Knees						
Legs						

As it emerges from the tables, TCC comprises various groups of recipes related to diseases which are not included in N, pointing to a deeper knowledge of pharmacopeia of the user of TCC and to their commitment to dealing with a greater variety of medical conditions. By contrast, the categories of recipes peculiar to N are those dealing with generic topics, such as 'evil in the body' or 'complexion', texts previously labelled as being in between medicine and folkloristic beliefs, and remedies against women's ailments, which will be discussed later.

Table 8.2 portrays the co-occurrent categories of recipes in the two codices, for which I have recorded the number of texts in each manuscript and the related number of correspondences I have found.

Table 8.2. Co-occurrent categories of recipes in the two manuscripts and relative correspondences.

		TCC	N	CORRESPONDENCES
TOPICAL CONDITIONS	Head	12	14	2
	Eyes	22	14	2
	Ears	11	6	2
	Teeth	14	8	1
	Face	6	6	1
	Mouth	5	1	/
	Abdomen, stomach, intestine	32	11	2
	Chest			
	Breasts	31	7	/
	Joints	2	6	1
	Back	2	3	/
		2	2	/
NON-LOCALIZED CONDITIONS	Blood	9	5	1
	Urination	5	4	3
	Wounds	15	1	/
	Thorn extraction	3	2	/
	Pestilence			
	Worms	1	2	/
		1	3	/
SKIN CONDITIONS	Warts	4	1	/

This table demonstrates that in most cases, TCC displays a higher number of recipes for each category: N seldom exceeds it, and, when it does, it is always with a slight difference, except in the case of remedies for ailments of breasts, of which there are six in N compared with two in TCC. Such numerical discrepancies may be explained simply by the fact that the Cambridge manuscript contains a richer corpus of recipes. However, a closer look at the texts also reveals that the nature of such recipes is usually more specific in TCC. For example, while among the recipes against diseases affecting teeth N transmits remedies for toothache only (which is the commonest disorder), TCC also offers cures against periodontitis and worms in the teeth, as well as instructions for the preparation of a toothpaste. The same can be said for other categories of ailments, such as those affecting the mouth, where TCC includes remedies for halitosis, pimples, and a tumour, whereas N deals exclusively with halitosis. Furthermore, among the recipes for disorders of the abdomen, stomach, and intestine, the Neapolitan manuscript presents remedies for generic problems, such as constipation, stomach-ache, or thirstiness, while TCC covers more specific and serious diseases as well, for example diarrhoea, intestinal worms, colic, and disorders of the spleen. In addition, in TCC it is also common to find references to surgical operations, as in the recipe 'For to drawe oute broken bones of a mannys hede that is woundyd' (fol. 126^{r}), which gives instructions for the preparation of a plaster to be applied on the sore, probably after bone extraction.

By contrast, N is more detailed than TCC as far as remedies for diseases of the breasts are concerned: the Naples manuscript includes recipes to counter the swelling of the breasts (possibly due to breastfeeding), discharging nipples, nagging aches, and ulcerous sores on nipples, while TCC deals with breast swelling only. Clearly this shows a much greater interest in women's health on the part of the compiler and, consequently, of the users of N. This is also evidenced by references to treatments for gynaecological disorders. Apart from the recipes concerning breasts, N also includes six recipes for childbirth, among which are the 'Maria peperit' charm and five medical remedies for menstruation.[30] In TCC there are only a few recipes which refer to women's illnesses, and only incidentally: among the various conditions they were meant to treat, the recipe for 'The V water of seynte Gyle' (fol. 97^{v}) also favours the appearance of menstruation; the recipe for the 'Oyle of hille wortte' (fol. 102^{v}) is useful against ailments of the uterus; and the 'Oyle of pulyoll ryall' and the 'Oyle of junipere' (both of fol. 101^{r}) are said to help a woman become pregnant. In other cases, such as the recipe for 'The IV water of seynte Gyle' (fol. 97^{v}), potential side effects of the medicament for pregnant women are explained. However, as it is evident from the titles of these recipes, which can be classified as recipes for medicaments, the main emphasis is placed on the name or the kind of the medicine rather than on the typically female ailments they were meant to cure.[31]

Among the shared categories of recipes, I have identified fifteen correspondences, each of them presenting discrepancies of various nature. I will now present three illustrative cases. The first, shown in Table 8.3, is a remedy against deafness or poor hearing:[32]

---

30 On the 'Maria peperit' charm in Irish tradition, see the chapter by Deborah Hayden in this volume.

31 It is worth noticing that a reverse situation is found in the Latin collection of thirteen recipes on fols 140^{r}–44^{r}, where there are three remedies against gynaecological conditions (concerning menstruation, disturbances of the uterus, and childbearing). The presence of a Latin *receptarium* in a mainly Middle English manuscript points to the high level of literacy of its user. An in-depth study of this collection, also aiming at detecting its source and its authoritativeness, would help to better understand its function in the codex and possibly to comprehend why typically female disorders are dealt with only in Latin. Because these recipes are not in the vernacular they have not been included in this study.

32 The transcriptions of both manuscripts offered in this essay are mine. I have followed the principles of semi-diplomatic transcriptions, reproducing all the scribes' practices, but silently expanding abbreviations and hyphenating words that are written separately in the manuscripts but form a single word in contemporary writing.

Table 8.3. Recipes for deafness.

TCC	N
A-nother for the same	ffor thik hiryng þat is rotid
Take the grece of a rostyd ele and medell it with the jous of singrene or of rubarbe of eche lyche moche and sethe hem to-geder and put it leuke in the hole ere and do ther-with as it is sayde be-fore · probatum est per certo (fol. 116r).	Take the grece of an Ele and the juse of Syngrene of eche liche moche and put it oft in-to thyne Ere and it schalle be thi bote (fol. 10r).
(Another for the same Take the grease of a roasted eel and mix it with the juice of houseleek or of rhubarb, of each in equal quantity, and boil them together, and put it warm in the ear, as it has been said before. This is well proved.)	(For rooted poor hearing Take the grease of an eel and the juice of houseleek, of each in equal quantity, and put it often in your ear. It will be of help.)

A first major difference is evident in the scope of the two remedies: to heal deafness in TCC and to mitigate poor hearing in N.[33] This slight divergence notwithstanding, other more significant discrepancies that testify to the more elaborate form of the recipe in TCC can be observed. First, the Cambridge manuscript provides details which are not included in N: (1) the specification that the eel to be used should be roasted, (2) the juice of rhubarb as an alternative ingredient to that of houseleek (*singrene*), (3) a passage in the procedure ('and sethe hem to-geder'). Moreover, the text in TCC contains additional information for a good outcome of the remedy: 'medell it with the juse' and 'put it leuke in the hole ere'. Interestingly, in TCC the phrases 'or of rubarbe' and 'and sethe hem to-geder and put it leuke in the hole ere' are interlinear additions by the same hand that copied the entire text. It is possible that the scribe wanted to complete this version of the remedy with elements directly derived from his own experience, producing a more accurate and effective remedy. Finally, it may be noted that the efficacy phrase at the end of the recipe in TCC is in Latin, whereas in N is in English. There is no doubt that such expressions are not necessarily an indicator of Latin literacy, since by the fifteenth century they constituted formulaic phrases which were commonly understood. However, I posit that the preference of TCC's scribe for Latinate expressions over vernacular ones, here and elsewhere in the manuscript, is indicative of a higher level of education.

The second recipe I discuss, in Table 8.4 is a remedy to quench thirst:

33 The title in TCC alludes to the previous remedy, 'For hym that maye not heyr' (fol. 116r).

Table 8.4. Recipes for thirstiness.

TCC	TCC	N
ffor him that is alwey thrysty	ffor hym that hath moche thurst	ffor hem that haue moche thurst
Take centorye or the rote loueache · stampe it and temper it vp with wyne or with warm water and drynke ther-of III nyghtes whan thu goste to bedd (fol. 124^{v})	Take the rote of louache · stampe it and temper it with water and yeue seke to drynke III nyȝtes and he schall be hole (fol. 150^{v})	Take the rote of loveache stamp it and temper it with watir and yeve the sike to drink therof III nyghtis and he schal be hole bi god-is grace (fol. 6^{v})
(For him that is always thirsty Take centaury or the root of lovage, crush it and mix it with wine or warm water and drink it for three nights when you go to sleep.)	(For him that has much thirst Take the root of lovage, crush it and mix it with water, and give it to the sick to drink for three nights, and he shall recover.)	(For them who have much thirst Take the root of lovage, crush it and mix it with water, and give it to the sick to drink for three nights, and, with God's grace, he shall recover.)

The recipe is the same in all three cases. As is visible in Table 8.4, this remedy occurs twice in TCC, where it appears in two different collections of recipes. The text of the second occurrence is identical to the one transmitted in N, except for the addition, in the Neapolitan version, of an invocation ('bi god-is grace'). The same phrasing of the recipe can be considered indicative of the wide circulation of these remedies among a broad range of medical practitioners. The other version of the recipe in TCC demonstrates once again a higher degree of specificity by adding some alternative ingredients ('centorye or the rote of loueache' and 'with wyne or with warm water'), and by providing more details both regarding the water's suitable temperature ('warm water') and the exact moment when the medicament should be administered ('whan thu goste to bedd').

The last example, Table 8.5, is a recipe for swelling of the breasts:

Table 8.5. Recipes for swelling of the breasts.

TCC	N
ffor suellynge of tetis	ffor swelling of tetits
Take oke appellis and stampe hem with oyle of Roses and ley it to the sore (fol. 120^{r})	Take oke apliis and stamp ham with oyle of Rosis and ley it to thi sore (fol. 4^{v})
(For the swelling of breasts Take oak's galls and crush them with oil of roses and spread it on the sore.)	(For the swelling of breasts Take oak's galls and crush them with oil of roses and spread it on your sore.)

This recipe is clearly the same in both manuscripts, but a small, and apparently meaningless, detail could be crucial to our understanding of the intended readership of the two codices. In the application section of the recipe, where in TCC it is written 'ley it to the sore', with the definite article that conveys an impersonal style, N reports 'ley it to thi sore' with the second person singular possessive pronoun, thus not only unveiling an overt reference to a female reader, but also suggesting that the performer of this treatment is herself a woman practising self-healing. Another case in which a recipe's instructions are explicitly directed to a woman is represented by the recipe for a plaster to be used after childbirth, which states 'ley it hote ther-to as *ye wymmen* wol finde'.[34] The mere presence of a discrete number of remedies for specifically women's diseases is not sufficient to demonstrate the female readership of a *receptarium*. As demonstrated by Monica Green, women's health was not exclusively women's business; on the contrary, male physicians were often involved in their healthcare, including gynaecological matters.[35] However, the use of such linguistic devices overtly addressing the intended audience can be taken as evidence for a female readership of the Neapolitan manuscript.

The comparative analysis of the two manuscripts can be concluded by outlining other clues that highlight the different degree of education and expertise of the audiences of these *receptaria*, demonstrating a more specialized readership for TCC — convincingly made for a trained practitioner — and a female readership for N, which was possibly produced for a woman in charge of her family's healthcare. The first significant element is the recurrence among the recipes of TCC of theoretical annotations describing ailments, such as the definition of the *scietica passio* on fol. 127^{r} or explaining the kinds of medicines to be used on a specific body part. Secondly, there is a wider use of Latin in TCC for some expressions, as well as for names of medical preparations, ingredients, and sicknesses, whereas it is never used in N's medical recipes.[36] A third relevant point is the higher degree of accuracy in the use of units of measures: while the Cambridge manuscript makes extensive use of precise units of measures, such as 'vnce', 'pennyweyght', or 'gallon', N favours vaguer expressions as 'a hondfull' or 'a good quantite'. As we can see from the list of ingredients in two recipes for migraine, shown in Table 8.6:

34 My emphasis. The recipe mentioned here is 'ffor the disease aftir hur travaile' (Naples, NL, MS XIII.B.29, fol. 2^{r}).

35 Green, 'Women's Medical Practice', p. 457.

36 The use of Latin occurs elsewhere in the codex, especially in formulaic endings of texts and in the colophon signed by Harry More.

Table 8.6. Recipes for migraine.

TCC	N
ffor demygreyne	ffor the megryme
Take *halfe an vnce* of galingale · *an vnce* of ginger · *halfe an vnce* of nottmugges · *a quartorn of an vnce* of clowes · *a peny weyȝte* of anyse · *a quartorn of an vnce* of enull campane · *halfe an vnce* of lycoryse and *an vnce* of sugr [...] (fol. 125ᵛ)	Take *an hondful* of Celidony *a-nothir* of betayne and *a litil* of camamyl [...] and cast ther-to *a sponeful* of comyn [...] (fol. 3ᵛ)
(For the migraine Take half an ounce of galangal, an ounce of ginger, half an ounce of nutmeg, a quart of an ounce of cloves, a pennyweight of anise, a quart of an ounce of Elecampane, half an ounce of liquorice and an ounce of sugar [...])	(For the migraine Take a handful of celandine, another of betony, a little camomile [...] and add to it a spoonful of cumin [...])

Finally, it is worth noticing the references to medieval medical authorities exclusive to TCC, where there are references to the 'leches of salern' that allude to the famous medical School of Salerno, and to a 'pouder wauter', a medicinal powder whose creation was attributed to the thirteenth-century physician Walter Agilon. Such mentions clearly point to a target audience with a considerable knowledge of influential medical figures of the time. On the contrary, N mentions only the universally known Hippocrates ('and the sike schalbe hole on warranties as seieth ypocrase þe good leche', fol. 3ʳ).

Conclusion

This chapter has discussed the intended readership of two little-studied fifteenth-century English manuscripts — Cambridge, Trinity College Library, MS R.14.32 and Naples, National Library, MS XIII.B.29 — by investigating the collections of medical recipes they contain. Codicological scrutiny, as well as the examination of the overall structure of these *receptaria*, have revealed the different nature of the two codices, and this has been further demonstrated by a comparative analysis of their texts. If the identification of fifteen recipes recurring in both manuscripts confirms that practical medical knowledge circulated widely in late medieval England, the discrepancies found among such recipes highlight the different degrees of specificity in these books, and consequently their diversified target audience.

On the one hand, TCC deals with a larger variety of typologies of medical recipes and diseases: its texts display more details, a wider use of technical vocabulary, and greater reliance on medieval medical authorities, which demonstrate a higher degree of specialization. Therefore, it is possible to conclude that it was written for a trained practitioner. On the other hand, N deals with more generic medical disorders and, along with the medical recipes, also contains non-medical items, suggesting a domestic usage. In addition, the presence of a fair number of recipes specifically for illnesses related to women, and of linguistic expressions overtly addressing a woman, corroborates the hypothesis of a female readership of this manuscript proposed by Weldon. The fact that N is not an exclusively medical compendium, but an anthology also transmitting texts of other genres, is proof that laywomen in charge of a household were also expected to have some medical competence in order to provide for their family's healthcare.

This study shows that, in order to respond to their users' needs, texts that are usually considered highly standardized, such as medical recipes, required diversified writing strategies according to the different levels of education and expertise of their intended audience.

Works Cited

Manuscripts

Cambridge, Trinity College Library, MS R.14.32

Naples, National Library, MS XIII.B.29

Primary Sources

Un ignoto ricettario medico inglese del XIV secolo trovato nella Biblioteca Nazionale di Napoli, Testo originale, trascrizione a fronte, introduzione, note e glossario, ed. by Tarquinio Vallese (Naples: A. G. D. A., 1940)

Lybeaus Desconus, ed. by Maldwin Mills, Early English Text Society, o.s., 261 (London: Oxford University Press, 1969)

Lybeaus Desconus, ed. by Eve Salisbury and James Weldon, TEAMS: Middle English Texts Series (Kalamazoo: Medieval Institute Publications, 2013)

La novella del chierico di Oxford: da un codice inglese inedito del XV secolo di G. Chaucer, testo originale con trascrizione a fronte, varianti e introduzione, ed. by Tarquinio Vallese (Naples: A. G. D. A., 1939)

Sir Bevis of Hampton: da un antico manoscritto inedito inglese, ridotto a miglior lezione e commentato, ed. by Tarquinio Vallese (Naples: Libreria Internazionale di Leo Lupi, 1941)

Three Receptaria from Medieval England, ed. by Tony Hunt with the collaboration of Michael Benskin, Medium Aevum Monographs New Series, 21 (Oxford: The Society for the Study of Medieval Languages and Literatures, 2001)

Secondary Studies

Andreani, Angela, 'Of Saint Alex of Rome. A Middle English Version of the Life of the Saint', *Linguistica e Filologia*, 28 (2009), 29–56

Benskin, Michael, Margaret Laing, Vasilios Karaiskos, and Keith Williamson, *An Electronic Version of a Linguistic Atlas of Late Medieval English* <http://www.lel.ed.ac.uk/ihd/elalme/elalme.html>

Braekman, Willy, *Studies on Alchemy, Diet, Medicine and Prognostication in Middle English* (Brussels: OMIREL, 1986)

Carroll, Ruth, 'Middle English Recipes: Vernacularisation of a Text-type', in *Medical and Scientific Writing in Late Medieval English*, ed. by Irma Taavitsainen and Päivi Pahta (Cambridge: Cambridge University Press, 2004)

Connolly, Margaret, 'Evidence for the Continued Use of Medieval Medical Prescriptions in the Sixteenth Century: A Fifteenth-century Remedy Book and its Later Owner', *Medical History*, 60.2 (2016), 133–54

Crossgrove, William, 'Introduction', in *Early Science and Medicine: A Journal for the Study of Science, Technology and Medicine in the Pre-modern Period*, 3.2, Special Issue: *The Vernacularization of Science, Medicine, and Technology in Late Medieval Europe*, ed. by William Crossgrove, Margaret Schleissner, and Linda E. Voigts (1998), pp. 81–87

De la Cruz Cabanillas, Isabel, 'A Medicine for the Vanity in the Head', *SELIM*, 21 (2015–2016), 157–66

Green, Monica, 'Women's Medical Practice and Health Care in Medieval Europe', *Signs*, 14.2 (1989), 434–73

Jones, Peter M., 'Information and Science', in *Fifteenth Century Attitudes: Perceptions of Society in Late Medieval England*, ed. by Rosemary Horrox (Cambridge: Cambridge University Press, 1994), pp. 97–111

Keiser, George R., *Manual of the Writings in Middle English, 1050–1500, vol. 10: Works of Science and Information*, ed. by Albert E. Hartung (New Haven: The Connecticut Academy of Arts and Science, 1998)

——, 'A Middle English Rosemary Treatise in Verse and Prose', *ANQ: A Quarterly Journal of Short Articles, Notes and Reviews*, 18.1 (2005), 9–18

Khalaf, Omar and Raffaele Cioffi, 'Un progetto di trascrizione ed edizione digitale del codice Napoli, Biblioteca Nazionale, MS XIII.B.29', *Umanistica Digitale*, 2.2 (2018), 139–59

Leemans, Annemie D. G., *Contextualizing Practical Knowledge in Early Modern Europe* (Berlin: Peter Lang, 2020)

Manly, John M., and Edith Rickert, *The Texts of the Canterbury Tales: Studied on the Basis of all Known Manuscripts*, 1 (Chicago: The University of Chicago Press, 1940)

Poggesi, Laura, *Farmacopea inglese tardomedievale. Edizione e traduzione delle ricette mediche dal MS R.14.32 (Cambridge, TCL)*, Collana della Scuola di Alta Formazione Dottorale (Bergamo: Università degli Studi di Bergamo, 2024)

Siraisi, Nancy G., *Medieval and Early Renaissance Medicine: An Introduction to Knowledge and Practice* (Chicago: The University of Chicago Press, 1990)

Taavitsainen, Irma, 'Discourse Forms and Vernacularisation Processes in Genres of Medical Writing 1375–1550', in *Translation – Interpretation: COLLeGIUM, University of Helsinki*, ed. by Anneli Aejmeiaeus and Päivi Pahta (Helsinki: Helsinki Collegium for Advanced Studies, 2012), pp. 91–112

——, 'Genres and the Appropriation of Science: *Loci communes* in English Literature in Late Medieval and Early Modern Periods', in *Opening Windows on Texts and Discourses of the Past*, ed. by Janne Skaffari, Matti Peikola, Ruth Carroll, Risto Hiltunen, and Brita Wårvik (Amsterdam: Benjamins, 2005), pp. 179–96

——, 'Middle English Recipes: Genre Characteristics, Text-type Features, and Underlying Traditions of Writing', *Journal of Historical Pragmatics*, 2.1 (2001), 85–113

Taavitsainen, Irma, and Päivi Pahta, 'Vernacularisation of Medical Writing in English: A Corpus-Based Study of Scholasticism', in *Early Science and Medicine: A Journal for the Study of Science, Technology and Medicine in the Pre-modern Period*, 3.2, Special Issue: *The Vernacularization of Science, Medicine, and Technology in Late Medieval Europe*, ed. by William Crossgrove, Margaret Schleissner, and Linda E. Voigts (1998), pp. 157–85

Voigts, Linda E., 'Medical Prose', in *Middle English Prose: A Critical Guide to Major Authors and Genres*, ed. by Anthony S. G. Edwards (New Brunswick: Rutgers University Press, 1986), pp. 315–35

Voigts, Linda E., and Robert P. Hudson, 'A Drynke that Men Callen Dwale to Make a Man to Slepe Whyle Men Kerven Him: A Surgical Anesthetic from Late Medieval England', in *Health, Disease and Healing in Medieval Culture*, ed. by Sheila Campbell, Bert Hall, and David Klausner (New York: Macmillan, 1992), pp. 34–56

Weldon, James, 'The Naples Manuscript and the Case for a Female Readership', *Neophilologus*, 93.4 (2009), 703–22

BRIGID MAYES

9. The *Materia medica* of the Gaelic Physician Tadhg Ó Cuinn (1415)

At the Interface of Theory and Practice

Introduction

The *Materia medica* is a compendium, in Irish, of the materials of medicine, compiled by Tadhg Ó Cuinn in 1415. Ó Cuinn was one of a number of Gaelic physicians who engaged with contemporary European learning, translating and adapting a corpus of Latin texts in a deliberate and concerted project to provide a high-quality education for physicians in Ireland, in their own language.[1] These physicians were working in a tradition established centuries before their time. Physicians were among the service kindred of Gaelic chieftaincies. They ranked with smiths, having the status of craftsmen. Senior, learned physicians could attain the highest rank of *ollamh leighis*. Their profession was well-developed: a number of physicians maintained schools and were well connected to the world outside Ireland.[2] As I discuss in this chapter, at least some physicians would already have been familiar with many non-native elements of the pharmacopoeia of the *Materia medica*.

The only complete translation into English of Ó Cuinn's *Materia medica* is by Micheál Ó Conchubhair. It is entitled *An Irish Materia Medica*[3] and is based on a fifteenth-century copy of the *Materia medica* now held in the library of

1 'Gaelic' is the term used to describe communities and territories in Ireland still ruled by Gaelic chieftains, between the Norman invasion of 1169 and the sixteenth-century Tudor reconquest: Simms, *Medieval Gaelic Sources*, p. 9.

2 Hayes, 'Irish Medical Links with the Continent'; Nic Dhonnchadha, 'The Medical School of Aghmacart'.

3 Accessible online at <https://celt.ucc.ie/published/G600005/index.html>. Throughout this chapter, references with page numbers refer to Ó Conchubhair's introduction to his work, entitled *An Irish Materia medica*, with his name in English, Michael O'Connor. References to Ó Cuinn's chapters carry the footnote 'Tadhg Ó Cuinn, *Materia medica*' with the chapter number. The same chapter numbers apply to the Irish text, the section on Latin sources, and the English translation of the Irish text. My study is based on Ó Conchubhair's translation.

Brigid Mayes • University College Dublin; mayesbrigid@gmail.com

Medicine in the Medieval North Atlantic World: Vernacular Texts and Traditions, ed. by Deborah Hayden and Sarah Baccianti, KSS, 5 (Turnhout, 2025), pp. 211-224
BREPOLS PUBLISHERS DOI 10.1484/M.KSS-EB.5.143987

Trinity College Dublin.[4] This copy has 292 chapters, set out in the standard European format of one material per chapter.[5] Two hundred and thirty-eight of the chapters are based on plants or plant-derived substances or products; sixteen on animal substances; twenty-five on mineral substances, and thirteen on general topics. The discussion below will focus on Ó Cuinn's sources, influences, and associates; the wide range of plants and plant derivatives featuring in the work; the framing of the work in Galenic theory; and the historic continuum in which the *Materia medica* sits.

Sources, Influences, and Associates

The following concluding words of Ó Cuinn's work offer a starting point for exploring the role of Ó Cuinn, and other Gaelic physicians, in grasping the breadth and depth of tradition and scholarship from which their European contemporaries were able to draw:

> Gurab aml*aidh* fagmait crich chumair tarbach arin leabur so noch do tairrngead a hainntetairib & a herbulairibh catrach Salernetane & da reir sduideir comaentaig*the* doctuireadh Sleibe Pisalani & adubradar na maigistreacha sin gach ni tinnscaintear *a n*-ainm Dia gurab dingmala a crichnug*adh a n*-ainm Dia.
>
> Gurab amlaigh sin da cricnaigead an leabar o Tadg O Cuinn .i. baistillerach a fisiceacht a mi Octimpir a sollain Lucais suibisceil & is*eadh* da bud slan an Tigerna an tan sin . m. cccc. & . x . u. in su*mm*o. Finit, amen.
>
>> (So we have achieved a succinct and beneficial fulfilment of this, drawn from the Antidotaries and Herbals of the city of Salerno, according to the united *studium* of the doctors of Montpellier. Those masters have stated that everything that is begun in the name of God deserves to be completed in the name of God.
>>
>> And that is how this book was completed by Tadhg Ó Cuinn, bachelor in physic, in the month of October, on the feast day of St Luke, the Apostle, in the year of Our Lord one thousand, four hundred and fifteen, to be precise. The End, Amen.)[6]

Here Ó Cuinn acknowledges his sources. Twenty standard compound medicines are named in his *Materia medica*, of which seventeen appear in the

4 Dublin, TCD, MS 1343 (H 3. 22).

5 This format was set by Dioscorides in his *De materia medica*, compiled in the first century AD, and has persisted through to the herbals of today: see Riddle, *Dioscorides on Pharmacy and Medicine*, p. 47.

6 Tadhg Ó Cuinn, *An Irish Materia medica*, ed. and trans. by Ó Conchubhair, pp. 275 (text) and 646 (trans.).

Salernitan *Antidotarium Nicolai*.[7] The herbal of Salerno is considered to have been the *Liber de simplici medicinae*, also known by its opening words as the *Circa instans*, attributed to Matthaeus Platearius and compiled in the twelfth century.[8] It was widely diffused throughout Europe both in manuscript and later in printed form, and it was Ó Cuinn's principal source. Besides Platearius, Ó Cuinn also draws on Macer Floridus, and to a lesser extent, Isaac Iudaeus.[9] Salerno was the bridgehead through which ancient Greek medical learning came back to Europe, enriched by the scholarship and practice of Arabic physicians. From Arabic texts translated into Latin, a body of works formed the *Articella*, the basis of medical education first in Salerno itself, and later in universities founded in the thirteenth century, including Montpellier.[10] By Ó Cuinn's time, Graeco-Arabic texts in Latin translation were well integrated into western European medical education, and commentaries and manuals of practice had been drawn up by master physicians to support practitioners.[11]

Moreover, Ó Cuinn states that his learning was supported by the 'united *studium* of the doctors of Montpellier'. This statement carries weight, and also allows to surmise that his qualification as bachelor in physic may have been awarded by the university of Montpellier. Several manuals associated with Montpellier are among the works translated into Irish by Ó Cuinn and his contemporaries. Ó Cuinn himself translated a commentary on Book Nine of the *Almansor* (a treatise on pathology, diagnostics, and therapy) written by Geraldus de Solo, *maître-régent* at the medical faculty of Montpellier in the mid-fourteenth century.[12]

There is no record of where Tadhg Ó Cuinn lived and worked, or to which Gaelic chieftaincy he was attached, but the supportive role played by two Munster physicians, Niocól Ó hIceadha and Aonghus Ó Callanáin, suggests he was senior to them and perhaps head of a school with which they were associated. Niocól Ó hIceadha acted as amanuensis for his translation of Geraldus de Solo's work in 1400,[13] and Aonghus Ó Callanáin is said, by a later scribe, to have written down the *Materia medica* from Ó Cuinn's dictation in 1415.[14] These two men were translators in their own right, and

---

7 O'Connor, *An Irish Materia medica*, pp. 51–56.

8 Tobyn and others, *The Western Herbal Tradition*, p. 9.

9 Additions to the *Circa instans* were made in later copies, including verses from the *De viribus herbarum* by Macer Floridus and chapters from a tenth-century treatise on dietetics by Isaac Iudaeus.

10 Porter, *The Greatest Benefit to Mankind*, p. 108.

11 Ausécache, 'Manuscrits d'antidotaires médiévaux'.

12 The work known as the *Almansor* was a compendium written by al-Razi (Latinized to Rhazes) in the tenth century. In it, Rhazes, one-time director of a hospital in the town of Rayy in present-day Iran, attempted to summarize all medical knowledge, dedicating his work to al-Mansor, governor of Rayy.

13 Ní Shéaghdha, *Catalogue*, p. 67.

14 This is recorded in a copy made by Seosamh Ó Longáin in 1848 (Dublin, RIA MS 24 B 2 [461], p. 122). He states that the copy made by his grandfather in 1761 was transcribed from the original.

together they translated a commentary on the *Aphorisms* of Hippocrates, a work which outlined a vision and philosophy of healthcare, in 1403. It has been suggested that Ó hIceadha and Ó Callanáin also collaborated in a translation of the Salernitan manual *Regimen sanitatis*.[15] This work is also associated with Montpellier.[16]

Further translations later in the fifteenth century were made by Cormac Mac Duinnshléibhe, a member of the Dunlevy family who were hereditary physicians to the O'Donnells of Tír Chonaill. The legacy of Montpellier is evident in Mac Duinnshléibhe's work too. Among other works, he translated the *Lilium medicine* and two other works by Bernard of Gordon, the *Rosa Anglica*[17] and the *Anathomia Gydo* (the first book of the fourteenth-century *Chirurgia magna* by Guy de Chauliac).[18]

The Range of Plants

Ó Cuinn's *Materia medica*, like its main sources, linked a contemporary understanding of plant pharmacology and human anatomy, physiology, pathology, and therapeutics within an encompassing theoretical framework. The range of plants discussed in the *Materia medica* is remarkably wide. It includes plants which are native to Ireland and grow in the wild, naturalized plants which were possibly or certainly introduced by human agency,[19] plants associated with cultivation, and exotic plants which could not be grown in our Irish climate. A number of the introduced plants are likely to have been brought to Ireland through monastic orders associated with care of the sick. Excavations at the Cistercian Bective Abbey in Co. Meath carried out from 2009 to 2012 included an archaeobotanical study.[20] Of the twenty archaeophytes (plants introduced before the year 1500) found, seven are well embedded in Ó Cuinn's *Materia medica*, and his discussion of them suggests a familiarity with their use. Among the exotic plants included in the *Materia medica* are materials associated with Arabic pharmacy, such as gums and resins, liquorice, sugar, rose, and spices; the exotics would have been obtained

15 *Regimen na Sláinte*, ed. by Ó Ceithearnaigh, I, pp. xxvi–xxviii.

16 The *Regimen sanitatis* was annotated and edited by Arnald of Villanova (d. 1311), a medical student and later a lecturer at Montpellier.

17 The *Rosa Anglica* is a manual by Englishman John of Gaddesden based on Bernard's *Lilium medicine*. It was edited and translated into English by Winifred Wulff in 1923.

18 Bernard of Gordon began to write his *Lilium medicine* in 1303 after his twentieth year of lecturing in the faculty of medicine in Montpellier. It was intended for 'young colleagues' and was required reading for medical students there: see Demaitre, *Doctor Bernard de Gordon*, pp. 51–55. Guy de Chauliac was also associated with Montpellier; the Irish version of his work, *Anathomia Gydo*, was edited and translated into English by Eithne Ní Ghallchobhair in 2014.

19 Identified in Parnell and Curtis, *Webb's An Irish Flora*, p. xxv.

20 Foley, 'The Botanical Legacy of Bective Abbey'.

through trade.[21] To help the practitioner, Ó Cuinn notes where they came from, how to recognize good quality, and how long they can be expected to retain their therapeutic potential. Whether the full range would have been available in Ireland is debatable.

In *Bretha crólige*, an Irish medico-legal text on sick-maintenance from the seventh century, the primary function of a garden was said to be for the care of the sick.[22] It is clear from reading the *Materia medica* that for it to be useful, the practitioner would have had to have access to a garden. In that garden, there would have to be food plants used as medicine, and plants associated with cultivation that are not found in the wild. It would also have been useful to have wild plants at hand in the garden, as the following extract from Ó Cuinn's chapter on the strawberry shows:

> Fragaria: .i. lus na sum tal*man*; fu*ar* tir*im* ata in luibh so & is mor fodnus da crectaib na scaman & na heasl*ainte* re n-abur tisis .i. *gabh* pre*m* madra & prem niamnaiti & lus na sum t*alman* & prema cru*aiche* Pa*draig* co mor d*a gach* n*i* bristear na l*uibhe* so & dentar praiseac dib & tobuir ar fin bog da ol & cneasaig*id* cr*eacht*a na scaman & foir*id* flux bronn.
>
> > (Fragaria: i.e. the strawberry plant; this plant is cold and dry; it serves well for lesions of the lungs [consumption] and the illness called phthisis: take the root of madder, root of tormentil, the strawberry plant, and roots of plantain, equal amounts of each, pound these herbs, make a soup of them, and give it in warm wine to drink, and this will heal lesions of the lungs, and it will help with flux of the abdomen.)[23]

The majority of recipes are simples, using only one plant ingredient. Compounds vary in complexity from two or three to many ingredients. Surprisingly, some plants which we consider commonplace, such as comfrey, ox-eye daisy, and common daisy, are included in recipes of mind-boggling complexity.[24]

The range of plants in the *Materia medica* includes nourishing food at one end of the spectrum, ranging through to flavourings with medicinal properties, to medicines varying in strength from mild to potentially dangerous. Many of the preparations could have been made and used by a lay person in a domestic setting. However, the work is written for practitioners familiar with Galenic theory. On the practical side, the user would have to know his materials, be skilled in preparing and compounding medicines, and aware of safety issues. A small number of strong and potentially toxic medicines, with a narrow therapeutic index, are for the skilled practitioner only and carry

---

21 Of the exotics discussed in the *Materia medica*, about twenty-five remain prominent in Ayurvedic pharmacy today; see Pole, *Ayurvedic Medicine*.

22 'Bretha crólige', ed. and trans. by Binchy, pp. 38–40 (§ 49).

23 Tadhg Ó Cuinn, *Materia medica*, ed. and trans. by Ó Conchubhair, § 128.

24 Tadhg Ó Cuinn, *Materia medica*, ed. and trans. by Ó Conchubhair, §§89–91.

cautions and contraindications. The following extract from the chapter on black hellebore (*Eleborus nider, in tathaba dub*), where dosage is specified, is given by way of illustration:

> Is mor foghnus an aig*id* mainia & melangcoil*ia* & don luct ara mbi vertigo & scotomia do-nitear o l*inn* d*ubh* & curtar isna purgadaib lac*tacha* hi mar so .i. ʒ da p*udur* premh na luibe so & madh e a b*earbadh* na l*uibhe* so da gentar ar fin no ar lind no ar midh fitear da ʒ *no* a tri da tobairt di mar sin. Et adeir Plaitiairius nac dl*eaghar* an luib so da tobairt dan lucht aga mbi easl*ainte* cleibh na don lucht aga mbidh corp cael anmann.
>
> (It serves well against mania and melancholia, and for people who have vertigo and dizziness arising from the melancholic humour; this is how it is put in the laxative purgatives, i.e. a drachma of the powder of the root of this herb, and if this herb is boiled in wine, ale or mead, two or three drachmas of it may be given in this way. Platearius says that this herb should not be given to people who have illness of the chest, or to those who have a thin, weak body.)[25]

The Underpinning of Galenic Theory

Galenic theory underpins the work and gives it coherence, as it underpins medical practice in general in medieval times. With Aristotle, Galen considered the constituents of living matter to be the elements earth, water, air, and fire, associated with the qualities dry, moist, cold, and warm. In the body the elements were believed to materialize in four fluids, known as 'humours': blood (warm and moist), yellow bile (warm and dry), phlegm (cold and moist), and black bile (cold and dry). The mixture and proportion of the qualities and humours accounted for the 'complexion' or 'temperament' of every living being. Galen categorized the qualities of individual medicines in terms of whether they dried or moistened, heated or cooled. The individual temperament of a person, in both physical and psychological terms, was shaped by the prevalence or predominance of one or other humour. Disease manifested as impaired physiological function and was understood in terms of an imbalance of humours.[26]

Emphasis was placed on the prevention of disease and the maintenance and restoration of health. The Salernitan *Regimen sanitatis* outlined guidelines for the maintenance of health, as mentioned above. A person's natural temperament could be kept in balance by managing lifestyle elements termed the six 'non-naturals': fresh air, food and drink, exercise and rest, sleep and wakefulness, timely bodily evacuations and state of mind. While

25 Tadhg Ó Cuinn, *Materia medica*, ed. and trans. by Ó Conchubhair, § 113.

26 Temkin, *Galenism*, pp. 13–19; see also the chapter by Conan Doyle in this volume.

discussion of regimen is not within the remit of a *Materia medica*, there is a clear therapeutic principle evident in discussion of the nutritional value of certain foods. Indeed, there is no clear demarcation between food and medicine, and easily digested and nourishing foods are seen as essential in the treatment of a patient in a debilitated state. Fergus Kelly has pointed out that in Old Irish there was no distinction between vegetable and herb: the word *luib* included plants eaten as part of a normal diet and plants used for medicine or flavouring.[27] *Cainnenn* (thought to be onion) and *imus* (thought to be celery) were mentioned particularly as being valuable in nursing. As well as onion and celery, all of the edible wild plants identified by Kelly in manuscript sources are the subject of chapters in the *Materia medica*: wild garlic, hazelnuts, watercress, nettles, sorrel, pignuts, silverweed, and brooklime. One of Ó Cuinn's sources was Isaac Iudaeus, the author of a tenth-century treatise on dietetics,[28] and the chapters of the *Materia medica* derived from Isaac Iudaeus discuss alexanders, hazelnuts, figs, almonds, barley, and wheat. The idea of nourishment is often present in Ó Cuinn's vehicles for the administration of medicine. Many preparations are infusions or decoctions of pounded plant material in water, milk, wine, honey, or butter.[29] Several recipes indicate that plant material could be given added value by boiling it in nutritious barley water. Part of the ease with which the Gaelic physicians took on the transmission of European medical knowledge must have been due to the fact that elements of Galenic theory were not unfamiliar. The regimen recommended for convalescents in the Old Irish law-tract on sick-maintenance, *Bretha crólige*, is remarkably reminiscent of elements of the Galenic non-naturals.

Chapters of the *Materia medica* open with the Galenic categorization of the plant or plant-derived product to be discussed according to its primary qualities: hot or cold, dry or moist, and in what degree. The example of *Plantago major*, greater plantain, can serve to illustrate how this plant categorization sits at the interface of theory and practice. Greater plantain is described as cold in the first degree and dry in the second degree. If we think of the four qualities hot, cold, dry, and moist as processes rather than states, hot becomes heating (stimulating); cold becomes cooling (calming and anti-inflammatory); dry becomes drying (reducing secretions); moist becomes moistening (soothing, softening). The cooling and drying actions of greater plantain make sense in these applications:

> as mait da glanad & do slanug*adh* na cneadh an luib so da brisidh & mil da cur triti & pot*aiste* da denam don l*uibh* so ar eanbruiti meth caeireach *no* ar leamnacht & foirigh flux na bronn. Item, bristear & coimiltear ar leamnacht an l*uibh* so & foirig an seili fola & an cosactach tic o teasaideacht.

27 Kelly, *Early Irish Farming*, p. 250.

28 See p. 213 above.

29 Butter made in the month of May was especially valued.

> Item, ceirin don luibh cetna da cur arin cneid> coiscidh a sileadh fola. Item, ceirin don l*uibh cet*na da cur arin cneid & coiscidh a sil*eadh* fola. Et an l*uibh cet*na da brisid & a cur tri *geal*an uigi & foirigh loscadh teineadh co cumhachtacht. [...] Item, an aig*id* tinnis na fiacul & aitt a feola & a teasbaigh an l*uibh* so da cognamh & icaidh.
>
> (To clean and heal wounds, it is good to pound this herb and to put honey through it; if a pottage be made of this herb in a rich mutton soup or in milk, it will help with flux of the abdomen. Item, pound this herb and put it in milk, and it will help with the spitting of blood and with the coughing that comes from hotness. Item, if a plaster of this herb be put on a wound, it will stop its bleeding. If the same herb be pounded and put through the white of egg, it will help powerfully with a burn. [...] Item, against toothache, swelling of the gums and their heating, if this herb be chewed, it will cure it.)[30]

The idea that an imbalance of humours is implicated in disease is well embedded in the *Materia medica*. The objective of the physician is to support the restoration of harmony in conditions of excess or imbalance. Six hundred years later, our world view and our understanding of human physiology, disease, and therapeutics are very different from those of Ó Cuinn and his contemporaries. Our grasp of the application of humoral theory in medieval medical practice can never be complete. That need not, however, prevent us from engaging as best we can. The following short discussion and examples illustrate the association of respiratory system disorders with an imbalance of phlegmatic humour.

The underlying cause of many chest complaints was understood to be cold and damp, the qualities of phlegmatic humour which, if present in excess, gave rise to disease. The majority of plants used in the treatment of such excess in respiratory conditions were classified as warm and dry in varying degrees, thereby suitable to counter the excessive cold and damp associated with phlegm. The organ most associated with phlegm was the brain. Catarrh was seen as a defluxion of phlegm from the head to the lungs. In the examples given below, the actions of the plant medicines indicated are what we would today call mucolytic and expectorant.

> Black pepper: *an sraedach noch is cuis da glannugh na hincinne ona* leann*aib reamra* (sneezing that results in the cleaning from the brain of the gross humours)[31]

---

30 Tadhg Ó Cuinn, *Materia medica*, ed. and trans. by Ó Conchubhair, § 52, entitled *Barba filicana, plantago maigheor: .i. an cruac Padraic*. The same attributes apply to *Plantago lanceolata*, the subject of § 166, entitled *Lansiolata: . i. in slanlus*, where it is noted that 'as inann brigh & oibriughadh do & don cruat Padraig' (it has the same efficacy and operation as plantain).

31 Tadhg Ó Cuinn, *Materia medica*, ed. and trans. by Ó Conchubhair, § 220.

Alexanders: *glanaig an t-uct & an scamhan o adbar reamur* leanna *find* (it cleans the chest and lungs of gross phlegmatic matter)[32]

Wild garlic: *glanaidh na baill spiradalta o* linn *finn reamur* (it will clear the breathing organs of the viscous phlegmatic matter)[33]

The Work of Ó Cuinn in a Historic Continuum

The elements of the *Materia medica* briefly discussed above reflect strands of influence which informed Ó Cuinn and gave him his place as both a European and an Irish physician of his time. Many of his entries are faithful, indeed slavish, renderings of his principal sources, who in their turn reached back to much older sources, some of whom are mentioned explicitly by Ó Cuinn: Rhazes, Avicenna, Galen, Gilbertinus, Hippocrates, John son of Mesue, Isaac, Averroes, Constantine, Dioscorides.

The work also reflects contemporary Ireland. Primarily, it reflects a deep history of learning and expression in the medium of the Irish language. In an examination of the medical terms found in the second paragraph of the *Rosa anglica* used in Winifred Wulff's translation, Liam Mac Mathúna found that they had been embedded in the Irish language, some for many centuries, with nuances of meaning evolving and adapting to changing concepts. In conclusion, he is able to place the work of Gaelic physicians in a new frame, saying that they had both the professional confidence and lexicographical resources to give expression to medical concepts encountered in the Latin works whose translation they undertook.[34] Medical texts were translated into other European languages at the same time, but haphazardly, and only in Ireland was there a systematic project to translate a full range of Latin texts into the vernacular, indicating the readiness of the language and the competence of the individuals who undertook the work.[35]

The patronage of the Gaelic aristocracy, evidence of which dates back to legal texts of the seventh or eighth century, gave a certain status to the physicians, as well as the security of hereditary landholding and all that entailed in terms of enabling the establishment and maintenance of schools and gardens. The influence of the patronage by the Gaelic aristocracy of monasteries in the Anglo-Norman period may be visible in the inclusion of introduced plants in the *Materia medica*. There must have been conversations on medical matters between physicians and those people in religious orders charged with medical care. Unfortunately, there are neither extant copies nor records of medical

32 Tadhg Ó Cuinn, *Materia medica*, ed. and trans. by Ó Conchubhair, § 19.

33 Tadhg Ó Cuinn, *Materia medica*, ed. and trans. by Ó Conchubhair, § 11.

34 Mac Mathúna, 'Terminology in the *Rosa Anglica*', pp. 68–74; see also the chapter by Sharon Arbuthnot in this volume.

35 Crossgrove, 'Vernacularization', p. 47; Harris, 'Latin Learning and Irish Physicians', pp. 18–19.

books held in monastic houses in Ireland.[36] They must have existed, and they may have served as exemplars for translations into Irish.

The use of plant medicines as advocated in the *Materia medica* must in some respects have represented a continuity with previous practices in Ireland, both lay and professional. To what extent is largely unknowable. In writing within the formulaic model of the European herbal, Ó Cuinn may have been validating existing use by placing it in a theoretical framework and making reference to authorities. He may also have been putting forward new applications and understanding of materials already in use, as well as introducing new medicines.

In the six centuries that have elapsed since the compilation of this landmark work, Ó Cuinn's *Materia medica* has maintained a presence, in many respects elusive. It has never appeared in a printed edition. Manuscript copies made up to and including the sixteenth century were made by and for physicians. There are no known extant copies from the turbulent seventeenth century, which brought the collapse of the Gaelic order. Quite apart from this collapse, developments in the sciences meant that Galenic paradigms were no longer adequate to accommodate evolving medical knowledge. Prolific copying of older manuscripts in the eighteenth and nineteenth centuries, including seven copies of the *Materia medica* made by members of the Ó Longáin family, were motivated at least in part by the desire to preserve and promote the Irish language and to validate Gaelic culture.[37]

John K'eogh's herbal, *Botanologia universalis Hibernica* or 'A General Irish Herbal', was printed in Cork in 1735.[38] Writing at a time when the market for proprietary medicines was growing, K'eogh advocated the use of 'simple herbs, the products of our own kingdom, whose qualities and virtues are by long experience known to us'. Echoing the principles of Galenic therapeutics, K'eogh deferred to 'our Native Physicians' who are 'the Proper Persons to administer these Herbs, according to the different Distempers, Constitutions, Tempers, way of living, etc., of the Patient'. Although K'eogh was writing long after the collapse of the Gaelic order, it is possible that the 'Native Physicians' he refers to were physicians in the Gaelic tradition. Of the plants discussed by K'eogh, many share similar indications with Ó Cuinn. This need not surprise us, as herbals drew from common sources, but it is possible that K'eogh drew at least partly from the *Materia medica*. Unlike his contemporary Caleb Threlkeld, he names no English sources.[39]

Thomas More Madden (1839–1902), obstetrician, writer, and member of the Royal Irish Academy, engaged Seosamh Ó Longáin to produce a translation of a portion Ó Cuinn's *Materia medica*. More Madden produced

36 Personal communication, Colman Ó Clabaigh, 2018.

37 See Ní Úrdail, 'On the Colophons, Correspondence and Notes'.

38 See John K'Eogh, *Botanalogia universalis Hibernica*, ed. by Scott.

39 Mitchell, 'The Sources of Threlkeld's Synopsis stirpium Hibernicum'.

some extracts of the translation in an essay entitled 'Medical Knowledge of the Ancient Irish'. In spite of the many developments in medicine between Ó Cuinn's day and his, plant-based medicine was still prominent enough for More Madden to see the *Materia medica* as a work in the lineage of European medicine recorded in texts. He comments on Ó Cuinn's account of water crowfoot, saying it is not now employed in medicine, implying that other plants he discusses were still in use in his day.[40] More Madden's allusions to Ó Cuinn's sources and to the continuing use of elements of the *Materia medica*, which can be confirmed in pharmacopoeias of the nineteenth century, belong to the visible spectrum of the history of medicine, recorded in writing. Observing social changes that had taken place in Ireland before the writing of his essay, he saw the need to 'collect any fragments of our popular leechdoms before they become lost in the course of the next few years'.[41] As Catherine Cox has observed, More Madden and his contemporaries, such as Henry Samuel Purdon and William Wilde — all medical practitioners in the established mainstream — combined overlapping interests. They looked, as antiquarians, at the learning of the Gaelic physicians; they sought to discover the cures belonging to 'popular leechdoms of their day'.[42] What still connected those two worlds with each other was the continuing presence of plant-based medicine in both mainstream and vernacular use.

In 1938 the Irish Folklore Commission initiated a Schools' Project. Children in primary schools all over Ireland were asked to speak to older people about customs and stories that were seen to be in decline. One of the categories of information recorded was the medicinal use of plants: this was like a fulfilment of More Madden's wish made fifty years previously. Many of the children's findings reveal remarkable echoes of the *Materia medica*, compiled over five hundred years before. Not surprisingly, simple remedies that can be made in a domestic setting are the ones that persist. The example below, a compilation of several entries written by children in different schools, may be compared with the passage from Ó Cuinn's chapter on plantain quoted above. In this case, the children are talking about ribwort, *Plantago lanceolata*, credited by Ó Cuinn with the same properties as Plantago major:

> It (ribwort, *slanlus, slanessis*) is used to stop bleeding, to cure a burn (applied to the wound, the leaf sticks on like sticking plaster, draws and heals at the same time); to cool down cuts and ease the pain; for putting on cuts as it cleans them out; for sores (put it inside a cloth and keep round the sore); to cure burns; to cure a swelling.[43]

40 More Madden, 'On the Medical Knowledge of the Ancient Irish', p. 13.

41 More Madden, 'On the Medical Knowledge of the Ancient Irish', p. 10.

42 Cox, 'The Medical Marketplace and the Medical Tradition'.

43 The Schools' Collection, vols 719.622–23; 722.52, 110 and 202; 724.159 and 326; 725.402.

Allen and Hatfield's analysis of the findings recorded in the Schools' Collection in their book *Medicinal Plants in Folk Tradition* would no doubt have been different if they had been aware of the corpus of work translated by the Gaelic physicians, in particular the *Materia medica* of Tadhg Ó Cuinn.[44] The absence of the *Materia medica* from any recent ethnobotany can be explained in several ways. Most obviously, the inaccessibility of the medieval texts has been an important reason: they are gradually becoming more available through English translations and publications. Peter Wyse Jackson, in a chapter on historical plant use, notes that he regrets not having been able to include material from early manuscript sources because it is inaccessible to him.[45] Vernacular medicine has not been associated directly with a learned European tradition. The view once held, by Francis Shaw and others, of the body of works translated by Gaelic physicians as scholastic, alien, derivative, divorced from real life and real practice, may have inhibited any impulse to make connections between those works and the later vernacular use of plant medicine.[46] Of all the medieval medical texts in Irish, Ó Cuinn's *Materia medica* is possibly the one to which Shaw's description least applies. It carries its Galenic framework lightly, and as medicine moved beyond that paradigm in Ireland and elsewhere, medicinal use of plants continued in many forms and settings. Recent and ongoing research in the field of medicine in the medieval world is extending beyond the European learned tradition to which Ó Cuinn and the Gaelic physician-translators belonged. Notably, it includes translation and study of previously unedited medical glossaries and remedy collections which are as numerous as academic texts in the Irish medical manuscripts.[47] Remedy collections include remedies, charms, and prayers, three elements which have persisted in vernacular medicine in Ireland to the present day.[48] This research is leading, and will lead, to a more inclusive and comprehensive understanding of the practice of medicine in medieval Ireland and beyond.

Plants have a central place in the history of medicine, as themselves or their products or derivatives, and as a basis for the discovery and isolation of phytochemicals, leading to their incorporation into pharmaceutical products. When we look at the materials of medicine of the medieval world, handed down to us through the texts we study, we are looking at a history which is very much alive.

---

44 Allen and Hatfield, *Medicinal Plants in Folk Tradition*, pp. 337–47.

45 Wyse Jackson, *Ireland's Generous Nature*, p. 12.

46 Shaw, 'Medicine in Ireland in Medieval Times', p. 11.

47 On Irish medical glossaries, see the chapter by Siobhán Barrett in this volume.

48 See Kingston, *Ireland's Hidden Medicine*, pp. 16–22, as well as Hayden, 'Old English in the Irish Charms' and 'A Sixteenth-Century Irish Collection'.

Works Cited

Manuscripts

Dublin, Royal Irish Academy, MS 24 B 2 (461)
Dublin, Trinity College, MS 1343 (H 3. 22)

Primary Sources

Anathomia Gydo, ed. and trans. by Eithne Ní Ghallchobhair, Irish Texts Society, 66 (London: Irish Texts Society, 2014)
'Bretha crólige', ed. and trans. by D. A. Binchy, *Ériu*, 12 (1938), 1–77
K'Eogh, John, *Botanalogia universalis Hibernica, or, A General Irish Herbal (1735)*, ed. by Michael Scott (Wellingborough: The Aquarian Press, 1986)
Regimen na Sláinte. Regimen sanitatis Magnini Mediolanensis, ed. by Séamus Ó Ceithearnaigh (alias James Carney), 3 vols (Dublin: Stationery Office, 1942–1944)
Rosa Anglica seu Rosa medicinae Johannis Anglici, ed. and trans. by Winifred Wulff, Irish Texts Society, 25 (London: Irish Texts Society, 1929)
The Schools' Collection <https://www.dúchas.ie> [accessed 6 February 2023]
Tadhg Ó Cuinn, *An Irish Materia medica (interim version*, 1991), ed. and trans. by Mícheál Ó Conchubhair (alias Michael O'Connor) <https://celt.ucc.ie/published/G600006/index.html> [accessed 6 February 2023]

Secondary Studies

Allen, David, and Gabrielle Hatfield, *Medicinal Plants in Folk Tradition: An Ethnobotany of Britain and Ireland* (Portland, OR: Timber Press, 2004)
Ausécache, Mireille, 'Manuscrits d'antidotaires médiévaux: quelques exemples du fonds latin de la bibliothèque nationale de France', *Médiévales*, 52 (2007), 55–74
Cox, Catherine, 'The Medical Marketplace and Medical Tradition', in *Folk Healing and Healthcare Practices in Britain and Ireland*, ed. by Ronnie Moore and Stuart McLean (New York: Berghahn Books, 2010), pp. 56–74
Crossgrove, William, 'The Vernacularization of Science, Medicine and Technology in Late Medieval Europe: Broadening our Perspectives', *Early Science and Medicine*, 5.1 (2000), 47–63
Demaitre, Luke, *Doctor Bernard de Gordon: Professor and Practitioner* (Toronto: Pontifical Institute of Medieval Studies, 1980)
Foley, Lorraine, 'The Botanical Legacy of Bective Abbey from the Twelfth to the Sixteenth Century', in *The Bective Abbey Project, Co. Meath: Excavations 2009–12*, ed. by Geraldine Stout and Matthew Stout (Dublin: Wordwell, 2016), pp. 202–13
Harris, Jason, 'Latin Learning and Irish Physicians, c. 1350–1610', in *Rosa Anglica: Reassessments*, ed. by Liam P. Ó Murchú, Irish Texts Society Subsidiary Series, 28 (London: Irish Texts Society, 2016), pp. 1–25
Hayden, Deborah, 'Old English in the Irish Charms', *Speculum*, 97.2 (2022), 349–76

——, 'A Sixteenth-Century Irish Collection of Remedies for Ailments of the Male Reproductive Organs', *Celtica*, 33 (2021), 248–76

Hayes, Richard, 'Irish Medical Links with the Continent', in *What's Past is Prologue. A Retrospect of Irish Medicine*, ed. by William Doolin and Oliver Fitzgerald (Dublin: Monument Press, 1952), pp. 23–28

Kelly, Fergus, *Early Irish Farming*, Early Irish Law Series, 4 (Dublin: Dublin Institute for Advanced Studies, 2016)

Kingston, Rosarie, *Ireland's Hidden Medicine* (London: Aeon Books, 2021)

Mac Mathúna, Liam, 'Terminology in the *Rosa Anglica*', in *Rosa Anglica: Reassessments*, ed. by Liam P. Ó Murchú, Irish Texts Society Subsidiary Series, 28 (London: Irish Texts Society, 2016), pp. 57–84

Mitchell, M. E., 'The Sources of Threlkeld's *Synopsis stirpium Hibernicarum*', *Proceedings of the Royal Irish Academy, Section B: Biological, Geological, and Chemical Science*, 74 (1974), 1–6

More Madden, Thomas, 'On the Medical Knowledge of the Ancient Irish', *Dublin Journal of Medical Science*, 71 (1881), 464–76

Nic Dhonnchadha, Aoibheann, 'The Medical School of Aghmacart, Queen's County', *Ossory, Laois and Leinster*, 2 (2006), 11–43

Ní Shéaghdha, Nessa, *Catalogue of Irish Manuscripts in the National Library of Ireland, Fasciculus I: MSS G1–G14* (Dublin: Dublin Institute for Advanced Studies, 1967)

Ní Úrdail, Meidhbhín, 'On the Colophons, Correspondence and Notes in the Ó Longáin Manuscripts', in *Medieval Insular Literature between the Oral and the Written: Continuity of Transmission*, ed. by Hildegard Tristram (Tübingen: Narr, 1997), pp. 221–47

Parnell, John, and Tom Curtis, eds, *Webb's An Irish Flora* (Cork: Cork University Press, 2012)

Pole, Sebastian, *Ayurvedic Medicine: The Principles of Traditional Practice* (London: Singing Dragon, 2013)

Porter, Roy, *The Greatest Benefit to Mankind, a Medical History of Humanity from Antiquity to the Present* (London: Harper Press, 1999)

Riddle, John M., *Dioscorides on Pharmacy and Medicine* (Austin: University of Texas Press, 1985)

Shaw, Francis, 'Medicine in Ireland in Medieval Times', in *What's Past is Prologue. A Retrospect of Irish Medicine*, ed. by William Doolin and Oliver Fitzgerald (Dublin: Monument Press, 1952), pp. 10–14

Simms, Katharine, *Medieval Gaelic Sources* (Dublin: Four Courts Press, 2009)

Temkin, Owsei, *Galenism – Rise and Decline of a Medical Philosophy* (Ithaca: Cornell University Press, 1973)

Tobyn, Graeme, Alison Denham, and Margaret Whitelegg, *The Western Herbal Tradition. 2000 Years of Medicinal Plant Knowledge* (Edinburgh: Churchill Livingstone, 2011)

Wyse Jackson, Peter, *Ireland's Generous Nature: The Past and Present Uses of Wild Plants in Ireland* (St Louis: Missouri Botanical Garden Press, 2014)

CHRISTIAN ETHERIDGE

10. The Role of Cathedrals in the Reception and Dissemination of Medical Knowledge in Medieval Scandinavia

During the Middle Ages, cathedrals throughout Latin Christendom functioned as centres of book learning due to their associated schools, libraries, and scriptoria. This same function existed in the twenty-seven cathedrals located in the three Scandinavian archdioceses. Previous research on these cathedrals has exposed many facets of their rich cultural and literary life.[1] This chapter aims to look at one particular aspect of this intellectual life, namely the role cathedrals in Scandinavia played in the reception and dissemination of medical knowledge. There were no universities in Scandinavia until the late fifteenth century. However, many scholars from Scandinavia, active in the cathedral environment, studied, and in some cases taught, at universities abroad from the thirteenth century onwards, as well as at foreign cathedrals and monastic schools during the preceding century. Therefore, cathedrals were among the largest repositories of learned material in the Middle Ages in Scandinavia and employed the greatest number of university-trained clerics. This study aims to look at the scholarly activity of these cathedrals by looking at the variety of medical volumes held within their libraries. These libraries provide a remarkable amount of information on the reading choices and habits of the literate members of cathedrals and especially, in the context of this essay, their use of medical literature. The study is divided into four periods: 1100–1250, 1250–1400, 1400–1475, and 1475–1525. Each period focuses on medical works connected to Scandinavian cathedrals, which are collated in Appendix 1.

1 For an excellent analysis of the Scandinavian archbishoprics as centres of learning at the turn of the thirteenth century, see Mortensen, 'The Nordic Archbishoprics'. Individual studies are too numerous to list in full here, but noteworthy essays include Keskiaho, 'Bortom fragmenten' on the cathedral of Turku; Ciardi, 'Some Reflections on the Canons of Lund' on the cathedral of Lund; and Myking, 'The French Connection' on Norwegian cathedrals.

Christian Etheridge • University of Southern Denmark;
christian.etheridge@nationalmuseum.se

Medicine in the Medieval North Atlantic World: Vernacular Texts and Traditions, ed. by Deborah Hayden and Sarah Baccianti, KSS, 5 (Turnhout, 2025), pp. 225-266
BREPOLS PUBLISHERS DOI 10.1484/M.KSS-EB.5.143988

Methodological Approaches

Given the different and varied types of sources available for medical volumes in Scandinavian cathedrals, a suitable methodology is vital. Michael Lapidge, in his critical work on Anglo-Saxon libraries, identifies three primary types of evidence that he uses in reconstructing lost book collections: manuscripts, inventories, and citations.[2] Internal evidence in manuscripts often gives a clue as to the institution they once belonged to, while inventories can provide detailed information on the books kept in libraries. Finally, citations can give an idea of what volumes an author had access to when composing their work. Lapidge's methodology provides the researcher with valuable tools to analyse and partially recover lost libraries and can be used in the context of medieval Scandinavian cathedrals and their scattered book collections. Considering the different source materials available for studying inventories in medieval Scandinavia compared to Anglo-Saxon England, other types of source materials also need to be considered. Therefore, in the context of the current study, fragments and printed books will be considered along with manuscripts, inventories will be supplemented with last wills and testaments, while citations will focus on volumes written by medieval Scandinavian authors as well as on the evidence of texts used in their teaching schemes at universities during the Middle Ages. Two important case studies given below emphasize the need for such work.

In her key study of canon law books from medieval Sweden, Mia Korpiola expressed positive surprise at the large number of volumes she could trace through her exploration of fragmented manuscripts, as well as from wills and other sources. This showed her that there was a far greater corpus of law books in medieval Sweden than previous research, which had primarily engaged with complete manuscript sources, had indicated.[3] Meanwhile, Wolfgang Undorf, in his magisterial work on early printed volumes from medieval Scandinavia, worked extensively with inventories and booklists as well as surviving incunabula and early prints.[4] Using these additional sources, he revealed that a much larger number of printed volumes were available in Scandinavia during the Middle Ages than survive today. Undorf further noted that many more manuscripts have survived from medieval England than Scandinavia. The difference in survival rate, he explained, can lead the unwary scholar to make assumptions, amplified by Scandinavia's peripheral geographical position, of a lack of interest in book learning in the medieval North. Undorf instead points out that many more manuscripts and early printed books have survived from England than from Scandinavia because of the political and scholarly environment during the Reformation and Early

---

2 As described in Lapidge, *The Anglo-Saxon Library*, p. 53.

3 See Korpiola, 'Literary Legacies and Canonical Book Collections', pp. 102–03.

4 See Undorf, 'From Gutenberg to Luther'.

Modern period. England had a stable environment of university and college libraries, with early antiquarian interest, which allowed for a greater rate of preservation.[5] Conversely, Scandinavia has a much larger survival rate of church art and ecclesiastical furnishings from the Middle Ages than England due to the different effects of the Reformation in these two places, with Lutheranism being less iconoclastic.[6] Due to the lack of medieval manuscripts from Scandinavia, albeit balanced by recent outstanding work on manuscript fragments, it is therefore paramount to look at other forms of evidence to find out more about volumes owned by Scandinavian cathedrals.[7] Consequently, this essay looks at a wide variety of source material but first briefly addresses the history of cathedrals in Scandinavia during the Middle Ages.

A Short History of the Dioceses of Scandinavia

The first dioceses in Scandinavia were established by the first half of the tenth century when the Danish cities of Ribe, Aarhus, and Schleswig became episcopal seats under the archdiocese of Hamburg-Bremen (Fig. 9.1). The other Danish dioceses of Roskilde, Odense, Viborg, and Børglum followed in the subsequent centuries. The twelfth century saw the creation of the first Scandinavian archbishoprics. Bishop Asser of Lund (d. 1137) became the first Metropolitan of all Scandinavia in 1104 after Pope Paschalis II (1099–1118) consecrated him as the new Archbishop of Lund. This Archbishopric of all Scandinavia lasted until the arrival of the English Augustinian papal legate, Nicholas Breakspear, later Pope Adrian IV (1154–1159). From 1152 to 1154, Nicholas Breakspear was in Scandinavia, where he organized a new Norwegian archbishopric based in Nidaros (Trondheim) and set the arrangements in motion which would result in recognition of the city of Uppsala as the seat of the Swedish metropolitan a few years later in 1164.[8] The Archbishopric of Nidaros was responsible for the dioceses of Nidaros, Skálholt, Bergen, Oslo, Orkney, and Kirkjubøur in the Faroe Islands. These were all founded in the eleventh century. The dioceses of Hólar and Garðar in Iceland, Sodor and Man, Stavanger, and Hamar followed in the twelfth century. The Archbishopric of Uppsala consisted of the dioceses of Skara and Uppsala, both founded in the eleventh century, with Linköping, Västerås, Strängnäs, and Växjö all created in the twelfth century. Finally, the

5 Described in Undorf, 'Print and Book Culture in the Danish Town of Odense', p. 231.

6 See Clausen, 'Reformation and the Monastery Inventory'.

7 Thousands of fragments from medieval Scandinavia have been the subject of recent studies. At the current point in time, it is still not possible to directly trace many of these fragments to a particular institution. For some of the most recent work on Scandinavian fragments, see the collected essays in Ommundsen and Heikkilä, eds, *Nordic Latin Manuscripts Fragments*. For Swedish and Finnish medical fragments, see Etheridge, 'Medieval Scientific Book Fragments'.

8 Waddingham, *Breakspear: The English Pope*, pp. 51–78.

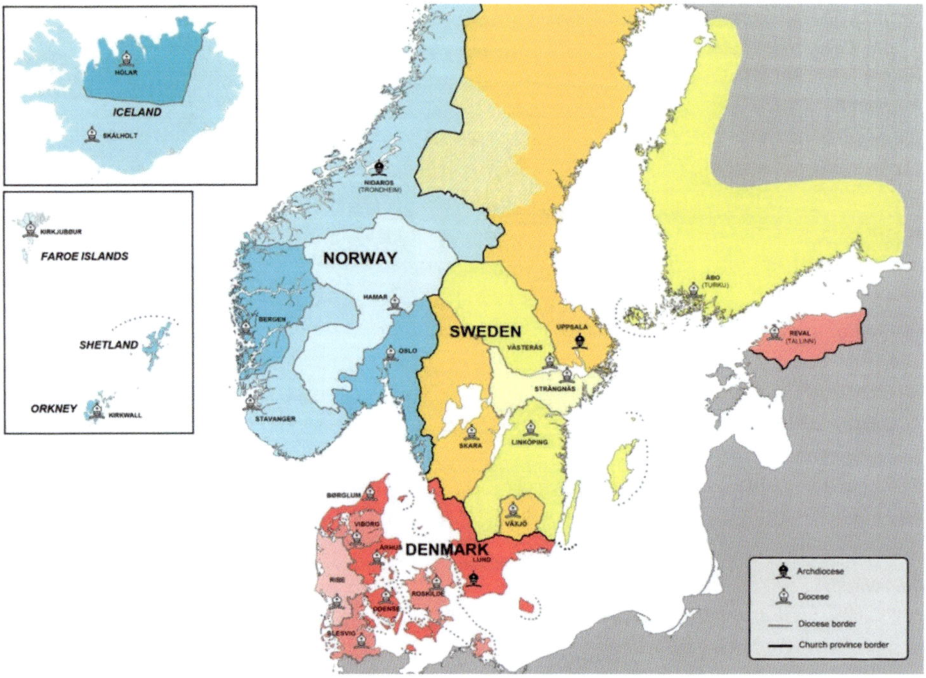

Figure 10.1. Dioceses of Scandinavia (with Iceland, Faroes, and Orkney). Image courtesy of Johnny Grandjean Gøgsig Jakobsen.

dioceses of Åbo (Turku), which came under Uppsala, and Reval (Tallinn), which came under Lund, were founded in the thirteenth century.

These cathedrals were the most important centres of learning from the twelfth century onwards in Scandinavia. Each cathedral church was part of a complex of buildings that included a scriptorium, library, chapter, and school, amongst other buildings devoted to the practical running of the diocesan structure. The three archbishoprics naturally contained Scandinavia's most important scriptoria, libraries, and schools. The archbishops, bishops, and canons often studied abroad and were among the most learned scholars in the diocese. The clerical community had its core in the chapter that was responsible for the spiritual and temporal running of the cathedral and for electing new bishops.[9] The canons there lived a communal life around the cathedral, with the bishop resident nearby.[10] Many of the canons had a university education funded by a benefice or financial support from family or a patron.[11] David Lepine, in his essential book on medieval canonical life, estimated that in the

9 Ciardi, 'Some Reflections on the Canons of Lund', pp. 65–66.

10 Galbon, 'The Canons Regular of St Augustine', pp. 253–54.

11 Lepine, *A Brotherhood of Canons Serving God*, p. 56.

early fourteenth century, around sixty per cent of English canons had received a university education.[12] In a similar study of the canons of Laon Cathedral in France from the late thirteenth to early fifteenth century, Lepine found that forty-eight per cent of them had achieved the university level of magister or a higher degree.[13] A contemporary Scandinavian comparison is given below due to the well-preserved evidence of the canons of Bergen Cathedral during the early fourteenth century.

The Canons of Bergen Cathedral

In the year 1309, during the episcopacy of Bishop Árni Sigurðsson (r. 1305–1314), there were twelve known canons that made up the chapter of Christchurch Cathedral in Bergen. There they resided in a building known as *Kannikeberget*. The biggest cathedral chapter in Norway was that serving the archbishopric of Nidaros, with twenty-four canons. Norwegian chapters tended to be quite small compared to their English counterparts. The smallest secular English cathedral, Exeter, had twenty-four canons, while the largest, Lincoln, had fifty-eight.[14] Like other cathedral chapters, the Bergen canons advised and aided the bishop in his duties. The canons were also involved in other tasks on the cathedral's behalf, whether liturgical, administrative, or legal.[15]

Canons had priests who would help them and substitute for them when they were away from the cathedral. The canons were frequently used in royal missions or ecclesiastical duties outside of the cathedral and might also be away for personal reasons, study, or private commitments. According to a document dated to Thursday 10 April 1309, less than half of the canons were at the cathedral in Bergen: two of them on this date were in France, studying at the University of Paris, another was at an English university, two were in service to the monarch, King Hákon V Magnússon (r. 1299–1319), another canon was busy with the archbishop's business in Nidaros, and the final canon was on a pilgrimage to the shrine of St Thomas Becket in Canterbury.[16] As learned canons, the chapter at the cathedral included many of the most educated and influential figures in Bergen's intellectual society.

12 Lepine, *A Brotherhood of Canons Serving God*, p. 57.

13 Moraw, 'Careers of Graduates', p. 257.

14 Lepine, *A Brotherhood of Canons Serving God*, p. 3.

15 Vihovde, *Kirkesenteret på Holmen*, p. 23 and Helle, *Bergen bys historie*, pp. 603–04. See also Etheridge, 'Canon, Dominican and Brother'.

16 From a copy of a lost codex, printed in DN VI nr. 72, 'duoque ex eis sunt jam Parysiis in studio et unus in Anglia, nec non et alii duo sunt in continuo servitio magnifici principis Haquini regis Norwegiæ illustris, ac unus in negotiis dicti domini archiepiscopi constitutus, prout hoc per numerum residentium manifeste constabat, qui non remanent nisi sex, quorum tamen unus propter votum quo astrictus est ad sanctum Thomam in Anglia' (discussed in Helle, *Bergen bys historie*, p. 598).

In the early fourteenth century, one of the most influential figures in Bergen was the aforementioned Bishop Árni Sigurðsson. Árni studied law and theology at the University of Orléans and was a member of the chapter in Bergen until his election to the bishopric in 1305.[17] His brother Auðfinn Sigurðsson also studied theology and law at Orléans and was also a member of the chapter until his own election to the bishopric of Bergen in 1314. Auðfinn's successor as bishop was Hákon Erlingsson, who most likely studied at the University of Paris or Orléans. He was a member of the chapter until he became bishop in 1332. Hákon's clerk, Arnfinn Tordsson, was university-educated, having studied at Cambridge in 1329.[18] As well as the bishops, the circle of canons at Bergen included other highly educated scholars, such as Magister Solve Ivarsson, canon in 1315, and Magister Árni, canon and cathedral schoolmaster from 1319–1320.[19] Of these clerics, maybe the most notable was Jón Halldórsson, canon *c.* 1310–1320, who studied at the universities of Paris and Bologna.[20] While the magisters and later bishops, Árni Sigurðsson, Auðfinn Sigurðsson, and Hákon Erlingsson, were all elected by the chapter, they were all previously canons. Evidence for manuscript production itself in Bergen in this time can be seen in the record of the visit of the Papal nuncio Petrus Gervasii, who, on 4 August 1333, bought six skins of parchment from a parchmenter in Bergen for the sum of four Gros Tournois.[21] Substantial evidence also exists of a library associated with one of the bishops.

This library is associated with Bishop Árni Sigurðsson and dates from 1313/1314. It can be found in a list in the manuscript Uppsala, Universitetsbibliotek, MS C 564, which details thirty-six works.[22] Of the thirty-six books, five were on canon law, ten on theology, two on liturgy and hagiography, five on grammar, three on logic, and two on computus. The collection also included six histories, of which four were in Old Norse, and three law books in Old Norse. The booklist represents a high degree of learning on the part of Árni, in both Latin and Old Norse, and is an excellent example of bilingual learning and scholarship in the learned circles of Bergen at this time. The works on computus are an unknown *Compotum cum tabulis* and a *Compotum manualem in parva forma*, maybe that of Johannes de Pulchro Rivo.[23]

The above example of the intellectual life of the cathedral of Christchurch in Bergen during the early fourteenth century shows a concentration of

---

17 Bagge, *From Viking Stronghold to Christian Kingdom*, pp. 272–73; Etheridge, 'Canon, Dominican and Brother', pp. 25–27.

18 Helle, *Bergen bys historie*, p. 601.

19 *Diplomatarium Norwegicum*, ed. by Lange and others (henceforth DN), Found in DN II, nr. 71, DN V, nr. 61, DN VIII, nr. 51–52. See also Bagge, 'Norge', p. 146 and Helle, *Bergen bys historie*, pp. 599–602.

20 The career of Jón Halldórsson is the subject of Etheridge, 'Canon, Dominican and Brother'.

21 *Pavelige Nuntiers Regnskabs- og Dagbøger*, ed. by Munch, pp. 67–134.

22 Most recently edited in Etheridge, 'The Booklist of Bishop Arne Sigurdsson'.

23 See Nothaft, 'John of Pulchro Rivo and John of Saxony'.

learned scholars, many of whom had reached the level of magister. Therefore, they would have studied the *quadrivium* in depth and been taught such scientific texts as Sacrobosco's primer on astronomy, *De sphaera*, and works of Aristotelian natural philosophy. They may have taught these subjects, too, and returned to Bergen with volumes of these texts. These clerical scholars attended universities as varied as Orléans, Paris, Bologna, and Cambridge. They were highly mobile and involved in networks connected all around Norway and to their universities. The library connected to Árni Sigurðsson shows the high degree of learning available to the Bergen clergy. There are no medical texts that appear in the booklist, but Árni Sigurðsson studied law and not medicine. To assess further medical texts available to other clergy at Scandinavian cathedrals and to try to understand the role medicine played there, it is necessary to look at the four periods mentioned above in the introduction in turn.

Period One: 1100–1250

A dramatic event occurred in Roskilde Cathedral in *c.* 1158 that was recorded in the *Gesta Danorum* of Saxo Grammaticus a few decades later. The event concerned the rector of the cathedral school, Arnfast, who was ill with a deadening weakness in his muscles. In an attempt to cure this, he drank some medicine ('potione per incuriam sumpta'). Unfortunately, the treatment did not have the desired effect. Instead, it induced lethargy, followed by a more violent reaction that burst Arnfast's liver and forced him to vomit up the pieces. A doctor collected fragments of Arnfast's liver for inspection and then showed them to Bishop Absalon (*c.* 1128–1201) when he came to visit the patient ('quas a medico pelui exceptas maximus pontifex Absalon'). The doctor could not cure Arnfast, and he died three months later.[24]

This passage tells us several things about Roskilde Cathedral during the twelfth century. Firstly, it had a cathedral school; indeed, the school in Roskilde was among the oldest in Scandinavia. During the twelfth century, many cathedral schools were founded in Scandinavia, where they became the most important centres of education there until the respective foundations of Uppsala University in 1477 and the University of Copenhagen in 1479. The second thing to notice here is that Arnfast had both access to medicine and that a doctor was at the cathedral to inspect him when he became ill. It is unsure whether the doctor was personally attached to Bishop Absalon or the cathedral. We know that one of Absalon's colleagues in Paris, Bishop Stephan of Tournai (1128–1203), sent the Roskilde bishop an ampule of the potent medical mixture called theriac in around 1180 when Stephan was Abbot of St Geneviève.[25] This recipe was possibly taken from the twelfth-century pharmaceutical treatise known as the *Antidotarium Nicolai*.

24 Saxo Grammaticus, *Gesta Danorum*, ed. and trans. by Fisher and Friis-Jensen, pp. 836–39.

25 Møller-Christensen, *Middelalderens lægekunst i Danmark*, p. 68.

The third important thing to realize is that Bishop Absalon had spent many years abroad learning in some of the great schools associated with the cathedrals and monasteries in the twelfth century. Specifically, Absalon studied in Paris from the mid-1140s to the 1150s.[26] He most likely studied at the school at St Genevieve in the city. Birger Munk Olsen notes that the teachers there were connected to the great scholars of the nearby Abbey of St Victor. Absalon, therefore, could have attended both St Victor and St Genevieve before he returned to Denmark.[27] Finally, the scribe who wrote the passage on Arnfast, Saxo Grammaticus, was a learned scholar with access to a library of books. He had connections to Lund Cathedral and possibly Roskilde Cathedral, both of which had libraries. Karsten Friis-Jensen points out that a large selection of learned sources used in the compilation of Saxo's *Gesta Danorum* are encyclopaedic works with medical chapters. These include the *Naturalis historia* of Pliny and the *Naturales quaestiones* of Seneca.[28] These encyclopaedic texts were used in the Parisian schools and other Northern French schools, such as the cathedral school at Chartres. It would seem likely that Saxo studied in France and either obtained those books there or that they were brought back to Denmark by Absalon. Norwegian clerics were also connected to these Parisian schools.

Learning Abroad in the Cathedral Schools: Learned Archbishops of Nidaros and Lund Cathedrals

The advanced education available in the French cathedral schools of the twelfth century is shown in the learned sources used by the Norwegian writer Theodoricus in the compilation of his *Historia de antiquitate regum Norwagiensium*.[29] Egil Kraggerud has pointed out the identity of Theodoricus as Þórir Gudmunarsson, archbishop of Nidaros (r. 1206–1214), who wrote the *Historia de antiquitate regum Norwagiensium* around 1180–1183, probably also at the cathedral.[30] Theodoricus or Þórir Gudmunarsson was born sometime after 1150 and studied in Paris in the early 1170s at St Victor. His Victorine influence appears when he writes 'Hugo bone memorie canonicus Sancti Victoris Parisiis, uir undecunque doctissimus' (Hugh of blessed memory, canon of St Victor in Paris, a man skilled in all branches of learning) at the

26 On Absalon in Paris, see Olsen, 'Absalons studier i Paris', p. 57.

27 Olsen, 'Absalons studier i Paris', pp. 70–71.

28 Friis-Jensen, *Saxo og Vergil*.

29 See the editions Theodoricus, *De antiquitate regum Norwagiensium*, ed. and trans. by Kraggerud, and Theodoricus Monachus, *Historia de antiquitate regum Norwagiensium*, ed. and trans. by McDougall and McDougall. For twelfth-century cathedral schools, see Bagge, 'Nordic Students at Foreign Universities until 1660', pp. 3–4.

30 Theodoricus, *De antiquitate regum Norwagiensium*, ed. and trans. by Kraggerud, pp. xxx–xxxv and l–li; Myking, 'The French Connection', pp. 98 and 107.

beginning of his work and uses treatises written by Hugh and Richard of St Victor.[31] Encyclopaedias that include medical texts that Theodoricus uses are the *Etymologiae* of Isidore of Seville and the *Naturalis historia* of Pliny. The library of St Victor contained all these works.[32] As Theodoricus composed his work after leaving St Victor, there is some debate as to whether he had access to the above volumes in Norway. Still, it is certainly possible, as Nidaros was an important centre of learning.[33] This supposition is strengthened by evidence from two fragmentary twelfth-century copies of Isidore's *Etymologiae* that are likely to have been in the cathedral chapter of Nidaros. The first (Oslo, Riksarkivet, MS NRA lat. fragmenter 2, 1–8; 1, 1–11; 3, 1–13) most likely comes from France, with the other example coming from England (Oslo, Riksarkivet, MS NRA lat. fragmenter 113b, 1–2).[34] It is tempting to suggest that the French transmission of Isidore's *Etymologiae* originated in the learned environment of St Victor. At the same time, the English manuscript points to the solid intellectual connections between England and Norway in the twelfth century.

A parallel figure to Theodoricus in twelfth-century intellectual cathedral life was the Danish cleric Anders Sunesen (*c.* 1167–1228), who later became Archbishop of Lund (1201–1223), following the reign of his relative Absalon. Lund Cathedral in the twelfth century was one of the most important centres of learning in Scandinavia. The manuscripts that we can trace to Lund or that were possibly used by archbishops and canons there are representative of texts used in the cathedral schools of Northern France.[35] It is possible that the Victorine milieu in Paris is the ultimate source of this. Anders Sunesen, like Absalon, travelled to Paris to study there in the 1180s at around the same time as his brother Peder. It seems most likely that Anders studied at St Geneviève, as we know Peder was there.[36] Anders Sunesen wrote his *Hexaëmeron*, a work in a genre of similarly titled theses of theological and scientific commentaries on the six days of creation, probably in Paris around the early 1190s. The *Hexaëmeron* uses the *Etymologiae* of Isidore of Seville.[37] As with Theodoricus,

31 Theodoricus Monachus, *Historia de antiquitate regum Norwagiensium*, ed. and trans. by McDougall and McDougall, p. 1. For Hugh, see pp. 91 n. 210 and for Richard, see pp. 56 n. 9, 67 n. 68 and possibly 67 n. 71.

32 Theodoricus Monachus, *Historia de antiquitate regum Norwagiensium*, ed. and trans. by McDougall and McDougall, pp. 56, 70, 77–99 and 111. See Theodoricus, *De antiquitate regum Norwagiensium*, ed. and trans. by Kraggerud, pp. 5, 7; 17: 1; 18: 13, 15, 21; 20: 5–8; 26: 8, as well as Myking, 'The French Connection', p. 106.

33 Myking, 'The French Connection', p. 90.

34 Karlsen, 'Fragments of Patristic and Other Ecclesiastical Literature in Norway', pp. 229–30. The French manuscript of Isidore is found in the fragments of Oslo, Riksarkivet, MS NRA lat. fragmenter 2, 1–8; 1, 1–11; and 3, 1–1, while the English Isidore is in Oslo, Riksarkivet, MS NRA lat. fragmenter 113b, 1–2.

35 Nielsen, *Danmarks Middelalderlige Haandskrifter*, pp. 27–48.

36 See Anders Sunesen, *Andreae Sunonis filii Hexaemeron*, ed. by Ebbesen and Mortensen; see also Olsen, 'Anders Sunesen og Paris', p. 86.

37 Pedersen, 'Stof og form de fire første dage', pp. 117–28.

we must explore the possibility that Anders took some of his books back with him to Lund and that they ended up in the library there.

The Library and Scriptorium of Lund Cathedral

The cathedral of Lund was preeminent among the cathedrals of twelfth-century Scandinavia. It was the archdiocesan church for all of Scandinavia for the first half of the century. Even after the creation of the archdioceses of Nidaros and Uppsala, it was still the centre of the richest archdiocese in Scandinavia. Such a wealthy cathedral would naturally have a substantial library, referred to as the *armarium librorum* in the twelfth century. According to the *Consuetudines Lundenses*, written before 1123, the care and supervision of the books in the library was the duty of the cantor,[38] who also recorded the titles of the books and the names of the people who loaned them.[39] Those canons of Lund who did not travel abroad to study were, therefore, able to be educated using the volumes in the library. Among the biblical commentaries, Patristic texts, and works of classical authors, were works of science. The earliest example that is recorded is from the testament of Archbishop Asser (1089–1137), who in 1131 donated his book collection to Lund cathedral; this included 'multos etiam phisicales' (many books on medicine).[40] The cathedral at Lund was also of great importance in producing and distributing manuscripts.[41]

Medical Texts at Uppsala Cathedral

Siward (d. 1157) was bishop of Uppsala in the 1140s, a couple of decades before the cathedral became an archdiocese. He left twenty-six volumes in his testament to the Benedictine monastery of Rastede in Lower Saxony, where he had become abbot of Rastede after a period of exile from Sweden, partially spent in England.[42] It is impossible to say where his volumes came from: they could date from his episcopacy in Uppsala, his sojourn in England, or his tenure as abbot of Rastede Abbey. Among the books are several medical texts. These include an entry that reads *Herbarium, lapidarium in uno volumine*. This entry is most likely the *De viribus herbarum* attributed to Macer Floridus and the popular *Liber lapidum* of Marbod of Rennes (*c.* 1035–1123) combined in one manuscript. Also included in the list is a *Medicinales sex*, which would refer to six untitled medicinal works. This entry could refer to the popular

38 Ciardi, 'Some Reflections on the Canons of Lund', pp. 75–76.

39 Christensen, 'Scandinavian Libraries in the Late Middle Ages', p. 482.

40 Møller-Christensen, *Middelalderens lægekunst i Danmark*, p. 66.

41 Rydén, 'Dalbyboken'.

42 Kleberg, *Medeltida Uppsalabibliotek I*, pp. 9–24.

medical compilation known as the *Articella*, which in its later transmission often consisted of six medical texts.[43]

The Medical Career of Henrik Harpestreng

The best-known Scandinavian who worked with medicine in the Middle Ages is undoubtably the Danish canon Henrik Harpestreng, who passed away at Roskilde Cathedral on 2 April 1244, where he is noted as 'Medicus canonicus Roskildensis'.[44] Harpestreng was titled *mester* or magister and so would have obtained this title abroad, possibly at the learned schools of Salerno.[45] Later sources found in two fifteenth-century manuscripts (Copenhagen, Det Kongelige Bibliotek, MS GKS 3656 8vo and Linköping, Stadsbibliotek, MS Grensholmensis Saml. I) record that Harpestreng was the royal physician to the Danish King Erik IV (r. 1241–1250). They further mention that he bled the king at the astrologically correct times.[46] There are three treatises associated with Henrik Harpestreng. *De simplicibus medicinis laxativis* is a Latin text with thirty-five herbs arranged alphabetically.[47] With each herb, recipes are given for medicines with exact doses, accompanied by a passage containing advice for use and storage. The only version of this treatise is found in the manuscript Copenhagen, Det Kongelige Bibliotek, MS GKS 1654 4to, from the fifteenth century. *De simplicibus medicinis laxativis* was probably written at the end of the twelfth century.[48] The second treatise, the *Liber herbarum*, is a Latin herbal possibly composed around 1200 that contains a catalogue of fifty-three different herbs, with qualities and instructions for medical use. The book uses the humoral-pathological system, as used by the Salerno school. According to this system, illness is caused by disharmony of the humours in the body.[49] The *Regimen sanitatis Salernitanum* was a key influence on this treatise, while the occurrence of the northern plants *Angelica, Benedicta alba*, and *Benedicta ruffa* points to a Scandinavian author rather than a direct copy.[50] The final treatise, the Old Danish *Den danske urtebog* (The Danish Book of Herbs), is a reference pharmacopoeia, with herbs and precious stones alphabetically arranged according to their Latin names. This treatise also shows the influence of the school in Salerno concerning the causes and cures of diseases. The major sources here are Constantinus Africanus' *De gradibus liber* and the *De viribus herbarum* of Macer Floridus. These last two

43 Kleberg, *Medeltida Uppsalabibliotek I*, pp. 24–37.
44 Henrik Harpestreng, *Liber herbarum*, ed. by Hauberg, pp. 9–13.
45 Holck, 'Middelalderens danske lægebog', p. 97.
46 These texts are not edited; see Jørgensen, 'Henricus Harpestreng'.
47 Henricus Dacus, *Liber de simplicibus medicinis laxativis*, ed. by Johnsson.
48 Jørgensen, 'Henricus Harpestreng'.
49 See the chapter by Conan Doyle in this volume.
50 Jørgensen, 'Henricus Harpestreng'.

treatises of Henrik Harpestreng proved to be two of the most important works of medicine in medieval Scandinavia and were eventually translated into all the Scandinavian vernaculars.[51]

The examples given above show that medical texts were in circulation in Scandinavian cathedrals from the twelfth century until the mid-thirteenth century. Scandinavians travelled abroad and were a part of the intellectual network of European scholarship. Furthermore, the Scandinavian cathedrals had libraries that contained medical texts and hosted important scriptoria. Finally, Scandinavian scholars were also writing treatises influenced by the scientific trends of the time, which included medicine.[52]

Period Two: 1250–1400

From 1250 to 1400, there was an increased mobility among bishops and canons from Scandinavia as they travelled to the newly founded universities in Europe. There is also a corresponding increase in the number of manuscripts of a scientific nature known in Scandinavia. A good example is a manuscript now known by the shelfmark Uppsala, Universitetsbibliotek, MS C 55, which, although containing no treatises on medicine, is very enlightening as its transmission is so well understood. UUB C 55 includes several university texts on medieval science, including works by Aristotle, Averroes, and Johannes de Sacrobosco.[53] The manuscript was made in Prague in the early fourteenth century and purchased by a Sigismund, a priest at Ösmo Church, a village now on the outskirts of modern-day Stockholm, sometime before 1327. Sigismund later became a canon in Uppsala and a member of the chapter of the cathedral of Strängnäs. He would end his career as the bishop of Strängnäs. An Ulpho Holmgersson later owned the UUB C 55 manuscript. He was also a canon at Uppsala Cathedral and later at Västerås Cathedral. The book probably passed from Sigismund to Ulpho at the end of the 1320s, when both were canons in Uppsala. Ulpho died in 1335, and no further owners are known after him; it is unknown how or when the manuscript made its final journey to the Birgittine Vadstena Abbey. However, it was there by the time of the librarian Brother Andreas Lydekini (1387–1410).[54] The UUB C 55 manuscript demonstrates the fluidity of movement that a single manuscript could have, passing from Prague to Ösmo Church, then to Uppsala Cathedral, from there to Västerås Cathedral, and eventually to Vadstena Abbey all in the course of a century.

51 Jørgensen, 'Henricus Harpestreng'.

52 For more see Bauer, *Laienastrologie im nachreformatorischen Island*; Ohrvik, *Medicine, Magic, and Art in Early Medieval Norway*; and Cucina, 'Il computo del tempo nella Scandinavia medievale'.

53 *Mittelalterliche Handschriften der Universitätsbibliothek Uppsala: Katalog über die C-Sammlung: Bd. 2. C 51–200*, ed. by Andersson-Schmitt and Hedlund, pp. 15–18.

54 Walta, 'Libraries, Manuscripts and Book Culture in Vadstena Abbey', p. 60.

Medical Texts at Uppsala and Lund Cathedrals

In 1369, Archbishop Birger Gregersson made an official inventory of the books in Uppsala Cathedral. He was aided by several canons, including Magister Mathias (later bishop in Västerås), who studied in Paris from 1335 to 1352, and Magister Ulpho Gislonis, who was at the same university in the 1340s. The inventory included medical texts and encyclopaedias such as the *Etymologiae* of Isidore of Seville, the *De proprietatibus rerum* of Bartholomeus Anglicus, the *De medicina equorum* of Jordanus Ruffus, and the translation by Leo Tuscanus of Abu Bakr Muhammad ibn Sirin's *Interpretaciones sompniorum* into Latin. These four texts were part of a total of ninety-six volumes held in both the cathedral library (*liberaria ecclesie*) and the archbishop's library. This latter library was found in a stone house (*domus lapidea*) belonging to the cathedral. In 1377, a further inventory also listed a copy of *De proprietatibus rerum*, which could be the same as the 1369 version. This volume was placed along with a couple of other books in the archbishop's library.[55] As the inventory of the cathedral library survives from this time, it gives us an insight into the books available to those at the cathedral. As expected, medical volumes make up only a tiny percentage of those available, but it is a significant number. A library inventory only records a snapshot in time, and library collections constantly fluctuate, as shown below in the case of Lund Cathedral.[56]

From the second half of the thirteenth century, we have a single incidence of a donation of scientific works to the library of Lund by Magister Knud, a canon at the cathedral. He died 12 June 1260 and donated unknown books on *scientia naturali* to the chapter.[57] There are more surviving wills from canons of Lund Cathedral that show them leaving encyclopaedic works with medical chapters to the cathedral library during the fourteenth century. Nicolaus Bunkeflod, a canon of Lund and Roskilde, donated a medical book with the title *Thesaurus pauperum* to Peter Svenssen, canon and cellarer in Lund, in his will from 28 September 1346.[58] Tucho Thuronis, from Malmö, was also a canon of Lund who, according to his will from 11 March 1352, donated the *De proprietatibus rerum* of Bartholomeus Anglicus and the *De viribus herbarum* of Macer with an attached lapidary.[59] The Lund canon Benechinus Henrici of Åhus, who had studied canon law in Paris and civil law in either Bologna or Orléans, passed away on 9 March 1358. He donated in his will the Hippocratic *Physiognomy* and the *De utensilibus* by Alexander Neckam.[60] The

---

55 Kleberg, *Medeltida Uppsalabibliotek II*, pp. 84–107.

56 For astronomical works in Lund, see Etheridge, 'Astronomy at Lund Cathedral in the Middle Ages', p. 206.

57 Møller-Christensen, *Middelalderens lægekunst i Danmark*, p. 68.

58 Møller-Christensen, *Middelalderens lægekunst i Danmark*, p. 71.

59 *Testamenter fra Danmarks middelalder*, ed. by Erslev, pp. 113–16.

60 *Testamenter fra Danmarks middelalder*, ed. by Erslev, pp. 118–24; for analysis of the whole will of Benechinus Henrici, see Mornet, 'Le testament du chanoine Benechinus Henrici de Åhus'.

most prominent collection of medical texts belonging to any cleric connected to the cathedral is that of Archbishop Jens Grand (*c.* 1260–1327).

The Collection of Medical Texts Belonging to Archbishop Jens Grand

Jens Grand had studied at the University of Paris in his youth and, on his return to Denmark, worked his way up the ladder of ecclesiastical power until he was finally elected archbishop of Lund in 1289. He was involved in an investiture conflict with King Erik VI (r. 1286–1319), which resulted in the archbishop excommunicating the king. In return, Jens Grand was arrested under the king's orders and imprisoned in Søborg Castle, around 50km north of Copenhagen, in 1294. Erik VI's brother Christopher (later King Christopher II) ransacked Jens Grand's apartments and apparently found a book on the Black Arts that the archbishop was supposed to have frequently studied.[61] According to an account of the trial of Jens Grand in 1294, the archbishop complained that his library had been plundered. Erik VI replied that the only book that had been confiscated was a '*liber necromanticus*'.[62] Jens Grand managed to escape his prison in 1295 and fled Denmark. After a colourful career path, including being Prince-Archbishop of Bremen, Jens Grand eventually ended up at the papal court in Avignon, where he died in 1327 at around the age of eighty. Papal commissioners then acquired his eighty-two-volume library.

Vilhelm Møller-Christensen noted that this extensive medical collection is likely to have come from his time as Archbishop of Lund in Denmark, rather than after this time, as Jens Grand was involved with his struggles against King Erik VI and had further problems throughout his later career that left him little time to collect books.[63] Of course, there were other opportunities for Jens Grand to pick up books during his subsequent career. However, if he had studied and possibly taught medicine while at the University of Paris, which seems likely due to his extensive collection of medical books, then his library may well have travelled with him from France to Denmark before he began his career in Lund. Indeed, almost all the works he owned were written earlier than around 1270, which would fit in with this timeline.

The library of Jens Grand contained nine volumes that were of a medical nature, with some encyclopaedias and other books.[64] As Cornelius O'Boyle points out, one book contained the Hippocratic *Aphorisms* and may have been a copy of the whole *Articella*.[65] In contrast, another contained a copy of the

61 Møller-Christensen, *Middelalderens lægekunst i Danmark*, p. 69.

62 Christensen, 'Scandinavian Libraries in the Late Middle Ages', p. 496.

63 Møller-Christensen, *Middelalderens lægekunst i Danmark*, pp. 70–71.

64 Møller-Christensen, *Middelalderens lægekunst i Danmark*, pp. 68–70; see also Appendix 1.

65 O'Boyle, *Medical Teaching at the University of Paris*, pp. 174–75.

Antidotarium Nicolai and may have been a copy of the subsidiary collection. Jens Grand also owned the three most popular and largest encyclopaedias of the Middle Ages, these being the *Etymologiae* of Isidore of Seville, the *De proprietatibus rerum* of Bartholomeus Anglicus, and the *Speculum maius* of Vincent of Beauvais. Together with these medical and encyclopaedic works he also owned works on computus and a digest on Aristotle and other philosophers. The final entry concerns various books on alchemy.[66] It seems possible therefore that Jens Grand practised alchemy and that this could also have included practising elements of magic, if the claims of Erik VI above were correct. The anonymous books noted in the inventory represent an unknown number of volumes. The collection of medical works owned by Jens Grand was extensive compared to other contemporaries. O'Boyle gives the examples of the Benedictine Abbot William of St-Paul-outside-the-Walls in Rome, who died during the residence of Pope Urban V (1362–1370) in 1367–1370 and left fifty-eight volumes, with one being a medical volume. Another example is Matthew Della Porta, the Franciscan Archbishop of Palermo, who died in 1377; when the papal commissioners collected his 114-book library, it was found to contain three medical works.[67]

Period Three: 1400–1475

In the fifteenth century, the great astronomical clock in Lund was placed inside the cathedral, next to the shrine of the Virgin Mary.[68] The astronomical clock, which was constructed *c.* 1422, was a triumph of fifteenth-century science and technology.[69] The clock is believed to have been made by the German clockmaker Nikolaus Lilienfeld, who represents one of the most important aspects of science and also medicine in fifteenth century Scandinavia: namely, the influence of the German-speaking world, especially that of the Hanseatic League.[70] Whereas in previous centuries, intellectual currents from France and England had been the most influential on science in Scandinavia, this changed in the fifteenth century. The Hanseatic League had important mercantile bases in all the major Scandinavian cities. Scandinavian merchants likewise conducted most of their trade through Hanseatic cities. It was not just trade items that sailed around Scandinavia with the Hanseatic ships but also culture and ideas. In the fifteenth century, the centre of Scandinavian intellectual life also shifted from the University of Paris to the universities in the Holy Roman Empire.

---

66 Mitchell, *Witchcraft and Magic in the Nordic Middle Ages*, p. 48.

67 O'Boyle, *Medical Teaching at the University of Paris*, pp. 174–75.

68 Axel-Nilsson, *Thesaurus Cathedralis Lundensis*, pp. 70–72.

69 Mogensen, 'Urets gamla och nya fasad' and Schukowski, 'Astronomiska ur i Hansatidens kyrkor', p. 126.

70 Andrén, 'Världen från Lunds horisont', pp. 126–27; Hamel, 'Nikolaus Lilienfeld'; Schukowski, 'Astronomiska ur i Hansatidens kyrkor', pp. 123–27; Etheridge, 'The Evidence for Islamic Scientific Works in Medieval Iceland', pp. 49–53.

The Library of Skara Cathedral

The manuscript Uppsala, Universiteitsbibliothek, MS C 622, containing the *Parvulus naturalis* of Petrus de Dresden from 1468, was written in Skara and was part of the cathedral library until it was moved at some point to Vadstena Abbey and given the shelfmark J 2 xvi.[71] The cathedral library was partially destroyed in the Danish invasions in 1566 during the Northern Seven Years' War and again in 1612 during the Kalmar War, when the collection was scattered.[72] According to the testament of Stockholm, Riksarkivet, MS SDHK nr 29337, the cathedral library of Skara received the personal library of 138 volumes of Bero Magni, lecturer at the University of Vienna, at some time between his death in 1465 and 1475.[73] By the end of the medieval period, the cathedral library in Skara had between three hundred and five hundred volumes, of which Bero's books formed between about a quarter and a half of the total collection.[74] Scientific works formed seventeen per cent of the total of Bero's books and included two copies of Bartholomeus Anglicus: *De proprietatibus rerum*, five unidentified books on medicine, and a treatise on chiromancy.

Bengt Knutsson and Västerås Cathedral

Benedictus Kanuti or Bengt Knutsson (d. 1462) was briefly Bishop of Västerås from 1461. He had practised medicine at the University of Montpellier and is mentioned in the Latin version of his work as 'medicine expertissimi professoris'. It is not clear when or where Bengt Knutsson wrote his treatise on the plague. Still, between 1450–1455, a virulent recurrence of the plague killed tens of thousands in Sweden, possibly providing the impetus for the treatise. The Latin treatise was titled *Regimen contra pestilentiam* and was first printed in Paris in 1480. It was reprinted three times in Antwerp in 1484, 1486, and 1491. A Middle English version was printed in London in 1485, titled *A litil boke for the Pestilence*.[75] This is the only Scandinavian scientific treatise known to have been published in Middle English. In 1546 Thomas Phaer made an English translation of the French version of the *Regimen sanitatis Salerni*. This was titled *the regiment of lyfe* and had the *A litil boke for the Pestilence* of Bengt Knutsson attached to it. This combined work went through several editions throughout the sixteenth century. The part relating to the plague was still being published in London as late as 1722.[76]

71 *Mittelalterliche Handschriften der Universitätsbibliothek Uppsala: Katalog über die C-Sammlung: Bd. 6. C 551–935*, ed. by Andersson-Schmitt, Hallberg and Hedlund.

72 Kihlman, 'Bero Magni de Ludosia: Student and Teacher', p. 123.

73 Kihlman, 'Bero Magni de Ludosia: Student and Teacher', p. 90.

74 Kihlman, 'The Inventory of Bero's Library', pp. 146–70.

75 Bengt Knuttson, *A litil boke for the Pestilence*, pp. xxxi–xxxvi.

76 Bengt Knuttson, *A litil boke for the Pestilence*, p. xxxvi.

Medical Texts at Roskilde Cathedral

At the beginning of the fifteenth century, the Roskilde Cathedral library was moved by deacon Laurids Jensen (1397–1419) into Saint Sigfrid's chapel in the north tower. The *Liber daticus Roskildensis* records the loans from the cathedral library to the canons in the years 1459 and 1460. In this list, sixty-three volumes were loaned in 1459 and sixty-six in 1460. This was during the bishopric of Oluf Daa (*c.* 1400–1461). He matriculated from the University of Rostock in 1423 and was elected to the bishop's throne in 1448. Of the cathedral's thirty-five canons, thirteen loaned books in 1459 and 1460.[77] Six of those thirteen loaned medical texts from the library, so around one in six of the canons. This provides the clearest picture from medieval Scandinavia of book loans of medical texts. The texts borrowed are shown in Table 10.1.

Table 10.1. Medical texts loaned from Roskilde Cathedral Library, 1459–1460.

Author	Title	Borrower	Dates
Bartholomeus Anglicus	*De proprietatibus rerum*	Tuco Johannis	1459
Bernardus Provincialis	*Commentarius in tabulas Salernitanus*	Olauus Boetii	1459–1460
Bernard de Gordon	*Lilium medicinae*	Jacobus Petri	1460
		Lauricius Petri	1460
Constantinus Africanus	*Viaticum*	Johannes Syndonis	1459–1460
Johannes Platearius	*Practica brevis*	Johannes Syndonis	1459–1460
		Olauus Boetii	1459–1460
Matthaeus Platearius	*Circa instans*	Johannes Syndonis	1459–1460
		Olauus Boetii	1459–1460
Matthaeus Platearius	*Glossae in Antidotarium Nicolai*	Johannes Syndonis	1459–1460
		Olauus Boetii	1459–1460
Petrus Hispanus	*Thesaurus pauperum*	Lauriencius Olaiij	1459
Pseudo-Galen	*Fortior medicinarum*	Olauus Boetii	1459–1460

Period Four: 1475–1525

An interesting correspondence has been preserved between Hans Brask (1464–1538), the Bishop of Linköping, and Margareta Eriksdotter Vasa (1497–1536), the sister of the Swedish king Gustav Vasa. On 9 March 1524, Hans Brask wrote a letter in Swedish to Margareta, where he expressed his thanks to her for sending him a medical book, the identity of which he, unfortunately, does not reveal. This medical book might have been a copy of a printed edition of the *Hortus sanitatis*. The letter states:

77 Møller-Christensen, *Middelalderens lægekunst i Danmark*, pp. 78–80.

> Vi tacke eder … för then läkesbok vi nu finge […] Tha vi vore senest til samtal pa Stegeborg var pa tall om monge böker tydzsche oc swensche saa at oss ey fullelica drager til minnes ther om edra begäre doch sende vi eder nu med thetta samme bud eth tyst passional til tiid fördriiff i thenne helge tiid nu är inne.
>
> > (We thank you for the medical book we now got […] During our last conversation at Stegeborg we talked about so many German and Swedish books that we cannot fully remember which books you desired so we send you by return of post a German Passionale to pass this holy time we are in now.)[78]

Hans Brask refers to his latest visit to Stegeborg castle, just outside of Söderköping, and to the literary conversations between him and Margareta. They then talked about the German and Swedish books Margareta wanted to acquire; there were so many of these that afterward, Hans Brask could not remember them all. Unfortunately, no more of this correspondence has survived. It shows, however, the learned nature of Margareta Vasa, who was fluent in Swedish and German and most likely knew Latin. She sent her daughters to the Cistercian Nunnery of Skokloster, as it was an important school for the daughters of the nobility. It is possible she was taught there as well.[79]

The Library of Christiern Pedersen

The Danish canon of Lund, scholar and bookseller Christiern Pedersen was influential in the early sixteenth-century book trade and wrote his own scientific treatises. Pedersen's collection of printed works recorded by Undorf contained several scientific works, which can be placed in several groups. There was a work of astrology that was either the *Epistola astrologiae defensiva* of Jean Ganivet from a 1508 Lyons edition or the *Adversus prognosticatorum astrologiae defensio* of Albertus Pighius from a 1519 Paris edition. There were several medical works, including the *Hortus sanitatis* of Jacob Meydenbach, possibly from a Strasbourg 1517 edition; the *Regimen contra pestilentiens* of Johannes Jacobi, possibly from either a Hagenau 1500 or Paris 1519 edition; the *Regimen sanitatis Salerni*, possibly from a Paris 1519 edition; and finally, three separate copies of the *De viribus herbarum* of Macer Floridus, possibly from a Paris 1515 edition. The collection was completed by encyclopaedic material, including the *Margarita philosophica* of Gregor Reisch, possibly from a Basel 1517 edition, and four copies of the most popular encyclopaedia in medieval

78 Undorf, 'From Gutenberg to Luther', p. 443.
79 Undorf, 'From Gutenberg to Luther', p. 443.

Scandinavia, the *De proprietatibus rerum* of Bartholomeus Anglicus, possibly from a Basel 1517 edition.[80]

Uppsala Cathedral Library

The cathedral library of Uppsala has a substantial collection of incunabula of a scientific nature surviving from the late fifteenth century, including two copies of the *Speculum naturale* by Vincent of Beauvais from the Strasbourg 1481 edition (Uppsala, Universitetsbibliotek, MSS Inc. 1492 and Inc. 1493). Ericus Erici, the economic administrator, owned a copy of the *De proprietatibus rerum* by Bartholomeus Anglicus in a possible Heidelberg 1488 version. Ericus Johannis (d. 1512), another economic administrator, also owned a copy of the *De proprietatibus rerum* by Bartholomeus Anglicus in a possible Heidelberg 1488 version; it seems likely that this is the same volume as that possessed by Ericus Erici.[81] The Uppsala Cathedral library had a substantial collection of Aristotelian commentaries and one or possibly two copies of the *De proprietatibus rerum*. The cathedral staff enhanced the library, which would have had strong connections to the university next door.

The Donation of Nicholas Senior to Roskilde Cathedral

In 1480, King Christian I's (r. 1448–1481) doctor Nicolaus Senior donated the following medical works contained in one volume to pay for a requiem at Roskilde Cathedral.[82] These were a plague book by Gentile de Foligno; a fever treatise of Bernard Alberti; the *Practica oculorum* of Beneventus Grapheus; Guglielmo da Saliceto's *Chirurgi* in five books; and a plague treatise written in 1376 by Johannes Jacobus.

Västerås Cathedral and Peder Månsson

Peder Månsson (*c.* 1460–1534) became a brother at the Birgittine abbey of Vadstena in 1499. In 1507, he left Vadstena for the Birgittine house in the Campo di Fiori in Rome to organize the Order's business as procurator, overseeing the rebuilding of the church there in 1513. In 1524, he left Rome to become Bishop of Västerås and was influential in spreading the Reformation for the next decade before dying in 1534. Peder Månsson was responsible for many scientific works that he wrote in Old Swedish. His *Konstbok* is found in his autograph manuscript

80 Undorf, 'From Gutenberg to Luther', pp. 131–57.
81 Undorf, 'From Gutenberg to Luther', p. 374.
82 Møller-Christensen, *Middelalderens lægekunst i Danmark*, p. 80.

Linköping J8 and concerns chemistry and various aspects of technology such as steel manufacture and silver gilding. Peder Månsson was also very interested in alchemy and translated alchemical texts into Old Swedish in this manuscript, including the *De secretis naturae* of Raymond Lully. Also found in Linköping J8 was his *Läkebok* (Medical Book), mainly a translation of Johannes de Rupescissa's *De consideratione quintæ essentiæ*.[83]

Schleswig Cathedral

The booklist of the library of the lecturer in theology at Schleswig cathedral (*Domum lectoris ordinarii Slesvvicensis*) from 1519 has been preserved. The inventory indicates that 80 per cent of the collection at this time were printed books and 20 per cent were manuscripts. The inventory was divided into three sections. *In sacris literis* contained 142 book titles and thirty-nine manuscript titles. *In jure* contained twenty-two book titles and five manuscript titles. *In naturalibus, historiis, artibus humanitatis et aliis* contained thirty-one book titles and four manuscript titles. Of the 243 titles in the booklist, the eight scientific titles listed make up around 3 per cent of the total, including three encyclopaedias with medical chapters. These are the *De proprietatibus rerum* of Bartholomeus Anglicus, from an unidentified edition; the *Etymologiae* of Isidore of Seville, from a Strasbourg 1473 edition; and the *Speculum Naturale* of Vincent of Beauvais, from an unidentified edition.[84]

Odense Cathedral Inventory

Numerous books were recorded in an inventory from 1530–1532 from the palace of the Bishop of Odense, during the episcopacy of Bishop Knud Henrikssen Gyldenstjerne (r. 1529–1534). Clerics in dioceses all over Scandinavia were engaged in the book trade, especially as commissioners of liturgical literature. They were also important as distributors and sellers of all kinds of mainly religious literature, as seen in Canon Christiern Pedersen's example above.[85] Three of the twenty-seven books in the Odense inventory were medical books. These were Antonio Gazio's *Florida corona que ad sanitatis hominum conservatione ac longevam vitam perducendam sunt pernecessaria*, published between 1491–1516 in either Venice or Lyons; Petrus de Montagnano's *Fasciculus medicinae*, printed 1513 by Gregorius de Gregoriis in Venice; and the *De disciplina medicina* of Symphorien Champier, from a Lyons 1508 edition.[86]

---

83 Peder Månsson, *Peder Månssons Skrifter på Svenska*, ed. and trans. by Geete.

84 Undorf, 'From Gutenberg to Luther', p. 238.

85 Undorf, 'From Gutenberg to Luther', p. 280.

86 Undorf, 'From Gutenberg to Luther', pp. 281–82.

Conclusion

Looking at the sources available to us, as demonstrated above and shown in Appendices 1 and 2 below, it is possible to see a wide interest in medical treatises on the part of Scandinavian clerics during the Middle Ages. The great encyclopaedias, such as the *Etymologiae* of Isidore of Seville, the *De proprietatibus rerum* of Bartholomeus Anglicus, and the *Speculum naturale* of Vincent of Beauvais, of course only contain a single chapter on medicine each. Their appearance in the collections of the cathedrals is not indicative of medical use, as they would have had many other functions in reference to theology, history, etc. However, they were also used for their medical information and so have been included here.

Comparing scientific literature in general owned by clerics in cathedrals in Scandinavia and England provides an interesting point of comparison. Scandinavian canons differed from their English counterparts in that they had access to more scientific texts, including medical ones, than the English canonry. Few of the great scholars of the late medieval period in England were active at cathedrals: most were instead based at universities or in episcopal households. Lepine notes that English canons had at least a shelf of books, and some owned small libraries containing from twenty-four to one hundred and fifty volumes, in the case of Martin Collins at York cathedral.[87] However, he cautions that, 'Science is hardly represented beyond Bartholomew the Englishman's encyclopaedia *De proprietatibus rerum* which was relatively widespread'.[88] Medical books were also found, but less frequently than most other genres. The English clergy used these libraries, but records for borrowing, like in Scandinavia, are rare. Cathedral libraries rarely received large gifts of books, as such collections typically went to the colleges of Oxford and Cambridge. Few English canons were authors.[89] In comparison, it seems that Scandinavian libraries were often more extensive than their English counterparts and had more scientific material.

Science was taught in the universities in England so those with a scientific bent could satisfy their careers with a position at Oxford or Cambridge. This option was not available for Scandinavians. Some individuals, like Bero Magni at Vienna, spent their entire career at a foreign university and died there. Others returned to Scandinavia, maybe for the greater choice of careers they would have as part of the learned elite there. Scientific manuscripts in England were generally held at Oxford or Cambridge. There was no such similar repository in Scandinavia until the late fifteenth century, and so the libraries of the cathedrals

87 See also the studies of McLachlan, *The Scriptorium of Bury St Edmunds*; Coates, *English Medieval Books*; and Leedham-Green and Webber, eds, *The Cambridge History of Libraries in Britain and Ireland*.

88 Lepine, *A Brotherhood of Canons Serving God*, p. 162.

89 Lepine, *A Brotherhood of Canons Serving God*, pp. 161–73.

and larger religious houses fulfilled this function. Nearly all the bishops in the Nordic dioceses were graduates of foreign universities, as were many canons, and they brought books to Scandinavia. This process changed with the arrival of the universities of Copenhagen and Uppsala. These universities only functioned in Scandinavia for a few decades before the Reformation. Perhaps if the universities had been established earlier, they would have followed the pattern of the English universities and functioned as repositories of texts, and the Scandinavian cathedral libraries and canons would have had fewer scientific works to hand. Further comparison with other clerics in places such as France and Italy would prove of great interest but is outside the scope of this essay. There are only a few physicians connected to Scandinavian cathedrals that we know of. These include the anonymous doctor recorded at Roskilde Cathedral in the mid-twelfth century, Henrik Harpestreng at the same institution in the following century, and Bengt Knutsson at Västerås Cathedral in the fifteenth century. These three lonely figures would not be able to enlighten us much about medicine at Scandinavian cathedrals if it was not possible to look at other source material. The numerous encyclopaedias found in these cathedrals' libraries contain chapters on medicine and could have been used in that context. There exists, however, a much more solid foundation of specialized medical treatises found in testaments and booklists, especially from the fourteenth century onwards. These medical books would point to somebody having a use for them. They could indeed have been trained in medicine and maybe working at an infirmary connected to the cathedral. The remarkable evidence from Roskilde Cathedral in the fifteenth century shows that the same clerics repeatedly borrowed books from the library on medicine. The canons Johannes Syndonis and Olauus Boetii stand out here and must surely have had an education in medicine. Finally, the letters of Bishop Hans Brask to Margareta Vasa show a lively correspondence between a cathedral cleric with a laywoman about medical books. All in all, cathedrals in Scandinavia held a very important function in being repositories of medical texts that would be borrowed and used by the various clerics who worked there. The assembling of the medical treatises here will, I hope, provide impetus for further investigation in more detail on these texts. The list is far from complete and further investigation of wills, inventories and fragmented manuscripts will, I am sure, expand our knowledge of the use of medical treatises in the cathedral environments of medieval Scandinavia.

Appendix 1

Medical Works Found in Scandinavian Cathedrals, 1100–1525

Appendix 1 is a summary of all medical texts and encyclopaedias with chapters on medicine associated with Scandinavian cathedrals in the Middle Ages. These appear in the form of surviving manuscripts, fragments, or printed books. Others are found listed in wills, donations, and booklists. These latter have the abbreviation BL for booklist. Finally, medical texts that were used in the compilation of works by Scandinavian clerics are also included, even though some of these must be considered tentative. The format lists the author's name alphabetically with their associated texts. The cathedrals owning these texts are then listed alphabetically along with the documentation. Printed books, where known, are given the place and year(s) of publication. Appendix 2 lists this information by each cathedral.

Booklists

Andreas Strangonis BL from 1432.[90]
Asser Thorkilsson BL from 1137.[91]
Benechinus Henrici BL from 1358.[92]
Bero Magni BL from 1465–1475.[93]
Birger Gregersson BL from 1369.[94]
Birger Gregersson BL from 1377.[95]
Christiern Pedersen BL from 1520.[96]
Ericus Erici BL from 1500.[97]
Ericus Johannis BL from 1512.[98]
Hemming of Turku BL from 1354.[99]
Hólar BL from 1396.[100]
Jacobus Petri BL from 1460.[101]
Jens Grand BL from 1327.[102]
Johannes Syndonis BL from 1459–1460.[103]

---

90 *Testamenter fra Danmarks middelalder*, ed. by Erslev, pp. 203–04.
91 Møller-Christensen, *Middelalderens lægekunst i Danmark*, p. 66.
92 *Testamenter fra Danmarks middelalder*, ed. by Erslev, pp. 118–24.
93 Kihlman, 'The Inventory of Bero's Library', pp. 135–74.
94 Kleberg, *Medeltida Uppsalabibliotek II*, pp. 84–107.
95 Kleberg, *Medeltida Uppsalabibliotek II*, pp. 84–107.
96 Undorf, 'From Gutenberg to Luther', pp. 131–57.
97 Undorf, 'From Gutenberg to Luther', p. 446.
98 Undorf, 'From Gutenberg to Luther', p. 446.
99 Klockars, *Biskop Hemming av Åbo*, p. 76.
100 *Diplomatarium Islandicum: Íslenzkt fornbréfasafn Vol. 3*, p. 613.
101 *Liber daticus Roskildensis*, ed. by Otto, pp. 127–31 and 139–41.
102 Møller-Christensen, *Middelalderens lægekunst i Danmark*, pp. 68–70.
103 *Liber daticus Roskildensis*, ed. by Otto, pp. 127–31 and 139–41.

Lauriencius Olaiij BL from 1459.[104]
Lauricius Petri BL from 1460.[105]
Master Knud of Lund BL from 1260.[106]
Nicolaus Bunkeflod BL from 1346.[107]
Nicolaus Kroogh BL from 1389.[108]
Nicolaus Senior BL from 1480.[109]
Niels Jensen Bild BL from 1379.[110]
Odense BL from 1532.[111]
Olauus Boetii BL from 1459–1460.[112]
Schleswig BL from 1519.[113]
Semundus Johannis BL from 1386.[114]
Siward BL from 1157.[115]
Skara BL from 1519.[116]
Tuco Johannis BL from 1459.[117]
Tucho Thuronis BL from 1352.[118]

Manuscripts and Printed Books

MS NRA lat. fragmenter 113b, 1–2.[119]
MS NRA lat. fragmenter 2, 1–8; 1, 1–11; 3, 1–13.[120]
MS UUB C 53.[121]
MS UUB C 55.[122]
MS UUB C 565.[123]

104 Møller-Christensen, *Middelalderens lægekunst i Danmark*, p. 71.
105 *Liber daticus Roskildensis*, ed. by Otto, pp. 127–31 and 139–41.
106 Møller-Christensen, *Middelalderens lægekunst i Danmark*, p. 68.
107 Møller-Christensen, *Middelalderens lægekunst i Danmark*, p. 71.
108 Møller-Christensen, *Middelalderens lægekunst i Danmark*, p. 81.
109 Møller-Christensen, *Middelalderens lægekunst i Danmark*, p. 80.
110 *Testamenter fra Danmarks middelalder*, ed. by Erslev, pp. 147–52.
111 Undorf, 'From Gutenberg to Luther', pp. 280–87.
112 *Liber daticus Roskildensis*, ed. by Otto, pp. 127–31 and 139–41.
113 Undorf, 'From Gutenberg to Luther', p. 238.
114 *Testamenter fra Danmarks middelalder*, ed. by Erslev, pp. 153–54.
115 Kleberg, *Medeltida Uppsalabibliotek I*, pp. 24–37.
116 Undorf, 'From Gutenberg to Luther', pp. 347–49.
117 *Liber daticus Roskildensis*, ed. by Otto, pp. 127–31 and 139–41.
118 *Testamenter fra Danmarks middelalder*, ed. by Erslev, pp. 113–16.
119 Karlsen, 'Fragments of Patristic and Other Ecclesiastical Literature in Norway', pp. 229–30.
120 Karlsen, 'Fragments of Patristic and Other Ecclesiastical Literature in Norway', pp. 229–30.
121 *Mittelalterliche Handschriften der Universitätsbibliothek Uppsala: Katalog über die C-Sammlung: Bd. 2. C 51–200*, ed. by Andersson-Schmitt and Hedlund, pp. 9–12.
122 *Mittelalterliche Handschriften der Universitätsbibliothek Uppsala: Katalog über die C-Sammlung: Bd. 2. C 51–200*, ed. by Andersson-Schmitt and Hedlund, pp. 15–18.
123 *Mittelalterliche Handschriften der Universitätsbibliothek Uppsala: Katalog über die C-Sammlung: Bd. 6. C 551–935*, ed. by Andersson-Schmitt, Hallberg and Hedlund, pp. 27–29.

MS UUB C 587.[124]
MS UUB C 622.[125]
MS UUB C 654.[126]
UUB Inc. 1492.[127]
UUB Inc. 1493.[128]

Treatises

Anders Sunesen, *Hexaëmeron*.[129]
Bengt Knutsson, *Parvum regimen sanitatis valde utile*.[130]
Bengt Knutsson, *Regimen contra pestilentiam*.[131]
Bjarni Bergþorsson, *Rimbegla*.[132]
Henrik Harpestreng, *De simplicibus medicinus laxativis*.[133]
Henrik Harpestreng, *Liber herbarum*.[134]
Peder Månsson, *Bergmanskonst*.[135]
Peder Månsson, *Bondakonst*.[136]
Peder Månsson, *Konstbok*.[137]
Peder Månsson, *Läkebok*.[138]
Peder Månsson, *Stenbok*.[139]
Saxo Grammaticus, *Gesta Danorum*.[140]
Theodoricus, *Historia de Antiquitate Regum Norwagiensium*.[141]

Albertus Magnus
De mineralibus
Skara Cathedral, published Augsburg 1519, found in Skara BL from 1519.

124 *Mittelalterliche Handschriften der Universitätsbibliothek Uppsala: Katalog über die C-Sammlung: Bd. 6. C 551–935*, ed. by Andersson-Schmitt, Hallberg and Hedlund, pp. 68–70.
125 *Mittelalterliche Handschriften der Universitätsbibliothek Uppsala: Katalog über die C-Sammlung: Bd. 6. C 551–935*, ed. by Andersson-Schmitt, Hallberg and Hedlund, pp. 141–43.
126 *Mittelalterliche Handschriften der Universitätsbibliothek Uppsala: Katalog über die C-Sammlung: Bd. 6. C 551–935*, ed. by Andersson-Schmitt, Hallberg and Hedlund, pp. 220–23.
127 Undorf, 'From Gutenberg to Luther', p. 984.
128 Undorf, 'From Gutenberg to Luther', p. 984.
129 Anders Sunesen, *Andreae Sunonis Filii Hexaemeron*, ed. by Ebbesen and Mortensen.
130 Bengt Knutsson, *A litil boke for the Pestilence*.
131 Bengt Knutsson, *A litil boke for the Pestilence*.
132 *Alfræði Íslenzk II: Rímtol*, ed. by Beckman and Kålund.
133 Henricus Dacus, *Liber de simplicibus medicinis laxativis*, ed. by Johnsson.
134 Henrik Harpestreng, *Liber herbarum*, ed. by Hauberg.
135 Peder Månsson, *Peder Månssons Skrifter på Svenska*, ed. and trans. by Geete, pp. 591–654.
136 Peder Månsson, *Peder Månssons Skrifter på Svenska*, ed. and trans. by Geete, pp. 189–364.
137 Peder Månsson, *Peder Månssons Skrifter på Svenska*, ed. and trans. by Geete, pp. 377–454.
138 Peder Månsson, *Peder Månssons Skrifter på Svenska*, ed. and trans. by Geete, pp. 575–88.
139 Peder Månsson, *Peder Månssons Skrifter på Svenska*, ed. and trans. by Geete, pp. 455–98.
140 Friis-Jensen, *Saxo og Vergil*, p. 81.
141 Theodoricus, *De antiquitate regum Norwagiensium*, ed. and trans. by Kraggerud.

Västerås Cathedral, used in Peder Månsson, *Bergmanskonst*.
Västerås Cathedral, used in Peder Månsson, *Bondakonst*.

Antonio Gazio
Florida Corona
Odense Cathedral, published Lyons/Venice 1491–1516, found in Odense BL from 1532.

Avicenna
Canon
Ribe Cathedral, found in Nicolaus Kroogh BL from 1389.
Roskilde Cathedral, used in Henrik Harpestreng, *De simplicibus medicinus laxativis*.

Bartholomeus Anglicus
De proprietatibus rerum
Lund Cathedral, found in Jens Grand BL from 1327.
Lund Cathedral, found in Tucho Thuronis BL from 1352.
Lund Cathedral, found in Niels Jensen Bild BL from 1379.
Lund Cathedral found in Andreas Strangonis BL from 1432.
Lund Cathedral, published Basel 1517, found in Christiern Pedersen BL from 1520 (a).
Lund Cathedral, published Basel 1517, found in Christiern Pedersen BL from 1520 (b).
Lund Cathedral, published Basel 1517, found in Christiern Pedersen BL from 1520 (c).
Lund Cathedral; published Basel 1517, found in Christiern Pedersen BL from 1520 (d).
Roskilde Cathedral, found in Tuco Johannis BL from 1459.
Schleswig Cathedral, found in Schleswig BL from 1519.
Skara Cathedral, found in Bero Magni BL from 1465–1475 (a).
Skara Cathedral, found in Bero Magni BL from 1465–1475 (b).
Turku Cathedral, found in Hemming of Turku BL from 1354.
Uppsala Cathedral, found in Birger Gregersson BL from 1369.
Uppsala Cathedral, found in Birger Gregersson BL from 1377.
Uppsala Cathedral, published Heidelberg 1488, found in Ericus Erici BL from 1500.
Uppsala Cathedral, published Heidelberg 1488, found in Ericus Johannis BL from 1512.
Västerås Cathedral, MS UUB C 654.

Bartholomeus of Salerno
Practica
Roskilde Cathedral, used in Henrik Harpestreng, *De simplicibus medicinus laxativis*.

Benevenutus Grapheus Hierosolymitanus
Practica oculorum
Roskilde Cathedral, found in Nicolaus Senior BL from 1480.

Bengt Knutsson
Parvum regimen sanitatis valde utile
Västerås Cathedral.

Regimen contra pestilentiam
Västerås Cathedral.

Bernardus Provincialis
Commentarius in tabulas Salernitanus
Roskilde Cathedral, found in Olauus Boetii BL from 1459–1460.

Bernhard Gordon
Lilium medicinae
Roskilde Cathedral, found in Jacobus Petri BL from 1460.
Roskilde Cathedral, found in Lauricius Petri BL from 1460.

Bernardus Alberti
Introductorium in practicam pro provectis in theorica
Roskilde Cathedral, found in Nicolaus Senior BL from 1480.

Camillius Leonardus
Speculum lapidum
Västerås Cathedral, used in Peder Månsson, *Stenbok*.

Constantine the African
De gradibus liber
Roskilde Cathedral, used in Henrik Harpestreng, *Liber herbarum*.
Roskilde Cathedral, used in Henrik Harpestreng, *De simplicibus medicinus laxativis*.

Viaticum
Roskilde Cathedral, found in Johannes Syndonis BL from 1459–1460.

Copho the Younger
De modo medendi
Roskilde Cathedral, used in Henrik Harpestreng, *De simplicibus medicinus laxativis*.
Lund Cathedral, found in Jens Grand BL from 1327.

Cristoforo Barzizza
Introductorium in medicinam
Skara Cathedral, published Augsburg 1519, found in Skara BL from 1519.

Dioscorides
De materia medica
Roskilde Cathedral, used in Henrik Harpestreng, *De simplicibus medicinus laxativis.*

Gabriele Zerbi
De cautelis medicorum
Skara Cathedral, published Venice 1495, found in Skara BL from 1519.

Galen
De simplicium medicamentorum
Roskilde Cathedral, used in Henrik Harpestreng, *De simplicibus medicinus laxativis.*

Geber
De Alchimia
Västerås Cathedral, used in Peder Månsson, *Konstbok.*

Gentile de Foligno
Consilium contra pestilentiam
Roskilde Cathedral, found in Nicolaus Senior BL from 1480.

Gregor Reisch
Margarita philosophica
Lund Cathedral, published Basel 1517, found in Christiern Pedersen BL from 1520.

Guillelmus de Saliceto
Chirurgi
Roskilde Cathedral, found in Nicolaus Senior BL from 1480.

Henrik Harpestreng
De simplicibus medicinis laxativis
Roskilde Cathedral.

Den danske urtebog
Roskilde Cathedral.

Liber herbarum
Roskilde Cathedral.

Hippocrates

Aphorisms

Lund Cathedral, found in Jens Grand BL from 1327.

Roskilde Cathedral, used in Henrik Harpestreng, *De simplicibus medicinus laxativis*.

Physiognomy

Lund Cathedral, found in Benechinus Henrici BL from 1358.

Prognostica

Roskilde Cathedral, used in Henrik Harpestreng, *Liber herbarum*.

Ibn Butlān

Tacuinum sanitatis

Aarhus Cathedral, MS UUB C 587.

Ibn Sirin

Interpretaciones sompniorum

Uppsala Cathedral, found in Birger Gregersson BL from 1369.

Isidore of Seville

Etymologiae

Hólar Cathedral, used in Bjarni Bergþorsson, *Rimbegla*.

Hólar Cathedral, found in Hólar BL from 1396.

Lund Cathedral, used in Anders Sunesen, *Hexaëmeron*.

Lund Cathedral, found in Jens Grand BL from 1327.

Nidaros Cathedral, used in Theodoricus, *Historia de Antiquitate Regum Norwagiensium*.

Nidaros Cathedral, MSNRA lat. fragmenter 113b, 1–2.

Nidaros Cathedral, MS NRA lat. fragmenter 2, 1–8; 1, 1–11; 3, 1–13.

Schleswig Cathedral, published Strasbourg 1473, found in Schleswig BL from 1519.

Uppsala Cathedral, found in Birger Gregersson BL from 1369.

Jacob Meydenbach

Hortus Sanitatis

Lund Cathedral, published Strasbourg 1517, found in Christiern Pedersen BL from 1520.

Jean Ganivet

Epistola astrologiae defensiva

Lund Cathedral, published Lyons 1508, found in Christiern Pedersen BL from 1520.

Johannes de Ketham
Fasciculus medicinae
Odense Cathedral, published Venice 1513, found in Odense BL from 1532.

Johannes de Rupescissa
De consideratione quintæ essentiæ
Västerås Cathedral, used in Peder Månsson, *Läkebok.*

Johannes de Toledo
Conservanda sanitate
Strängnäs Cathedral, MS UUB C 565.

Johannes Jacobi
Regimen contra pestilentiens
Lund Cathedral, published Hagenau 1500 / Paris 1519, found in Christiern Pedersen BL from 1520.
Roskilde Cathedral, found in Nicolaus Senior BL from 1480.

Johannes Platearius
Practica brevis
Roskilde Cathedral, found in Olauus Boetii BL from 1459–1460.
Roskilde Cathedral, found in Johannes Syndonis BL from 1459–1460.

John of Milan
Regimen sanitatis Salernitanum
Lund Cathedral, found in Jens Grand BL from 1327.
Lund Cathedral, published Paris 1519, found in Christiern Pedersen BL from 1520.
Roskilde Cathedral, used in Henrik Harpestreng, *Liber herbarum.*

Jordanus Ruffus
De medicina equorum
Uppsala Cathedral, found in Birger Gregersson BL from 1369.

Macer Floridus
De viribus herbarum
Lund Cathedral, found in Tucho Thuronis BL from 1352.
Lund Cathedral published Paris 1515, found in Christiern Pedersen BL from 1520 (a).
Lund Cathedral, published Paris 1515, found in Christiern Pedersen BL from 1520 (b).
Lund Cathedral, published Paris 1515, found in Christiern Pedersen BL from 1520 (c).
Roskilde Cathedral, used in Henrik Harpestreng, *Liber herbarum.*
Uppsala Cathedral, found in Siward BL from 1157.

Marbod of Rennes
Liber lapidum
Linköping Cathedral, MS UUB C 53.
Lund Cathedral, found in Tucho Thuronis BL from 1352.
Uppsala Cathedral, found in Siward BL from 1157.

Matthaeus Platearius
Circa instans
Roskilde Cathedral, used in Henrik Harpestreng, *De simplicibus medicinus laxativis*.
Roskilde Cathedral, found in Johannes Syndonis BL from 1459–1460.
Roskilde Cathedral, found in Olauus Boetii BL from 1459–1460.

Glossae in Antidotarium Nicolai
Roskilde Cathedral, found in Nicolaus Senior BL from 1480.
Roskilde Cathedral, found in Olauus Boetii BL from 1459–1460.

Mesue
De simplicibus
Roskilde Cathedral, used in Henrik Harpestreng, *De simplicibus medicinus laxativis*.

Nicholas of Salerno
Antidotarium Nicolai
Lund Cathedral, found in Jens Grand BL from 1327.
Roskilde Cathedral, Henrik Harpestreng, *De simplicibus medicinus laxativis*.

Peter of Limoges
De oculo morali
Skara Cathedral, found in Bero Magni BL from 1465–1475.

Peder Månsson
Bergmanskonst
Västerås Cathedral.

Bondakonst
Västerås Cathedral.

Konstbok
Västerås Cathedral.

Läkebok
Västerås Cathedral.

Stenbok
Västerås Cathedral.

Petrus de Dresden
Parvulus naturalis
Skara Cathedral, MS UUB C 622.

Petrus Hispanus
Thesaurus pauperum
Lund Cathedral, found in Jens Grand BL from 1327.
Lund Cathedral, found in Nicolaus Bunkeflod BL from 1346.
Roskilde Cathedral, found in Lauriencius Olaiij BL from 1459.

Pliny
Naturalis Historia
Lund Cathedral, used in Saxo Grammaticus, *Gesta Danorum*.
Nidaros Cathedral, used in Theodoricus, *Historia de Antiquitate Regum Norwagiensium*.
Roskilde Cathedral, used in Henrik Harpestreng, *De simplicibus medicinus laxativis*.
Västerås Cathedral, used in Peder Månsson, *Stenbok*.

Pseudo-Galen
Fortior medicinarum
Roskilde Cathedral, found in Olauus Boetii BL from 1459–1460.

Ramon Llull
De secretis naturae
Västerås Cathedral, MS Lin J8.

Rhazes
Liber medicinalis Almansoris
Roskilde Cathedral, used in Henrik Harpestreng, *De simplicibus medicinus laxativis*.

Roger of Salerno
Practica Chirurgiae
Roskilde Cathedral, used in Henrik Harpestreng, *Liber herbarum*.

Seneca
Naturales quaestiones
Lund Cathedral, used in Saxo Grammaticus, *Gesta Danorum*.

Symphorien Champier
De disciplina Medicina
Odense Cathedral, published Lyons 1508, found in Odense BL from 1532.

Vincent of Beauvais
Speculum Naturale
Lund Cathedral, found in Jens Grand BL from 1327.
Schleswig Cathedral, found in Schleswig BL from 1519.
Uppsala Cathedral, published Venice 1483, found in UUB Inc. 1492.
Uppsala Cathedral, published Strasbourg 1481, found in UUB Inc. 1493.

Unknown
Libellus Arquimie
Lund Cathedral, found in Jens Grand BL from 1327.

Libellus de medicina
Lund Cathedral, found in Jens Grand BL from 1327.

Libellus medicine
Lund Cathedral, found in Jens Grand BL from 1327.

Libelus [sic] de medicina
Lund Cathedral, found in Jens Grand BL from 1327.

Liber scientia naturali
Lund Cathedral, found in Master Knud of Lund BL from 1260.

Librum de medicinis
Lund Cathedral, found in Semundus Johannis BL from 1386.

Medicinales sex
Uppsala Cathedral, found in Siward BL from 1157.

Multos etiam phisicales
Lund Cathedral, found in Asser Thorkilsson BL from 1137.

Questiones medicine
Lund Cathedral, found in Jens Grand BL from 1327.

Quinque parvi libri in medicinis
Skara Cathedral, found in Bero Magni BL from 1465–1475.

Appendix 2

Medical Works Found in Scandinavian Cathedrals, 1100–1525

Aarhus Cathedral
Ibn Butlān *Tacuinum Sanitatis*

Hóιar Cathedral
Isidore of Seville *Etymologiae*
Isidore of Seville *Etymologiae*

Linköping Cathedral
Albertus Magnus *De mineralibus*
Marbod of Rennes *Liber lapidum*

Lund Cathedral
Alexander Neckam *De utensilibus*
Anders Sunesen *Hexaëmeron*
Bartholomeus Anglicus *De proprietatibus rerum*
Bartholomeus Anglicus *De proprietatibus rerum*
Bartholomeus Anglicus *De proprietatibus rerum*
Bartholomeus Anglicus *De proprietatibus rerum*
Bartholomeus Anglicus *De proprietatibus rerum*
Bartholomeus Anglicus *De proprietatibus rerum*
Bartholomeus Anglicus *De proprietatibus rerum*
Bartholomeus Anglicus *De proprietatibus rerum*
Copho the Younger *De modo medendi*
Gregor Reisch *Margarita philosophica*
Hippocrates *Aphorisms*
Hippocrates *Physiognomy*
Isidore of Seville *Etymologiae*
Isidore of Seville *Etymologiae*
Jacob Meydenbach *Hortus Sanitatis*
Jean Ganivet *Epistola astrologiae defensiva*
Johannes Jacobi *Regimen contra pestilentiens*
John of Milan *Regimen sanitatis Salernitanum*
John of Milan *Regimen sanitatis Salernitanum*
Macer Floridus *De viribus herbarum*
Macer Floridus *De viribus herbarum*
Macer Floridus *De viribus herbarum*
Macer Floridus *De viribus herbarum*
Marbod of Rennes *Liber lapidum*
Nicholas of Salerno *Antidotarium Nicolai*
Nicolas Chappuis *De mente et memoria libellus utilissimus*

Petrus Hispanus *Thesaurus pauperum*
Petrus Hispanus *Thesaurus pauperum*
Pliny *Naturalis Historia*
Pseudo-Aristotle *Liber de causis*
Seneca *Naturales quaestiones*
Themistius *De anima*
Unknown *Liber scientia naturali*
Unknown *Librum de medicinis qui incipit Ego*
Unknown *Multos etiam phisicales*
Unknown *Questiones medicine*
Unknown *Quidam libellus Arquimie*
Unknown *Quidam libellus de medicina*
Unknown *Quidam libellus medicine*
Unknown *Quidam libelus [sic] de medicina*
Vincent of Beauvais *Speculum Naturale*

Nidaros Cathedral
Isidore of Seville *Etymologiae*
Isidore of Seville *Etymologiae*
Isidore of Seville *Etymologiae*
Pliny *Naturalis Historia*

Odense Cathedral
Antonio Gazio *Florida Corona*
Johannes de Ketham *Fasciculus medicinae*
Symphorien Champier *De disciplina Medicina*

Ribe Cathedral
Avicenna *Canon*

Roskilde Cathedral
Anders Sunesen *Hexaëmeron*
Avicenna *Canon*
Bartholomeus Anglicus *De proprietatibus rerum*
Bartholomeus of Salerno *Practica*
Benevenutus Grapheus Hierosolymitanus *Practica oculorum*
Bernardus Alberti *Introductorium in practicam pro provectis in theorica*
Bernardus Provincialis *Commentarius in tabulas Salernitanus*
Bernhard Gordon *Lilium medicinae*
Bernhard Gordon *Lilium medicinae*
Constantine the African *De gradibus liber*
Constantine the African *Viaticum*
Copho the Younger *De modo medendi*
Dioscorides *De materia medica*
Galen *De simplicium medicamentorum*

Gentile de Foligno *Consilium contra pestilentiam*
Guillelmus de Saliceto *Chirurgi*
Henrik Harpestreng *De simplicibus medicinis laxativis*
Henrik Harpestreng *Den danske urtebog*
Henrik Harpestreng *Liber herbarum*
Hippocrates *Aphorisms*
Hippocrates *Prognostica*
Johannes Jacobi *Regimen contra pestilentiens*
Johannes Platearius *Practica brevis*
Johannes Platearius *Practica brevis*
John of Milan *Regimen sanitatis Salernitanum*
Macer Floridus *De viribus herbarum*
Matthaeus Platearius *Circa instans*
Matthaeus Platearius *Circa instans*
Matthaeus Platearius *Circa instans*
Matthaeus Platearius *Glossae in Antidotarium Nicolai*
Matthaeus Platearius *Glossae in Antidotarium Nicolai*
Mesue *De simplicibus*
Nicholas of Salerno *Antidotarium Nicolai*
Petrus Hispanus *Thesaurus pauperum*
Petrus Hispanus *Thesaurus pauperum*
Pliny the Elder *Naturalis Historia*
Pseudo-Galen *Fortior medicinarum*
Rhazes *Liber medicinalis Almansoris*
Roger of Salerno *Practica Chirurgiae*
Sacrobosco *Computus*

Schleswig Cathedral
Bartholomeus Anglicus *De proprietatibus rerum*
Isidore of Seville *Etymologiae*
Vincent of Beauvais *Speculum Naturale*

Skara Cathedral
Albertus Magnus *De minerabilus*
Bartholomeus Anglicus *De proprietatibus rerum*
Bartholomeus Anglicus *De proprietatibus rerum*
Cristoforo Barzizza *Introductorium in medicinam*
Gabriele Zerbi *De cautelis medicorum*
Peter of Limoges *De oculo morali*
Petrus de Dresden *Parvulus naturalis*
Unknown *Quinque parvi libri in medicinis*

Strängnäs Cathedral
Johannes de Toledo *Conservanda sanitate*

Turku Cathedral
Bartholomeus Anglicus *De proprietatibus rerum*

Uppsala Cathedral
Bartholomaeus Anglicus *De proprietatibus rerum*
Bartholomaeus Anglicus *De proprietatibus rerum*
Bartholomeus Anglicus *De proprietatibus rerum*
Bartholomeus Anglicus *De proprietatibus rerum*
Ibn Sirin *Interpretaciones sompniorum*
Isidore of Seville *Etymologiae*
Jordanus Ruffus *De medicina equorum*
Macer Floridus *De viribus herbarum*
Marbod of Rennes *Liber lapidum*
Unknown *Medicinales sex*
Vincent of Beauvais *Speculum Naturale*
Vincent of Beauvais *Speculum Naturale*

Västerås Cathedral
Albertus Magnus *De animalibus*
Albertus Magnus *De minerabilus*
Bartholomeus Anglicus *De proprietatibus rerum*
Bengt Knutsson *Parvum regimen sanitatis valde utile*
Bengt Knutsson *Regimen contra pestilentiam*
Camillius Leonardus *Speculum lapidum*
Geber *De Alchimia*
Johannes de Rupescissa *De consideratione quintæ essentiæ*
Peder Månsson *Läkebok*
Pliny *Naturalis historia*
Raymond Lully *De secretis naturae*

Works Cited

Manuscripts

Copenhagen, Det Kongelige Bibliotek, MS GKS 1654 4to
Copenhagen, Det Kongelige Bibliotek, MS GKS 3656 8vo
Linköping, Stadsbibliotek, MS Grensholmensis Saml. I
Oslo, Riksarkivet, MS NRA lat. fragmenter 2, 1–8; 1, 1–11; 3, 1–13
Oslo, Riksarkivet, MS NRA lat. fragmenter 113b, 1–2
Stockholm, Riksarkivet, MS SDHK nr. 29337
Uppsala, Universitetsbibliotek, MS C 53
Uppsala, Universitetsbibliotek, MS C 55
Uppsala, Universitetsbibliotek, MS C 564
Uppsala, Universitetsbibliotek, MS C 587
Uppsala, Universitetsbibliotek, MS C 622
Uppsala, Universitetsbibliotek, MS C 654
Uppsala, Universitetsbibliotek, MS Inc. 1492
Uppsala, Universitetsbibliotek, MS Inc. 1493

Primary Sources

Alfræði Íslenzk II: Rímtol, ed. by Natanael Beckman and Kristian Kålund (Copenhagen: S. L. Møllers Bogtrykkeri, 1916)

Anders Sunesen, *Andreae Sunonis Filii Hexaemeron*, ed. by Sten Ebbesen and Lars Boje Mortensen (Copenhagen: Det Danske Sprog- og Litteraturselskab, 1985–1988)

Bengt Knutsson, *A litil boke for the Pestilence*, intro by Guthrie Vine, John Rylands Facsimiles, 3 (Manchester: Manchester University Press, 1910)

Diplomatarium Islandicum: Íslenzkt fornbréfasafn. Vol. 3.: 1269–1415 (Copenhagen: S. L. Möllers, 1896)

Diplomatarium Norwegicum, ed. by Christian Christoph Andreas Lange, Carl Richard Unger, Henrik Jørgen Huitfeldt-Kaas, and Gustav Storm, 22 vols (Christiana/Oslo: Riksarkivet, 1847–1997)

Henricus Dacus (Henrik Harpestreng), *De simplicibus medicinis laxativis*, ed. by J. W. S. Johnsson (Leiden: Brill, 1917)

Henrik Harpestreng, *Liber herbarum*, ed. by Poul Hauberg (Copenhagen: Hafnia, 1936)

Liber daticus Roskildensis: Roskilde gavebog & domkapitlets anniversarieliste, ed. by Alfred Otto (Copenhagen: Levin and Munksgaard, 1933)

Mittelalterliche Handschriften der Universitätsbibliothek Uppsala: Katalog über die C-Sammlung: Bd. 2. C 51–200, ed. by Margarete Andersson-Schmitt and Monica Hedlund, Acta Bibliothecae R. Universitatis Upsaliensis, 26.2 (Stockholm: Almqvist u. Wiksell International, 1989)

Mittelalterliche Handschriften der Universitätsbibliothek Uppsala: Katalog über die C- Sammlung: Bd. 6. C 551–935, ed. by Margarete Andersson-Schmitt, Håkan

Hallberg, and Monica Hedlund, Acta Bibliothecae R. Universitatis Upsaliensis, 26.6 (Stockholm: Almqvist u. Wiksell International, 1993)
Pavelige Nuntiers Regnskabs- og Dagbøger: førte under Tiende-Opkrævningen i Norden 1282–1334, ed. by Peter Andreas Munch (Christiania: Brögger & Christies Bogtrykkeri, 1864)
Peder Månsson, *Peder Månssons Skrifter på Svenska*, ed. and trans. by Robert Geete (Stockholm: P. A. Norstedt & Söner, 1913–1915)
Saxo Grammaticus, *Gesta Danorum: The History of the Danes Volume II*, ed. and trans. by Peter Fisher and Karsten Friis-Jensen, Oxford Medieval Texts (Oxford: Oxford University Press, 2015)
Testamenter fra Danmarks middelalder indtil 1450, ed. by Kristian Erslev (Copenhagen: Den Gyldendalske Boghandel, 1901)
Theodoricus, *De antiquitate regum Norwagiensium: On the Old Norwegian Kings*, ed. and trans. by Egil Kraggerud (Oslo: Novus Press, 2018)
Theodoricus Monachus, *Historia de antiquitate regum Norwagiensium: An Account of the Ancient History of the Norwegian Kings*, ed. and trans. by David McDougall and Ian McDougall (London: Viking Society for Northern Research, 1998)

Secondary Studies

Andrén, Anders, 'Världen från Lunds horisont', in *Metropolis Daniae: Ett stycke Europa*, ed. by Claes Wahlöö (Lund: BTJ Tryck, 1998), pp. 116–29
Axel-Nilsson, Göran, *Thesaurus Cathedralis Lundensis: Lund domkyrkas medeltida skattsamling* (Gothenburg: Kungl. Vetenskaps- och Vitterhets-Samhället, 1989)
Bagge, Sverre, *From Viking Stronghold to Christian Kingdom: State Formation in Norway, c. 900–1350* (Copenhagen: Museum Tusculanum Press, 2010)
——, 'Nordic Students at Foreign Universities until 1660', *Scandinavian Journal of History*, 9.1 (1984), 1–29
——, 'Norge', in *Ur nordisk kulturhistoria: studiebesöken i utlandet före 1660, XVIII nordiska historikermötet i Jyväskylä: mötesrapport I*, ed. by Mauno Jokipii and Ilkka Nummela (Jyväskylä: Jyväskylän Yliopisto, 1981), pp. 141–66
Bauer, Alessia, *Laienastrologie im nachreformatorischen Island* (Munich: Herbert Utz Verlag, 2015)
Christensen, Claude H., 'Scandinavian Libraries in the Late Middle Ages', in *The Medieval Library*, ed. by James Westfall Thompson (Chicago: University of Chicago Press, 1939), pp. 477–508
Ciardi, Anna Minara, 'Some Reflections on the Canons of Lund and their Tradition of Law and Learning in the First Quarter of the Twelfth Century', in *Law and Learning in the Middle Ages: Proceedings of the Second Carlsberg Academy Conference on Medieval Legal History 2005*, ed. by Helle Vogt and Mia Münster-Swendsen (Copenhagen: DJØF Publishing, 2006), pp. 63–78
Clausen, Svend, 'Reformation and the Monastery Inventory: Structures of Reuse in the Kingdom of Denmark', in *The Dissolution of Monasteries: The Case of Denmark in a Regional Perspective*, ed. by Per Seesko, Louise Nyholm Kalles-

trup, and Lars Bisgaard, Studies in History and Social Sciences, 580 (Odense: University of Southern Denmark Press, 2019), pp. 327–56

Coates, Alan, *English Medieval Books: The Reading Abbey Collections from Foundation to Dispersal* (Oxford: Clarendon Press, 1999)

Cucina, Carla, 'Il computo del tempo nella Scandinavia medievale. Riflessioni sulla memoria lineare e ciclica dalle genealogie ai calendari runici', in *Figure della memoria culturale*, ed. by Massimo Bonafin (Alessandria: Edizioni dell'Orso, 2013), pp. 245–86

Etheridge, Christian, 'Astronomy at Lund Cathedral in the Middle Ages', in *Lund Domkyrka: Idéer och Världsbilder*, ed. by David Dunér, Sveriges Kyrkor, 245 (Gothenburg: Makadam förlag, 2023), pp. 201–08

——, 'The Booklist of Bishop Arne Sigurdsson', in *Dominican Resonances in 14th Century Iceland: The Legacy of Bishop Jón Halldórsson of Skálholt*, ed. by Gunnar Harðarson and Karl-Gunnar Johansson, The Northern World, 91 (Leiden: Brill, 2021), pp. 303–16

——, 'Canon, Dominican and Brother: The Life and Times of Jón Halldórsson in Bergen', in *Dominican Resonances in 14th Century Iceland: The Legacy of Bishop Jón Halldórsson of Skálholt*, ed. by Gunnar Harðarson and Karl-Gunnar Johansson, The Northern World, 91 (Leiden: Brill, 2021), pp. 7–40

——, 'The Evidence for Islamic Scientific Works in Medieval Iceland', in *Fear and Loathing in the North. Jews and Muslims in Medieval Scandinavia and the Baltic Region*, ed. by Cordelia Heß and Jonathan Adams (Berlin: De Gruyter, 2015), pp. 49–72

——, 'Medieval Scientific Book Fragments Held in Swedish and Finnish Archives: The Tantalizing Remains of a Greater Scientific Corpus', in *Medieval Science in the North: Travelling Wisdom, 1000–1500*, ed. by Christian Etheridge and Michele Campopiano, Knowledge, Scholarship, and Science in the Middle Ages, 2 (Turnhout: Brepols, 2021), pp. 111–40

Friis-Jensen, Karsten, *Saxo og Vergil: en analyse af 1931-udgavens Vergilparalleller* (Copenhagen: Museum Tusculanum Press, 1975)

Galbon, Clemens Timothy, 'The Canons Regular of St Augustine: A Priestly Vision', in *Locus Celebris: Dalby kyrka, kloster och gård*, ed. by Stephan Borgehammar and Jes Weinberg, Centrum för Danmarksstudier, 28 (Gothenburg: Makadam Förlag, 2012), pp. 253–54

Hamel, Jürgen, 'Nikolaus Lilienfeld – ein norddeutscher Astronom des späten 14. Jahrhunderts?', *Acta Historica Astronomiae*, 9 (2008), 15–25

Helle, Knut, *Bergen bys historie, Vol. 1: Kongssete og kjøpstad* (Bergen: Alma Mater Forlag, 1982)

Holck, Jakob Povl, 'Middelalderens danske lægebog. Et kontaktfænomen' (unpublished doctoral thesis, University of Copenhagen, 2001)

Jørgensen, Karen Dreyer, 'Henricus Harpestreng', in *Medieval Nordic Literature in Latin: A Website of Authors and Anonymous Works c. 1100–1530* <https://wiki.uib.no/medieval/index.php/Henricus_Harpestreng> [accessed 20 November 2022]

Karlsen, Espen, 'Fragments of Patristic and Other Ecclesiastical Literature in Norway from *c.* 1100 until the Fifteenth Century', in *Latin Manuscripts of Medieval*

Norway: Studies in Memory of Lilli Gjerløw, ed. by Espen Karlsen (Oslo: Novus Press, 2013), pp. 215–70

Keskiaho, Jesse, 'Bortom fragmenten: Handskriftsproduktion och boklig kultur i det medeltida Åbo stift', *Historisk tidskrift för Finland*, 93.3 (2008), 209–52

Kihlman, Erika, 'Bero Magni de Ludosia – Student and Teacher', in *Swedish Students at the University of Vienna in the Middle Ages*, Sällskapet Runica et Mediævalia. Scripta minora, 20 (Stockholm: Sällskapet Runica et Mediævalia, 2011), pp. 89–133

——, 'The Inventory of Bero's Library: An Edition with Analysis, Teacher', in *Swedish Students at the University of Vienna in the Middle Ages: Careers, Books and Preaching*, ed. by Olle Ferm and Erika Kihlman (Södertälje: Mandarin AB, 2011), pp. 135–74

Kleberg, Tönnes, *Medeltida Uppsalabibliotek I: Biskop Siward av Uppsala och hans bibliotek* (Uppsala: Almqvist & Wiksells Boktryckeri AB, 1968)

——, *Medeltida Uppsalabibliotek II: Bidrag till deras historia till 1389* (Uppsala: Almqvist & Wiksells Boktryckeri AB, 1972)

Klockars, Birgit, *Biskop Hemming av Åbo* (Helsinki: Svenska litteratursällskapet i Finland, 1960)

Korpiola, Mia, 'Literary Legacies and Canonical Book Collections: Possession of Canon Law Books in Medieval Sweden', in *Law and Learning in the Middle Ages: Proceedings of the Second Carlsberg Academy Conference on Medieval Legal History 2005*, ed. by Helle Vogt and Mia Münster-Swendsen (Copenhagen: DJØF Publishing, 2006), pp. 79–104

Lapidge, Michael, *The Anglo-Saxon Library* (Oxford: Oxford University Press, 2006)

Leedham-Green, Elisabeth, and Teresa Webber, eds, *The Cambridge History of Libraries in Britain and Ireland, Volume 1* (Cambridge: Cambridge University Press, 2006)

Lepine, David, *A Brotherhood of Canons Serving God: English Secular Cathedrals in the Later Middle Ages*, Studies in the History of Medieval Religion, 8 (Woodbridge: The Boydell Press, 1995)

McLachlan, Elizabeth Parker, *The Scriptorium of Bury St Edmunds in the Twelfth Century* (New York: Garland, 1986)

Mitchell, Stephen A., *Witchcraft and Magic in the Nordic Middle Ages* (Philadelphia: University of Pennsylvania Press, 2011)

Mogensen, Lone, 'Urets gamla och nya fasad', in *Det underbara uret i Lund*, ed. by Lone Mogensen (Lund: Wallin & Dalholm, 2008), pp. 89–122

Møller-Christensen, Vilhelm, *Middelalderens lægekunst i Danmark* (Copenhagen: Ejner Munksgaard, 1944)

Moraw, Peter, 'Careers of Graduates', in *A History of the University in Europe: Volume I. Universities in the Middle Ages*, ed. by Hilde De Ridder-Symoens (Cambridge: Cambridge University Press, 2003), pp. 244–79

Mornet, Élisabeth, 'Le testament du chanoine Benechinus Henrici de Åhus, chantre de Lund et la culture de clercs nordiques au XIV siècle', in *Les élites nordiques et l'Europe occidentale, XII–XV siècle*, ed. by Tuomas M. S. Lehtonen and Élisabeth Mornet (Paris: Publications de la Sorbonne, 2007), pp. 197–220

Mortensen, Lars Boje, 'The Nordic Archbishoprics as Literary Centres around 1200', in *Archbishop Absalon of Lund and his World*, ed. by Karsten Friis-Jensen and Inge Skovgaard-Petersen (Roskilde: Roskilde Museums Forlag, 2000), pp. 133–58

Myking, Synnøve Midtbø, 'The French Connection: Norwegian Manuscript Fragments of French Origin and their Historical Context' (unpublished doctoral thesis, University of Bergen, 2017)

Nielsen, Lauritz, *Danmarks Middelalderlige Haandskrifter* (Copenhagen: Gyldendal, 1937)

Nothaft, C. Philipp E., 'John of Pulchro Rivo and John of Saxony: A Mise au Point', *Journal for the History of Astronomy*, 45.2 (2014), 227–42

O'Boyle, Cornelius, *Medical Teaching at the University of Paris, 1250–1400* (Leiden: Brill, 1998)

Ohrvik, Ana, *Medicine, Magic, and Art in Early Modern Norway* (London: Palgrave Macmillan, 2018)

Olsen, Birger Munk, 'Absalons studier i Paris', in *Absalon: fædrelandets fader*, ed. by Frank Birkebæk, Tom Christensen, and Inge Skovgaard-Petersen (Roskilde: Roskilde Museums Forlag, 1996), pp. 57–72

——, 'Anders Sunesen og Paris', in *Anders Sunesen: stormand, teolog, administrator, digter*, ed. by Sten Ebbesen (Copenhagen: GEC Gad, 1985), pp. 75–97

Ommundsen, Åslaug, and Tuomas Heikkilä, eds, *Nordic Latin Manuscripts Fragments. The Destruction and Reconstruction of Medieval Books* (Abingdon: Routledge, 2019)

Pedersen, Fritz Såby, 'Stof og form de fire første dage', in *Anders Sunesen: stormand, teolog, administrator, digter*, ed. by Sten Ebbesen (Copenhagen: GEC Gad, 1985), pp. 115–36

Rydén, Thomas, 'Dalbyboken: En omvärdering av attributionskriterierna', in *Locus Celebris: Dalby kyrka, kloster och gård*, ed. by Stephan Borgehammar and Jes Weinberg, Centrum för Danmarksstudier, 28 (Gothenburg: Makadam Förlag, 2012), pp. 425–36

Schukowski, Manfred, 'Astronomiska ur i Hansatidens kyrkor', in *Det underbara uret i Lund*, ed. by Lone Mogensen (Lund: Wallin & Dalholm, 2008), pp. 123–27

Undorf, Wolfgang, 'From Gutenberg to Luther – Transnational Print Cultures in Scandinavia 1450–1525' (unpublished doctoral thesis, Humboldt-Universität zu Berlin, 2012)

——, 'Print and Book Culture in the Danish Town of Odense', in *Print Culture in Early Modern Europe: A Contribution to the History of Printing and the Book Trade in Small European and Spanish Cities*, ed. by Benito Rial Costas Library of the Written World, 24 (Leiden: Brill, 2013), pp. 227–48

Vihovde, Anne Brit, *Kirkesenteret på Holmen* (Bergen: Bryggens Museum, 1998)

Waddingham, R. A. J., *Breakspear: The English Pope* (Cheltenham: The History Press, 2023)

Walta, Ville, 'Libraries, Manuscripts and Book Culture in Vadstena Abbey' (unpublished doctoral thesis, University of Helsinki, 2014)

Part II

Language and Lexicography

JOSEPH J. FLAHIVE

11. Celtic-Latin Medical Vocabulary

This chapter is a not a contribution from a medical historian, but rather from a linguist, presenting research on behalf of a lexicographical project.[1] It will examine the so-called Celtic fringe, the area in which I research, attempting to distil evidence regarding the practice of medicine in those regions from the vocabulary of their Latin-language literature.

A sizeable corpus of medical texts from the historically Celtic-speaking nations survives. Of particular note is the large and rather under-investigated corpus of Irish and Scottish medical manuscripts from the later Middle Ages through to the seventeenth century. These occasionally copy the canonical Latin texts of the authors read in continental universities, such as Galen, Cassius Felix, Avicenna, and 'the Arabians'; but more often translate them into Irish. Works such as John of Gaddesden's *Rosa Anglica*, which circulated in an early-modern Irish translation, testify to the prominence of mainstream European interests and wider connexions of the Gaelic medical families. Commentaries, recipes, and personal notes abound, and some of the grander late-medieval codices, such as the Book of the O'Lees, fancifully called the Book of Hy Brasil,[2] are well known. However much basic work remains to be done in this field, the outlines of the later phase of Gaelic medical culture are known,[3] as are later medieval Welsh and Breton medicine, for which

1 I thank my colleague Anthony Harvey, for the help and support of the Dictionary of Medieval Latin from Celtic Sources in all phases of the research presented here, and for the advice and insight he provided in discussing a draft of this chapter, which is based on a paper read to the Conference 'Medicine in the Medieval North Atlantic World', hosted by Maynooth University and Queen's University Belfast on 13 May 2021.

2 Dublin, RIA, MS 23 P 10 [ii] (453).

3 Ó Corráin, *Clavis Litterarum Hibernensium*, III, pp. 1707–12, § 1318, provides the standard bibliography on this subject for Ireland. The proceedings of a recent symposium *Rosa Anglica: Reassessments*, ed. by Ó Murchú, provides a narrative account of recent scholarship on the material in Ireland; for Scotland, Nicolson, 'The McBeths — Hereditary Physicians of the Highlands', provides a classic introduction; and more in-depth, Bannerman, *The Beatons*.

Joseph J. Flahive • Royal Irish Academy, Dublin; j.flahive@ria.ie

Medicine in the Medieval North Atlantic World: Vernacular Texts and Traditions, ed. by Deborah Hayden and Sarah Baccianti, KSS, 5 (Turnhout, 2025), pp. 269-286
BREPOLS PUBLISHERS DOI 10.1484/M.KSS-EB.5.143989

summaries of this type could also be presented.[4] What preceded this in the early Middle Ages has scarcely come down to us. Professional handbooks, manuals, or extended tracts of medical learning, whether in the vernacular or Latin, do not survive apart from a few fragments or items of questionable origin, and it is hardly possible to guess the range of materials that circulated. Furthermore, although a few eighth- and ninth-century codices containing Graeco-Roman Latin medical texts written in Insular script do survive on the continent, it appears that most of this activity can be attributed to expatriates, and it testifies to the intellectual pursuits of the Carolingian Renascence. Nevertheless, there remains a possibility for Insular origins of a very few items.[5] One curious and decidedly international item is the bifolium fragment (now Leiden, Universitätsbibliothek, MS Vossianus in folio 96A) dated post-850 by McKee, that was later inserted into a larger compendium at Fleury. It comprises four medical fragments written in Insular script, each in a different hand. The texts are a section from a health regimen, miscellaneous cure recipes in two different hands, and part of an herbarium (some of the contents of which parallel Anglo-Saxon medical books) in which the herb names are largely in some form of Neo-Brittonic apart from one in Irish (and there is also an additional phrase and a *prima manus* gloss in Old Irish).[6] Other textual sources, such as law and literature (especially hagiographical accounts of healings), provide less direct evidence for the state of medical culture when they touch upon medical matters. There are fundamental questions that remain practically unanswerable: to what extent (if any) did antique medical treatises circulate in the Celtic fringe; did they serve as textbooks and references for medical education and practice or merely as scholarly curiosities; and, to what extent did Latin, the international language of learning in medieval Europe, serve as a vehicle for the transmission of professional medical knowledge?

This chapter is rooted in the on-going work of the Dictionary of Medieval Latin from Celtic Sources (DMLCS) at the Royal Irish Academy. The central

4 Concerning the former, an overview is provided by Owen, 'Medics and Medicine'. Further attention is drawn to the texts in *Medieval Welsh Medical Texts*, ed. and trans. by Luft; and Parina, 'Medical Texts in Welsh Translation'.

5 E.g., St Gallen, Stiftsbibl., MS 759, in fully Insular script with uncertain origins, dated. *c.* 800. Palaeographical and codicological analysis (in particular of the type of membrane and gatherings) will be required to establish the origins of these manuscripts. Other medical manuscripts, such as St Gallen, Stiftsbibl., MS 761 (ninth century, Insular script influenced by Caroline minuscule), and BnF, MS lat. 9332 (a Fleury manuscript containing works by Oribasius penned by a hand with Insular symptoms) raise additional questions regarding the interest of Irish *perigrini* in medicine. Thanks are due to Conan Doyle for suggesting the discussion of these manuscripts; his own contribution to this volume provides discussion of Oribasius in English manuscripts and continental sources.

6 *Editio prima* 'A Celtic Leechbook', ed. by Stokes; edition and commentary in *The Leiden Leechbook*, ed. by Falileyev and Owen; see especially the manuscript description in the Introduction, pp. 1–10; the evaluation of the Brythonic vocabulary, pp. 74–87; and a palaeographical appendix by McKee, 'The Script of the Leiden Leechbook'.

task of this project is to compile a lexicon for the medieval Latin of the historically Celtic-speaking countries: Ireland, Scotland, Mann, the Brythonic regions of the former Roman Britain that retreated to become Wales and Cornwall, and Brittany. Its remit extends from the introduction of literacy through to *c.* 1200, with some additions up to *c.* 1400. From an early date, all of the Celtic regions had significant literatures in their own vernaculars in addition to Latin. Latin arrived in classical antiquity with Roman trade — followed by conquest — in Armorican Gaul and then Britain, where it established itself as the spoken and written language of prestige. Some Latin undoubtedly reached Ireland, Scotland, and Mann as a trade language in antiquity, and the development of ogham script bears witness to the transfer of the concept of literacy and the Latin alphabet.[7] Nevertheless, no evidence for widespread literacy, which would be a pre-requisite for any Latin literary culture, predates Christian conversion in the Gaelic world.[8] The Latin that circulated in early-Christian Atlantic Europe was a foundational package, largely confined to the late-Latin grammarians and Christian texts; strictly classical literary learning appears to have been quite limited until the ninth century, probably derived from excerpts and florilegia:[9] nearly everything that circulated was either educational or devotional. When St Isidore of Seville's works began to circulate in seventh-century Ireland, they were embraced with enthusiasm as a large-scale expansion to the learning available, and his shadow in Hiberno-Latin is especially long.[10]

For reasons of audience, prestige, or religious custom, authors in Celtic nations frequently chose to write on many different subjects in Latin, and the

7 See McManus, *A Guide to Ogam*, chs 1–3. Harvey provides a discussion of the state of the question in 'Languages and Literacy in Mid-First-Millennium Ireland'; see further Harvey, 'Latin, Literacy, and the Celtic Vernaculars'. Certain archaic Irish-language texts also display traces of an early reception of Latin-alphabet orthography whose distinguishing characteristics derive from phonetic changes peculiar to Irish that occurred prior to and independent of the reception of Patrician Brythonic Latin. This trait implies continuity for writing in the Roman alphabet from the earliest introduction of literacy (when ogham was created) through to archaic Old Irish; this could imply a limited reception of Latin writing possibly as early as the second century: see Harvey, 'Reading the Genetic Code', pp. 163–64. The OG(H)AM Project at the Universities of Glasgow and Maynooth is compiling an online corpus of the inscriptions and scholarship (see ogham.glasgow.ac.uk).

8 See Johnston, *Literacy and Identity in Medieval Ireland*, ch. 1. She argues (pp. 14–15) for a late date of Christianization of the elites and introduction of literacy in the sixth century. Other scholars maintain that there was a gap between attaining Christian literacy in the fifth century and the later undertaking of active literary composition, as outlined in Ó Cróinín, 'Hiberno-Latin Literature to 1169', pp. 371–77.

9 Stanford, 'Towards a History of Classical Influences', pp. 17–18 and 72; Ó Cróinín, 'Hiberno-Latin Literature to 1169', pp. 374–77.

10 Ó Cróinín, 'Hiberno-Latin literature to 1169', p. 390. See further Bischoff, 'Die europäische Verbreitung der Werke Isidors', pp. 180–87, and Michael Herren, 'On the Earliest Irish Acquaintance with Isidore of Seville'. Irish use of Isidorian linguistic methods is considered in Harvey, 'Frankenstein in the Scriptorium', pp. 113–16.

areas of their composition were not confined to the genres of their inherited reading. This, of course, stretched the linguistic skills of people working through a second language. Medieval Celtic-Latin authors would naturally lack the advantage of the mental store of vocabulary that native speakers of early Romance would have acquired (if in an evolved form) through their vernaculars. Celts put their received Latin vocabulary to use, coined new words within Latin, borrowed from Greek and other languages.[11] They not infrequently had cause to re-appropriate or modify vocabulary for technical use in such subjects as grammar, rhetoric, law, astronomy and computus, and philosophy.[12] Closer to the nature of their foundational Latin sources, they wrote biblical exegesis, theology, and a great corpus of hagiography. Lapidge and Sharpe's *Bibliography of Celtic-Latin Literature 400–1200* provides a hand-list of the literary corpus. As the authors of Celtic Latin borrowed, stole, or re-appropriated words for their literary tasks, the traces of their struggle to write left distinctive traces: when established mainstream terminology is not followed, one finds evidence as to what the parameters of the inherited vocabulary were, and clues as to how writers dealt with gaps in the technical lexicon available to them.

As a Latin lexicographer, I have a distinctive viewpoint whence I can approach the earlier period, looking at vocabulary across the entire corpus of literature, to see what words are used for medical concepts such as anatomical structures, symptoms, and diseases, and then look for routes of transmission of vocabulary, and analyse new coinages. This contribution is based on an electronic search, using the complete A–H volume of *The Non-Classical Lexicon of Celtic Latinity* (*NCLCL*), its Supplement,[13] and the drafts of letters not yet in print[14] for the 'medical' tag, then following up some of the authors cited most frequently, checking each entry in which they are cited.[15] Following the parameters of *NCLCL*, on which this research is founded, classical vocabulary has been excluded from this discussion.[16] The texts are consulted and cited through the Project's database, the *Archive of Celtic Latin Literature* (*ACLL*).[17] Although there are no formally medical texts as such in the digitized corpus at present, there was a need to be clinically precise in writing about medical matters in other types of texts: there were more than fifty technical lexemes

---

11 See Harvey, 'The Non-Classical Vocabulary' and 'Frankenstein in the Scriptorium'.

12 As analysed in Harvey, 'Technical Vocabulary'.

13 Available online at journals.eeecs.qub.ac.uk.

14 The unpublished letters sufficiently complete as to be searchable at the time of writing were K–N, R, T–Z; some words have also been drawn from I.

15 See Harvey's note of caution in 'Technical Vocabulary', pp. 380–82, concerning some technical terms whose field is obvious remaining unlabelled in *NCLCL*; the search therefore falls slightly short of comprehensive.

16 For practical purposes classical Latin is defined here as comprising lexemes or variants found in *The Oxford Dictionary of Classical Latin*, ed. by Glare. Late-Latin vocabulary, although part of the inherited vocabulary, is included; this word-store is evaluated by the present author in '*Venialia et Ventositas*'.

17 Published online by subscription at <www.brepolis.net>.

tagged. Combing through dictionary entries that contained several of the authors cited elsewhere for medical vocabulary for further unflagged terms brought the total over sixty. In pursuing the linguistic origins and possible routes of transmission of this vocabulary, the most important tool is the Brepolis *Cross Database Searchtool*, which provides searchable access to thousands of the most important Latin authors from pre-classical to modern.[18] This search enables a quick comparison of the medical terms in Celtic Latin with those found elsewhere in Latinity, including medical treatises, but just as importantly, with the vocabulary of digitized texts of the Bible and the Fathers, since correspondences between these sources and Celtic texts would strongly imply transmission within the core package of basic Christian Latinity. In addition to the medical texts digitized by Brepols as part of the database, a further resource is found in lexicons that cover late Latin, several of which have excerpted additional medical treatises. Chief among these are Alexander Souter's *Glossary of Later Latin*, Albert Blaise's *Dictionnaire Latin–Français des auteurs chrétiens*, Gaffiot (the standard Francophone dictionary of Latin) as well as the monumental but unfinished *Thesaurus Linguae Latinae* (*TLL*). Together, these sources provide a check for word occurrence in the major medical treatises of the later Empire. If late-antique medical texts were in active circulation in the early-medieval Celtic fringe, their vocabulary should have left a trail. Although the Brepolis databases have not encompassed the entire corpus of literature yet, it can be seen at a glance whether a word is commonplace, rare, or unique to a single author among the hundreds of works already digitized; furthermore, the accumulation of such evidence provides some indications regarding the Latin language as a medium for transmission of medical knowledge. The medieval use of the words can also be consulted to determine whether they are mainstream across Europe in post-Patristic Latin.

One large group of words used for medical purposes comprises the linguistic inheritance from late Latin. When searching the databases, likely texts for transmitting the words are frequently recognisable. When a word is in the text of the Bible (and then in the Patristic commentators as well), it is no surprise when it recurs in Celtic texts: Columbanus' **confractio**,[19] in

18 An abbreviated database reference will be given for all Brepolis database citations, as the full bibliographical citation is provided there; authors or titles are mentioned when useful. Citations are from *ACLL* unless otherwise stated and appear in the format used in *NCLCL*. In them, references to *ACLL*, the initial letter of the code indicates the national origin of the text. Those found in this chapter are: A – Roman Britain, Wales, or Cornwall; B – Ireland (including early texts associated with Iona); C – Irish scholars writing on the continent; D – Brittany; E – Scotland. *LLT* and *eMGH* citations appear formatted as in the search results.

19 Latin lemmata in this paper will be presented in **bold** type; their declined forms and minor orthographical variants that are found in texts appear in *italics*. This policy, universally employed in DMLCS interpretative publications, avoids confusion by distinguishing whether a particular form cited is that which appears in the text or the standardized form

the sense 'a fracture',[20] appears in the Vulgate at Isaiah 24. 9, as well as in the active vocabularies of Augustine and Jerome. There are also instances where a particular Patristic source from which the word is overwhelmingly likely to be gleaned leaps out: Thomas of Monmouth's rather rare adjective **clinicus**, 'bedridden', appears in an epistle of Jerome.[21] **Colatorium**, 'a colander, sieve', is used by Eriugena, both in this basic sense[22] and for the vocal chords — the 'strainers' of the breath[23] (elsewhere in medieval Latin the same lexeme came to be used for the kidneys). The searchable corpus of late Latin provides only one author who employs the word in Eriugena's sense: Dionysius Exiguus, whose Latin translations of Gregory of Nyssa, in particular, *De opificio hominis*, in which this word appears twice,[24] would have been available to — and potentially of assistance to — Eriugena as an aid to reading the Greek original. Perhaps less esoterically, though as certain, **conualescentia**, 'recovery, being "on the mend"', in Gerald de Barri (known as Cambrensis or of Wales)[25] most often takes a spiritual sense in the Fathers, though it is used to denote physical recovery from illness by Isidore.[26] **Elephantiacus**, 'suffering from elephantitis, elephantiac',[27] appears in Jerome's commentary on Ezechiel,[28] which was quoted in later commentaries, and the word is later explained by Isidore.[29] **Epilentia**, 'epilepsy',[30] is a more assimilated variant of the classical-period Greek loanword **empilmpsia**; attested as early as Augustine in *Contra Iulianos*[31] and Gregory of Tours's *Liber vitae patrum*[32] and *Historiarum*;[33] this form spread widely in the works of authors such as these. Its related late-Latin adjective **epilempsicus/ epilenticus** appears with the same spelling variants in Celtic authors,[34] as well as some more unusual ones.[35] **Liuido**, 'a puce colour — and figuratively, the spite that causes one to turn such a hue',[36] extends in early Breton canons to

that appears as the dictionary headword. Variants of greater significance are lemmatized separately with cross-references to the basic lemma (whether they are classical Latin or lexemes included in *NCLCL*).

20 C640@98.

21 CPL 0620, *LLT*, epist. 77, vol. 55, par. 6, p. 44.

22 C708@75.

23 C698@219.

24 CPL 0652A(A), *LLT*, cap. 9, col. 359, linea. 29; and cap. 12, col. 362, l. 32.

25 A71@174; A71@242.

26 CPL 1186, *LLT*, lib. 4, cap. 7, par. 27.

27 B370@139; B409@292.

28 CPL 0587, *LLT*, lib. 6, cap. 18, l. 294.

29 CPL 1186, *LLT*, lib. 4, cap. 8, par. 12.

30 A115@302.

31 CPL 0356, *LLT*, lib. 6, par. 16.

32 Two times: *eMGH*, SS. rer. Merov. 1.1, lib. V, cap. 5, pag. 201, l. 16; and SS rer. Merov. 1.2, cap. 8, pag. 249, l. 1.

33 CPL 1023, *LLT*, lib. 5, cap. 5, pag. 201, l. 16.

34 D950@158; A70DIST1@69.

35 **epilencius**, A115@302; **epilentioticus**, E1018@212.

36 A39@397.

'a black-and-blue bruise'.[37] Although there are a number of authors, such as Paulinus of Nola, who use this word, Isidore's *De differentiis* makes a particular example of it: *Libido per b cupiditas est animi; livido per v livor est corporis*[38] (*Libido* with a b is 'longing of the spirit'; *livido* with a v is 'a dark discolouring of the body'). **Rabiare**, 'to be mad, be rabid', a late-Latin variant of classical **rabere**, 'to rage' was a grammatical example in Eutyches[39] — and probably thence Malsachanus[40] and Sedulius Scottus[41] — in addition to being a medical term in Eriugena,[42] as it had been in late Latin, e.g. five times in *Mulomedicina Chironis*.[43] The final example is particularly interesting: **ustura**, 'the property of cauterizing', leaves a distinct trail: Sedulius Scottus[44] quotes Pelagius,[45] who states the proverbial idea, similarly expressed in multiple Patristic biblical commentaries, that the more invasive treatment of cauterizing brings greater healing than a mere salve. In none of these cases was there any need to look beyond the basic Latin package to find the precise medical word required.

In other cases medical words had become completely mainstream, such as **dyscrasia**, 'a state of poor temperament', which was a commonplace of the early universities by the time of Gerald of Wales.[46] Likewise **hyposarca**, 'subcutaneous dropsy', had migrated from Roman medicine in the works of Caelius Aurelius, Celsus, and Oribasius[47] into the medieval mainstream by the time that Jocelyn of Furness used it.[48] There can be no certainty in such cases except that there was no great difficulty in finding the correct word. Likewise, **logicus** in the sense that characterizes one of the classical approaches to medicine or a doctor who follows it[49] is typical of late-antique treatises by authors such as Cassius Felix,[50] but more importantly it is described in Isidore's much-circulated *Etymologiae*[51] and consequently appears more widely. **Uenenosus**, '(full of) poison', frequently weakening to 'poisonous', has a specific medical sense 'deadly, fatal', as early on as Cassius Felix,[52] later becoming widespread; Celtic authors use it in this specialized way to describe plague (**pestis**).[53]

37 D995@138; D995@154; D995@156.
38 CPL 1187, *LLT*, par. 331, col. 44, l. 19.
39 LLA 704, *LLT*, p. 459, l. 7.
40 B306@251; B306@253.
41 C684@99.
42 C708@96.
43 LLA 513, *LLT*, lib. 3, par. 284, pag. 84, l. 14; lib. 4, par. 301, p. 90, l. 1; lib. 4, par. 302, p. 90, l. 16; lib. 5, par. 515, p. 168, l. 21; lib. 10, par. 982, p. 293, l. 11; lib. 10, par. 982, p. 293, l. 19.
44 C680@173.
45 A2@272.
46 A59DIST1@19.
47 Souter, *Glossary of Late Latin*; and *TLL*, s.n. **hyposarca**.
48 E1019@272.2.
49 C665@9.
50 LLA 721.1, *LLT*, cap. 46, p. 115, l. 4.
51 CPL 1186, *LLT*, lib. 4 cap. 4, par. 2.
52 LLA 721.1, *LLT*, cap. 46, p. 115, l. 4; cap. 46, p. 118, l. 13; cap. 51, p. 132, l. 1.
53 B305@332; B487@48; C702@228.

In some cases, especially in philosophical contexts explored by Eriugena, the appropriate late-Latin words are not so easily acquired and hint at specialist sources or glossaries. **Concasus**, 'meeting, coming together', the accusative of which he used to gloss *contractionem*,[54] is also used thrice more by him for 'a contraction, coming together',[55] a meaning close to the one found in Caelius Aurelius, for whom the action of closing the teeth could be described by this word,[56] though Eriugena could have applied the word the same way independently. **Meninga**, 'the meninges, membrane surrounding the brain, dura mater', appears in Pseudo-Theodorus Priscianus, Caelius Aurelius, and Cassius Felix;[57] though when Eriugena spells it *menigga* and *meninca*, forms of the original Greek μῆνιγξ (whence the late Latin had been borrowed) that he translates may be reflected or simply transliterated.[58] Another Eriugenian usage of a rare word that circulated with Caelius Aurelius is **reflatio**,[59] 'transpiration, evaporation'.[60] Eriugena also uses **respiratorius**, 'that pertains to breathing',[61] otherwise found in medical texts only, including the works of Oribasius[62] and Cassius Felix (who uses it to translate the transliterated Greek *anapneusticon morion*).[63] In having access to these words — and almost certainly their source-texts — the *peregrinus* Eriugena is a unique case among the first millennium Celtic authors, because he had the libraries of the Carolingian court, as well as many French and Rhineland cathedral schools, at his disposal.

In other instances, an existing Latin word has been re-appropriated for a particularly precise meaning or re-applied from another sphere of learning. The Latin translation of the Welsh laws used **attritio**, originally 'wearing away, rubbing against', later 'wasting away' and more vaguely, 'degradation, impairment; and "hard times"' (as attested in Walter Map),[64] translating Welsh *clais*, for 'abrasion of the skin, a weal'.[65] Late-Latin **confortatiuus**, 'that strengthens', was used in Patristic texts in a moral sense; Thomas of Monmouth and Gerald use it of the curative powers of medicine.[66] Gerald, if probably not the first, is early among those using **infectio**, 'dyeing, steeping', in the sense of its linguistic descendent: 'infection'.[67] Both Gerald and the Norman-based *Life* of Laurence O'Toole in the Codex Dublinensis make a medical metaphor of

54 C698@259.
55 C698@223.
56 *TLL*; Souter, *Glossary of Late Latin*; and Gaffiot, *Dictionnaire Latin-Français*, **concasus**.
57 *TLL*; and Souter, *Glossary of Late Latin*, **meninga**.
58 C704@3; C704@105; C698@222; C698@223; C700LIB1@122; C700LIB1@124.
59 *TLL*; and Souter, *Glossary of Late Latin*, **reflatio**.
60 C698@260.
61 C698@223.
62 Souter, *Glossary of Late Latin*, **respiratorius**.
63 LLA 721.1, LLT, cap. 39, p. 85, l. 17.
64 A76@231; A76@23.
65 A150@254; A153@462.
66 A43@72; A70DIST3@243.
67 A60EPIST@205; A60EPIST@296; A71@158.

the phrase **infernalis ignis**' 'hellfire', to mean 'septicaemia, blood poisoning'.[68] Late-Latin **latificare**, 'to make larger', is found non-medically in the works of Ambrose and Augustine when citing *latificet* in a *Vetus latina* text of Genesis 9. 27 where the Vulgate uses its synonym **dilatare**: *Dilatet Deus Japeth* (May God enlarge Japeth). Eriugena puts **latificare** to medical use in the sense to widen, dilate.[69] The properly classical medical term **mentagra**, 'skin-eruption on the chin', evolves in an hisperic direction; Cummian used it in the metaphorical description of the Britons and Irish as *mentagrae orbis terrarum*.[70] This was mis- (? dis-) understood as '(the tip of) a toe' in Laidcenn's *Lorica*[71] and later (spelt *mentegra*) in the *Life* of Baedán.[72] **Redditor**, 'he who returns (goods), in particular, most often God as dispenser of "just deserts"', is quasi-adjectival as 'restorative, healing' in *fons sanitatum redditor*, 'a health-restoring spring', in the later expansion of Rhygfarch's *Life* of David.[73]

Some further re-appropriations are not fresh coinages in Celtic Latin, but cribbed other medieval authors who had faced similar lexical gaps. **Distemperantia**, 'imbalance (of the humours)', as adopted by Gerald[74] was used in the universities, including by Albertus Magnus.[75] **Gutta cadiua/caduca**, literally 'epileptic essence',[76] which served as a medieval circumlocution for epilepsy, attested from the tenth century, is mainstream, not a Celtic coinage. **Moderantia**, 'self-control, restraint', was found in the Patristic phrase *moderantia animae*, 'governing/checking one's spirits';[77] the related **moderatio**, 'moderation', in the phrase *moderatio sanitatis*, 'restoration of health', is found in a miracle-story

68 A52@134; B491@177: it is questionable whether the *Life* of Laurence is sufficiently independent of the text written at Eu on which it is based to be considered among Celtic-Latin texts at all.

69 C698@223.

70 B289@72.

71 B294RIA@18. Laidcenn mac Buíth Bannaig (d. 661), a scholar based in Clonfert-Mulloe at Kyle in Co. Laois, wrote this poem, a prayer for God and the heavenly host to defend him, which catalogues the parts of the body on which he calls for protection in a deliberately mysterious hermeneutic Latin that makes use of Greek and Hebrew terminology. His scholarly tract *Ecologia de moralibus in Iob* (B293, not yet available on *ACLL*) also survives. The *ACLL* text of the *Lorica* used is not a capture of a previous printed edition, but a compilation that makes especial use of Michael Herren, 'The *Lorica of Laidcenn*' (see his *The Hisperica Famina II*, pp. 76–89) and David Howlett, 'Five Experiments in Textual Reconstruction and Analysis'. The *NCLCL* etymologies cited *infra* have made of use their commentaries. For editions, translations, commentary, and scholarship on the poem, see Ó Corráin, *Clavis Litterarum Hibernensium*, II, pp. 725–27, § 567.

72 B422@381.

73 A32@11.

74 A59DIST1@19.

75 *Commentarii in Quartum Librum Sententiarum*, *LLT*, distinctio 32E, articulus 13, vol. 30, p. 284, col. 1, l. 3; *De Praedicamentis*, *LLT*, tractatus 5, caput 2, p. 247, col. 1, l. 14; *De Sex Principiis*, tractatus 3, caput 2, p. 333, col. 2, l. 3.

76 A71@142.

77 Examples on CDS are: Ambrose, CPL 0143, *LLT*, lib.7, l. 1550; Augustine, CPL 0351, *LLT*, lib. 2, col. 680, l. 39; and col. 681, l. 38.

about St Ambrose of uncertain date.[78] Gerald, a frequent non-medical user of this word, also puts **moderantia** to use for 'lessening of the severity of disease, i.e. recovery',[79] reflecting the sense of the phrase that used its close relation. Likewise, his **recidiuare**, 'to relapse',[80] is as mainstream as his non-medical sense of 'backsliding into sin'.[81] Robertus Salopiensis has St Wenefreda miraculously set a broken neck (**resolidare**),[82] a term commonplace in the medical sense in hagiography, as well as simply 'to solidify (again)'. **Umidare/humidare**, 'to make soggy', appears early as the verb that describes what drinking does to the brain, weighing it down with somniferous fluid.[83]

One author's collection of examples frequently forms rather more of a linguistic game; many items within his anatomical vocabulary do not provide medical insight, as a few examples will demonstrate. Laidcenn's *femoralia* in the sense of 'thighs'[84] is the neuter plural of the late-Latin adjective **femoralis**, bearing various senses 'relating to the *femur* (thigh)', frequently as a substantive, 'trousers'. Laidcenn creates a full linguistic circle by applying the meaning of the noun **femur** to the substantive adjective whence it derives. **Femur** appears so many times in the Bible, Fathers, and other basic sources that it is inconceivable that the scholarly Laidcenn was not playing an hermeneutic game. {**gingis**},[85] a variant dative plural of the well-attested classical **gingiua**, is notable for reducing *–iuis* to *–ís* in a playful parallel to the syncopated perfect of fourth-conjugation verbs. Select examples of additional lexemes drawn from Laidcenn are discussed below where they appear to have been useful terms, or where the neologism is illustrative of a point or pattern of usage.

Like every language, Latin has internal tools for the creation of new coinages from the existing word-stock. **Adnexitas** (**annexitas**), 'the state of being bound up', which derives from the classical participle and adjective **adnexus**, 'tied up, bounden', in particular describes 'some intestinal affliction, perhaps constipation'.[86] Laidcenn's innovative **bucliamen**, coined from **bullire**, 'to bubble' — but influenced by the form of **buccula**, '"little cheek", i.e. a swelling' — seems to mean 'reflux'.[87] **Curatiuus**, 'remedial',[88] is an obvious and mainstream derivative of classical **curare**. Thomas of Monmouth added the prefix *e-* to mainstream late-Latin **mingere**, 'to urinate', making a transitive verb **emingere**, for which the object in this case was blood.[89] Donatus

78 Blaise, *Dictionnaire Latin–Français des auteurs chrétiens*, **moderatio**.
79 A71@74.
80 A59DIST1@14; A71@175.
81 A71@328.
82 A51P1@714.1.
83 C778@1298.
84 B294RIA@17.
85 B294RIA@12.
86 A70DIST1@59.
87 B294RIA@20.
88 A52@73.
89 A43@145.

Faesulanus's hapax <**foedere**>/**federe**, 'to be gangrenous',[90] is an interesting case. Classical **foetere**, 'to stink, smell ill', and **foedus**, 'repugnant', have different etymologies but converge in sense; this formation melds the two words. The hapax {**marsem**} (accusative) is an hisperic, and possibly corrupt word; the strongest possibility is that it is a back-formation from **marsuppium**, 'sack, purse', with the specialized sense 'scrotum'.[91] Eriugena's coinage **refluxio**, from classical **refluere**, is used by him and others for a destructive tidal surge,[92] but also for 'a swallowing (of liquid) again (? reflux)'.[93]

The coinages just listed are based on general vocabulary; in other cases, the base term is already part of the medical vocabulary. Eriugena's **circumrubescere**, 'to become inflamed',[94] builds on the prefix for 'around' and the verb for becoming red, which was already used of the skin, whether by blushing or burning. His **fellifer**, 'that secretes bile',[95] similarly builds on classical **fel**, the mainstream word for that humour. Jocelyn's <**lethargion**>/**letargion**, 'a sleeping-draught',[96] is a hellenizing derivative of **lethargia**, 'drowsiness'.

Often, however, the shift simply arises from the need to obtain a different part of speech with the word-building tools innate in the language (as Laidcenn had done playfully in the **femur** circle above). The neuter plural of the adjective **epidemius**, 'epidemic', was used as a noun in late Latin; later it came to be widely declined as a feminine a-stem. This led Gerald to re-coin an adjective, **epidemicus**, from the substantive as he knew it.[97] Gerald's **ictericius**, also **icteritius**, 'of jaundice',[98] forms an adjective from the widely attested late-Latin **icterícia** in the absence of knowledge of the rare classical adjective **ictericus**. Some coinages can be prompted by the gender of a noun. One such case is **minutrix**, 'a woman who bleeds (patients), a (therapeutic) bloodletter',[99] which derives from the verb **minuere**, 'to lessen', with reference to the earlier-attested medieval masculine noun **minutor,** 'he who bleeds (patients)'.

Providing a transition into the next group is **uuula/ugula**, 'uvula',[100] a mainstream word coined early in the medieval period. This is a diminutive of classical **uua**, which bore this medical meaning alongside its general meaning, 'a grape'; re-assigning the specific anatomical term to the diminutive was a useful way of making an explicit distinction. Thomas of Monmouth and

---

90 C693@104.

91 B294RIA@19.

92 C697@1220; A97@212.

93 C708@57.

94 C698@247.

95 C698@223.

96 E1018@163.

97 A71@142.

98 A54@103; A64@131; A64@165; A69@151; A69@171.

99 B491@177.

100 B337@7. On this word, see the discussion by Sharon Arbuthnot in this volume, pp. 291-92.

Gerald both use **gutturnosus** as the adjective for 'suffering from a swollen throat, goitred'.[101] This derives from classical **guttur**, 'a goitre', whence the standard — though rare — adjective **gutturosus**. Though it is probable that this is a (redundant) coinage from the root, it is hard to rule out the alternative, that it is a mere variant of the classical adjective. Simple variants of form or spelling provide another category; some of these are solecisms, but others were transmitted in reputable sources and became normalized. **Eemorrois**[102] is a slightly perverse spelling of standard **haemorr(h)ois**, 'piles'. **Erisipila**[103] is more respectable, being Isidore's form of the Greek-influenced **erysipelas**. **Leucoflancia**, 'leucophlegmatic dropsy',[104] is a variant or corruption of late-Latin **leucophlegmatia** — used by Caelius Aurelius among others[105] — one may wonder here about the possible influence of Norman (-French) pronunciation.[106] **Archites**[107] can be assigned to corruption: the *s* of the mainstream late-Latin (< Greek) **ascites**, 'abdominal dropsy', having been misread, probably in Insular script. {**disnoim**}[108] represents a confusion of the a-stem accusative of standard but rare classical **dyspnoea** or its late-Latin variant **dyspnia**. Laidcenn's **tolia**[109] blends synonyms, taking the root of the classical consonant-stem plural **toles**, but the a-stem declension of its synonym **tonsillae**. His **exugia**, 'body fat'[110] is a variant of (? or play on) classical **auxungia**, 'axle grease' — which was usually made of suet, the fat that protects the kidneys. These are hisperic, and Laidcenn clearly had an idea why he created the forms he did. The *hapax legomenon* glossary-word **lapifulta**, defined in Irish as *lecc an árain*, 'a kidney-stone',[111] resembles late-Latin **lapillulus**, 'a gravel stone', of which it may be a corruption.

There are a handful of words that derive from Greek for which there is no evidence for late-Latin transmission. Among these, **melanc(h)olia**, 'irrational perversity, a humour arising from too much black bile',[112] is quite mainstream; Isidore used it, and it was widely diffused long before the Norman-influenced authors cited here. The Cosmographer Pseudo-Jerome responsible for the so-called *Cosmographia Aethici Istrici*, who may or may not have been Irish, but certainly betrays Irish affinities in his hispericism, is a frequent source of Greek loans, few of which caught on. **Aspidiscus**, 'a clyster-pipe'[113] comes from

101 A43@86; A43@220; A43@250; A69@346.
102 A115@304.
103 B409@297.
104 E1019@272.2.
105 *TLL*; and Gaffiot, *Dictionnaire Latin–Français*, **leucophlegmatia**.
106 The word evolved in Old French as *leucofleumance* and Anglo-Norman *leucoflemancie*.
107 E1019@272.2.
108 A115@304.
109 B294RIA@20.
110 B294RIA@10.
111 B337@9.
112 A76@144; A76@201; A66@ParsI.649; A66@ParsII.757.
113 C647@63.

the Greek, where this definition falls within its broad range of meanings; the same word had been borrowed into late Latin denoting a boss, ornaments, but is not attested in this sense. The Cosmographer's word may be an independent borrowing. Adomnán's **lepri**, 'people afflicted with leprosy or other (stigmatizing) skin disease',[114] takes the expected form in borrowing Greek λεπροί (singular λεπρός). The word is part of a nexus of related borrowings and adjustments: late Latin, and many of the medieval Celtic writers of Latin, actively used the mainstream and biblical adjective **leprosus**; and the classical language already had **lepra** as a substantive, which continued in use through the Middle Ages. Adomnán's form later appears in another Irish source, the glosses in the Southampton Psalter at Psalm 38(37):20(21): *QUI RETRIBUNT MALA PRO BONIS DETRAHEBANT MIHI .i. dum 'resuscitarem mortuos eorum et lepros mundarem'* (THEY THAT RENDER EVIL FOR GOOD HAVE DETRACTED ME, that is, until 'I have revived their dead and cleansed their lepers').[115] Laidcenn frequently borrowed terms for basic anatomy. **Michinae**, 'nostrils',[116] which appears to be an altered or corrupt form of Greek μυκτήρ, may eliminate the ambiguity that Latin **naris**, 'nose', denotes 'nostrils' in the plural as well as 'noses'. More often, his borrowings are gratuitous. **Cephale**, 'skull, crown of the head',[117] uses the Greek form of a word frequently seen as a root-element in Latin, but not elsewhere alone. When he uses a Greek word, rather than Latin **caput**, he amplifies the mysterious polylinguistic construction of his prayer; his neologism adds nothing to the mundane anatomical meaning. The obscure, possibly corrupt accusative plural **{conas}**[118] could either derive from Greek κῶνος, 'pine-cone, point of a helmet', probably intending 'the cranium' — or be a corruption of *ainas* (**aina**), from the Hebrew for 'eyes', as suggested by the glossator, who interlineated *oculos*. **Cladum/caladum**, 'neck, throat, gullet',[119] is probably from Hebrew (though potentially affected by or playing on late-Latin and/or Greek words). **Senna**, the accusative plural of which is glossed *dentes*,[120] is a latinization of the Hebrew, but appears to bear no specialized meaning and hints at no specialized medical sourcebook. Michael Herren's commentary accompanying his edition of this *Lorica* draws attention to the fact that the roots of the Hebrew-derived vocabulary in the poem can be gleaned from biblical commentaries and Patristic resources, most especially Jerome's explanations of Hebrew biblical names.[121] Although Laidcenn's poem can potentially testify to words in circulation, he appears to

---

114 B305@348.

115 *Psalterium Suthantoniense*, ed. by O'Neill, p. 94, l. 62.

116 B294RIA@10; also in another hisperic poem, B314RIA@96.

117 B294RIA@10.

118 B294RIA@10.

119 B294RIA@10; B314RIA@96.

120 B294RIA@10.

121 *The Hisperica Famina: II. Related Poems*, ed. and trans. by Herren, pp. 76–89 (ed. and trans.), 113–37 (commentary).

be seeking an obscure substitute for an ordinary word rather than attempting to be technically precise. In this Laidcenn was not alone; **<lisana>/lisina**, an adaptation of the Hebrew for 'tongue', appears in his work and that of others: twice in the physical sense[122] and, by metonymy, 'word'.[123]

Finally, there are two borrowings that come from vernacular languages, a phenomenon much rarer than one would expect in an area where vocabulary was potentially lacking. **Bocium**, 'a lump, swelling', in the *Life* of Laurence O'Toole[124] is a straightforward latinization of Old-French *boce*; it is attested in a number of Anglo-Latin texts as well.[125] Only one medical word in the Latin of the Celtic countries has a possible Celtic element in its etymology. This is **tillum**, 'tree-bark (as a poison)', first attested in the *Vita prima* of Samson.[126] Du Cange spotted the similarity of this lexeme to Old-French *tille*, '(linden) bark' — < Latin **tilia**, 'a linden, lime-tree' — though he was cautious enough to set the mark of query before the suggestion.[127] There are two possible doubts, to wit, that lime-bast is medicinal, not toxic; and that the author of the *Life* was almost certainly Breton, and the text lacks other signs of French influence. Yet Old Breton also has this word in the form *till*, found in the *Leiden Leechbook* among other sources, and Owens and Falileyev propose that **tilia** is rather derived from or cognate with 'Gaulish *tillum*, "poison" (properly "lime"?) or "turpentine" and that the short *i* [cf. Modern-Breton *tilh*] makes it less likely to be a direct loan from Latin'.[128]

What, then, can be drawn forth from this data? Perhaps alignment of the attested vocabulary with that in particular non-Celtic texts might identify which Latin medical treatises were circulating or even in widespread use in the Celtic world or particular regions within it? This had been a hope at the beginning of this study. Having examined the evidence, the search for substantial alignment of medical terms that occur in Celtic-Latin literature with the terminology of popular antique medical treatises has largely been fruitless. Some of the terms did occur in these treatises as noted above, but it was not possible decisively to pin down particular authors whose vocabulary was being adopted widely, which would imply that they were in active professional circulation. Notably, words attested in Cassius Felix's vocabulary turn up somewhat more than other authors, though the lack of so many more of his terms that would have been useful suggests that their transmission was indirect, as words from a standard authority could circulate through vocabularies, possibly some short excerpts or quotations in florilegia, and through anecdotes of miraculous cures that are such a widespread element in hagiography across early-medieval Europe.

122 B294RIA@10; B314RIA@96.
123 B326@147.
124 B491@275.
125 Ashdown and others, *Dictionary of Mediaeval Latin from British Sources*, **botium**.
126 D950@116.
127 Du Cange, *Glossarium Mediae et Infimae Latinitatis*, **tillum**.
128 *The Leiden Leechbook*, ed. by Falileyev and Owen, p. 56.

Overall, words that found their way into the Vulgate or the Fathers surfaced most regularly, especially among the early-medieval authors.

Turning to the two most cited first-millennium Irish authors in this study, the coinages in Laidcenn's hyperlearned poem testifies more to his linguistic ingenuity than to the limits of his vocabulary. The other important case, Eriugena's use of rarer medical terminology, draws attention to the fact that he worked in the centre of the Carolingian Empire, with all its resources of learning at his disposal, whilst his countrymen — and other Celts — lacked access to such materials. Contreni has assembled wider evidence that Eriugena was the same as the Irish John who acted as a medical practitioner in the court of Charles the Bald.[129] Eriugena's works indicate deep interest in medical studies and texts in Greek as well as Latin, and some form of professional medical training in Francia is a distinct possibility. His medical vocabulary stands distinctly apart from others in the corpus of Celtic Latinity.

In all the nations of the Celtic fringe, there were times when an author simply did not have the precise Latin term he needed, and turned to re-appropriating, borrowing, or occasionally coining to say what he needed to get across. These authors certainly had an exact concept of what they were trying to say; there is no question of that. They gleaned the sources they had for words that they could use, adapt grammatically, or re-appropriate, so as to express their ideas. Increased faculty for adaptation of word forms occurs most among those twelfth-century authors who operated in elite circles in which French was spoken and the birth of university learning was making its mark: Walter Map, Jocelyn of Furness, Gerald de Barri (Kambrensis), and the anonymous translators of the Welsh laws; earlier authors were slightly more cautious, rather more likely to search through the standard devotional authors or to re-appropriate words, describing a medical phenomenon by extension or metaphorical use of their basic store of Latin. Nevertheless, the difference over time and nation is unexpectedly slight.

In the end, the medical vocabulary in the *Non-Classical Lexicon of Celtic Latinity* is a record of language use over more than 800 years in texts written across the Celtic-speaking regions of the Atlantic Archipelago and Brittany, as well as by expatriates from these lands. What is held in common is that prior to the influences of major European centres of learning that accompanied francophone elites who increasingly penetrated these regions, it appears quite unlikely that any significant quantity of Latin medical treatises circulated widely. Overall, the evidence suggests that Latin was not the main language of transmission of professional medical knowledge in any of the Celtic countries of the Atlantic fringe in the first millennium and did not become its primary language at any rate in the centuries following. Nevertheless, that did not mean that there was a tolerance for sloppiness or widespread vernacular borrowing

129 For Eriugena's involvement in specifically medical learning, see Contreni, 'Masters of Medicine in Northern France', pp. 270–77.

in the expression of medical ideas when one communicated them through the prestige medium of the Latin language.

Works Cited

Manuscripts

Dublin, Royal Irish Academy, MS 23 P 10 [ii] (453)
Leiden, Universitätsbibliothek, MS Vossianus latinus in folio 96a
Paris, Bibliothèque Nationale de France, MS lat. 9332
St Gall, Stiftsbibliothek, MS 759
St Gall, Stifitsbibliothek, MS 761

Primary Sources

Brepolis, *ACLL = Archive of Celtic Latin Literature* <clt.brepolis.net/acll/> [accessed 6 October 2021]

Brepolis, *eMGH = Monumenta Germaniae Historica* <clt.brepolis.net/eMGH/> [accessed 6 October 2021]

Brepolis, *LLT = Library of Latin Texts* <clt.brepolis.net/llta/> [accessed 6 April 2024]

'A Celtic Leechbook', ed. by Whitley Stokes, *Zeitschrift für celtische Philologie*, 1 (1897), 17–25

The Hisperica Famina: II. Related Poems, ed. and trans. by Michael Herren, Studies and Texts, 85 (Toronto: Pontifical Institute of Mediaeval Studies, 1987)

The Leiden Leechbook: A Study of the Earliest Neo-Brittonic Medical Compilation, ed. by Aleksandr I. Falileyev and Morfydd Owen, Innsbrucker Beiträge zur Kulturwissenschaft, 122 (Innsbruck: Institut für Sprachen und Litteraturen der Universität, 2005)

Medieval Welsh Medical Texts. Volume I: The Recipes, ed. and trans. by Diana Luft (Cardiff: University of Wales Press, 2020)

Psalterium Suthantoniense, ed. by Pádraig P. O'Neill, Corpus Christianorum Continuatio Mediaevalis, 240 (Turnhout: Brepols 2012)

Secondary Studies

Ashdown, Richard, David Howlett, and Ronald Latham, eds, *The Dictionary of Medieval Latin from British Sources*, 17 fasc. (Oxford: Oxford University Press, 1975–2013; reprint in 3 vols, 2018)

Bannerman, John, *The Beatons: A Medical Kindred in the Classical Gaelic Tradition* (Edinburgh: John Donald, 1986)

Bischoff, Bernhard 'Die europäische Verbreitung der Werke Isidors', in *Mittelalterliche Studien: Ausgewählte Aufsätze zur Schriftkunde und Literaturgeschichte*, ed. by Bernhard Bischoff, 3 vols (Stuttgart: Hiersemann 1966), I, pp. 171–94

Blaise, Albert, *Dictionnaire Latin–Français des auteurs chrétiens*, Corpus Christianorum (Brepols: Turnhout, 1967; reprint 1997)

Brepolis, *CDS: Cross Database Searchtool* <clt.brepolis.net/llta/> [accessed 6 October 2021]

Contreni, John J., 'Masters and Medicine in Northern France during the Reign of Charles the Bald', in *Charles the Bald: Court and Kingdom. Papers Based on a Colloquium Held in London in April 1979*, ed. by Margaret Gibson and Janet Nelson, 2nd revised edn (Aldershot: Variorum, 1990), pp. 267–82

Du Cange, Charles, *Glossarium Mediae et Infimae Latinitatis*, 10 vols, revised edn (Niort: Favre, 1883–1887)

Flahive, Joseph, '*Venialia et Ventositas*: Late-Latin Vocabulary in Medieval Ireland', *Journal of Medieval Latin*, 31 (2021), 159–89

Gaffiot, Felix, ed., *Dictionnaire illustré Latin–Français* (Paris: Hachette, 1934)

Glare, Peter G. W., ed., *Oxford Latin Dictionary*, 2 vols (Oxford: Oxford University Press, 1982; 2nd edn 2012)

Harvey, Anthony, 'Frankenstein in the Scriptorium: Bringing Latin to Life in Medieval Ireland', in *Code-Switching in Medieval Ireland and England*, ed. by Mícheál Ó Flaithearta, Münchner Forschungen zur historischen Sprachwissenschaft, 18 (Bremen: Hempen, 2018), pp. 105–19

——, 'Languages and Literacy in Mid-First-Millennium Ireland: New Questions to Some Old Answers', in *Transforming Landscapes of Belief in the Early Medieval Insular World and Beyond*, ed. by Nancy Edwards, Máire Ní Mhaonaigh, and Roy Flechner, Converting the Isles, 2 (Turnhout: Brepols, 2017), pp. 47–63

——, 'Latin, Literacy, and the Celtic Vernaculars around the Year AD 500', in *Celtic Languages and Celtic Peoples: Proceedings of the Second North American Congress of Celtic Studies, Held in Halifax, August 16–19, 1989*, ed. by Cyril J. Byrne, Margaret Harry, and Pádraig Ó Siadhail (Halifax [Nova Scotia]: St Mary's University, 1992), pp. 11–26

——, 'The Non-Classical Vocabulary of Celtic-Latin Literature: An Overview', in *Spoken and Written Language: Relations between Latin and the Vernacular Languages in the Earlier Middle Ages*, ed. by Mary Garrison, Arpad P. Orbán, and Marco Mostert, Utrecht Studies in Medieval Literacy, 24 (Turnhout: Brepols, 2013), pp. 87–100

——, 'Reading the Genetic Code of Early Medieval Celtic Orthography', in *LautSchriftSprache: Beiträge zur vergleichenden historischen Graphematik*, ed. by Elvira Glaser, Annina Seiler, and Michelle Waldispühl, Medienwandel – Medienwechsel – Medienwissen, 15 (Zurich: Chronos, 2011), pp. 155–66

——, 'Technical Vocabulary and its Identification in Medieval Celtic Latinity', *Archivium Latinitatis Medii Aevi (Bulletin Du Cange)*, 66 (2013), 377–88

Harvey, Anthony, and Angela Malthouse, *The Non-Classical Lexicon of Celtic Latinity. Supplement: Letters A to H* (2015; online at <journals.eecs.qub.ac.uk/dmlcs/supplmt.pdf>; print edition forthcoming)

Harvey, Anthony, and Jane Power, *The Non-Classical Lexicon of Celtic Latinity. Part I: A–H*, Royal Irish Academy Dictionary of Medieval Latin from Celtic

Sources Constituent Publications, 1 / Corpus Christianorum Continuatio Mediaevalis (Turnhout: Brepols, 2005)

Herren, Michael, 'On the Earliest Irish Acquaintance with Isidore of Seville', in *Visigothic Spain: New Approaches*, ed. by Edward James (Oxford: Clarendon, 1980), pp. 243–50; reprinted in Michael Herren, *Latin Letters in Early Christian Ireland* (Aldershot: Variorum, 1996), ch. 3

Howlett, David, 'Five Experiments in Textual Reconstruction and Analysis', *Peritia*, 9 (1995), 1–50

Johnston, Elva, *Literacy and Identity in Medieval Ireland*, Studies in Celtic History, 33 (Woodbridge: Boydell, 2013)

Lapidge, Michael, and Richard Sharpe, *The Bibliography of Celtic-Latin Literature 400–1200* (Dublin: Royal Irish Academy, 1985)

McKee, Helen, 'The Script of the Leiden Leechbook', in *The Leiden Leechbook: A Study of the Earliest Neo-Brittonic Medical Compilation*, ed. by Aleksandr I. Falileyev and Morfydd Owen, Innsbrucker Beiträge zur Kulturwissenschaft, 122 (Innsbruck: Institut für Sprachen und Litteraturen der Universität, 2005), pp. 88–94

McManus, Damian, *A Guide to Ogam*, Maynooth Monographs, 4 (Maynooth: National University of Ireland, Maynooth, Department of Early Irish, 1991)

Nicolson, Alexander, 'The McBeths — Hereditary Physicians of the Highlands', *Transactions of the Gaelic Society of Glasgow*, 5 (1958), 94–112

Ó Corráin, Donnchadh, *Clavis Litterarum Hibernensium*, Corpus Christianorum Claves, 3 vols (Turnhout: Brepols, 2017)

Ó Cróinín, Dáibhí, 'Hiberno-Latin Literature to 1169', in *A New History of Ireland, I: Prehistoric and Early Ireland*, ed. by Dáibhí Ó Cróinín (Oxford: Oxford University Press, 2005), pp. 371–404

Ó Murchú, Liam P., ed., *Rosa Anglica: Reassessments*, Irish Texts Society Subsidiary Series, 27 (London: Irish Texts Society, 2016)

Owen, Morfydd, 'Medics and Medicine', in *The Welsh King and His Court*, ed. by Thomas M. Charles-Edwards, Morfydd Owen, and Paul Russell (Cardiff: University of Wales Press, 2000), pp. 116–41

Parina, Elena, 'Medical Texts in Welsh Translation: *Y Pedwar Gwlybwr* and *Rhinweddau Bwydydd*', in *Crossing Borders in the Insular Middle Ages*, ed. by Aisling Byrne and Victoria Flood, Medieval Texts and Cultures of Northern Europe, 30 (Turnhout: Brepols, 2019), pp. 47–63

Souter, Alexander, *A Glossary of Later Latin* (Oxford: Oxford University Press, 1949)

Stanford, William B., 'Towards a History of Classical Influences in Ireland', *Proceedings of the Royal Irish Academy*, 70C (1970), 13–91

Thesaurus Linguae Latinae, ed. by Bayerische Akademie der Wissenschaften (Leipzig: Teubner; Munich: Saur; Berlin: De Gruyter [repr. of all previous fascs], 1900–, and online at <thesaurus.badw.de> [accessed 6 April 2024])

SHARON ARBUTHNOT

12. Late Medieval Irish Medicalese and its European Context

Although no medical texts, as such, are known from the Old or Middle Irish periods (conventionally defined as *c.* 700 – *c.* 1200), the Irish language of that time was not devoid of medical terminology.[1] Narrative literature, annals, legal and other texts produced prior to the thirteenth century refer to diseases, to organs of the body and to medical treatments and implements, using relatively consistent and/or transparent vocabulary. Based on descriptions of symptoms, on accounts of prevailing environmental factors and on the time-frame in which certain diseases are reported in Ireland, it has been possible to suggest that early Irish *blefed* denotes bubonic plague and that *bolgach* was smallpox.[2] Easily analysed anatomical terms include *macloc*, literally 'child-place', a name for the womb.[3] In a ninth-century gloss, *áru* is revealed as the Irish equivalent of Latin *rien* (a kidney).[4] Possibly of slightly later date, an explanatory comment on the rare word *gibne* identifies this as *adarc lege* (a physician's cupping-horn).[5] The appearance of the phrase *gae*

1 For the sake of convenience, I use the term 'Irish' to refer to the language of the texts under investigation in this chapter. This is in keeping with the usage in the historical dictionary (eDIL, see n. 2 below) on which this work relies heavily and which covers material of Scottish as well as Irish provenance.

2 Grace, 'From *blefed* to *scamach*', pp. 77–82 and 87. In what follows, references to published and manuscript examples of particular items of vocabulary are given only where these words are not recorded in the *electronic Dictionary of the Irish Language* (eDIL) or where specific attestations are useful to demonstrate points of date, application or context. To facilitate consultation, Irish terms have been cited according to the relevant eDIL headwords, despite the generally early orthography of those headwords and their occasional inconsistencies.

3 For an example in a Middle Irish text, see 'Niall Frossach's True Judgement', ed. and trans. by Wiley, p. 21.

4 *Thes.*, II, p. 138 (96b4).

5 '*Sanas Cormaic*: An Old-Irish Glossary', ed. by Meyer, § 732. The shorter recension of this glossary is often associated with Cormac mac Cuilennáin (†908), but the entry on *gibne* is found only in the longer, later recension.

Sharon Arbuthnot • University of Cambridge; sja50@cam.ac.uk

Medicine in the Medieval North Atlantic World: Vernacular Texts and Traditions, ed. by Deborah Hayden and Sarah Baccianti, KSS, 5 (Turnhout, 2025), pp. 287-305
BREPOLS PUBLISHERS DOI 10.1484/M.KSS-EB.5.143990

cró in early tales suggests that the monastic scholars who produced these narratives were aware of the practice of tenting wounds.[6]

Recently, it has become increasingly clear that, even in the earlier medieval period, there was some understanding of the key doctrines of classical and Arabic medicine. In the Irish-language context,[7] arguments for this have depended to some extent on interpretative readings of episodes in important tales. Thus, Ranke de Vries has suggested that the colours of the vomit produced by Caílte in late twelfth- or early thirteenth-century *Acallam na senórach* characterize this healing experience as an expelling of bodily humours, although that text makes no direct use of humoral theory as articulated by ancient Greek physicians and thinkers.[8] Other Old and Middle Irish texts sporadically bear witness not only to a basic knowledge of humourism but also to the linguistic terms needed to expound such concepts. Using *linn* (liquid) to provide an Irish equivalent of Latin *humor*, which has a similar primary meaning, a ninth-century collection of traditions associated with the Monastery of Tallaght describes nocturnal emissions in terms of the expulsion of *imarcraid lenda* (excess humour) that is in the body.[9] In what seems to be an alternative approach to the naming of humours in Irish, the word *dublaithe*, almost certainly derived from *dub* (black) and *laith* (liquid),[10] appears in the eleventh- or twelfth-century comic-satiric tale of *Aislinge Meic Con Glinne* and again in an early Irish vision poem attributed to Saint Fursa. On both occasions, 'melancholic' would provide a suitable sense for *dublaithe*,[11] and this interpretation can be supported if we assume that the black liquid in question here is black bile, the presence of which is associated with a melancholic temperament, according to humoral doctrine of the European Middle Ages.

It is easily demonstrated, then, that medical vocabulary was a feature of earlier medieval Irish and that this included at least a smattering of terms relevant to the expression of ideas which can be traced back to the likes of Hippocrates and Galen. Equally obvious is the fact that, sometime after the arrival of the French-speaking Normans in the country, medicine in Ireland

---

6 In the early Middle Irish tale of *Tochmarc Ferbe*, for example, one of the characters is said to have experienced such anger that the tents fell out of his wounds: see '*Tochmarc Ferbe*', ed. and trans. by Windisch, l. 735.

7 On a Latin-language expression of the principle that 'contraries heal contraries' in an Irish milieu, see McNeill, 'Medicine for Sin', pp. 17–18.

8 De Vries, 'Medieval Medicine and the Healing of Caílte', particularly pp. 61–68.

9 'The Monastery of Tallaght', ed. and trans. by Gwynn and Purton, p. 164 § 88. For discussion, see Arbuthnot, 'The Medieval Irish Vocabulary of Sex and Reproduction'.

10 For this analysis, see eDIL s.v. *dub* Compds II (dil.ie/18985).

11 'is dublathi díscir dian' (he is melancholic, bold, impetuous): *Aislinge Meic Con Glinne*, ed. by Jackson, p. 34, l. 1040, where the speaker is characterized as *fáithliaig* (a wise [or prophetic] physician); 'dublaithe a ndeouid an domain' (melancholic at the end of the world): 'Mitteilungen aus irischen Handschriften', ed. by Meyer, p. 168, l. 25. In both instances, it seems likely that the genitive case of a compound noun is functioning adjectively.

entered a new phase.[12] Perhaps around the mid-fourteenth century, extensive medical texts seem to be made available in Irish for the first time. These were substantially translations and adaptations of original Latin texts emanating from continental Europe and England. A manuscript held in the Royal Irish Academy, Dublin, which contains the Irish version of the *Trotula* texts on women's medicine, seems to have been copied, at least in part, from a book produced in 1352.[13] In the year 1400, an Irish treatise on pathology, based mainly on the *Practica super nono Almansoris* of Gerardus de Solo, was completed by Tadhg Ó Cuinn.[14] An Irish version of Magninus of Milan's *Regimen sanitatis* probably dates from around the same time.[15] John of Gaddesden's *Rosa anglica* came into Irish sometime before 1462.[16] Sections of Guy de Chauliac's *De anathomia* were translated and probably somewhat revised by Cormac Mac Duinnshléibhe before the mid-fifteenth century; the same scholar seems to have been responsible also for Irish versions of material from Bernard of Gordon's *Lilium medicinae*, from Gualterus Agilon's *De dosibus mediciarum* and of a number of other medical and metaphysical texts.[17] In sum, a core corpus of Latin medical material was transferred into Irish in a century and a half of intensive work between *c.* 1350 and *c.* 1500.

This burst of activity in Irish broadly coincides with the Europe-wide phenomenon of rendering medical and other scientific works into vernacular languages. Recently, the place of Irish in this movement, which included also English, French, German, Dutch, and Spanish, has been increasingly recognized. Notably, Jason Harris has proposed that Irish medical scholars were 'entirely in step with developments elsewhere in northern Europe, not within the scholastic, university-based discipline of medicine, but in the broader process of "vernacularisation" which has come to be seen as distinctive of medical and scientific history in this period'.[18] Beyond the mere fact of vernacularizing, certain similarities have been observed across the medical outputs of late medieval Europe: the same texts were being translated into diverse languages,[19] and analogous techniques were being employed to deal

12 Useful general accounts of the background can be found in Grace, 'Medicine in Gaelic Ireland and Scotland'; Ní Shéaghdha, *Translations and Adaptations*, pp. 5–9; Nic Dhonnchadha, 'Irish Medical Writing, 1400–1600' and 'Medical Writing in Irish'.

13 This date can be found in Dublin, RIA, MS 23 F 19, fol. 24^{v}a17–18.

14 See Nic Dhonnchadha, 'Some Words from *Almusór*', p. 15, and also the chapter by Brigid Mayes in this volume.

15 See *Regimen na sláinte*, ed. by Ó Ceithearnaigh, I, pp. xxvii–xxviii.

16 See Nic Dhonnchadha, 'The Irish *Rosa anglica*', p. 120.

17 See *Anathomia Gydo*, ed. and trans. by Ní Ghallchobhair, pp. 2 and 4.

18 Harris, 'Latin Learning and Irish Physicians', p. 19.

19 Pahta and Taavitsainen detail the many European languages (including Irish/Gaelic) into which Bernard of Gordon's *Lilium medicinae* and the *Trotula* texts had been translated in or by the fifteenth century: Pahta and Taavitsainen, 'Vernacularisation of Scientific and Medical Writing', p. 10.

with specialized medical terminology for which there were no readily available equivalents in English, French, and so on.

Studies of the methods adopted to translate Latin vocabulary into vernacular languages suggest that different scholars took different approaches, that multiple variants of certain terms existed simultaneously, and that a large proportion of the innovative forms generated in this context were extremely short-lived.[20] Looking at the processes by which the technical vocabulary of a Latin surgical text was rendered into Middle French, Howard Stone said of the translator: 'now he uses a folk-term, now he paraphrases in simple French; again he leaves the term intact, alone or with an explanation, a comment, or a French approximation. A common device was to formulate a French calque or close imitation of the Latin, usually by merely adapting the ending to French spelling'.[21] More than thirty years later, Tony Hunt mentioned 'calques, adoption of Latin terms with or without morphological adaptation to the target language, i.e. including encysts, and a variety of techniques of paraphrase, including glosses'.[22] Juhani Norri has discussed in great detail how new medical terms were created in English in the fourteenth to sixteenth centuries, citing additional translation-strategies such as semantic extension, equivalence (describing one and the same situation using completely different wording), and creating new affix formations.[23] Taavitsainen and Pahta, meanwhile, made the pertinent comment that methods employed by English translators and adaptors have models in 'the already established conventions and features of Latin scientific writing'.[24]

Looking back at uses of *linn* and *laith* to refer to a bodily humour: these are instances of calquing — well-established Irish words have been mapped onto roughly synonymous Latin *humor* — and they exemplify also how different scholars can take different approaches in their attempts to convert the same lexical item from one language to another. Such terms, dating from the pre-Norman period, are not necessarily indicative of how translators met the demand for new medical vocabulary on a much larger scale from the fourteenth century onwards, however. To date, there has been little consideration of the methods by which medical material in Latin was rendered into Irish or

20 The journal *Early Science and Medicine* has published a number of important studies on translation into different vernaculars, including Cifuentes, 'Vernacularization as an Intellectual and Social Bridge'; Crossgrove, 'The Vernacularization of Science, Medicine, and Technology in Late Medieval Europe'; Demaitre, 'Medical Writing in Transition'; Taavitsainen and Pahta, 'Vernacularisation of Medical Writing in English'. Other studies of relevance are mentioned in the references cited in those articles and throughout the notes below. On the points highlighted here, see in particular Norri, 'Translation from Latin and French', pp. 569, 608 and 611–12.

21 Stone, 'Puzzling Translations in the Thirteenth Century', p. 175.

22 Hunt, 'Old French Translations of Medical Texts', p. 350.

23 Norri, *Dictionary of Medical Vocabulary in English*, p. 1; 'Translation from Latin and French', especially pp. 573–74, 575, 578 and 585.

24 Taavitsainen and Pahta, 'Vernacularisation of Medical Writing in English', p. 157.

of the extent to which these methods align with patterns identified in other European vernaculars.[25] Two factors in particular seem to have contributed to this situation: Ireland's medical output from the late medieval period remains substantially unedited and unpublished, and the historical dictionary of the language was compiled mainly from literary texts. The main purposes of the rest of this chapter, then, are to document further the specialized vocabulary found in Irish medical texts of *c.* 1350–*c.* 1500 (though mostly surviving in later manuscript copies) and to take forward the work of examining techniques of vernacularization in the hope of bringing the Irish tradition more centrally into the emerging dialogue on the translation and adaptation of scientific writing in Europe in the latter part of the Middle Ages. With these objectives in mind, various features of the language of late medieval Irish medical texts are discussed below under separate headings.

Multiple Variants

The palatine uvula is perhaps an unlikely candidate to have produced one of the more interesting clusters of terminology in medieval Irish medical texts. In manuscripts of the fifteenth century and later, however, there are numerous different ways of alluding to this small, conical projection which hangs at the back of the throat.

- In the Irish version of *De anathomia*, the Latin term, itself a diminutive of *uva* (a grape), is borrowed to round off a list which is otherwise in Irish: 'tigim chum rann an bhéil ... uachtuir 7 īachtuir 7 an charbaid 7 in teangaidh 7 uula' (I come to the parts of the upper and lower mouth, the palate and the tongue and uvula).[26]
- A few paragraphs earlier, the same text refers to 'an carbad uachturach leath hsiar don tsine sidāin' (the upper palate behind the uvula).[27] Semantically, the Irish phrase in use here, *sine sidáin*, seems entirely appropriate for the organ in question: the word *sine* is used to describe a small flesh protuberance and is best-known in the sense 'teat' or 'nipple', while *sidén* or *sidán* can mean 'a blast of wind'.
- An intriguing variant of the above phrase, *sine Seáin*, apparently incorporates the proper name Seán. This occurs as a gloss on Latin in a sixteenth-century copy of an anatomical tract ('uvla .i. an sine Seaain'),[28] but the native name regularly stands alone. A well-preserved *materia medica* text in Dublin, Royal Irish Academy, MS C iv 2, for example, holds forth on the efficacy

25 Mac Mathúna, 'Terminology in *Rosa anglica*', has some useful remarks. See also Ní Shéaghdha, *Translations and Adaptations into Irish*, p. 9, and *Rosa anglica*, ed. and trans. by Wulff, pp. xxxiii–xxxviii.

26 *Anathomia Gydo*, ed. and trans. by Ní Ghallchobhair, pp. 80 and 81.

27 *Anathomia Gydo*, ed. and trans. by Ní Ghallchobhair, pp. 78 and 79.

28 Edinburgh, NLS, Adv. MS 72.1.33, p. 21.16. See also *Irish Glosses*, ed. by Stokes, p. 7 (§ 151).

of what seem to be mulberries 'a n-agaidh […] tuitim an tsine Sheaáin' (against […] prolapse of the uvula).[29]

- Despite dwelling at length on the functions and vulnerabilities of the uvula, a mid-fifteenth-century scholar at work on what is now London, British Library, MS Harley 546, gives no indication that he knows of any Irish term for the organ of interest. Instead, he ensures that his readers understand what is being discussed by reworking a statement made previously in Latin. According to this, the uvula is 'rét bís a cosmailius tsengan sa scornaigh' (a thing like a tongue in the throat).[30]
- Finally, in a medical catechism preserved in Edinburgh, National Library of Scotland, MS 72.1.2, the word *maelán* seems to indicate the uvula.[31] This term is immediately meaningful as 'small, rounded eminence' and is probably best regarded as an ad-hoc descriptive term. As a result, its exact meaning in the context in which it appears is not entirely certain.[32]

To refer to this one part of the body, then, we see the architects of Irish medical texts involved in a range of activities: using the Latin term with no concessions to readers who may not move so easily between the two languages; producing both Latin and Irish equivalents ('uvla .i. an sine Seaain'); glossing the Latin term with a longish explanatory statement in Irish ('rét bís a cosmailius tsengan sa scornaigh'); making use of one or other native term (*sine sidáin, sine Seáin*); and apparently eschewing names altogether in favour of a simple description of the physical appearance of the organ (*maelán*).

Borrowing

Medical terms borrowed from Latin into Irish occupy various points along a scale which includes, at one end, the Latin word taken over relatively unchanged and, at the other, the Latin term assimilated to the rules of Irish

29 Dublin, RIA, MS C iv 2, fol. 30^{v}b15–16. See also *Anathomia Gydo*, ed. and trans. by Ní Ghallchobhair, p. 78 n. 385; Dublin, King's Inns MS 15, fol. 115^{v}21. In a commentary on the Census of Ireland for the year 1841, the prolapse of the *Sineadh Seaain* is discussed as a cause of death: Wylde, 'Report upon the Tables of Deaths', p. 280. The English equivalent is given there as 'John's teat down'.

30 London, BL, Harley MS 546, fol. 28^{r}1–2; cf. O'Grady, *Catalogue of Irish Manuscripts*, pp. 187–88.

31 Edinburgh, NLS, Adv. MS 72.1.2, fol. 60^{v}4; Hayden, 'Observations on the "Doors of Death"', p. 32.

32 Hayden ('Observations on the "Doors of Death"', pp. 32–33) wondered if *malán* (which is the manuscript reading) might denote the epiglottis, for the text characterizes the organ in question as alternatively blocking the openings to the trachea and to the oesophagus. Other Irish texts of similar content clearly conceive of the uvula as performing this function, however: see, for example, Dublin, King's Inns, MS 15, fol. 115^{v}35–36; Edinburgh, NLS, Adv. MS 72.1.4, fol. 72^{v}4–11; London, BL, Harley MS 546, fol. 28^{r}2–3.

grammar. Sometimes, it is difficult firmly to assign a mid-scale word to one language or the other,[33] and we probably have to reckon also with garblings, pronunciation spellings, and forms already influenced by other European vernaculars in the process of transmission, especially English and Norman French. Extracts referring to the uvula cited above illustrate a number of the situations in which relatively unassimilated Latin vocabulary appears in otherwise Irish-language environments. In the main, the foreign term may be:

- consciously flagged in an introductory phrase: e.g. 'an comsuigigud re n-abar oxisacra' (the compound which is called *oxisacra*);[34]
- attributed to authorities such as Galen: e.g. 'dona srebhannaiph remhra dā ngoirionn Gailēan perecraneum' (of the fatty panicles which Galen calls *pericranium*);[35]
- explicitly identified as Latin and given alongside roughly equivalent words in Irish: e.g. 'is inann antrum tri Laidin 7 u[a]mha no clais a Gaedilg' (*antrum* in Latin is the same as *uamha* (a cave) or *clais* (a pit) in Irish);[36]
- incorporated into statements which combine Irish and Latin, without any linguistic signalling: e.g. 'gabh blath uióli 7 nenufar 7 casia fistula' (take the flower of *viola* and *nenuphar* and *Cassia fistula*);[37]
- accompanied by explanatory glosses: e.g. 'flux epaticus .i. flux doniter ona haeib' (*flux hepaticus*, i.e. a flux produced from the liver).[38]

There is scant consistency in how residual Latin words are spelt in the medical texts in question here. Corresponding to forms of Latin *fisticus* (pistachio), as a case in point, Aoibheann Nic Dhonnchadha has identified *le fistici* (with pistachios), *caitheadh fistisi* (eating pistachios), and *pistisi do cur na ninadh* (to substitute pistachios for them).[39] Clearly, some such oddities reflect attempts to make Latin originals conform to the orthographical conventions used to represent the phonology of Irish; more solid evidence for the assimilation of Latin borrowings into Irish are provided by forms which adhere to the rules of Irish grammar in that they take on case endings and show initial mutations. Typical of inflections of this kind is an instance of *dosis* (a dose) in an Irish version of *De dosibus medicinarum* which shows not only the Irish dative plural ending but also nasalization following the 3 pl. possessive adjective: *dá ndosisibh* (of their doses).[40] It is possible that the word which has nominative singular *puls* and *pulsa* in late medieval Irish

33 Cf. Hunt, 'The Languages of Medical Writing', p. 85; Norri, *Dictionary of Medical Vocabulary in English*, pp. 5–6.
34 'A Treatise on Fevers', ed. by Duncan, p. 30.
35 *Anathomia Gydo*, ed. and trans. by Ní Ghallchobhair, pp. 60 and 61 (my own italics).
36 *Rosa anglica*, ed. and trans. by Wulff, p. 210. The translation here is my own.
37 Nic Dhonnchadha, 'Some words from *Almusór*', p. 19.
38 'Tract on the Plague', ed. and trans. by Wulff, p. 147. The translation here is my own.
39 Nic Dhonnchadha, 'The Irish *Rosa anglica*', p. 142 (main text and n. 113).
40 O'Grady, *Catalogue of Irish Manuscripts*, p. 176.

is more closely related to English or Norman French forms than to Latin *pulsus*.[41] Nevertheless, attestations of the term neatly demonstrate how the endings of different native Irish stem classes could be attached to the same loanword, as both *dona pulsaib* and *dona pulsadhaibh* are evidenced around the same time to mean 'of the pulses'.[42]

Suffixes

The Irish adaptation of several chapters of Lanfranc of Milan's *Chirurgia magna* contains terms derived ultimately from Latin *chirurgia* (surgery) and *chirurgus* (surgeon), which has various case forms, including *chirurgi*. An agent noun, the nominative of which might be intended as *siruirce*, conforms mainly to the rules of Irish grammar: e.g. 'bí a fhis agad curob eigintech don tshiruirci aithne coimplex na mball [...] do bheith aige' (know that the surgeon needs to understand the physical constitution of the organs).[43] To allude to the practice of surgery, meanwhile, this text turns to freshly coined *siruircecht*: e.g. 'innstrumint na siruircecht' (an instrument of surgery).[44] The latter has the distinctive suffix *echt*, which is frequent in Irish abstract nouns and is one of a range Irish suffixes which fuse with foreign words to produce new hybrid forms. The adjectival ending *-ech/-ach* appears in *diuretech* and *diureticach*, variants which have their origins in Latin *diureticus* (diuretic). Some version of Latin *diaeta*, English *diet* or Norman French *diete* underlies the Irish verbal noun *dietugud* (dieting). From Latin *purgatio* or a related intermediary form, the Irish derived a noun *purgóit* (a purgation; a purgative). Through the addition of the verbal noun suffix *-ugud/-ugad*, they developed further *purgóidiugad* (purging). Accruing *-amlacht* turned *puls* into *pulsamlacht* (pulsating).[45]

Suffixes, then, helped to assimilate borrowings from other languages, but these were attached also to native Irish words to bolster the reserves of available medical vocabulary. A cluster of such forms serve to denote the four contraries, which pre-modern physicians endeavoured to keep in equilibrium. The abstract noun *tessaidecht* (heat) is on record from the Old Irish period; it is a predictable derivative of the adjective *tessaide* (hot). Similarly, as *tírmaide* (dry) and *fliuchaide* (moist) go back to Old Irish, abstract nouns *tírmaidecht* (dryness) and *fliuchaidecht* (moisture) can be regarded as organic extensions. The idea of 'coldness' is expressed in Irish, however, through the use of

41 For variant nominative singular forms in Irish, see e.g. '*De amore hereos*', ed. and trans. by Wulff, p. 178, ll. 13 and 16.

42 Edinburgh, NLS, Adv. MS 72.1.27, fol. 5^{r}b8; Dublin, RIA, MS 23 K 42, p. 380.4 (cited in eDIL s.v. *puls*, dil.ie/34656), respectively.

43 'On the Qualitees', ed. by Wulff, p. 264.

44 'On the Qualitees', ed. by Wulff, p. 260.

45 *Regimen na sláinte*, ed. by Ó Ceithearnaigh, III, p. 83.

fuitidecht and *fuaraidecht*.[46] These words seem to appear first in the medical arena and to be based on the simple adjectives *fuit* (cold) and *fuar* (cold) respectively. Presumably, then, novel forms ending in *-idecht* were generated on analogy with pre-existing terms to allow for a nicely balanced group of abstract nouns to refer to heat, coldness, dryness and moistness: *tessaidecht, fuitidecht/fuaraidecht, tírmidecht,* and *fliuchidecht*.[47]

Like *-idecht*, the termination *-amlacht*, as seen in *pulsamlacht*, is prevalent in medical texts and is attached to native as well as borrowed words. Normally, Irish abstract nouns in *-amlacht* have related adjectives ending in *-amail*, thus, *feramail* (manly) underlies *feramlacht* (manliness). Native medical terms incorporating the suffix *-amlacht* and first evidenced in the fourteenth to sixteenth centuries include: *bíadamlacht* (nourishment), *gáethamlacht* (flatulence),[48] *gláedamlacht* (coagulation), *gumamlacht* (stickiness, adhesiveness),[49] and *uiscemlacht* (moisture). With the exception of *uiscemail* (watery), corresponding adjectives ending in *-amail* are either lacking entirely or themselves confined to the language of medicine. Thus, it would seem that the suffix *-amlacht* was added to the likes of *gáeth* (wind), *gláed* (glue) and *gum* (gum) to create medically-focused abstract nouns from more general, concrete ones.[50]

In light of the frequency with which new abstract nouns in *-idecht* and *-amlacht* were formed, the appearance of doublets is not entirely unexpected. Irish medical vocabulary from the period under discussion includes semantic doublets, such as *uiscemlacht* and *fliuchidecht*, both of which mean 'moisture', and also etymological doublets like *gáethamlacht* and *gáethmairecht*, both based on *gáeth* (wind) and meaning 'flatulence'. Interestingly, as well as meaning flatulence, *gáethmaireacht* was used to refer to air in blood and in abscesses, and the flexibility of medieval Irish medical terminology is well-illustrated by the fact that, in these situations, *gáethmaireacht* is found paired with both *fliuchaidecht* and *uiscemlacht* to mean 'moisture and air'. On the matter of which abscesses are comprised, the Irish *Rosa anglica* mentions 'na 4 lenna, 7 uisgiamlacht 7 gaotmuirecht' (the four humours, and moisture and air),[51] whereas another Irish version of the same text opts for an alternative pairing to describe how grapes fill the blood 'do fliuchaidecht 7 do gaethmuirecht' (with moisture and air).[52]

---

46 For the latter, see eDIL s.v. *(f)úaraigecht* (dil.ie/42770).

47 The various terms often appear side-by-side. See, for example, *Regimen na sláinte*, ed. by Ó Ceithearnaigh, I, pp. 7, 8, 11 and 12.

48 There are several attestations in Edinburgh, NLS, Adv. MS 72.1.2, including fols 30r8, 31v18 and 32r9.

49 In addition to the single instance cited in eDIL s.v. (dil.ie/26824), see *An Irish Version of Gaulterus [sic] De dosibus*, ed. by Sheahan, §§41 and 48.

50 It is possible that the few corresponding adjectives we do find — such as *bíadamail* (nourishing) and *gláedamail* (glutinous, viscous) — are actually back-formations from relevant abstract nouns.

51 *Rosa anglica*, ed. and trans. by Wulff, p. 170. The translation here is my own.

52 'A Mediaeval Handbook', ed. by Wulff, p. 56.

Calques and Metaphors

When Latin words and phrases are accompanied by explanatory glosses in Irish, these often equate Latin and native terms: e.g. 'uvla .i. an sine Seaain'. Sometimes, however, such glosses offer word-for-word translations of the Latin into Irish. In the Irish version of *De anathomia*, a reference to the *os sacrum*, the large bone at the base of the spine, is immediately glossed with Irish '.i. cnāimh coisrica'.[53] This Irish phrase is comprised of *cnáim* (a bone) followed by a genitive of *coisrecad* (consecrating, blessing) and is a rough calque on Latin *os sacrum* (the holy bone).

It is unclear whether Irish *cnáim coisrectha* or the like was ever understood and used, even in narrow medical circles, as a name for the bone at the base of the spine.[54] Some obvious Irish calques on Latin names do appear independently, however. *Lingua avis*, the Latin name of the plant known in English as Greater Stitchwort, offers an example. The only medieval Irish references to this plant seem to be in medical and adjacent texts where we find *tengae énáin* or *tengae énán* — literally, 'the tongue of a little bird/of little birds' — as both a gloss on the Latin name and on its own, e.g.: 'ling[u]a auis .i. in teanga enan';[55] 'pimentaria, tenga enain, spica nardi' (Melissa, Greater Stitchwort, Spikenard).[56] It is difficult to establish the chronology of texts of interest here, but it does not seem unreasonable to suppose that use of Latin and Irish phrases side-by-side prepared the way for calques in Irish to stand alone.[57]

Lingua avis (bird's tongue), a name obviously inspired by the tongue-like anthers which are characteristic of Greater Stitchwort, is one of many metaphors which crop up in classical medical texts. These provide names for various features of human anatomy, as well as for birds and animals, and they generally involve novel combinations and applications of everyday words.

---

53 *Anathomia Gydo*, ed. and trans. by Ní Ghallchobhair, p. 88.

54 At least one such term is unlikely to have had any existence outside of the surgical text in which it is preserved. In the extract in question, the *ossa paris* (zygomatic bones; the bones forming the prominent parts of the cheeks) are mistakenly referred to as *ossa pacis* 'bones of peace' and this is glossed in Irish with synonymous 'cnāmha na sīchāna': *Anathomia Gydo*, ed. and trans. by Ní Ghallchobhair, p. 66. As *ossa pacis* was not a genuine Latin medical term in the first instance, it seems reasonable to assume that the Irish calque is nothing more than a linguistic exercise. Interestingly, given that it has been suggested that some Irish medical texts may have been transcribed from dictation (see Harris, 'Latin Learning and Irish Physicians', pp. 12–13), the error in question here points towards a written exemplar, short-stemmed *r* being mistakenly copied as *c*.

55 'On the *materia medica* of the Mediaeval Irish', ed. and trans. by Stokes, p. 242.

56 *Rosa anglica*, ed. and trans. by Wulff, p. 142.

57 In relation to the wagtail, Nic Dhonnchadha has examples of both 'an ten renabarur cauda tremula .i. erball ar crith' (the bird which is called *Cauda tremula*, i.e. *erball ar crith* [shaking tail]) and also 'in ten re nabar earboll ar crith' (the bird which is called *erball ar crith*): Nic Dhonnchadha, 'Some Words from *Almusór*', p. 21.

Irish calques on such terms are similarly based around common nouns and adjectives and, as a result, medical terminology often has a familiar feel. The *dura mater* and *pia mater*, for example, two of the membranes which surround the brain and spinal cord, are identified in Irish as 'an māthair chruaidh 7 an māthair bhuidh',[58] meaning literally 'the hard mother and the tender mother'. Irish *mesócach* (glandulous) is derived from *mesóc* (an acorn) and is an approximate loan-translation of Latin *glandulosus* (literally, 'full of kernels').[59] *Inar*, a word which generally denotes a tunic or a short garment, often worn next to the skin, provides a convenient means of reference to the fibrous tunic of the eye.[60]

Knowing the meaning of individual words is, of course, of little or no help in attempting to grasp the usage of *máthair*, *mesócach*, and *inar* in medical texts, but calquing on Latin was probably a reasonable enough response on the part of Irish scholars when confronted with metaphorical terms for which Irish had no call prior to contact with continental medicine. That said, there are some unusual — and seemingly unnecessary — calques. Irish has a long-established term for the pupil of the eye. As *mac imblissen*, this term was in use around the ninth century;[61] as *mac imreasan*, it continues in Modern Irish. The name means literally 'son of the iris' and like English *pupil*, which derives from Latin *pupilla* (orphan; pupil of the eye), it was probably inspired by the tiny image of a person which is reflected in the pupil of an onlooker. Despite the widespread use of *mac imblissen* in narrative texts and poetry, medical texts employ *dub* (black thing), *duibe* (blackness), and Latin *pupilla*,[62] and a medical catechism twice makes use of the word *dílechtae* to specify the pupil of the eye, e.g. 'a n-iarar an dīlechta ōn ūaine go ræle' (in the back of the pupil from one suture to the other).[63] *Dílechtae* is otherwise attested in Irish mainly as a word for an orphan. Although no Latin exemplar for the medical catechism in question has been identified, as Deborah Hayden has pointed out, it seems fairly clear what has happened here: *pupilla* in a Latin original, which could mean both 'orphan' and 'pupil of the eye', was rendered into Irish using the term for someone parentless.[64]

---

58 *Anathomia Gydo*, ed. and trans. by Ní Ghallchobhair, p. 60.

59 To the single example cited in eDIL s.v. *mesócach* (dil.ie/32070) add *Anathomia Gydo*, ed. and trans. by Ní Ghallchobhair, p. 142.

60 As the examples cited in eDIL s.v. *inar* (dil.ie/28219) are from the same manuscript, note also the attestations in Edinburgh, NLS, Adv. MS 72.1.2, fols 46^{v}15, 47^{v}17, 50^{v}16.

61 See, for example, *Thes.*, I, p. 103 (39c3).

62 For *dub* and *duibe*, see eDIL s.vv. (dil.ie/18985 and dil.ie/19067). The references given on both occasions are to Dublin, RIA, MS 23 P 10, but I have not been able to verify the readings as it is not clear what system of pagination or foliation is in use in the eDIL references. For *pupilla*, see Edinburgh, NLS, Adv. MS 72.1.2., fol. 50^{v}18. I am grateful to Dr Eystein Thanisch for supplying this last reference.

63 Hayden, 'On the Meaning of Two Medieval Irish Medical Terms', p. 10. Another example is provided on pp. 7–8.

64 Hayden, 'On the Meaning of Two Medieval Irish Medical Terms', p. 8 n. 28.

In another type of text, the application of *dílechtae* to the pupil of the eye might be regarded as a one-off bilingual play on words; however, a medical text is hardly the place for such recreations, especially if we assume that such a text might serve a practical purpose. There seem, then, to be two possible explanations: either *dílechtae* is the result of a genuine failure to associate Latin *pupilla* with Irish *mac imblissen*, or a new Irish term was deliberately generated, modelled on the Latin concept. If the latter, then it would seem that calquing on Latin was being used not just to fill gaps in the lexicon, but also to produce new items of vocabulary which were, to some extent, in competition with already-established terms. That *dub, duibe,* and *pupilla* were also employed in predominantly Irish-language environments as terms for the centre of the eye suggests that alternative terminology, specific to medical contexts, was being actively sought.

Repurposing

The issue of calquing leads us on to wider consideration of how established items of vocabulary were directed into specialized and extended senses in order to generate new medical terminology in Irish. This technique proved especially effective when dealing with verbs. *Táthaid* and *táthaigid* (joins) were pressed into service in the medical domain to express how wounds close and bones knit.[65] *Folmaigid* (empties) came to mean also 'purges',[66] while in other discourses relating to the bodily humours *pec(th)aigid* (sins) provided the sense usually indicated in English by 'corrupts'.[67] Other evidence for this kind of repurposing of common vocabulary can be gathered mainly from verbal nouns. Thus, *tuitim* — literally 'falling' — is used to convey the idea of prolapse,[68] and *imthelcud* or *imthelgun* (casting), which is used to mean defecation in earlier narrative texts, is given new life as a term for both giving birth and discharging bodily fluids.[69]

In the case of nouns too, similarities of function, composition or shape paved the way for context-specific uses of pre-existing terms. *Tenchor*, a long-established word for smiths' tongs, was recast in the medical arena to

65 For examples of short *táthaid* in the sense 'knits' (of bone), see Hayden, 'Observations on the "Doors of Death"', p. 40.

66 This extended sense is well-illustrated in eDIL s.vv. *folmaigid* (c) and *folmugud* (c) (dil.ie/23144 and dil.ie/23148).

67 Attestations of the active verb in this sense can be found in 'A Treatise on Fevers', ed. by Duncan, p. 27; Edinburgh, NLS, Adv. MS 72.1.33, p. 40.18. For the corresponding verbal noun, see also Edinburgh, NLS, Adv. MS 72.1.4, fol. 60ʳ12.

68 An occurrence of 'tuitim an tsine Sheaáin' (prolapse of the uvula) is cited on p. 292 above; for 'tuitim in maclaig' (prolapse of the womb), see 'A Mediaeval Handbook', ed. by Wulff, p. 26.

69 'A Mediaeval Handbook', ed. by Wulff, pp. 24 and 40.

denote lithotomy forceps.[70] *Ette* (a wing, a fin) does duty also as a name for a lob of the lung.[71] *Soithech* (a container for liquids) actually occurs in an early legal passage on miscarriage in cows, where it seems to signify the amniotic sac.[72] In later medical texts, it is applied to various fluid-filled vessels or sacs in the human body. The gall-bladder and the spleen are each described using the word *soithech* in the Irish version of *De anathomia*.[73] In an anatomical tract which pays tribute to the authority of Galen, the seminal vesicles are in question.[74] In the Irish version of *Rosa anglica*, the allusion is to blood vessels.[75]

The morphology of *tenchor*, *ette*, and *soithech* remained fundamentally unchanged even when these words were employed in medical writing to mean forceps, lobe of the liver, blood vessel, and so on. In other instances, new cognates of common items of vocabulary were coined to accommodate specialized meanings. *Lámann*, for example, is robustly attested as a term for a glove; related *lámannán* seems unique to the language of medicine, where it serves generally to mean 'bladder' and also specifically to mean 'the urinary bladder'.[76] Similarly, *bréit* was known since the Old Irish period as a term for a piece of cloth and in medical texts was used to denote the cloth on which a poultice is prepared and applied;[77] related *bréitín* appears with the meaning 'a veil' in a fifteenth-century religious text, but its main contribution to the Irish language is in the late medieval medical texts where it signifies a membrane.[78] Whereas *bréitín* crosses domains, referring to both a piece of textile and a biological barrier,[79] the adjective derived from it, *bréitínech*, seems to occur only with the sense 'membranous'.[80]

---

70 In instructions for the extraction of a bladder-stone, *tenchor* is actually paired with another repurposed term, *crommán*, which is usually a domestic or agricultural hook: 'tarraing hí le tenchair nó re cromán' (pull it with forceps or with a hook), O'Grady, *Catalogue of Irish Manuscripts*, p. 271.

71 See *Anathomia Gydo*, ed. and trans. by Ní Ghallchobhair, p. 112.

72 See eDIL s.v. *soithech* (b) (dil.ie/38397).

73 *Anathomia Gydo*, ed. and trans. by Ní Ghallchobhair, p. 132.

74 Edinburgh, NLS, Adv. MS 72.1.33, p. 9.16.

75 *Rosa anglica*, ed. and trans. by Wulff, p. 18.

76 This word is used to refer to the urinary bladder in, e.g. *Regimen na sláinte*, ed. by Ó Ceithearnaigh, II, p. 80, whereas in, e.g., *Anathomia Gydo*, ed. and trans. by Ní Ghallchobhair, p. 132, it denotes the gall-bladder.

77 For this usage, see Hayden, 'A Sixteenth-Century Irish Collection of Remedies', p. 273; Edinburgh, NLS, Adv. MS 72.1.27, fols 5ra40 and 5rb1.

78 For some examples, see Edinburgh, NLS, Adv. MSS 72.1.4, fol. 67v7, and 72.1.33, p. 10.6. The latter attests also to the use of the Latin phrases *dura mater* and *pia mater* rather than their equivalent calques in Irish: 'na breidine re naburtur dura mater agus pia mater' (the membranes called *dura mater* and *pia mater*).

79 The relationship between Irish *bréit* and *bréitín* may reflect that between Latin *pannum* (*lineum*) and its diminutive *panniculum*, the former denoting a (linen) cloth and the latter a membrane. My thanks to Dr Deborah Hayden for pointing this out to me.

80 A single instance of this adjective is listed in eDIL s.v. (dil.ie/6712), but see also *Anathomia Gydo*, ed. and trans. by Ní Ghallchobhair, p. 132.

Diminutives

It is not without relevance here that *bréitín* and *lámannán* are diminutives of *bréit* and *lámann* respectively. Latin *uvula* is also a diminutive, and diminutive suffixes feature regularly in the medical vocabulary in other vernaculars, including the likes of Middle English *almondins* (tonsils) and *annulet* (cartilage of windpipe).[81] Mention of the latter segues neatly into a brief look at another short-lived medical term from medieval Ireland: *scornachán*. In contrast to *bréitín* and *lámannán*, this diminutive was based on a word which was already employed in Irish as a term for a part of the body. Indeed, *scornach* (throat) turns up in that gloss which defines the uvula as 'a thing like a tongue in the throat' (*sa scornaigh*). *Scornachán* is of interest in the present discussion not merely on account of its diminutive suffix, but because it seems to have been applied differently by different medical scholars. A passage on the functions of the throat in the aforementioned medical catechism asks at one point 'cidh fódera nach tēit in biadh isin scornachán 7 go tēit isan [d]íbhechān' (why does food not go into the *scornachán* but does go into the *díbechán*?).[82] It seems reasonable to assume that, in this question, *scornachán* refers to the trachea or windpipe, while *díbechán* refers to the oesophagus. A separate text on wounds suggests, though, that the *scornachán* of an animal can be placed against intestinal injuries so that undigested food can run through this *scornachán* into the stomach.[83] In this instance, the *scornachán* serves as a replacement for the oesophagus.[84]

These irregular applications of *scornachán* are provoking but do not seem unduly problematic. Given the propensity for casting new medical terms as diminutives, it is not inconceivable that one translator coined *scornachán* as a term for one of the two pipes of the throat, while someone else used the same innovation to refer to the other. Equally, it would not be surprising if, particularly in the early stages of training, those responsible for rendering Latin medical texts into Irish were at times confused by the proliferation of technical vocabulary which had recently come into circulation and uncertain whether *scornachán* was intended to denote the oesophagus or the trachea. That neither *scornachán* nor *díbechán* had a firm foothold in medieval Irish medical vocabulary is suggested at any rate by the fact that Latin words in Irish dressing, such as *trachia* and *isophagus*, seem to appear more frequently than their native equivalents.[85]

---

81 Norri, *Dictionary of Medical Vocabulary in English*, pp. 40 and 47.

82 Hayden, 'Observations on the "Doors of Death"', p. 32.

83 'A Mediaeval Handbook', ed. by Wulff, p. 3. For a fuller discussion, see Hayden, 'Observations on the "Doors of Death"', pp. 32–35.

84 The two terms turn up also, in related material, in Dublin, King's Inns, MS 15, fol. 115^{v}33–36, where it is made explicit that *scornachán* refers to the trachea and *díbechán* to the oesophagus.

85 See, for example, *Anathomia Gydo*, ed. and trans. by Ní Ghallchobhair, pp. 84, 106 and 126; Edinburgh, NLS, MS 72.1.33, p. 21.19–20; Dublin, King's Inns, MS 15, fol. 115^{v}31–32.

Conclusion

In 2016, Liam Mac Mathúna proposed that the scholar-physicians of late medieval Ireland had 'the requisite lexicographical [*sic*] resources to hand — in the established vocabulary of Irish — to enable them to make their own of the new medical concepts' which they encountered in classical and Arabic medicine.[86] There is a good deal of truth in what he says.[87] The lexicon of the medical texts is not entirely unfamiliar territory to someone whose main interests might lie in literature, legal, or other material: *fuaraidecht* (coldness) may be an innovation in the language but *fuar* (cold) was and is an everyday word; *soithech* was abundantly attested as a term for a drinking-vessel before it was applied to a vessel of the body; knowing the meaning of *scornach* ensures that new *scornachán* can readily understood as a part of the throat. In the pursuit of new medical terminology, though, long-standing Irish words were stretched with suffixes, channelled into exceptional senses and augmented with straightforward borrowings, sometimes-strange calques and a clutch of hybrid terms. On a closer look, it becomes clear that considerable industry and ingenuity were required to convert the established vocabulary of Irish into functioning medicalese.

Further research into the linguistic strategies on display in the Irish medical texts might shed light on the extent to which alternative terms — like *dílechtae* (pupil) — were being sought in preference to common, native names and might encourage us to contemplate the role of medical schools, like that in Aghmacart, Queen's County,[88] in guiding and perhaps stabilizing the work of translation. However, these strategies need to be considered also in the context of the wider, contemporary European trend in producing vernacular versions of Latin medical texts. It is already apparent that the methods adopted in Irish to plug gaps in the vocabulary of this subject-area have much in common with those employed to translate similar material into the likes of English and French. Some are straightforward processes, such as borrowing and suffixation, which can be observed in the lexicon more generally and might have occurred independent of any particular models; some, such as the obvious proclivity for diminutives, were probably influenced by the underlying Latin texts. Given that the Irish material occasionally incorporates words in other vernacular languages,[89] there seems reason to think also

86 'Terminology in *Rosa anglica*', p. 83.

87 Grace, 'Medicine in Gaelic Ireland and Scotland', p. 209, oversimplifies in claiming that 'an Irish vocabulary already existed to represent the medical concepts of the texts being translated'.

88 See further Nic Dhonnchadha, 'The Medical School of Aghmacart'.

89 In the Irish version of *Rosa anglica*, for instance, an allusion to Latin *anthrax* is accompanied by the information that the English name for this ailment is *filun* ('is e a hainm tre Berla .i. filun': *Rosa anglica*, ed. and trans. by Wulff, p. 210). On the other hand, an isolated paragraph in a fifteenth- or sixteenth-century manuscript observes that 'antrax a Laidin is inann é 7

about the sources of those references and whether the scholars behind the first flourish of Irish medicalese found additional inspiration in solutions implemented by their English- and French-speaking counterparts. In short, although investigations might begin with the Latin texts, ultimately we may find that (to adapt a statement made by Tony Hunt with reference to medieval England) 'it is medicine which *par excellence* engages us with the languages' of late medieval Ireland.[90]

Works Cited

Manuscripts

Dublin, King's Inns, MS 15
Dublin, Royal Irish Academy, MS C iv 2
Dublin, Royal Irish Academy, MS 23 F 19
Dublin, Royal Irish Academy, MS 23 K 42
Dublin, Royal Irish Academy, MS 23 P 10
Dublin, Trinity College, MS 1436
Edinburgh, National Library of Scotland, Adv. MS 72.1.2
Edinburgh, National Library of Scotland, Adv. MS 72.1.4
Edinburgh, National Library of Scotland, Adv. MS 72.1.27
Edinburgh, National Library of Scotland, Adv. MS 72.1.33
London, British Library, MS Harley 546

Primary Sources

Aislinge Meic Con Glinne, ed. by Kenneth Hurlstone Jackson (Dublin: Dublin Institute of Advanced Studies, 1990)

Anathomia Gydo, ed. and trans. by Eithne Ní Ghallchobhair, Irish Texts Society, 66 (London: Irish Texts Society, 2014)

---

felún a Fraingcbérla' (*anthrax* in Latin is the same *felún* in French: Dublin, TCD, MS 1436, p. 360b30 and 32). In the translations here, I have retained the manuscript spellings of the English and French words.

90 Hunt, 'The Languages of Medical Writing in Medieval England', p. 96. A version of this chapter was first delivered in December 2018 at the conference 'Science and Medicine in the Insular Middle Ages', Queen's University, Belfast. I would like to thank those present on that occasion for their insightful and generous remarks. To help locate certain items of vocabulary, I have drawn on manuscript transcriptions prepared by Dr Eystein Thanisch and Dr Martina Maher for Faclair na Gàidhlig. I am grateful to have been allowed access to those resources. Finally, thanks to Dr Siobhán Barrett for sending me a pre-publication copy of her work on 'Multilingual Medicalese', which came to my attention only after this chapter had been completed but offers invaluable examples of the use of Latin in Irish medical texts, of coexisting parallel terms and of allusions to English and French plant-names in glossaries of Irish provenance.

'*De amore hereos*', ed. and trans. by Winifred Wulff, *Ériu*, 11 (1932), 174–81

Irish Glosses: A Mediæval Tract on Latin Declension, with Examples Explained in Irish…, ed. by Whitley Stokes (Dublin: The Irish Archæological and Celtic Society, 1860)

An Irish Version of Gaulterus [*sic*] *De dosibus*, ed. by Shawn Sheahan (Washington, DC: Catholic University of America, 1938)

'A Mediaeval Handbook of Gynaecology and Midwifery…', ed. by Winifred Wulff, *Irish Texts*, 5 (London: Sheed and Ward, 1934)

'Mitteilungen aus irischen Handschriften', ed. by Kuno Meyer, *Zeitschrift für celtische Philologie*, 9 (1913), 166–77

'The Monastery of Tallaght', ed. and trans. by Edward J. Gwynn and W. J. Purton, *Proceedings of the Royal Irish Academy: Archaeology, Culture, History, Literature*, 29 (1911–1912), 115–79

'Niall Frossach's True Judgement', ed. and trans. by Dan M. Wiley, *Ériu*, 55 (2005), 19–36

'On the *materia medica* of the Mediaeval Irish', ed. and trans. by Whitley Stokes, *Revue celtique*, 9 (1888), 224–44

'On the Qualitees, Maners, and Kunnynge of a Surgean, etc.', ed. by Winifred Wulff, *Zeitschrift für celtische Philologie*, 18 (1930), 249–86

Regimen na sláinte: Regimen sanitatis Magnini Mediolanensis, ed. by Séamus Ó Ceithearnaigh [James P. Carney], 3 vols, Leabhair ó Láimhsgríbhnibh 9, 11, 13 (Dublin: Stationery Office, 1942–1944)

Rosa anglica sev rosa medicinae Johannis Anglici: An Early Modern Irish Translation of a Section of the Mediaeval Medical Text-book of John of Gaddesden, ed. and trans. by Winifred Wulff, Irish Texts Society, 25 (London: Irish Texts Society, 1929)

'*Sanas Cormaic*: An Old-Irish Glossary', ed. by Kuno Meyer, *Anecdota from Irish Manuscripts*, 4 (Halle: Max Niemeyer, 1912)

Thes. = *Thesaurus Palaeohibernicus: A Collection of Old-Irish Glosses, Scholia, Prose, and Verse*, ed. and trans. by Whitley Stokes and John Strachan, 3 vols (Cambridge: Cambridge University Press, 1901–1910)

'*Tochmarc Ferbe*', ed. and trans. by Ernst Windisch, *Irische Texte mit Wörterbuch*, 3.2 (Leipzig: S. Hirzel, 1897), 445–556

'Tract on the Plague', ed. and trans. by Winifred Wulff, *Ériu*, 10 (1926–1928), 143–54

'A Treatise on Fevers', ed. by Lilian Duncan, *Revue celtique*, 49 (1932), 1–90

Secondary Studies

Arbuthnot, Sharon, 'The Medieval Irish Vocabulary of Sex and Reproduction: Insights from the *Trotula* and Other Medical Texts', *Kelten*, 89 (2022) <https://kelten.vanhamel.nl/k89-2021-arbuthnot-irish-literature-medieval-medicine> [accessed 28 October 2022]

Barrett, Siobhán, 'Multilingual Medicalese', in *Medieval Multilingual Manuscripts: Texts, Scribes and Patrons*, ed. by Nike Stam (forthcoming)

Cifuentes, Lluís, 'Vernacularization as an Intellectual and Social Bridge: The Catalan Translations of Teodorico's "Chirurgia" and of Arnau De Vilanova's "Regimen Sanitatis"', *Early Science and Medicine*, 4.2 (1999), 127–48

Crossgrove, William, 'The Vernacularization of Science, Medicine, and Technology in Late Medieval Europe: Broadening Our Perspectives', *Early Science and Medicine*, 5.1 (2000), 47–63

de Vries, Ranke, 'Medieval Medicine and the Healing of Caílte in *Acallam na Senórach*', *North American Journal of Celtic Studies*, 5.1 (2021), 49–82

Demaitre, Luke, 'Medical Writing in Transition: Between *Ars* and *Vulgus*', *Early Science and Medicine*, 3.2 (1998), 88–102

eDIL = eDIL 2019: *An Electronic Dictionary of the Irish Language*, based on the *Contributions to a Dictionary of the Irish Language* (Dublin: Royal Irish Academy, 1913–1976) <www.dil.ie 2019> [accessed 28 October 2022]

Grace, Pierce A., 'From *blefed* to *scamach*: Pestilence in Early Medieval Ireland', *Proceedings of the Royal Irish Academy: Archaeology, Culture, History, Literature*, 118C (2018), 67–93

——, 'Medicine in Gaelic Ireland and Scotland, *c.* 1350 – *c.* 1750', *Irish Historical Studies*, 44.166 (2020), 201–23

Harris, Jason, 'Latin Learning and Irish Physicians, *c.* 1350 – *c.* 1610', in *Rosa anglica: Reassessments*, ed. by Liam P. Ó Murchú, Irish Texts Society, Subsidiary Series, 28 (London: Irish Texts Society, 2016), pp. 1–25

Hayden, Deborah, 'Observations on the "Doors of Death" in a Medieval Irish Medical Catechism', in *Rosa anglica: Reassessments*, ed. by Liam P. Ó Murchú, Irish Texts Society Subsidiary Series, 28 (London: Irish Texts Society), pp. 26–56

——, 'On the Meaning of Two Medieval Irish Medical Terms: *derg dásachtach* and *rúad (fh)rasach*', *Ériu*, 64 (2014), 1–21

——, 'A Sixteenth-century Irish Collection of Remedies for Ailments of the Male Reproductive Organs', *Celtica*, 33 (2021), 249–76

Hunt, Tony, 'The Languages of Medical Writing in Medieval England', in *Medieval and Early Modern Literature, Science and Medicine*, ed. by Rachel Falconer and Denis Renevey, Swiss Papers in English Language and Literature, 28 (Tübingen: Narr, 2013), pp. 79–101

——, 'Old French Translations of Medical Texts', *Forum for Modern Language Studies*, 35.4 (1999), 350–57

Mac Mathúna, Liam, 'Terminology in *Rosa anglica*', in *Rosa anglica: Reassessments*, ed. by Liam P. Ó Murchú, Irish Texts Society Subsidiary Series, 28 (London: Irish Texts Society), 57–84

McNeill, John T., 'Medicine for Sin as Prescribed in the Penitentials', *Church History*, 1.1 (1932), 14–26

Nic Dhonnchadha, Aoibheann, 'Irish Medical Writing, 1400–1600', in *The Field Day Anthology of Irish Writing. Volume IV: Irish Women's Writing and Traditions*, ed. by Angela Bourke and others (Cork: Cork University Press, 2002), pp. 341–57

——, 'The Irish *Rosa anglica*: Manuscripts and Structure', in *Rosa anglica: Reassessments*, ed. by Liam P. Ó Murchú, Irish Texts Society Subsidiary Series, 28 (London: Irish Texts Society), pp. 114–97

——, 'The Medical School of Aghmacart, Queen's County', *Ossory, Laois and Leinster*, 2 (2006), 11–43

——, 'Medical Writing in Irish', *Irish Journal of Medical Science*, 169.3 (2000), 217–20

——, 'Some Words from *Almusór* (1400)', *Ossory, Laois and Leinster*, 7 (2019), 14–31

Ní Shéaghdha, Nessa, *Translations and Adaptations into Irish*, Statutory Lecture 1984, School of Celtic Studies (Dublin, Dublin Institute for Advanced Studies, 1984)

Norri, Juhani, *Dictionary of Medical Vocabulary in English, 1375–1550: Body Parts, Sicknesses, Instruments, and Medicinal Preparations, Part I & II* (London: Routledge, 2016)

——, 'Translation from Latin and French as a Source of New Medical Terms in Late Medieval England', *Romance Philology*, 71 (2017), 563–622

O'Grady, Standish Hayes, *Catalogue of Irish Manuscripts in the British Museum, Volume 1* (London: British Museum, 1926)

Pahta, Päivi, and Irma Taavitsainen, 'Vernacularisation of Scientific and Medical Writing in its Sociohistorical Context', in *Medical and Scientific Writing in Late Medieval English*, ed. by Irma Taavitsainen and Päivi Pahta (Cambridge: Cambridge University Press, 2004), pp. 1–22

Stone, Howard, 'Puzzling Translations in the Thirteenth Century: Multiple Equivalents in Early French Medical Terminology', *Romance Notes*, 10.1 (1968), 174–79

Taavitsainen, Irma, and Päivi Pahta, 'Vernacularisation of Medical Writing in English: A Corpus-Based Study of Scholasticism', *Early Science and Medicine*, 3.2 (1998), 157–85

Wylde, William Robert, 'Report upon the Tables of Deaths in the Census of Ireland for the Year 1841', *The Edinburgh Medical and Surgical Journal*, 63 (April 1845), 249–85

SIOBHÁN BARRETT

13. An Gilla Glas Ó Caiside and an Irish Version of Symoin Ianuensis' *Clavis sanationis**

During the medieval period, much of the activity of medical writers was devoted to the translation of Greek and Arabic works into Latin and to the copying of Latin treatises.[1] In order to have more manageable forms of this ever-expanding material, scholars constantly rearranged the existing body of scientific knowledge, often into abridged versions of medical works, resulting in compendia which were then further modified to suit the evolving needs of the medical curriculum. One such collection, known as the *Ars medicine*, consisted of five or six medical texts and was adopted throughout Europe as the basic canon of texts in medical education.[2] Nessa Ní Shéaghdha describes a medical manuscript from the Irish corpus, Dublin, NLI, MS G8, as 'a pocket-size medical encyclopaedia, containing texts, in a digested form, on almost every branch of medicine and medico-philosophy. It was perhaps intended as a teacher's note-book written with the collaboration of a whole medical school'.[3] The demand for compendia resulted in more practical summaries of weighty tomes which were more convenient to consult and more portable. Even in the seventh century, Paul of Aegina had observed that books of ready reference were particularly useful for physicians whose work often required speedy action, and in the case of physicians in outlying regions, where more detailed medical works were inaccessible, they were invaluable.[4] Such material was typically organized either topically or alphabetically to allow for quick consultation. A common and widespread example of this process of re-working existing scientific material developed in the form of medical

* The research for this article was funded by an Irish Research Council postdoctoral award for the project *A Triad of Medical Glossaries* (IRC/GOIPD/2020/341). I am grateful to the editors of this volume and the anonymous reviewers, whose many suggestions for improvements have been welcomed. I am responsible for any errors that remain.

1 MacKinney, 'Medical Dictionaries and Glossaries', p. 242.

2 O'Boyle, *The Art of Medicine*, p. 82.

3 Ní Shéaghdha, *Catalogue*, p. 42.

4 MacKinney, 'Medical Dictionaries and Glossaries', pp. 240–43.

Siobhán Barrett • Maynooth University; siobhan.barrett@mu.ie

Medicine in the Medieval North Atlantic World: Vernacular Texts and Traditions, ed. by Deborah Hayden and Sarah Baccianti, KSS, 5 (Turnhout, 2025), pp. 307-325
BREPOLS PUBLISHERS DOI 10.1484/M.KSS-EB.5.143991

glossaries or wordbooks, which provided synonyms in different languages for difficult or obscure words (often plant-names), sometimes alongside brief explanations of their meaning. This contribution will consider some examples of this genre of text from Irish manuscripts, focusing in particular on a quadrilingual text that draws substantially on the *Clavis sanationis* of the thirteenth-century scholar Simon of Genoa.

Alphabetical Arrangements of Medical Material

For practical reasons, standard classical works were sometimes rearranged into handy alphabetical forms. This was especially the case in the pharmaceutical handbooks, *materia medica*, glossaries, and lexicons. Between AD 1000–1500, new medical knowledge, both Arabic and Western material, was added to the existing body of classical learning with a consequent increase in the number of items and technical terms being used in medical texts. This expansion in medical vocabulary, much of which was unfamiliar to potential users of these translated texts, prompted a demand for glossaries, wordlists, lists of synonyms, and dictionaries to explain foreign and technical terms. The purpose of these kinds of texts was to clarify the meaning of a word without presenting any additional medical information. The earliest examples were Latin handbooks of Greek terms, referred to as *glossaria* and *hermenuemata*. Next, with the addition of translations of Arabic works in the twelfth and thirteenth centuries, Arabic terms were included in *synonyma*, or books of synonyms. Towards the end of the Middle Ages, polylingual lexicons appeared that served to interpret Latin, Arabic, and Greek terms in English, French, Italian, and German.[5] These wordlists were also found in Irish manuscripts of the same period, sometimes with headings, as in a text in Dublin, NLI, MS G11 that begins *Nomínair sisana* ([list of] names below).[6] Often, however, they are acephalous with nothing more than a large capital 'A', the initial letter of the first word of the text, to mark the beginning of the wordlist. Like their counterparts in other languages, there is very little information beyond lexicographic and they take the format 'Latin name .i. Irish name', for example, 'ambrocia .i. iub*ur* sleib*hi*' (*ambrocia*, that is, mountain sage).[7] The primary concern of these texts was to provide an Irish synonym for the Latin word.

5 MacKinney, 'Medical Dictionaries and Glossaries', pp. 242–44 and 262. See also Riddle, 'The Latin Alphabetical Dioscorides', pp. 204–08.

6 Dublin, NLI, MS G11, p. 98b28. In this quotation and other passages cited from unedited texts, expansions are indicated by italics. I have not added length marks to vowels in my transcriptions except for those included by the scribe. Where translations have been provided by editors of texts, I make use of them. Otherwise, translations of unedited passages are my own. Three Irish glossaries, two from Dublin, TCD, MS 1334 (H 3. 15), pp. 47–49 and the other from Manchester, JRL, Irish MS 35, fols 117–18 are edited in Stokes, 'Three Irish Medical Glossaries'.

7 Dublin, NLI, MS G11, p. 98b29.

Another type of list, sometimes referred to as a *materia medica*, was thought to originate from the *De materia medica* of Diascorides (fl. AD 40–65), the prototype for Western herbals. This alphabetical list of simples, or *materia medica*, the basic ingredients from which medicines are made, included much more information about the material than that found in synonym lists, such as, 'habitats-locations, medicinal virtues and preparations of around 850 plants, animal products, and minerals'.[8] Like other medical texts, collections in this format were revised and added to, resulting in many different versions. MacKinney refers to one of these, Platearius's *Liber de simplici medicina* (also known by its opening words, *Circa instans*) as 'the greatest single event in the evolution of medieval dictionaries of simples'.[9] This influential text was translated into Irish by Tadhg Ó Cuinn. Many copies of Tadhg Ó Cuinn's Irish *Materia medica* survive, with colophons in some of these copies referring to him as a 'Bachelor in Physic' and stating that he completed this work in Montpellier in 1415. His *Materia medica* contains 292 chapters, each one dedicated to a medical ingredient.[10]

An Gilla Glas Ó Caiside

Oxford, Corpus Christi College MS 129 is an early-sixteenth-century vellum manuscript of medical, astronomical, and veterinary texts.[11] It is the work of one scribe, who has identified himself in a number of colophons as 'An Gilla Glas Ó Caiside'. Ó Caiside is the family name of the physicians associated with the Maguires of Fermanagh and there are several occurrences of this name in the annals.[12] Two entries in the *Annals of Ulster* and in the *Annals of the Four Masters* under the year 1520 note the death of a physician with the same family name, Feidhlimidh, mac Taidg Ui Caisidi/O Caiside Feilim mac Taidhcc, who would have been a contemporary, and possibly a relative, of our scribe.[13]

---

8 Riddle, 'The Latin Alphabetical Dioscorides', p. 204. See also Hunt, *Plant Names*, pp. xxxvii–iii.

9 MacKinney, 'Medical Dictionaries and Glossaries', p. 258.

10 Edited and translated by Ó Conchubhair. On this text, see also Nic Dhonnchadha, 'Medical Writing in Irish', p. 218; Ní Shéaghdha, *Catalogue*, p. 70; Aoibheann Nic Donnchadha's catalogue of Dublin, TCD, MS 1323 (H 3. 4) (available on ISOS); and the chapter by Brigid Mayes in this volume.

11 Hereafter CCC 129. For a description of the contents of this manuscript, see Ó Cuív, *Catalogue*, pp. 281–97.

12 Ó Muraíle, 'The Hereditary Medical Families of Gaelic Ireland', pp. 86, 88 and 104.

13 AU, III.1520.3, p. 535: *O Caiside d'h-eg an bliadhain-si; .i. Feidhlimidh, mac Taidg Ui Caisidi, ollamh legha shlechta Pilib Mhég Uidhir & liaigh clumur, deghaithnech an Feidhlimidh-sin* (O'Caiside died this year: to wit, Feidhlimidh, son of Tadhg O'Caiside, chief physician of the descendants of Philip Mag Uidhir, and a reputable, well-informed physician was that Feidhlimidh); AFM, V.1520.11, pp. 1348-49: *O Caiside Feilim mac Taidhcc ollamh legha Sleachta Pilip* [...] *d'écc.* (O'Cassidy, Felim, the son of Teige, ollav to the descendants of Philip Maguire [...] died.)

In his scribal notes in CCC 129, An Gilla Glas Ó Caiside provides dates of writing between 1515 and 1527 and names four locations: Carraig O Chuanig, Cillin na nEala, Cill tSibneáin, and Mainisdir na nAcaidech in Caisel na Righ (Cashel).[14] These places are located in counties Limerick and Tipperary: *Carraig O Chuanig* can be identified as Carrigoguonagh in County Limerick; *Cillin na nEala* is now known as Killeenagallive, the site of a Franciscan Abbey near Emly, Co Tipperary;[15] *Cill tSibneáin* (also *Cill Teimhneáin*) is now called Kiltinan, Co Tipperary;[16] and *Mainisdir na nAcaidech* in *Caisel na Righ* is Hackett's Abbey, the Franciscan Friary in Cashel, Co Tipperary.[17] In his notes, he also makes a point of complaining three times about the poor condition of his exemplar.[18] These notes document that our scribe was moving around and working in different locations in the midwest of Ireland and he acknowledges that he has copied the work of other scholars, including Diarmaid O Siriden,[19] Seaan mac Math(g)amna mic Diarmada Duibh, Semuis mic Davidh mic Muiris, and Cormac Ua Duinlebi. Of these four, 'Cormac Ua Duinlebi' is the most well-attested translator of medical texts.[20] These scribal notes with their snippets of information are tantalizing but do not clarify if Ó Casaide was permanently based in this area or not.

An Alphabetical and Quadrilingual Text in Oxford CCC 129

The text of interest to this study is what Ó Cuív describes as a 'medico-botanical glossary alphabetically arranged'.[21] It is found on pp. 21^{v}–38^{r}18 and begins with an *incipit* in Latin, followed by an Irish translation:

> Hic incipiunt nomina herbar*um* cu*m* qualitatib*us* earundem *et* quarundum etciam aliarum re*rum* cum eo*rum* inte*r*petacionibus in Gaillco *pro* pa*r*ti 7 Latino 7 Ai*n*glico p*ro* alia pa*r*te.
>
> Is andso tin*ns*ga*ni*t*er* anman*n*a na luibi*n*d maill*e* *re* na coi*m*plexaib 7 anman*n*a neiti h*egin* *eile* maill*e* riu .i. a*n*man*n*a coda dib a Ladin 7 coda a Berla 7 coda *aile* a f*r*aincb*er*la.[22]

14 Ó Cuív, *Catalogue*, p. 283.
15 40 km west of Cashel.
16 23 km southeast of Cashel.
17 Established by Sir William Hackett in 1265.
18 Ó Cuív, *Catalogue*, pp. 290–96.
19 Also named as a translator in Dublin, TCD, MS 1299 (H 2. 8): see <https://www.isos.dias.ie/TCD/TCD_MS_1299.html> [accessed 7 February 2023].
20 The more usual spelling is 'Cormac Mac Duinnshléibhe'. For discussions on his work as a translator, see Nic Dhonnchadha, 'Medical Writing in Irish', p. 218; *Anathomia Gydo*, ed. and trans. by Ní Ghallchobhair, pp. 3–4; and Nic Dhonnchadha, 'Mac Duinnshléibhe [MacDonlevy], Cormac'.
21 Ó Cuiv, *Catalogue*, p. 291.
22 Edited in Ó Cuív, *Catalogue*, p. 291.

(Here begins names of the herbs with the qualities and with names of other things along with them, i.e. some of their names in Latin and some are in English and some others in Anglo-Norman.)

This quadrilingual text contains Latin, French, and English names for the medical materials but, surprisingly, there are very few Irish names for these substances.[23] The name for the category into which the material fits is provided in Irish, e.g. *planda* (plant), *deoch* (drink), *gum* (resin), *íasc* (fish), *cloch* (stone), *maide* (wood), and *crann* (tree), but the Irish word for the medical material is very rarely given. There are four possible exceptions noted so far, the first of which is the Irish gloss *.i. macall* over the Latin word *auancia*: 'Auancia i. macall gariofilata peis leporis sanamunda idem *calida* 7 *sicca* in 2° *gradu*' (*Auancia* i.e. avens also [called] *gariofilata, peis leporis, sanamunda,* hot and dry in the second degree).[24] The second example of an Irish plant name is *finemain coillidi* (vine of the wood), following the Latin word *lambrusca*: 'Lambrusca finemain coillidi idem Gallice uine sanagen' (*Lambrusca,* vine of the wood also, in French, wild vine).[25] In the entry for *pollicaria,* the third Irish plant name *gluineach* is preceded by the adjective *hibernice* (Irish), thus signalling that, according to this text, *gluineach* is the Irish equivalent for Latin *pollicaria*: 'Pollicaria cullí arabies persicarium idem *calida* 7 *sicca* in 4° *gradu Gallice* culraye[26] híbernice gluineach' (*Pollicaria,* also *cullí arabies, persicarium,* hot and dry in the fourth degree, French *culraye,* Irish *gluineach*).[27] In the fourth example, it is not

---

23 An acephalous copy this text, beginning with *Omentum,* is found in Dublin, TCD, MS 1334 (H 3. 15), pp. 37a1–44b21. A Latin glossary which bears close resemblances to this text is contained in the fourteenth-century London, BL, MS Add. 15236, a collection of botanical, medical, and prognostic texts. See British Museum, *Catalogue of Additions,* p. 117; Hunt, 'The Botanical Glossaries', p. 106; Hunt, *Popular Medicine* p. 217; Hunt, *Plant Names,* pp. xix–xx; Nic Dhonnchadha, 'Michael Casey's Medical Transcripts', p. 88, n. 104.

24 CCC 129, fol. 21v16.

25 CCC 129, fol. 27v20-1. *Sanagen* may be a copying error for *savage.* See Hunt, *Plant Names,* p. 153, s.v. *Labrusca* [*lambrusca*], where he cites the entry *gallice vine savage* (French *vine savage*), from the similar Latin glossary that he calls 'A3'.

26 *AND*², s.v., *culrage* 'water-pepper, smartweed, arsesmart'.

27 CCC 129, fol. 32r22-3. Nic Dhonnchadha, 'Michael Casey's Medical Transcripts', p. 88, has recorded *gluineach* as occurring in the acephalous copy of this text in Dublin, TCD, MS 1334 (H 3. 15), p. 38b7.
I suspect there may be some corruption in this entry. 'Pollicaria' is possibly an error for 'poligonia' or alternatively the words following 'pollicaria' have been omitted by the scribe. Forms of the word 'gluinech' are associated with several other Latin words in other glossaries and the best match, which omits 'pollicaria', is found in Hunt, 'The Botanical Glossaries, p. 131: 'Persicarium, gallice culerage, hibernice glunach'. Other instances of 'gluineach' are found in: 'Three Irish Medical Glossaries', ed. and trans. by Stokes, p. 333, § 13: 'Cardo Capalínus 7 paleonius.i. fed coille .i. gluineach'; p. 335, § 79: 'Corigeola .i. gluineach'; p. 329, § 114: 'Corrgieola [leg. Corrigeola] .i. in gluin[e]ach bec'; p. 329, § 103: 'Sinnodia [leg. Celidonia? Cinopodion?] .i. in gluinech bec'; p. 332, § 44: 'Cordieola uel lingua passerina .i. in gluin[e]ach bec'; as well as in Dublin, NLI, MS G11, p. 99b36: 'Fricaria .i. gluinech'; Dublin, King's Inns Library, MS 20 163 27: 'Poligonum knotgrass gluinech bec'; and Tadhg

entirely clear if the Irish words *pibar fada* are a plant description, or if this is the plant name in Irish: 'Macros [pibar] .i. longum Macropi pibar fada *calida* 7 *sicca* in 4° *gradu Gallice* nerpiber'[28] (Macros [pepper] .i. longum Macropi, long pepper, hot and dry in the fourth degree, *Gallice* black-pepper).

Aoibheann Nic Dhonnchadha has calculated that this text contains more than 680 headwords in Latin, 540 of which are *nomina herbarum*, with 275 French synonyms and 215 English synonyms. This makes it the longest Irish medico-botanical glossary identified to date, even though it contains more English and French names than Irish ones.[29] The text contains more than double the 292 items that are found in Tadhg Ó Cuinn's Irish translation of *Circa instans*, but it must be emphasized that in Ó Cuinn's text, the entries are much longer and more detailed.[30] The length of the entries in CCC 129 varies greatly: some are purely lexicographical, like the *lambrusca* example above, but most have more information included and some have long discussions. For example, nearly all of the entries provide a description of the quality of the ingredient, like the entry on *auancia* given above, which is simply described as 'calida 7 sicca in 2° gradu' (hot and dry in the second degree). At the other extreme is the discussion on *sambucus*, which takes up twenty-one lines of text.[31] Several Latin synonyms can be included under one heading and the *auancia* example above contains three, i.e. *gariofilata*, *peis leporis*, and *sanamunda*.

In spite of the absence of Irish names, there is a lot of Irish content, almost always composed of descriptions of the substance under discussion. Unlike the *Materia medica* texts, however, the CCC 129 text does not contain therapeutic information. For example, the following is the entry for *anabulla*, a variety of spurge:

> Anabulla spurgia id*em calida* in 3° *gradu sicca in* 2° A*nglice* olasi*n*gras G*allice* spurge 7 is do gneth*e* in titomall*us* é 7 bí a lurga r*amar* fada 7 moran duille a*r*na timu*r*gad ina barr 7 is é a bain*n*e is mó gnath*aightea*r dé.[32]
>
> (*Anabulla*, also *spurgia*, hot in the third degree and dry in the second. *Olasingras* in English, *spurge* in French, and it is a variety of *titomallus*

Ó Cuinn, *An Irish Materia medica*, ed. and trans. by Ó Conchubhair, § 96: 'Centinodia .i. in gluinech bec'. The following entry in CCC 129, fol. 32^{r}14, 'Poligonia, corrigiola, poliganum, linga pasirin*a*, geniculata, p*er*spinata, cintinodia id*em*' agrees substantially with many of the above glossary entries and reinforces my suspicion that 'pollicaria' does not belong with the synonyms 'cullí arabies' and 'persicarium'. This lack of clarity is common in all medieval glossaries due to regional differences and in some cases scribal error.

28 CCC 129, fol. 28^{v}12. Anglo-Norman Dictionary (*AND*² Online Edition), s.v., 'ner' <https://anglo-norman.net/entry/ner>.

29 Nic Dhonnchada, 'Michael Casey's Medical Transcripts', p. 88.

30 Tadhg Ó Cuinn, *An Irish Materia medica*, ed. and trans. by Ó Conchubhair.

31 CCC 129, fol. 33^{r}37-33^{v}20.

32 CCC 129, fol. 22^{r}28–22^{v}1. A similar description is contained in a glossary in MS London, BL, MS Add. 15236; see Hunt, 'The Botanical Glossaries', p. 123: 'Anabulla: species titimalli, idem spurge, oblonga habet folia versus terram, flores habet multos in summitatate parum croceos et latos.'

> and it has a long thick stem and lots of leaves gathered around the tip and it is its milk that is mostly used.)

This description includes two Latin synonyms, *anabulla* and *spurgia*, followed by the quality of the plant, and then by the English and French names. The English name *olasingras* is obscure but could be a mistake for *clansing-gras*, which is given as a synonym for *anabulla* in the comparable glossary in London, BL, MS Add. 15236.[33] If his scribal notes are to be believed, Ó Caiside's mistake could be due to the poor quality of his exemplar.[34] The plant is described as being a variety of *titimallus*, which is a Greek term associated with the group of plants called *euphorbia* or spurges. The entry includes a description of the leaves and draws attention to the fact that for medicinal purposes it is valued for its milk. There are many different varieties of spurge, all of which are characterized by having a milky juice or latex. Its caustic sap was used topically to remove warts from the skin; however, caution is advised because it is injurious to the surrounding skin.[35] It is toxic, but according to Tadhg Ó Cuinn's *Materia medica*, it could be mixed with honey and used as a purgative; he refers to it as *gerraneime* in Irish. There are some discrepancies between the two texts. The quality of *anabulla* as given in CCC 129 is 'hot in the third degree and dry in the second' and Ó Cuinn says it is 'hot and dry in the third degree'. As always, CCC 129 excludes therapeutic uses. Ó Cuinn does not include the Latin synonym *spurgia* but does include *titimaillus*:

> Anabulla, titimaillus: .i. gerraneime & is luib teasaide tirim sa treas ceim e da reir na ndochtuiredh & in luib so do tinol isna laeib re n-abur dieis cainicalareis & a cumusc a haitle a bristi re mil & a bearbadh no go mbia a tige meala & a taisci a mbucsa glan & geraidtear na leigis lactacha leis & folmuigid linn finn saillti & fiabrus morgaithi coididiana & ni dleagar an leiges so do tobairt acht dona dainibh aga mbia inne remurra & meadon feolmur oir da mbeitis na hinni tana daba egal flux disinteria da tiacht & as maith e bruith & as olc omh an luib so.
>
> > (Anabulla, titimaillus: i.e. spurge; according to the doctors, it is a herb that is hot and dry in the third degree; this herb should be gathered on the days called the dog days; having been pounded, it should be mixed with honey, boiled until it be of the thickness of honey, and kept in a clean box; the laxatives are sharpened by it; it purges the salty phlegmatic humour and corrupt quotidian fever; this medicine should not be given except to people who have gross intestines and a stout body, because if the intestines be slight, there would be danger of dysentery coming; this herb is good when cooked but bad when raw.)[36]

---

33 Hunt *Plant Names*, p. 22, s.v. *anabulla*; *clansing-gras* is found in the glossary that Hunt identifies as A3.

34 Ó Cuív, *Catalogue*, pp. 290–96.

35 Grieve, *A Modern Herbal*, II, pp. 765–66.

36 Tadhg Ó Cuinn, *An Irish Materia medica*, ed. and trans. by Ó Conchubhair, § 28.

Latin glossaries, upon which the Irish ones were modelled, also give multiple synonyms. An example of this is the collection of edited Latin glossaries known as *Alphita,* which often includes English and French synonyms alongside Latin ones. One of the Latin synonyms for *anabulla* in *Alphita* is *spurga* and it states that it is called *spurge* in both English and French, and here also it is stated that this plant is a variety of *titimallus*:

> Anabulla maior, spurga, mezereon, rapiens uitam, faciens uiduas, leo terre, species [est] titimalli, oblonga habet folia uersus terras, flores multos in summitate parum croceos, cuius semen uocatur catapucia. Gallice et angl. spurge.[37]
>
> > (Anabulla maior, spurga, mezereon, rapiens uitam, faciens uiduas, leo terre, a variety of titimallus, it has oblong leaves facing the ground, many flowers on the top which are slightly yellow-coloured, the seed is called catapucia. In French and English, spurge.)

Some of these Latin synonyms attest to the toxicity of the plant, e.g. *rapiens uitam* (life-snatcher) and *faciens uiduas* (widow-maker).[38] There are many cross-references within the CCC 129 text which provide additional information about the medicinal ingredients, for example, the entry below about *esula,* which is classified as another variety of *titimallus. Esula,* one of the smaller spurges, has a milky sap, while *linaria* (toadflax) also contains a disagreeable sap, but not a milky one:

> Esula gne don titamall*us* í 7 atait *dá* gne uirre .i. b*e*c 7 mór 7 gai*r*t*er* h*er*ba linaria don luib so .i. don esula m*ar* a *der* a M*acer.* Esula lactesit s*ine* lacte linaria c*r*esit .i. bid bain*ne* san esula 7 is aml*aid* fas*us* linaria gan bain*ne*.[39]
>
> > (Esula is a variety of titamallus and it has two varieties, i.e. little and big and this plant is called herba linaria i.e. as Macer says of the esula: 'esula with milke doth flow, toadflax without milke doth grow' i.e. there is milk in the esula and so toadflax grows without milk.)[40]

Linaria is found elsewhere in the text in CCC129 with further discussion on the similarities between it and *esula*:

---

37 'Alphita', ed. by Mowat, p. 9.

38 Indeed, one of the spurges is called 'widow-waile' in English (Gerard, *The Herball*, p. 1401).

39 CCC 129, fols $25^{v}35$–$26^{r}2$.

40 I have not located this verse in Macer Floridus, *De viribus herbarum*, ed. and trans. by Choulant (originally composed in the eleventh century) but it is possible that I have misinterpreted the text. This verse is also found in 'Alphita', ed. by Mowat, p. 60 ('Esula lactescit sine lacte linaria crescit'), and n. 2 on the same page says that it comes from the *Flos Medicinae* of the Schola Salernitana. However, I have not been able to find it there either. It is also quoted in Simon of Genoa's *Clavis sanationis*, dated to the thirteenth century. Additionally, Gerard's *Herball* (first published in 1597) explains that 'the one (esula) is hardly known from the other (linaria/toadflax), but by this old verse; esula with milke doth flow, toadflax without milke doth grow' (p. 551).

Linaria pl*anda* é ag a mbid*h* a duille a cosm*ailus* duille lín *nó* as coír a rad g*ur*ob e in lín fiad*hain* é 7 do cosm*ailidir* dro*ng* an*n* re hesula é gid*idh* an luib si*n* gabm*ais* m*ar* esula is g*ere* 7 is le*te* a duill*eabhar*.[41]

(*Linaria* is a plant whose leaves are like the leaves of flax or it is correct to say that it is the wild flax and some liken it to *esula*, the leaves of the plant we take for *esula* have shorter and wider leaves.)

Corresponding entries in other glossaries help to identify plants and demonstrate the interconnectedness of these texts. While they are not always word-for-word translations, it is clear from the above example of *esula* that this information has originally come from a common source. It can be inferred from the various scribal notes by An Gilla Glas Ó Caiside that he has copied most, if not all, of these texts from existing Irish translations. An acephalous copy of this text exists in the fifteenth-century manuscript Dublin, TCD, MS 1334 (H 3. 15), suggesting that it had already been translated into Irish and that An Gilla Glas Ó Caiside is not the translator.

References to Other Authors

As discussed earlier, An Gilla Glas Ó Caiside takes care to acknowledge the Irish scholars from whom he has copied texts. He also quotes many other well-known medical authorities; in addition to the aforementioned references to Macer, he cites Dioscorides, Serapion, Rogerus, Constantine, Alexander, Isidorus, Pliny, Avicenna, Gerardus, Johannes, and Simon of Genoa. These names are usually preceded by the words *do réir* (according to), as can be seen in this example, referring to the tendency of the seedheads or burs of greater burdock to stick to clothing:

Lapa maighior .i. b*ar*dana 7 g*artar* a te*n*gaid g*reg*a*ch* filanat*ro*pos di a*r* so*n* co lenand si edac*h* na ndai*ne* o*n* a gairb*he* do r*éir* Symoin Ia*nuensis* ysid*or*us sa 7 l*eabar* dh*eag*.[42]

(Lapa maighior .i. bardana and in the Greek language it is called *filanatropos* on account of its roughness, which causes it to cling to people's clothes, according to Simon of Genoa Isidore in his seventeenth book.)

In this example, the scribe has drawn a line through the name *Symoin Ianuensis* in order to correct the source of this information to the following passage in Isidore's seventeenth book:

Lappa dicta quod habeat caulem ingentem per terram dispositam. Haec herba a Graecis φιλάνθρωπος vocatur, quod vestibus hominum inhaereat ob asperitatem sui. Nascitur iuxta muros.

41 CCC 129, fols $27^{v}29$–32.

42 CCC 129, fol. $28^{r}20$.

> (Burdock (*lappa*) is so called because it has a huge stalk extending across the ground. This herb is called φιλάνθρωπος (*filantropos*, 'man loving') by the Greeks because it sticks to people's clothing due to its rough surface. It grows by walls.)[43]

There is another curious entry on the same page of CCC 129 about this same plant and, in this case, the reference to Simon of Genoa is correct:

> Lapa maigior gart*ar* o moran bardana dí 7 is lug*h*a cu fír*inea*ch a duille-si 7 bí an g*h*oire do be*t* cru*in*d m*ar* atr*i*plex. Et ad*er* Pl*inius* as i*n* gn*éth* do*n* lapa ac a mbí a bl*áth* 7 a síl a fola*c*h no gan faicsi*n* ac*h*t a be*th* m*ur* bis a toirrcis ac na hai*n*mi*n*tib do r*éir* Sy*moin* Ia*nuensis*.[44]
>
> > (*Lapa maigior* called *bardana* by many and truly its leaves are smaller and it is very close to being round like *atriplex*. And Pliny says that it is a kind of *lapa* whose flower and seeds are hidden or unseen like pregnancy in animals according to Simon of Genoa.)

The entry about *lappa maior* from a text known as *Clavis sanationis* by the thirteenth-century scholar Simon of Genoa is indeed similar in many respects:

> Lappa maior a multis vocatur bardana: minor vero folia habet obrotunda ut attriplex de qua Dya. sanction aut fagasmon quam multi aparine vocant et cetera. Pli. mirabile inquit in lappa que adherescit quod in ipsa flos nascitur non evidens sed intus occultus et intrat se seminat velut animalia que in se pariunt et cetera.[45]
>
> > (*Lappa maior* is called 'bardana' by many: the minor has smaller rounded leaves like *atriplex*, for which reason Dyascorides calls it *sanction* or *fagasmon*, what many people call *aparine*, etc. Pliny marvels at how the *lappa* clings, because a flower grows in it that is not evident but hidden within it, and it enters and sows itself, like animals that bear offspring inside themselves, etc.)[46]

Dioscorides' section on *xanthion*, with the suggested Latin synonym, *lappa minor* (lesser burdock), seems to be the source for the reference to round

---

43 Isidore of Seville, *Etymologiae*, XVII.ix.66–68 (ed. by Lindsay, II, p. 264; trans. by Barney and others, p. 353).

44 CCC 129, fol. 28r10.

45 Simon of Genoa, *Clavis sanationis*. This and all Latin quotations from the *Clavis sanationis* follow the transcriptions in Simon Online, a collaborative edition of Simon of Genoa's *Clavis sanationis*, a medical dictionary from the late-thirteenth century. Unless stated otherwise, the English translations are my own.

46 The corresponding entry in Pliny is: 'In the *lappa*, too, which clings so tenaciously, there is this remarkable peculiarity, that within it there grows a flower, which does not make its appearance, but remains concealed and there produces the seed, like those among the animals which produce within themselves' (Pliny the Elder, *Natural History*, ed. by Bostock and Riley, XXI.64).

leaves of *lappa minor* and their similarity to the leaves of *atriplex*, which is mentioned in the entry on *Lapa maigior* in the Irish text:

> *Xanthion: Xanthium* [...] *lappa minor* [...] grows in fertile places and marshes that are dried up; it has a cornered stalk a cubit long, clean, and many stings upon it. It has leaves like atriplex having incuts, close in scent to nasturtium, but a round fruit as a great olive, prickly, like the balls of the plane tree taking hold of clothes after you touch it.[47]

The above examples of descriptions of *lappa maigior* and *lappa minor* and their parallels in various sources demonstrate a very common problem of conflation of descriptions from different texts. In this case, the distinction between greater and lesser burdock seems to rest mainly on the difference in size of the varieties and may not have any implications as to its therapeutic effect.

Simoin Ianuensis' *Clavis sanationis*

Although there are many authorities listed in the Irish glossary in CCC 129, Simoin Ianuensis (Simon of Genoa in English) — whose name is usually shortened by the scribe to Sy.Ia. — is mentioned at least sixty-two times, far outnumbering any other author in the Irish text. Most of the other authorities named in the text are acknowledged as being Simon of Genoa's sources, as in this example, where the Irish text quotes Simon quoting Dioscorides, Serapion, and Pliny:[48]

> Acasia sug*h* na n-air*nidh* ide*m* f*rigida* 7 *sicca* i*n* 3° *gradu* Gall*ice* acacsie. Acasia an*n*sa n-Eigift is mó do gab*ad* torad*h* i*n* cr*aind* da ndent*ar* é 7 d'esb*ad* *na* cr*ann* di fagb*al* a coitci*n*de do*niter* acasia do tsug*h* na n-airn*idh* coill*idi* ina th*egmann* brig*h* acasia do b*eth* m*ar* ad*er* S*ymoin* Ia*uenensis* a hud*aras* Dy*oscorides* 7 Serapio 7 Plíni*us*.[49]
>
> > (*Acasia*, the juice of sloes, the same, cold and dry in the third degree. French *acacsie*. *Accasia*, it is in Egypt mostly that the fruit of the tree from which it is made is found, and due to scarcity of the trees *acasia* is commonly made from juice of wild sloes and the efficacy of *acacia* is found in it, as Simon of Genoa says on the authority of Dioscorides, Serapion and Pliny.)

Simon of Genoa is the author of the extraordinary text known as *Clavis sanationis* (Key of Healing). What is known of him and his life is taken from the *incipit* and preface to his *Clavis*:

47 Dioscorides, *De materia medica*, trans. by Osbaldeston, p. 687 (§ 4-138).

48 For further comments on authority in Irish medical texts see Hayden, 'Attribution and Authority'.

49 CCC 129, fols $21^{v}27$–$22^{r}2$.

> Incipit clavis sanationis elaborata per venerabilem virum magistrum Simonem Ianuensem domini pape subdyaconum et capellanum medicum quondam felicis recordationis domini Nicolai pape quarti qui fuit primus de ordine minorum.
>
> > (Here begins the *Clavis Sanationis* ['Key of Healing'], laboured on by the venerable man, Master Simon of Genoa, subdeacon and medical chaplain to the lord pope, at one time to lord Pope Nicholas IV of auspicious memory who was foremost from among the Order of Friars Minor.)[50]

From this *incipit* it can be understood that Simon of Genoa worked in the papal-court of Pope Nicholas IV (1288–1292) and his role of subdeacon and medical chaplain would have included the medical care of the pope. In his preface, he refers to Campano of Novara (d. 1296), who was an astrologer, astronomer, and physician and who seems to have motivated Simon to compile the *Clavis*. It is said that this compilation took thirty years, during which time he made visits to Roman monasteries, commissioned copies of manuscripts, and studied medical treatises in Latin, Greek, and Arabic. Simon's sources are thought to be mainly Latin translations of the Greek and Arabic texts but along with manuscript sources, there is evidence in his *Clavis* that he travelled extensively and engaged with local people to help him in his quest to identify plants. He mentions a Saracen woman from Aleppo twice and an Arab soldier.[51] The *Clavis* is not simply a glossary of synonyms but is more in the character of a medical dictionary, containing 6500 entries arranged in alphabetical order and including names of medicines, parts of the body, plants, animals, minerals, diseases, and spices. He includes more information than that found in a glossary or synonym list but does not include the therapeutic information that is typical of a *materia medica* such as the *Circa Instans*. Simon's interest was in the names for and descriptions of medical substances rather than in their healing properties. He compared texts from Latin, Greek, and Arabic traditions in his mission to correctly identify as much medical terminology as possible.[52] In contrast to other thirteenth-century authors, Simon of Genoa is not just an epitomizer; rather, much of the material is substantiated by his own comments, which provided apothecaries and physicians with essential details.[53] By collating these words into one text, the *Clavis sanationis*, he provided a useful resource for physicians and apothecaries with the safety of their patients in mind. As stated in his preface:

> Sunt medicinarum simplicium ciborum ve multa peregrina vocabula: quorum quedam a greca: quedam vero ab arabica lingua deducta sunt. Nonulla et quamquam latina varietate idiomatum dubia: ad quorum

50 Text and translation from *Clavis sanationis* (Simon Online), s.v. *Incipit*.

51 Zipser, 'Simon Online, an Alternative Approach', pp. 150-51.

52 Petit, 'Galen's Pharmacological Concepts', p. 130.

53 Bouras-Vallianatos, 'Simon of Genoa's *Clavis sanationis*', p. 33.

omnium agnitionem non opus est assertione facili sed deliberato iudicio: ne ut neglectu medico grave et irreparabile occurat dispendium.

> (There are many foreign terms for simple medicines and foodstuffs. Some of these are derived from the Greek language, some from the Arabic language. A few words are also unclear in the Latin language. To recognize all of these, we do not need easy claims, but reasoned judgement, so that a physician does not meet grave and irreparable damage through negligence.)[54]

Although the Irish translator of the text in CCC 129 seems to have used Simon's *Clavis* as his primary source, there are differences, besides language, between the entries found in both. The translator has not simply composed an Irish translation of sections of the *Clavis* but has reworked it to include the qualities, in Latin, of the substances, which are not a feature of the *Clavis*. He has also incorporated French or English synonyms, and very often both, into many of the entries, likewise not a feature of the Latin original.[55] Whether this is an element of the exemplar from which the Irish translation was made or an innovation on the part of the Irish translator is impossible to say. The content of the *Clavis* in this Irish text is most clearly seen in the descriptions of the plants and medical materials. The Irish text's discussion of *cyclamen* with its English translation is followed below by Simon's Latin discussion of the same plant. The similarities are obvious:

> Ciclam*in* porcin*us* malum t*er*re cassm*us* id*em* *Anglice* aythnecte a d*er* dy*ascorides* gur*o*b cosmail a duille re duille eidin*n* 7 ata exam*nacht* ina ndat*h* 7 bi bl*áth* an d*ath* rosa 7 an d*ath* purpure i*n* a ba*rr* 7 prem d*u*b aigi dor*éir* *symoin* ia*nuensis*.[56]

> (*Ciclamin porcinus malum terre cassmus* also, English *aythnecte*, Dioscorides says that its leaves are like the leaves of ivy and there is variety in their colour and there are pink flowers and purple flowers on its top and it has black roots according to Simon of Genoa.)

Simon's Latin parallel:

> Ciclamen Dya. ciclaminus folia habet similia ciso .i. edere sed vario colore ... habens in summo flores roseos vel purpureos cuius radix nigra est.[57]

54 Simon of Genoa, *Clavis sanationis* (Simon Online), Preface.

55 The fourteenth-century London, BL, MS Add. 15236 contains two glossaries with many similarities to our text. The first one, on fols 2r–9r, gives Latin names with French and English equivalents. The second one, a copy of the first, is found on fols 172v–87v and provides the qualities of each item. See Hunt, 'The Botanical Glossaries', pp. 102–03 (§ 2) and p. 106 (§ 27). It could be suggested that the exemplar for our text was based on a fusion of two glossaries like these.

56 CCC 129, fol. 23v19.

57 Simon of Genoa, *Clavis sanationis* (Simon Online), s.v. *ciclamen*.

(Ciclamen Dioscorides. Ciclamen has leaves like *cisa* i.e. ivy but with various colours … having pink or purple flowers on top and its root is black.)[58]

The Irish text contains only about one-tenth of the entries of the *Clavis* and it is difficult to understand the rationale behind the choices made by the Irish translator or by the compiler of his exemplar. The chosen items are mostly plant names and Simon's zeal to identify the substance accurately and to call attention to incorrect information found elsewhere manifests itself in the Irish text, as seen in the following example:

> Coconidium sem*en* lauriola c*alida* 7 *sicca* G*allice* sem*en*te de lauriol 7 do *réir* S*ymoin* Ia*nuensis* a hug*ur*d*u*ras Alaxand*er* 7 morai*n* *ele* is breg sin *acht* is é sil i*n* pl*and*a renab*ur* semelia [*sic*] é do *réir* S*ymoin* Ia*nuensis*.[59]
>
> > (Coconidium, seed of laureola, hot and dry, French, laurel seed, and according to Simon of Genoa through the authority of Alexander and many others, this is false, but it is the seed of the plant called semelia? [camelea?] according to Simon of Genoa.)

The corresponding information in Simon's entry about this substance is:

> Cocognidum est semen plante dicte grece camelea […] et per Alex […] Inquit camelea unde cocognidium colligitur, et est lacticinium, folia olive habens […] arabice dicitur mezerion, qui dicunt cocognidium semen esse laureole non noverunt veritatem.[60]
>
> > (*Cocognidum* is the seed of a plant called *camelea* in Greek […] and according to Alex […] he says that is from *camelea* that *cocognidium* is collected and it is milky, it has leaves like olive […] in Arabic *mezerion* […] those who say *cocognidium* is seed of laurel do not know the truth.)

Mezerion is the Arabic for *camelia* if this tentative translation is correct. Echoes of this are found under the heading *mesereon* in CCC 129. While the Irish entry, cited below, is not explicitly quoting Simon, it repeats his statement that *coconidum* does not come from the *lauriola* but from *mezerion*, also called *camelea* in Greek:

> Meserion esti lactecíninum bid a duille cosm*ail* re duille na holiva 7 is e torad in cocoíniduín 7 ní he torad in lauriola é.[61]

---

58 This is very similar to the text found at the beginning of the section on *Cyclaminus* in Dioscorides, but as is Simon's practice, the long discussion on the therapeutic effects of this plant is not included in the *Clavis* nor subsequently in the Irish glossary. See Dioscorides, *De materia medica*, trans. by Osbaldeston, pp. 323–24 (§ 2–194).

59 CCC 129, fol. 24v2.

60 Simon of Genoa, *Clavis sanationis* (Simon Online), s.v. *cocognidum*.

61 CCC 129, fol. 29v7-9. *Mezerion* is also mentioned above as a synonym of *anabulla* in 'Alphita', ed. by Mowat.

> (Meserion is milky, its leaves are like leaves of the olive and [its] fruit is the *cocoíniduín* and it [*cocoíniduín*] is not the fruit of the *lauriola*.)

Simon's statement that 'Alexander and many others' consider *coconidium* to be 'the seed of the bay laurel' rather than 'the seed of the mesereon' and his intimation that there may be confusion surrounding its identity seems to be justified as this confusion is found in Irish texts too. Out of three examples I have found, one seems to be for the seed of laurel and the other two are for the seed of spurge laurel:[62] the entry 'contonidium [*sic*] .i. sil lauiri' (*contonidium* i.e. bay laurelseed) is found in a glossary in Dublin, TCD, MS 1334 (H 3. 15).[63] Tadhg Ó Cuinn's *Materia medica* contains the entry 'conconidum .i. sil in labriola' (*conconidum*, i.e. seed of spurge laurel).[64] A third entry is found in a *quid pro quo*, or list of substitutes, also included in CCC 129. This states: 'coconidium .i. sil lauriola gab .i. coiriandrum arason' (*coconidium* i.e. seed of spurge laurel, use coriander instead of it).[65]

Although the vast majority of entries in the Irish text are plant names, some of the more engaging snippets are for non-plant items, for example this one describing a seal:

> Foca g*rece* iasc é renab*ur* vitol*us* marin*us* 7 bit cosa aigi m*ar* cat 7 clum gab*air* aigi 7 be*r*it clan*n* m*ar* na hai*n*minntib c*ethair* cosac*h*a *ele* 7 sast*ar* 7 oilt*er* é o luib*ib* a tal*am* 7 a (a) m*uir* dor*éir* Sy*moin* Ia*nuensis*.[66]
>
> (*Foca*, Greek, is a fish called a sea calf and it has feet like a cat and it has fur like a goat and it gives birth like other four-legged animals and it is nourished and fed from herbs from the land and from the sea according to Symoin Ianuensis.)

On the same page, near a pointing index finger in the margin that compellingly draws the reader's attention, there is a discussion on a drink called *focha* in Arabic:

> Focha u*el* fucha*ch* ainm *ar*aip*each é* 7 is i*nann* e 7 deoc*h* a*r*na denam le heorna 7 le n*eithe ele* 7 is gne dí in ce*r*uisia 7 gnath*aidh*it d*r*onga imda a*r* so*n* fína é 7 ad*eir* Sy*moin* Ia*uensis* is i*nann* he 7 eorna a*r*na dail 7 do*n*itir le

---

62 Spurge laurel is also called *daphne laureola*. According to Tadhg Ó Cuinn (*An Irish Materia medica*, ed. and trans. by Ó Conchubhair, [§ 777]), 'Some confusion was caused in the past by reason of the fact that Daphne was the Greek name for the bay laurel, and the myth was that she was a nymph who ran away from Apollo, and, just as he caught up with her, she appealed to Mother Earth for help. The help took the form of turning her into a shrub, the bay laurel.'

63 'Three Irish Medical Glossaries', ed. and trans. by Stokes, p. 332 (§ 48; = Dublin, TCD, MS 1334 [H 3. 15], p. 49b25).

64 Tadhg Ó Cuinn, *An Irish Materia medica*, ed. and trans. by Ó Conchubhair, § 74.

65 CCC 129, fol. 39^r5–6.

66 CCC 129, fol. 26^v12-15.

> *c*ruithnech*t*a é a*r* an adb*ar* sin is i*m*da m*o*d a*r* a ngnath*aidtear* a g*h*enam 7 is edir daine do *cur* a*r* meisgi leis do *réir* Sy*moin* Ia*uensis ina* sinon*i*ma fein a hugd*uras* dy*ascorides*.[67]
>
> > (*Focha* or *fuchach* is an Arab name and it is the same as a drink made from barley and other things and it is a kind of beer and many people use it instead of wine and Simon of Genoa says it and barley are the same after [?] and it is made with wheat. On that subject, there are many ways in which it is regularly produced and it is possible for people to become intoxicated with it according to Simon of Genoa in his own synonyma by the authority of Dioscorides.)

The corresponding entry in Simon of Genoa refers to this drink being made from wheat in Ireland and Britain:

> Focha vel fuchah ut arabes est potus factus ex ordeo et aliis rebus et cervisia est species eius Dyascorides, furca vocat fit inquit ex ordeo [...] suci tales fiunt in ybernia et britania, conficiuntur aut et de tritico unde pultes fieri solent et cetera [...] potest autem inebriare [...]
>
> > (*Focha* or *fuchah* according to the Arabs is a drink made from barley and other ingredients and it is a kind of beer that Diascorides refers to as *furca* and he says it is made from barley [...] such beverages are made in Ireland and Britain and are usually made from wheat, which is used to make porridge etc [...] however, it can intoxicate [...])

These quirky entries aside, the most remarkable aspect of this entire text is the almost complete absence of Irish names for the *materia medica*. Someone has taken the care to transcribe and translate the text into Irish, but clearly did not feel a need to include the Irish equivalents for the names of plants and other materials. Although much of the descriptive content translated into Irish draws strongly on Simon of Genoa, there are other elements in the Irish text that are not found in the *Clavis*, most notably the qualities of the materials and the English and French names. A close examination of the similar glossaries in London, BL, MS Add. 15236 could be key to finding parallel texts. The names and places mentioned by An Gilla Glas Ó Caiside could be another starting point for more research beyond the scope of this study. It could be speculated that Simon of Genoa's close connection to Pope Nicholas IV, the first Franciscan pope, could account for a Franciscan allegiance to the *Clavis sanationis* particularly, and perhaps this explains why at least some of the texts in CCC 129 were copied in Irish Franciscan houses.

---

67 CCC 129, fol. 26^{v}6-11. I am not certain about *arnadail/arna dail/ar nadail/arnad ail* in this context.

Works Cited

Manuscripts

Dublin, National Library of Ireland, MS G8
Dublin, National Library of Ireland, MS G11
Dublin, Trinity College, MS 1299 (H 2. 8)
Dublin, Trinity College, MS 1323 (H 3. 4)
Dublin, Trinity College, MS 1334 (H 3. 15)
London, British Library, MS Additional 15236
Manchester, John Rylands Library, Irish MS 35
Oxford, Corpus Christi College, MS 129

Primary Sources

AFM = *Annala Rioghachta Eireann: Annals of the Kingdom of Ireland by the Four Masters*, ed. and trans. by John O'Donovan, 7 vols (Dublin: Hodges Smith, 1856) <https://celt.ucc.ie/published/T100005E/index.html> [accessed 4 July 2022]

'Alphita, a Medico-Botanical Glossary from the Bodleian Manuscript, Selden B. 35', ed. by John Lancaster Gough Mowat, *Anecdota Oxoniensia Vol. 1, Part 11* (Oxford: Clarendon Press, 1887)

Anathomia Gydo, ed. and trans. by Eithne Ní Ghallchobhair, Irish Texts Society, 66 (London: Irish Texts Society, 2014)

AU = *Annala Uladh: Annals of Ulster otherwise Annala Senait, Annals of Senat: A Chronicle of Irish Affairs from A.D. 431 to A.D. 1540*, ed. by W. M. Hennessy and Bartholomew Mac Carthy, 4 vols (Dublin: Royal Irish Academy, 1887–1901; repr. with new introduction and bibliography by Nollaig Ó Muraíle, Dublin: De Búrca, 1998) <https://celt.ucc.ie/published/T100001C/index.html> [accessed 4 July 2022]

CELT = Corpus of Electronic Texts <https://celt.ucc.ie> [accessed 2 November 2022]

Dioscorides, *De materia medica*, trans. by Tess Anne Osbaldeston (Johannesburg: IBIDIS Press, 2000) <http://www.cancerlynx.com/dioscorides.html> [accessed 2 July 2022]

Gerard, John, *The Herball, or, Generall Historie of Plantes* (London: Adam Islip, Joice Norton and Richard Whitakers, 1636)

Isidore of Seville, *The Etymologies of Isidore of Seville*, trans. by Stephen, A. Barney, W. J. Lewis, J. A. Beach, and Oliver Berghof (Cambridge: Cambridge University Press, 2006)

——, *Isidori Hispalensis Episcopi Etymologiarvm sive originvm libri XX*, ed. by W. M. Lindsay, 1st edn (Oxford: Oxford University Press, 1911)

ISOS = Irish Script on Screen <www.isos.dias.ie> [accessed 2 November 2022]

Macer Floridus, *De viribus herbarum*, ed. by Ludwig Choulant (Leipzig: Leopold Voss, 1832)

Pliny the Elder, *The Natural History of Pliny, Volume 4*, ed. by John. Bostock and H. T. Riley (London: Henry G. Bohn, 1856) <https://www.gutenberg.org/files/61113/61113-h/61113-h.htm#BOOK_XXI_CHAP_64> [accessed 7 February 2023]

Simon of Genoa, *Clavis sanationes* (Simon Online) <http://www.simonofgenoa.org/index.php?title=Simon_Online> [accessed 4 July 2022]

Tadhg Ó Cuinn, *An Irish Materia medica* (*interim version*, 1991), ed. and trans. by Mícheál Ó Conchubhair (alias Michael O'Connor) <https://celt.ucc.ie/published/G600006/index.html> [accessed 4 July 2022]

'Three Irish Medical Glossaries', ed. and trans. by Whitley Stokes, *Archiv für Celtische Lexicographie*, 3 (1899), 325–47 <https://archive.org/details/b21465745/page/n1/mode/2up> [accessed 23 April 2024]

Secondary Studies

*AND*² = *Online Anglo-Norman Dictionary*, 2nd edn <https://anglo-norman.net> [accessed 2 November 2022]

Bouras-Vallianatos, Petros, 'Simon of Genoa's *Clavis sanationis*: A Study of Thirteenth-Century Latin Pharmacological Lexicography', in *Simon of Genoa's Medical Lexicon*, ed. by Barbara Zipser (Berlin: de Gruyter, 2013), pp. 1–48

British Museum, *Catalogue of Additions to the Manuscripts in the British Museum in the Years 1841–1845* (London: British Museum, 1850)

Demaitre, Luke, *Medieval Medicine: The Art of Healing, from Head to Toe* (Santa Barbara, CA: Praeger, 2013)

Grieve, Maud, *A Modern Herbal*, 2 vols (New York: Harcourt, Brace & Co, 1931; repr. New York: Dover Publications, 1971)

Hayden, Deborah, 'Attribution and Authority in a Medieval Irish Medical Compendium', *Studia Hibernica*, 45 (2019), 19–51

Hunt, Tony, 'The Botanical Glossaries in MS London B. L. Add. 15236', *Pluteus*, 4 (1986), 101–50

——, *Plant Names of Medieval England* (Cambridge: D. S. Brewer, 1989)

——, *Popular Medicine in Thirteenth-century England: Introduction and Texts* (Cambridge: D. S. Brewer, 1990)

MacKinney, Loren C., 'Medieval Medical Dictionaries and Glossaries', in *Medieval and Historiographical Essays in Honor of James Westfall Thompson*, ed. by James Lea Cate and Eugene N. Anderson (Chicago: University of Chicago Press, 1938), pp. 240–68

Nic Dhonnchadha, Aoibheann, 'An Irish Medical Treatise on Vellum and Paper from the 16th Century', in *Paper and the Paper Manuscript: A Context for the Transmission of Gaelic Literature*, ed. by Pádraig Ó Macháin (Cork: Cló Torna, 2019), pp. 111-25

——, 'Mac Duinnshléibhe [MacDonlevy], Cormac (fl. c. 1459), Physician and Translator of Medical Texts', *Oxford Dictionary of National Biography* <https://doi.org/10.1093/ref:odnb/17456 (2004)> [accessed 18 January 2023]

——, 'Medical Writing in Irish', in *2000 Years Irish Medicine*, ed. by John B. Lyons (Dublin: Eireann Healthcare Publications, 1999), pp. 21–26 (repr. in *Irish Journal of Medical Science*, 169.3 [2000], 217–20)

——, 'Michael Casey's Medical Transcripts in Gilbert MS 147', *Éigse*, 40 (2019), 43–114

Ní Shéaghdha, Nessa, *Catalogue of Irish Manuscripts in the National Library of Ireland, Fasciculus 1* (Dublin: Dublin Institute for Advanced Studies, 1967)

O'Boyle, Cornelius, *The Art of Medicine: Medical Teaching at the University of Paris, 1250–1400*, Education and Society in the Middle Ages and Renaissance, 9 (Leiden: Brill, 1998)

Ó Cuív, Brian, *Catalogue of Irish Language Manuscripts in the Bodleian Library at Oxford and Oxford College Libraries. Part 1: Descriptions* (Dublin: Dublin Institute for Advanced Studies, 2001)

Ó Muraíle, Nollaig, 'The Hereditary Medical Families of Gaelic Ireland', in *Rosa Anglica: Reassessments*, ed. by Liam P. Ó Murchú, Irish Texts Society Subsidiary Series, 28 (London: Irish Texts Society, 2016), pp. 85–113

Petit, Caroline, 'Galen's Pharmacological Concepts', in *Simon of Genoa's Medical Lexicon*, ed. by Barbara Zipser (Berlin: de Gruyter, 2013), pp. 129-48

Riddle, John M., 'The Latin Alphabetical Dioscorides Manuscript Group', in *Proceedings of the 13th International Congress for the History of Science, Acts Section IV* (Moscow: Nauka, 1974), pp. 204–09 (repr. in John M. Riddle *Quid pro quo: Studies in the History of Drugs* (Great Yarmouth: Galliard, 1992), Section IV)

Zipser, Barbara, 'Simon Online, an Alternative Approach to Research and Publishing', in *Simon of Genoa's Medical Lexicon*, ed. by Barbara Zipser (Berlin: de Gruyter, 2013), pp. 149-56

MATTEO TARSI

14. Lexical Pairs in the Old West Norse Medical Manuscript Tradition

Introduction

This chapter is derived from my doctoral research,[1] in which I investigated the coexistence and competition of loanwords and their native synonyms in Old and Middle Icelandic prose literature (about 40 texts produced between the twelfth century and 1550), whose medical texts are subsumed under 'Treatises'. Other examples of this genre are the four grammatical treatises and texts which deal with astronomy and computus.

Since the overarching aim of the research was to understand the lexical and textual dynamics of the phenomenon, a taxonomical model was envisaged (Fig. 14.1), according to which the excerpted material was categorized. The categories in the taxonomy are explained as follows:

- Loanwords: **integral loans**, i.e. loans which do not show adaptation on the phonological and/or morphological level, and **loanwords** proper, which feature characteristic traits of the recipient language.
- Endogenous (or native) words: **semantic calques**: words which calque a foreign term in meaning; **structural calques**: words which calque a foreign term in meaning and structure; **neoformations** (native coinages): lexical items formed within a given language which show a high degree of formal independence from their purported foreign model (if any), even though they still render the same semantics; finally, **inherited lexemes**:

1 The project was funded by the University of Iceland Research Fund from 2018–2020. For a compact overview of the project, its methodology, and main findings see Tarsi, 'Loanwords and Native Words in Old and Middle Icelandic'. A more thorough discussion is offered in Tarsi, *Loanwords and Native Words in Old and Middle Icelandic*. Although the methodology and data displayed in this paper is the same as in Tarsi, *Loanwords and Native Words in Old and Middle Icelandic* (see the relevant section of Ch. 3 for data), the philological explanation of the word *heranzrifon* is laid out with additional details.

Matteo Tarsi • Uppsala University, Sweden; matteo.tarsi@nordiska.uu.se

Medicine in the Medieval North Atlantic World: Vernacular Texts and Traditions, ed. by Deborah Hayden and Sarah Baccianti, KSS, 5 (Turnhout, 2025), pp. 327-336
BREPOLS PUBLISHERS DOI 10.1484/M.KSS-EB.5.143992

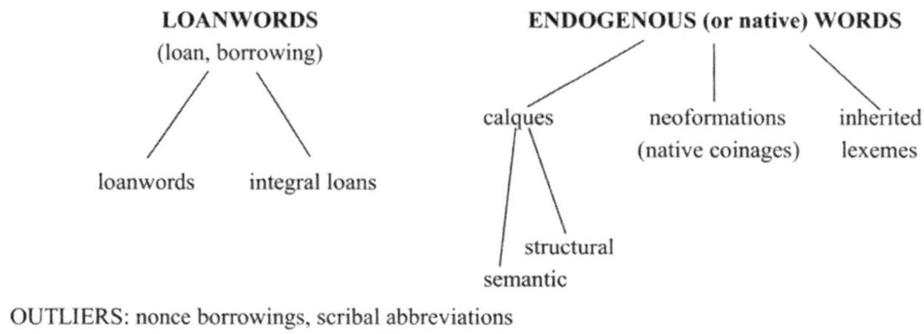

Figure 14.1. Taxonomy of loanwords and native words. Drawing by the author.

words which, like semantic calques, are part of the native lexical stock but whose meaning, unlike those of semantic calques, is not dependent on foreign influence.

- Outliers: **nonce borrowings**: integral loans which never appear as used independently but occur instead in a pattern where they are followed by an explanatory phrase (cf. the term 'explicative insertion') in which the corresponding native term occurs; and **scribal abbreviations** (not relevant in the present discussion).

The analytical model shown above was implemented by research of three types: 1) with reference to texts and manuscripts; 2) with regard to the typology of loanwords and native words; and 3) with respect to the etymology of loanwords.

The first type of research has demonstrated that loanwords and native words can occur in four ways:

1. In the same *locus* in different manuscripts (intrastemmatic variation):
   Licorcia er sæti-vidur[2]

   (Licorice is sweet-tree)

   Liq*ue*ricia e*r* ligoriz[3]

   (Licorice is ligoriz)

2. In simple alternation in a given text (in the majority of manuscripts):
   Vid haufud-verk siod pulegium in oleo

   (In case of a headache, boil some pennyroyal in olive oil)

   Vid sar legg vid sallt ok gef honum vid-smior med vine at drecka[4]

   (In case of a wound, add salt and give him to drink olive oil mixed with wine)

2 *Den islandske lægebog*, ed. by Kålund, p. 34.

3 *An Old Icelandic Medical Miscellany*, ed. by Larsen, p. 75.

4 *Den islandske lægebog*, ed. by Kålund, pp. 17 and 18, respectively.

3. As a synonymic dittology, i.e. in pairs conjoined by the conjunction *ok* (and) or *eða/eðr* (or); that is:
   Cjriaca diathesaron heit*ir* eitt antidonu*m* er kalla ma lækning eda mote gipt þ*eir*ra sotta er h*en*nar nat*ura* er j moti skipath[5]

   (Ciriaca diathesaron is named a cure which could be called medicine or antidote of those diseases to which it has an opposite nature)

4. In an explicative insertion, i.e. whenever a loanword is immediately followed by its endogenous equivalent (or *vice versa*), which is introduced by an explanatory clause such as *þat er* (that is), *er vér kǫllum* (that we call), *vel sim.*:
   Artaticu*m* [*sic*!, recte: *cartaticum*] imperiale heit*ir* en lausn er kalla ma aa noræ nu keis*ar* lausn.[6]

   (Cartaticum imperiale is named a remedy which could be called cure of the emperor in [West] Norse.)

The second type of research was focused on categorizing the word pairs according to semantic field and on understanding the relationship between loanword and native word typologies, between so-called necessity and prestige loans on one side, and calques, semantic and structural, neoformations, and inherited lexemes on the other.

The third type of research was devoted to improving, whenever necessary, earlier etymologies (especially for loanwords) and to establishing a relative chronology between loanword and native synonyms, which took their typology into consideration. Two main findings emerged from this research:

1. A set of rules (with relative exceptions) which describe the relationship between loanwords, native word typology, and their relative chronology.
2. A 'law of semantic specificity' which establishes a direct proportionality between the number of terms specific to a given genre and the number of word pairs in that genre.

Lexical Pairs in the Old West Norse Medical Manuscript Tradition

Only two medical books were circulating in the Old West Norse-speaking area during the Middle Ages, both of which can ultimately be traced back to Latin sources: a West Norse translation of Henrik Harpestræng's herbarium (b1), and a compilation from several different sources (b2).[7] The lexical material presented here was excerpted from four manuscripts: AM 655 XXX

5 *An Old Icelandic Medical Miscellany*, ed. by Larsen, p. 106.
6 *An Old Icelandic Medical Miscellany*, ed. by Larsen, p. 108.
7 Schwabe, 'Den norrøne legemiddelboktradisjonen'.

4to (1250–1300, Copenhagen, Den Arnamagnæanske Samling)[8] —which only contains b2; AM 194 8vo (1387, Copenhagen, Den Arnamagnæanske Samling);[9] AM 434a 12mo (1475–1525, Copenhagen, Den Arnamagnæanske Samling);[10] and RIA 23 D 43 (1475–1500, Dublin, Royal Irish Academy).[11] The other manuscripts, of which RIA 23 D 43 is the neatest, preserve instead both works together, although to a significantly varying extent. AM 194 8vo and AM 434a 12mo witness a mixture of b1 and b2, named b3. The surveyed material was collated with two other manuscripts, which are Norwegian but pertain nevertheless to the same stemma, namely AM 696 I 4to (1325–1375, Reykjavík, Stofnun Árna Magnússonar í íslenskum fræðum),[12] pertaining to b1, and AM 673a II 4to (*c.* 1370, Copenhagen, Den Arnamagnæanske Samling),[13] pertaining to b2. Moreover, a comparison of the excerpted material with its sources was carried out according to the information provided by Schwabe and Larsen.

In this section, I list the word pairs found in the Old West Norse medical manuscript tradition belonging to the semantic fields which are specific to their genre: 1) medical terminology and 2) nature-related terminology (see Table 14.1). For further discussion, the reader is referred to Chapter 3 in Tarsi, *Loanwords and Native Words in Old and Middle Icelandic.*

Table 14.1. Lexical pairs in the Old West Norse medical manuscript tradition: Medical Terminology and Nature-related Terminology.

Semantic field	Word pair	Typology	Dynamics	Source
Medical Terminology	antidotum – mótgift (antidote)	necessity loan – structural calque	synonymic dittology	*An Old Icelandic Medical Miscellany*, p. 106
	antidotum – lækning (antidote)	necessity loan – neoformation	simple alternation, synonymic dittology	*An Old Icelandic Medical Miscellany*, pp. 106 (SD) and 107 (SA)
	athanasia – ódauðleg (lækning) (immortal (cure))	nonce loan – structural calque	explicative insertion	*An Old Icelandic Medical Miscellany*, p. 107
	cartaticum imperiale – keisarlausn (an imperial remedy)	nonce loan – structural calque	explicative insertion	*An Old Icelandic Medical Miscellany*, p. 108

8 Edited by Gíslason in *Fire og fyrretyve for en stor del forhen utrykte prøver af oldnordisk sprog og literatur.*

9 Edited by Kålund in *Alfræði Íslenzk I.*

10 *Den islandske lægebog*, ed. by Kålund.

11 *An Old Icelandic Medical Miscellany*, ed. by Larsen.

12 *Gamalnorsk fragment af Henrik Harpestræng*, ed. by Hægstad.

13 *Eit stykke av ei austlandsk lækjebok fraa 14 hundradaaret*, ed. by Hægstad.

Semantic field	Word pair	Typology	Dynamics	Source
	heranzrifon – steinbrot (stone-piece [a cure for kidney stones])	nonce loan – neoformation	explicative insertion	*An Old Icelandic Medical Miscellany*, p. 105
	matrix – barnsleg (womb)	nonce loan – neoformation	explicative insertion	*An Old Icelandic Medical Miscellany*, p. 105
	michlete – reynd lækning (a tested cure)	nonce loan – neoformation	explicative insertion	*An Old Icelandic Medical Miscellany*, p. 107
	stomachus – matmagi (stomach)	nonce loan – neoformation	explicative insertion	*An Old Icelandic Medical Miscellany*, p. 104
	unguentum – smyrsl (unguent)[a]	prestige loan – inherited term	synonymic dittology	*An Old Icelandic Medical Miscellany*, p. 97
Nature-related Terminology	arnoglossa – læknisblað (curing leaf [a plant of the Plantago genus])	nonce loan – neoformation	explicative insertion	*An Old Icelandic Medical Miscellany*, p. 55
	artemisia – búgras (farm-grass? [common mugwort; wormwood])	nonce loan – neoformation	explicative insertion	*An Old Icelandic Medical Miscellany*, p. 54
	camomilla – baldrsbrá (Baldur's eyelash) [b]	nonce loan – neoformation	explicative insertion	*An Old Icelandic Medical Miscellany*, p. 69
	fraxinus – askr (ash-tree)	nonce loan – inherited term	explicative insertion	*An Old Icelandic Medical Miscellany*, p. 73
	gariophilus – naglagras (nail-grass)	nonce loan – neoformation	explicative insertion	*An Old Icelandic Medical Miscellany*, p. 74
	juniper – einir (juniper-tree)	prestige loan – inherited term	explicative insertion	*Alfræði Íslenzk I*, p. 68 = *An Old Icelandic Medical Miscellany*, p. 74
	lappacium – borrablað (burdock-leaf)	nonce loan – neoformation	explicative insertion	*An Old Icelandic Medical Miscellany*, p. 76

a The word *smyrsl* also alternates in my data with Lat. *balsamum*. The word pair is found in the oldest version of *Dínus saga* (Tarsi, *Loanwords and Native Words in Old and Middle Icelandic*, pp. 248–50).

b Probably a folk etymology (ÁBM, s.v.).

Semantic field	Word pair	Typology	Dynamics	Source
	lappacium – hævindla (origin unknown)	nonce loan – neoformation	explicative insertion	*An Old Icelandic Medical Miscellany*, p. 76
	licoricia – sœtiviðr (sweet-wood)	nonce loan – neoformation / structural calque	explicative insertion	*Den islandske lægebog Codex Arnamagnæanus 434 a, 12 mo*, p. 34
	ligoriz – sœtiviðr (sweet-wood)	necessity loan – neoformation / structural calque	intrastemmatic variation	*Den islandske lægebog Codex Arnamagnæanus 434 a, 12 mo*, p. 34 (*sœtiviðr*); *An Old Icelandic medical miscellany*, p. 75 (*ligoriz*)
	oleum – viðsmjǫr (wood-butter)	prestige loan – neoformation	simple alternation	*Den islandske lægebog Codex Arnamagnæanus 434 a, 12 mo*, p. 18 (*oleum*), pp. 17, 20 (*viðsmjǫr*)
	papaver – svefngras (sleep-grass)	nonce loan – neoformation	explicative insertion	*An Old Icelandic Medical Miscellany*, p. 84
	pinum – grǫn (pine tree)	nonce loan – inherited term	explicative insertion	*An Old Icelandic Medical Miscellany*, p. 86
	plantago – læknisblað (curing leag [a plant of the Plantago genus])	nonce loan – neoformation	explicative insertion	*An Old Icelandic Medical Miscellany*, p. 55
	populus – bjǫrk (poplar tree)	nonce loan – inherited term	explicative insertion	*An Old Icelandic Medical Miscellany*, p. 87
	rhamnus – fúlviðr (stinky wood)	nonce loan – neoformation	explicative insertion	*An Old Icelandic Medical Miscellany*, p. 87
	rubea – roðagras (red grass)	nonce loan – neoformation	explicative insertion	*Fire og fyrretyve for en stor del forhen utrykte prøver af oldnordisk sprog og literatur*, p. 472 = *Den islandske lægebog Codex Arnamagnæanus 434 a, 12 mo*, p. 27

Semantic field	Word pair	Typology	Dynamics	Source
	sal – salt (salt)	nonce loan – inherited term	explicative insertion	*Den islandske lægebog Codex Arnamagnæanus 434 a, 12 mo*, p. 35 = *Alfræði Íslenzk I*, pp. 66–67, *An Old Icelandic Medical Miscellany*, p. 90
	scamonia – hrossaþistill (horse thistle)	nonce loan – neoformation	explicative insertion	*An Old Icelandic Medical Miscellany*, p. 90
	senecio – hrossaþistill (horse thistle)	nonce loan – neoformation	explicative insertion	*An Old Icelandic Medical Miscellany*, p. 90

A Philological Exercise: *Heranzrifon* (*recte: Herontrifon*)

The following cure for kidney stones is described in Dublin, RIA MS 23 D 43:

> Heranz*r*ifon heit*ir* ein lækni*n*g. ein stein brot ma kalla. þviat hun bryt*ur* b*rutt* stein *ok* hvo*rt* *sem* ha*nn* er j lendu*m* eda blodru.[16]
>
> > (A cure is called heranzrifon, which could be named stone-breaker, because it breakes away stones, be they in the kidneys or bladder.)

The word *heranzrifon* (recte: *herontrifon*, see Figs 14.2, 14.3, and 14.4) is without a doubt a misread word. The source for the text where it is found is the so-called *Antidotarium Nicolai*,[17] a medical book from the late eleventh / early twelfth century written in the circles of the Salernitan School. The recipe for this cure in the *Antidotarium* is as follows:

> Litontripon pertundens lapidem interpretatur. hoc proprie lapidem frangit et expellit s vescica vel in renibus fuerint.[18]

The Icelandic text is an exact translation of the Latin. Hence, the solution for the original name of the cure is clear: *litontripon* (existing beside *lithontripton vel sim.*), which is in turn a common Medieval Latin misspelling for *lithont(h)rypton*, a word compounded by Gk *λίθος* (stone) and *θρύπτω* (to break in pieces), and not *τρίβω* (to rub, pound, crush), cf. the phrase '(φάρμακα τῶν ἐν

16 *An Old Icelandic Medical Miscellany*, ed. by Larsen, p. 105.

17 Schwabe, 'Den norrøne legemiddelboktradisjon', p. 3.

18 London, BL, MS Harley 4983, fol. 14v, abbreviations silently expanded.

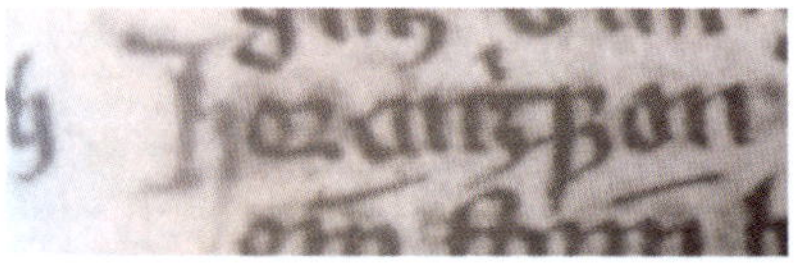

Figure 14.2. *Heranzrifon* (recte: *Herontrifon*)

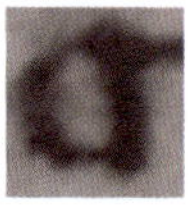

Figure 14.3. ⟨o⟩ in *brot*

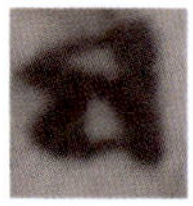

Figure 14.4. ⟨a⟩ in *ma*

All figures courtesy of the Árni Magnússon Institute for Icelandic Studies, Reykjavík.

νεφροῖς) λίθων θρυπτικά' ([drugs] comminutive of stones [in the kidneys]) (OED, s.v. *lithontriptic, lithontryptic*).

It remains, however, to be explained how a purportedly original *litontripon* (and not any other variant) came to be corrupted into *heranzrifon*. The process can be broken down into two stages:

1. The former constituent of the compound, *liton*, is misread as ⟨Heron⟩ due to similarity between ⟨H⟩ and ⟨L⟩ in the script on the one hand and *t* and *r* rotundae on the other. Lending support to this is a possible influence from Med. Lat. *hiera* (medicine, remedy; Gk *ἱερά* (*ἀντίδοτος*), Med.Gal., s.v. *ἱερά*), a common word occurring in names of medicines (also spelled *yera vel sim.*). This also establishes that the original word began *liton-* and not *lithon-*. The final ⟨n⟩ remained.
2. The latter constituent of the compound, *tripon*, was corrupted into ⟨*trifon*⟩. The z in Larsen's edition is possibly a misreading (although the letter is, as it appears, modified at a later time in the manuscript). The *f*, a misreading for *p* rather than *b* for paleographic reasons, testifies to the fact that the original word ended with *-pon* (less likely *-bon*) and not *-pton*.

Concluding Remarks

Research on lexical synonymic (and quasi-synonymic) pairs gives an insight into lexical dynamics. More precisely, it makes it possible to understand the mechanisms behind the enlargement of the lexicon. In the extensive study of this phenomenon,[19] it has been shown that the prose genre 'Treatises' ranks high in required semantic specificity and hence number of word pairs. The native terms coined testify to the effort made in adapting foreign knowledge to Icelandic and hence expanding its domains of use.

---

19 Tarsi, *Loanwords and Native Words in Old and Middle Icelandic*.

In the case of medical texts, it can be said that the overwhelming appearance of one type of dynamic, explicative insertions, which correlates with nonce borrowings, points to a high degree of dependence from the source text. This is readily explained by saying that the authority of the sources clearly gave a path to follow for what concerns the terminology involved, even when this was well-established, as in the case of phytonyms.

Works Cited

Manuscripts

Copenhagen, Den Arnamagnæanske Samling, MS AM 194 8vo
Copenhagen, Den Arnamagnæanske Samling, MS AM 434a 12mo
Copenhagen, Den Arnamagnæanske Samling, MS AM 655 XXX 4to
Copenhagen, Den Arnamagnæanske Samling, MS AM 673a II 4to
Dublin, Royal Irish Academy, MS 23 D 43
London, British Library, MS Harley 4983
Reykjavík, Stofnun Árna Magnússonar í íslenskum fræðum, MS AM 696 I 4to

Primary Sources

Alfræði Íslenzk I, ed. by Kristian Kålund, STUAGNL XXXVII (Copenhagen: S. L. Møller, 1908)

Fire og fyrretyve for en stor del forhen utrykte prøver af oldnordisk sprog og literatur, ed. by Konráð Gíslason (Copenhagen: Gyldendal, 1860)

Gamalnorsk fragment af Henrik Harpestræng, ed. by Marius Hægstad, Videnskabs-Selskabets Skrifter. II. Hist.-Filosof. Klasse 1906, no. 2 (Christiania: Dybwad, 1906)

Den islandske lægebog Codex Arnamagnæanus 434 a, 12 mo, ed. by Kristian Kålund (Copenhagen: Bianco Luno, 1907)

An Old Icelandic Medical Miscellany: MS Royal Irish Academy 23 D 43 with Supplement from MS Trinity College (Dublin) L-2-27, ed. by Henning Larsen (Oslo: Norske videnskaps-akademi i Oslo, 1931)

Eit stykke av ei austlandsk lækjebok fraa 14 hundradaaret, ed. by Marius Hægstad, Kristiania Videnskapsselskaps Forhandlinger for 1913, no. 8 (Christiania: Dybwad, 1913)

Secondary Studies

ÁBM = Ásgeir Blöndal Magnússon, *Íslensk orðsifjabók*, 3rd edn (Reykjavík: Orðabók Háskólans, 2008)

Med.Gal. = Durling, Richard J., *A Dictionary of Medical Terms in Galen*, Studies in Ancient Medicine, 5 (Leiden: Brill, 1993)

OED = *Oxford English Dictionary* <http://www.oed.com> [accessed 16 May 2022]

Schwabe, Fabian, 'Den norrøne legemiddelboktradisjonen', in *Translation – Adaptation, Interpretation, Transformation: Proceedings from the 28th Study Conference of IASS, Lund 3–7 August 2010*, ed. by Claes-Göran Holmberg and Per Erik Ljung (Lund: Lunds Universitet, 2011), pp. 1–13

Tarsi, Matteo, *Loanwords and Native Words in Old and Middle Icelandic*, Studies in Viking and Medieval Scandinavia, 4 (Turnhout: Brepols, 2022)

——, 'Loanwords and Native Words in Old and Middle Icelandic (12th c.–1550): Doctoral Defense', *Íslenskt mál og almenn málfræði*, 43 (2021), 137–51

EYSTEIN THANISCH

15. Knowing through Defining

Collections of Scientific Definitions in Gaelic Medical Manuscripts*

Introduction

Several medieval Gaelic medical manuscripts contain structured collections of definitions, propositions, and aphorisms. This chapter considers the structure and function of definitions in this sort of text and beyond with reference to two manuscript collections, which were both compiled in Ireland for use in Scotland. The definitions involved are not linguistic in nature. Instead, they are scientific classifications of key concepts and phenomena relevant to medicine, made with reference to species, genus, and properties. As well as offering analysis of much of the subject-matter of medicine, with a particular focus on pathology and anatomy, they also contextualize medicine within wider human thought and the human person within the cosmos. It is argued that these collections are attempts to encapsulate the essentials of medicine, which is to an extent supported by the circumstances of their compilation. It is also shown that some of the scientific definitions found in the collections are important to argumentation in other medical texts, from which the collections were apparently culled. As a result, such collections emerge as a valuable source of insight into the study of medicine in the medieval Gaelic world.

Collections of Definitions

At the outset, it should be stated that the definitions with which this chapter is concerned are scientific definitions of concepts and phenomena, not lexical

* I conducted the research for this contribution while working on the Faclair na Gàidhlig Manuscripts Corpus. In this context, it benefitted considerably from comments by William Gillies and Martina Maher. I am also grateful to Deborah Hayden for sharing pre-publication copies of her work with me and to Daniel Watson for his bibliographical advice. I take full responsibility for any errors or omissions in what is presented here.

Eystein Thanisch • Independent Scholar; eystein.thanisch@gmail.com

Medicine in the Medieval North Atlantic World: Vernacular Texts and Traditions, ed. by Deborah Hayden and Sarah Baccianti, KSS, 5 (Turnhout, 2025), pp. 337-364
BREPOLS PUBLISHERS DOI 10.1484/M.KSS-EB.5.143993

definitions such as those found in a glossary. This distinction will be explained in more detail presently, after we have introduced the manuscripts in which the two collections we will be examining are found, namely Edinburgh, NLS, Adv. MSS 72.1.4 and 72.1.2.[1]

The NLS Adv. 72.1.4 collection (**M**) of around 245 items was written out by Maol Sheachlainn mac Iollain Mac an Leagha Ruaidh (fl. 1512). The Mac an Leagha Ruaidh family provided physicians for the Mac Diarmada and Mac Donnchaidh lords of Sligo and Roscommon.[2] As Maol Sheachlainn tells us via notes in the manuscript, he was writing for Niall Óg Mac Bheathadh (Neil Og Beaton). Multiple branches of the Beaton family were active in medicine across Scotland's western seaboard in the premodern era. Niall Óg was from the branch based at Kilelane, in Islay.[3]

Bannerman has speculated that Niall Óg was studying under Maol Sheachlainn in Sligo when the latter wrote out this text.[4] NLS Adv. 72.1.4 opens with Psalm 118 in the hand of Niall Óg's father, Niall. This psalm is associated with fathers teaching sons and Niall Óg seems to have been significantly younger than Maol Sheachlainn.[5] Bannerman therefore suggests that Niall Óg's father inscribed the psalm for Niall Óg upon his departure for Ireland and that Maol Sheachlainn then added the collection of definitions, which takes up the rest of the manuscript's pages, during or upon completion of Niall Óg's studies. This is possibly supported by an inscription in Niall Óg's own hand in the manuscript: 'hic est liber unius scolaris qui uocatur Negelus' (this is a book belonging to a student who is called Niall).[6] As Maol Sheachlainn also refers to him in a closing note as *mo sesi* (my companion),[7] implying parity of status, the production of the volume could have straddled Niall Óg's completion of his education. Hands that also appear in other Beaton manuscripts of the same period have made secondary additions within Maol Sheachlainn's portion of the manuscript, suggesting that NLS Adv. 72.1.4 soon returned to Scotland, presumably with Niall Óg.[8]

---

1 Both manuscripts are catalogued in Black, *Catalogue*, and digitized on *Irish Script on Screen* (ISOS), where versions of Black's catalogue entries are also reproduced.

2 Walsh, *Irish Men of Learning*, pp. 206–18; Hayden, 'A Sixteenth-century Irish Collection', pp. 250–51.

3 Bannerman, *The Beatons*, pp. 44–46.

4 Bannerman, *The Beatons*, p. 45. Later tradition holds that the Beaton and Mac an Leagha Ruaidh families were distantly related (Bannerman, *The Beatons*, p. 8). Even if not historically accurate, the existence of this tradition implies a close relationship of some sort between the families.

5 Maol Sheachlainn dates his own work on Dublin, King's Inns, MS 15, to 1512. His son, Iollan Buidhe, died in 1531 as a mature professional (*The Annals of Loch Cé*, ed. by Hennessy, s.a. 1531). Niall Óg, meanwhile, was apparently still alive in 1541 (Bannerman, *The Beatons*, p. 45).

6 Edinburgh, NLS, MS Adv. 72.1.4, fol. 25^{r}3–5.

7 Edinburgh, NLS, MS Adv. 72.1.4, fol. 100^{r}6. Maol Sheachlainn uses the same word to refer to his brother, Connla ('De febre efemera', ed. by Wulff, p. 126).

8 Black, *Catalogue*.

NLS Adv. 72.1.2 is a large, composite manuscript assembled from diverse physical components by the Mull Beatons in the seventeenth century. The collection of definitions with which we are interested (**E**) is found in Section 4 (fols 27–70).[9] As it is now, **E** contains around ninety-five items, but it appears to be acephalous. Most of Section 4, including **E**, was written out by a scribe who names himself Eoin mac Domhnaill (Black's Hand 14). As well as some secondary additions by Mull Beatons, Section 4 also includes a medical catechism and a version of the Old Irish gnomic collection, *Tecosca Cormaic*, both in the hand of a scribe identified only as 'Tadhg' (Hand 22).[10] Eoin mac Domhnaill has been identified with a member of the Ó Conchubhair family of Lorne (another Scottish medical family) who was active in the early seventeenth century.[11] Eoin states in a colophon that he is writing in the house of the Earl of Howth.[12] Why he was there, what sources he was using, and how his scribal work relates to that by Tadhg are questions requiring further investigation, but, as in the case of **M**, Eoin seems to have been using Irish sources to produce a manuscript for use in Scotland.[13]

Other premodern Gaelic manuscript collections of definitions are extant. The Maol Sheachlainn who produced **M** also produced a much larger collection, Dublin, King's Inns, MS 15.[14] Another collection appears in Edinburgh, EUL, Laing MS III.21,[15] a volume commissioned by Eoin Mac Bheathadh (John Beaton; fl. 1563) of Ballenabe, Islay, from the Connacht-based scribe, Cairbre Ó Ceannmháin,[16] in yet another example of such a collection travelling northwards across Sruth na Maoile. These merit examination in the context of a wider study, and the sizeable, under-explored corpus of premodern Irish medical manuscripts may well contain yet more examples. In order to offer some initial general thoughts on the philosophical workings, purpose, and influence of such collections, however, this chapter is largely about **M** and **E**.[17]

---

9 Edinburgh, NLS, MS Adv. 72.1.2, fols $44^{r}1$–$48^{r}6$.

10 For the medical catechism, see Hayden, 'Observations'.

11 Bannerman, *The Beatons*, pp. 144–46; Black, *Catalogue*.

12 Edinburgh, NLS, MS Adv. 72.1.2, fol. $42^{v}6$.

13 Black (*Catalogue*) suggests that Tadhg may be identifiable with a scribe of the same name active in Ossory in the late sixteenth century and associated with other members of the Ó Conchubhair family.

14 'De febre efemera', ed. by Wulff, pp. 126–27. King's Inns, MS 15 can be viewed in its entirety alongside a detailed catalogue entry on ISOS.

15 Edinburgh, EUL, Laing MS III.21, fol. $10^{r}a1$–$23^{r}b6$.

16 Bannerman, *The Beatons*, pp. 116–17.

17 Tables summarizing the contents of **M** and **E** are presented in Appendix 1. Itemized references to these texts refer to rows in these tables. In text quoted from **M** and **E**, word division, capitalization, and punctuation are editorial, and all abbreviations have been expanded silently. Where a length mark in Gaelic text is scribal, it is represented by an acute accent; where supplied, it is represented by a macron. Otherwise, spelling is scribal. Supplied words and characters are in square brackets. Translations of quotations from **M** and **E** are my own.

The Workings of a Definition

In both collections, following a structure typical for pre-modern Gaelic medical writing,[18] each definition is given in Latin, followed by a Gaelic translation, which can expand considerably upon the Latin. **M** introduces each definition by stating what is being defined, often also including the name of the authority to whom the definition is attributed and sometimes even the work from which it is purportedly taken, while such information is only occasionally provided in **E**. The following is a typical example of a definition from **E** (§ 62):[19]

> Oculus componitur ex septeim tunisi et tribus humoribus .i. is ed is súil and ball cruin deallragthach tsuighidhter ō .7. ninaribh agus ō .3. leannaibh.
>
> > (The eye is composed of seven membranes and three humours. i.e. The eye is a round, shining organ composed of seven membranes and three humours.)

And the following is illustrative of definitions in **M** (§ 122):

> Et do-berar in difinicon so ō Geralldus ar in tennes. Dolor est mutacon cito facta in membro .i. is ed is tinnes and claochlōd obund do-nīter isin ball.
>
> > (And this definition of pain is given by Gerard [de Solo]. Pain is swift change wrought in an organ. i.e. Pain is swift change wrought in the organ.)

While the medieval study of medicine required direct or indirect engagement with Graeco-Latin technical terminology,[20] the definitions under discussion are not about glossing this terminology in Gaelic.[21] The focus is on defining essences rather than words, on 'real' rather than on nominal definitions.[22] This is most clearly evidenced by an essence being apparently equally denotable and definable in both Latin and Gaelic. Furthermore, multiple definitions are often provided of the same lemma; for example, **M** contains four definitions of pain (*dolor / tinnes*; §§ 122–25).[23] The lemmata being defined do not have

18 Harris, 'Latin Learning', pp. 3–6.

19 The Gaelic version of **E** § 62 better matches the Latin of **M** (§ 142), which begins 'Oculus est membrum rotundum splendosum compositum' and thereafter basically follows **E** § 62.

20 Ní Shéaghdha, *Translations*, pp. 6, 10; Harris, 'Latin Learning', pp. 15–18.

21 The definitions discussed here can be contrasted with, for example, the collections of definitions edited by Whitley Stokes as 'Three Irish Medical Glossaries', which do seem to be about explicating Latin terminology. For a study of such glossaries, see the contribution by Siobhán Barrett in this volume. For consideration of lexical issues more generally in the context of medieval medicine, see the contributions by Sharon Arbuthnot, Joseph Flahive, and Matteo Tarsi.

22 For discussion of different types of definition, see Gupta, 'Definitions'.

23 In this article, where not quoted from a specific primary source, Gaelic terms are given in the form of their headword in eDIL for ease of reference.

fixed, straightforward meanings, but are instead subjects of investigation. **M** (§§ 236–37) presents a detailed account of the type of definition at work here:

> Qu[a]libus pars difiniti est maius sub toto .i. is mō gach rann don dēnum inā in dēnum fēin co huilidi. Esimimpláir dó sin ann so: Homo est animal racionale mortale [risibile] .i. is ed is duine ann ainmide rēsūnta somarbtha sotibrach.
>
> > (Each part of what is defined is greater than the whole. i.e. Each part of the definition is greater than the entire definition itself. Here is an example of that: a human is a rational, mortal animal [capable of laughter]. i.e. A human is a rational, mortal animal capable of laughter.)

The Gaelic commentary (**M** § 237) on this commonplace definition of human goes on to explain the opening paradox by pointing out that there are many other species (*gné*) of animal — the genus (*cenél*) — besides humans, that these animals are all also mortal, and that angels are also rational. Except for risibility, each of the properties that define humans also define other species. A definition is thus a kind of verbal Venn diagram that defines a species as an intersection of more broadly predicable properties.

Genus and species form the framework for many of the definitions.[24] They are referenced explicitly another extended commentary in **M** (§ 77), this time on definitions of medicine itself. Having provided three such definitions (§§ 74–76), all of which describe medicine as a type of knowledge (*scientia / fis*), **M** goes on to explain knowledge:

> Mīnigim in difinision. Mar adeir scientia .i. fis, is ē sin is cinēl don leigis agus dealagthar é ona haibidib aile nach fis, mar atā intellectus .i. tuicsin, prudensia .i. glicas, sapiensia .i. hegna, opinio .i. in baramail. Et atā deichfir [eter] intellectus agus scientia .i. intellectus timcill na tosaigid amāin agus scientia timcill na concluised, mar aderar a ndered an cētlebuir do Posterioris agus in .6. Eticorum.
>
> > (I summarize the definition. When one says *scientia* (i.e. knowledge), that is the genus of medicine. It differs from other habits that are not knowledge, such as *intellectus* (i.e. understanding), *prudentia* (i.e. cleverness), *sapientia* (i.e. wisdom), and *opinio* (i.e. opinion). And there is a difference between *intellectus* and *scientia*: *intellectus* is concerned

24 This analytical system is derived from Porphyry's so-called universal predicables. While fundamental to later medieval scholastic logic (Arlig, 'Medieval Mereology'), it was not new to Gaelic learned tradition. It is employed in the early medieval grammatical text *Auraceipt na nÉces* (Poppe, 'The Latin Quotations', pp. 299–300), which was also studied by later medieval medical scholars (Hayden, '*Auraicept na nÉces*'). Elsewhere in Section 4 of Edinburgh, NLS, MS Adv. 72.1.2 (fols $35^{r}1$–$37^{v}21$), Eoin mac Domhnaill writes out a text derived from Boethius' translation of Porphyry's *Isagoge*, which focuses on the predicables and was a standard introduction to logic in the Middle Ages.

> with principles only, while *scientia* is concerned with conclusions. So it is said at the end of the first book of *On Posterior Analytics* and in the sixth book of *Ethics*.)

M has previously identified three different species of medicine (§§ 71–73) — conservation, prognostication, and recuperation — making medicine both a species of knowledge and a genus under which further species are grouped, just as knowledge is both a genus that contains medicine and a species of *habitus*.[25]

Turning back to our collections' definitions of medical phenomena, we find many of them are implicitly cross-referenced through this kind of genus and species relationship. For example, **E**'s definition of eye (§ 62), quoted above, defines it as an organ ([*membrum*] / *ball*) with certain properties. **E** has already defined *membrum* / *ball* at § 40:[26]

> Meamrum est firma et solgita parsa anmalis .i. adeir Betrus Mustinus gur beith is ball and rand danghan lāidir an nanmigh arna cōrugud ō nēithibh cosmuil agus ēagcosmuil, agus is uime adurmur ēgcosmuil, ōir, mun beith ēgcosmuil, do ētfaid dūil do rādha ris.
>
> > (An organ is a firm and solid part of an animal. i.e. Petrus Mustinus says that an organ is a firm and solid part in an animal that has been set in place by things similar and dissimilar. And this is why we say 'dissimilar', since, if it were not for what is dissimilar, we could say it was [all] a single thing.)

M includes versions of both these definitions (§§ 142, 65). **M** also happens to include detailed discussion of the concept of animal (*animal* / *ainmide*) through its explanation of the definition of human at § 241. While their ordering in the collections might not always imply as much, the definitions of different essences in these collections are further explicated when cross-referenced with each other.

Different definitions of the same essence may also be intended to complement one another. For example, in the four definitions of pain in **M** (§§ 122–25) mentioned above, § 123 and § 124 class pain as a sensation (*sensus* / *cétfaid*), while § 125 classes it as an impact (*tactus* / *tadall*) and § 122 classes it as a change (*mutatio* / *cláechlód*). These seem to represent a range of perspectives and levels of analysis, and they are, indeed, attributed to four different authorities. In this instance, pain might be said to have a composite definition, which the reader is expected to synthesize.

Occasionally, the Gaelic text goes beyond translating and expanding on the Latin definition to offer a more distanced sort of commentary. For

25 On *habitus* and knowledge, see Faucher and Roques, 'The Many Virtues'.

26 Again, the Gaelic version of **E** § 40 more fully matches the Latin in **M**, with **M** § 65 adding 'ex particleicleibus similibus et disimilibus'.

example, **E** § 40, quoted above, offers a nested comment on the concept of dissimilarity in the context of anatomy. **E** § 74 goes further and flags up an apparent contradiction in its definition of *materia prima*:

> Materia prima est meidium inter ensa et non ensa .i. atā in cētadhbar innmedōnach ider beith and agus gan beith and, agus atā sin contra, mas ed ní ní é mas ed ní tosach é.
>
> > (*Materia prima* is between being and not being. i.e. *Materia prima* is between being and not being. And that is contradictory, as it is not a thing if it is a thing of beginnings.)

Such interventions are rare, and definitions are usually offered as apparently straightforward sources of truth. Yet even the occasional presence of such commentary, the inclusion of multiple definitions of the same essence, and the implicit cross-referencing between definitions all suggest that these collections are not simple lexica but the products and intended objects of scholastic study.

The collections seem to have been structured according to a conscious scheme, further implying that the definitions are designed to be read in the context of one another. Thematic grouping of and progression between subjects will be apparent from the outlines presented in Appendix 1. **M** includes occasional commentary to mark the transition from one group of definitions to another. For example, after defining conservation, recuperation, and prognostication (**M** §§ 71–73), the compiler states (§ 74) 'o do luadima don leigis ina gnetib, labrum anois do cinel in leigis' (since we have spoken of medicine in its species, let us speak now of the genus of medicine), which introduces the definitions of medicine as *scientia* discussed above. Francis Shaw has compared **M** to certain major scholastic encyclopaedias, namely *De proprietatibus rerum* by Bartholomaeus Anglicus (d. 1272) and *Speculum maius* by Vincent de Beauvais (d. *c.* 1264).[27] These works also arrange their material according to an overarching understanding of cosmology and sacred history respectively.

The Purpose of the Collections

With at least four substantial collections of definitions extant from the medieval Gaelic world, what might the purpose of this kind of compilation have been? As we have seen, there is evidence that Maol Sheachlainn may have written **M** for Niall Óg during or upon completion of the latter's medical training, perhaps implying that it was meant to encapsulate the medical curriculum.

27 Shaw, 'Medieval Medico-Philosophical Treatises', pp. 156–57. On the reception of *De proprietatibus rerum* in medieval Ireland, see Ní Shéaghdha, *Translations*, p. 11.

While it is difficult to match up the contents to what is known about the medical curriculum at the time,[28] Maol Sheachlainn himself provides some evidence to support this. He suggests in his opening comments (**M** § 1) that he sees definitions as having pedagogical value:

> dob áil lim in compendium so ar difinicion gach aonneith da ficfithir duin do scrībad, uair is tre difinicion na nethed ticmait docum a naithne agus a tuicsina.
>
> (I desire to write this compendium for the purpose of defining each thing that has come to my attention, since it is through defining things that we come to know and understand them.)

Introducing his larger collection of definitions in Dublin, King's Inns, MS 15, he states that he is writing 'do lucht in studēir' (for students).[29] His compilation, he claims, provides everything that students of medicine might seek in a single volume, and he has deliberately avoided including much theory for the sake of readability. He comes across as concerned with the process and practicalities of learning when producing each of these collections.

A relationship between collections of definitions and education is also implied by some of the other texts that appear with **E** in Section 4 of Edinburgh, NLS, MS Adv. 72.1.2. Deborah Hayden has examined a medical catechism that is found later in the section, although not in the hand of Eoin mac Domhnaill. Due to its question-and-answer structure and the introductory nature of its subject-matter, she has suggested that it may be primarily didactic in purpose.[30] Indeed, the text alludes to topics it will not cover, on the grounds that these constitute *airdeólus* (advanced knowledge),[31] echoing Maol Sheachlainn's pragmatic concern for the immediate needs of his novice readers. Eoin mac Domhnaill himself writes out two short texts consisting of riddling questions on medical texts, one in Section 4 in which the questions are followed by answers and one in Section 10 in which they are not,[32] suggesting he drew on a comparable sort of material.

There is no positive evidence to suggest that the collection in Edinburgh, EUL, MS Laing III.21 was produced with an especially pedagogical purpose in mind. It is perhaps noteworthy, however, that this manuscript plus Eoin mac Domhnaill's component of Edinburgh, NLS, MS Adv. 72.1.2 and **M** were produced in Ireland in the probable knowledge that they would be taken to Scotland. Definitions of and brief commentary on key concepts may have been seen as the most concise and efficient way to package the essentials of the expansive scholastic medical

28 Shaw, 'Irish Medical Men', p. 81; O'Boyle, *The Art of Medicine*, chs 3 and 4.

29 'De febre efemera', ed. by Wulff, p. 127 (my translation).

30 Hayden, 'Observations', pp. 27–28. A didactic purpose is further implied, Hayden suggests, by the text being followed in Section 4 by *Tecosca Cormaic*, a collection of more general gnomic pronouncements framed within a dialogue between the legendary king, Cormac mac Airt, and his son, Cairpre Lifechair.

31 Hayden, 'Observations', pp. 46–48.

32 Edinburgh, NLS, MS Adv. 72.1.2, fols 50^{r}21–27 (with answers) and 114^{v}2–9 (without answers).

literature available in Ireland at the time.[33] The satisfaction expressed by Maol Sheachlainn in Dublin, King's Inns, MS 15 at having fitted the curriculum into a single volume further suggests that this was the perceived benefit of the form.[34]

The collections under discussion cannot be said to represent the period's medical learning or training in its entirety, as neither **M** nor **E** provide any coverage of cures or any other sort of active intervention in which a physician might be expected to have been trained. Both are concerned with anatomy, ailments, the human person's place within the created cosmos, and medicine's place within philosophy. While they do cover diseases (especially fevers), they provide little practical detail on diagnosis, prognosis, and the like. They thus provide at best a conceptual grounding in medicine. The Dublin, King's Inns, MS 15 collection differs in this respect, in that it combines definitions of ailments and related concepts with cures.[35]

Both **M** and **E** also offer more general aphorisms on the ethos of medicine as a profession, which may also be intended as part of basic professional grounding. **E** §§ 53–59 especially stress the importance of medicine being founded on studied understanding. § 56 is illustrative:

> Credere expermento absge recione fallax est .i. gach neach creidis d'urcosc ag nach bī rēsūn, nach increidi hē.
>
> > (It is fallacious to believe experience in the absence of reason. i.e. Anyone who believes in a treatment that does not have [a basis in] reason, they are not themselves to be believed.)

This gnomic aspect to **E** is echoed by *Tecosca Cormaic*, which, as noted above, appears later in Section 4 of Edinburgh, NLS, Adv. MS 72.1.2.

M takes a different angle. Early on, it provides a series of definitions and aphorisms on philosophy, knowledge, the human soul, and other related concepts (§§ 29–36). These stress the crucial role of rational knowledge in the formation of the human soul and humanity's natural aptitude for knowledge. The latter point is made most exuberantly in § 36, which comprises a passage from the Hermetic text, *Asclepius*, beginning 'Magnum miraculum est homo' (the human is a great miracle; see Appendix 2).[36] **M** § 37 then introduces

---

33 Definitions seem to have been the subject of active interest in learned circles in Islay at the time, as several hands associated with the Islay Beatons add further definitions and aphorisms to Edinburgh, NLS, MS Adv. 72.1.4: see fols 24^{r}1–10, 25^r–25^{v}5 and 81^{r}1–82^{r}10 (§§ 183–84). For the hands, see Black, *Catalogue*.

34 As Siobhán Barrett explores elsewhere in this volume (pp. 307–09), condensing and arranging the medical literature's content for convenient use was a long-standing concern of medieval medical scholars generally, not just of those writing teaching texts.

35 de Brún, *Catalogue*, pp. 36–43. Interestingly, cures are very much the focus of a remedy book produced by Connla Mac an Leagha Ruaidh, Maol Sheachlainn's brother: Hayden, 'Attribution and Authority', pp. 26–30; Barrett, 'Varia I'; Hayden, 'A Sixteenth-Century Irish Collection'.

36 *Asclepius*, § 6 (ll. 1–19), ed. by Nock and Festugière, pp. 301–02 (trans. [English] by Copenhaver, § 5, pp. 69–70). The passage is said in **M** to come from a commentary by

medicine and suggests that, as the art of preserving human life, it is the noblest of all the arts:

> Nobilitas scientiarum arguit nobilitatem subiectorum .i. is ī uaisli na suibidechta do-beir in hegna uasal. Agus, ō nach fuil eter na corpurdachta cumuscda dūilita suibidecht is uasli nā suibidecht in duine, is ī in elada comēdus a shlāinti elada is uaisle ann.
>
> > (The nobility of sciences proves the nobility of subjects. i.e. The nobility of the subject gives rise to noble knowledge. And, since there is no subject among the con-mixed, elemental corporealities that is nobler than the human subject, it is the art that maintains the human subject's health that is the noblest.)

The items cited from **E** stress that, if medical practice is to have consistently acceptable outcomes, then it must be founded in reason. Those cited from **M** present reason as both directly beneficial to the human soul and the basis of medicine, which preserves the human body. This is re-emphasized in **M** § 77, cited above, where medicine is defined as a species of knowledge.

Both collections go beyond providing definitions of key concepts within medicine. They attempt to contextualize it as a discipline, while also considering the implications for those studying and aspiring to practice it. This may in some cases have been required in the kind of pedagogical context implied by the background to the production of **M**. In general, collections of interrelated definitions and other aphorisms seem to have been seen as a way of structuring and packaging up detail and encapsulating medicine as a whole, an interest also reflected in the more general aphorisms on the subject. This could have been needed in a variety of contexts.

Definitions in Medieval Medical Texts

While definitions are important throughout philosophy and science, they can be pivotal to the dialectical reasoning that characterizes medieval scholasticism. Scholasticism is concerned with commenting on and reconciling conflicting

Thomas Aquinas on Boethius' *De consolatione philosophiae*. It is found in a commentary by Pseudo-Aquinas (William Wheatley, 'In Boethii De consolatione philosophiae', ed. by Busa, I, 3), which is thought to have been composed in the mid-fifteenth century (Minnis, 'Aspects', p. 354) and which was printed in 1473 (King, 'Boethius', pp. 46–47). If **M** did derive the passage thence, it would be the latest identifiable source used in either collection. **M** also states that the passage is found in the *Almagest*. The Greek original of this astronomical work, composed by Claudius Ptolemy (second century AD; *Ptolemy's Almagest*, trans. by Toomer), does not contain anything corresponding to the 'Magnum miraculum est homo' passage. However, the *Almagest* was translated multiple times into Latin from both Arabic and the original Greek in the Middle Ages, so some resulting version might contain it. Verifying this is beyond the scope of the present study.

authorities,[37] and the route to such reconciliation often lay through examining the authorities' terminology and the possible definitions thereof.[38] Conversely, the formation of a definition could itself be the subject of a disputation.[39] The logic and appropriate use of definition was the subject of philosophical analysis by the tradition's authorities and commentators, with one of the most influential discussions occurring in Aristotle's *Posterior Analytics*.[40] In scholastic medical writing, definitions often form the jumping-off points for discussion or information on a subject. In Gaelic translations and re-compilations of such writing, these definitions are often similar in style to those that appear in collections like **M** and **E** and can resemble them closely in wording. This underlines the importance of collections of definitions vis-à-vis medieval Gaelic medical writing more widely and perhaps provides some clues as to how the collections were produced and used.

In the later fifteenth-century Irish translation of John of Gaddesden's *Rosa anglica*, discussion of an ailment and its cures often begins with a definition. For example, *ephemera* is defined as follows:[41]

> Is edh is efemera ánd .i. fiabras tic o ainmesurdacht oirida na spirut nach teid do reir a nadura fein tar 4 huairib .xx.
>
> > (Ephemera is a fever resulting from exceptional immoderation of the spirits which does not last beyond twenty-four hours, as regards its own nature.)

E § 77 offers a similar definition:

> Efemira est febiris ex distemparancia spiritum procediens et ultra diem naturaleim suam crisim non extendiens .i. is ed is efemira and fiabras tosgius ō ainmesaracht na spirad agus nach lēigind an fantham tar a lā nādūra gan crīchad.
>
> > (Ephemera is a fever proceeding from distemper of the spirits whose crisis does not extend beyond one natural day. i.e. Ephemera is a fever that begins as a result of immoderation of the spirits and that does not extend the crisis beyond a natural day without ending.)

Rosa anglica, however, goes on to use this definition to distinguish between true ephemera (*efemera fíri*) and false ephemera (*efemera nach fír*): the former complies with the definition and recedes within a day, while the latter seems to recede within a day but soon returns. The definition is thus used as the basis for further refinement of the subject under discussion.

---

37 Hayden, 'Attribution and Authority', pp. 19–22.

38 O'Boyle, *The Art of Medicine*, pp. 190–95.

39 O'Boyle, *The Art of Medicine*, pp. 214–22; Novikoff, *The Medieval Culture of Disputation*, pp. 141–42.

40 Bronstein, *Aristotle on Knowledge*, pp. 69–222.

41 *Rosa anglica*, ed. and trans. by Wulff, pp. 48–49.

Discussion of paralysis in *Rosa anglica* begins with a definition that is then used in a similar way:[42]

> Et is edh is pairilis and da reir sin .i. bogach na feithid ar mbuain a ngluasachta 7 a ratuighte astu.
>
> > (According to that, paralysis consists in the softening of the nerves [sinews?] by taking from them their movement and perception.)

M § 127 provides a reasonably close parallel:

> Parilis est mollicon neruorum cum impeticione motus et sensibilis .i. is ed is parilis ann bogad na fēted maille re hasbrain cumscaigti agus rāthaigthi.
>
> > (Paralysis is the softening of nerves with an adverse impact on movement and perception. i.e. Paralysis is the softening of the nerves with an adverse impact on motion and sensation.)

Again, *Rosa anglica* goes on to use this definition to distinguish paralysis from other conditions such as cramp, with the distinction often being based around the loss of both movement and sensation in cases of 'true' paralysis.

An unedited tract in Edinburgh, NLS, MS Adv. 72.1.48 details the benefits of delivering medicine by means of an electuary (*lictuáire*), that is, by mixing it with something sweet.[43] As the tract explains, the digestive system needs to be fooled into treating the medicine as nourishment that is to be preserved and distributed to the members, not as waste to be excreted. In support of this explanation, a definition of digestion attributed to Avicenna (Ibn Sina, d. 1037) is quoted:[44]

> DEGESTIO EST calitas faciens sesare putredinim .i. gurub eadh is dílegud and cáil noch coischis in morgud.
>
> > (Digestion is the quality of making putrefaction cease. i.e. digestion is the quality that prevents putrefaction.)

This somewhat resembles **M** § 115, although this is attributed to Galen:

> Et do-beir Galen a Lebur na Cuis[l]inn in dēnum so ar in dīlegud. Digestio est alteracon faciens cesare putredinem manente substancia .i. is ed is dīlegud ann claechlōdh coiscis in morgad agus in tsubstaint ar marthain.
>
> > (And Galen gives this definition of digestion in *On Veins*. Digestion is change that makes putrefaction cease while substance remains. i.e. Digestion is change that prevents putrefaction, with the substance remaining.)

42 *Rosa anglica*, ed. and trans. by Wulff, pp. 246–47.

43 Edinburgh, NLS, MS Adv. 72.1.48, fol. $1^{r}a1$–$1^{v}b26$.

44 Edinburgh, NLS, MS Adv. 72.1.48, fol. $1^{v}a45$–46.

In each of the above examples, a definition familiar from our collections is treated as a single authoritative source. There are other situations where definitions of the same concept require reconciliation with each other. A treatise on fevers edited by Lilian Duncan from fifteenth-century manuscripts opens by defining disease and then moves on to present two definitions of fever.[45] One, attributed to Galen, traces the cause of fever to an overall hot complexion affecting the body. The other, attributed to 'other doctors', describes fever as originating in the heart and arteries and then spreading to other members. Definitions akin to these appear in **M** as §§ 108 and 110 (**E** § 75) respectively. The treatise then proceeds to synthesize its opening definitions by quoting several more definitions of different sorts of fever.[46] These show that, while different fevers originate in different parts of the body, they all come to affect the body as a whole. Galen's definition is thus right about fever in general, while the other doctors are right about one sort of fever.

It seems likely that collections like **M** and **E** were compiled by culling Latin definitions and Gaelic explications from continuous texts,[47] where they would have been encountered as the building blocks of larger and more complex arguments. This process of culling seems to have been far from uncritical, however, with the definitions being selected and arranged to explain and reinforce each other or else to represent different learned viewpoints on the concept in question. It is possible that the resulting collections were then used as a source of building blocks for new medical tracts, although no examples of this have been identified and any such identification would likely require a great deal more editorial work on the medieval Gaelic medical corpus.

Conclusion

Collections of definitions have emerged from this brief study as an important type of source for understanding medical learning in the medieval North Atlantic, in terms of both subject-matter and concrete intellectual history. They are attempts at encapsulating the fundamentals of medicine, or at least certain sub-divisions thereof, and thus show what was considered key to understanding the human body and its place in the cosmos. The collections also address broader issues, such as the classification of medicine within *scientia* or the logic of definition itself. Considered alongside their occasional critical commentary on definitions and the placing of antithetical definitions alongside one another, they yield insights into the processes of reading and reasoning by which medical learning was pursued. Their manuscript and

45 'A Treatise on Fevers', ed. and trans. by Duncan, pp. 1–4 and 57–58.

46 'A Treatise on Fevers', ed. and trans. by Duncan, pp. 4–7 and 58–59.

47 Shaw, 'Medieval Medico-Philosophical Treatises', pp. 156–57; Ní Shéaghdha, *Translations*, p. 7.

social context implies that they had a practical, pedagogical purpose, further implying the material's centrality to the discipline and profession.

There are various possible avenues for further enquiry relating to collections of definitions. Identifying sources of definitions could help identify the texts available in the medieval Gaelic world, although this will always be complicated by the potential for definitions to circulate independent of particular texts. The philosophical influences evidenced by the method of definition employed and exposited within the collections might yield insights into the intellectual resources on which medical learning in the medieval world drew. The textual history of the collections themselves also merits attention; this would determine whether all the collections stem from the same tradition or whether multiple independent collections were made, with implications for how important the form was for medical learning.

Appendix 1

Table Summarizing the Contents of M and E

The tables given below summarize the contents of the **M** and **E** collections respectively. Where an item is a definition, its lemma is given under 'Subject'.[48] When it is some other sort of aphorism, the incipit of the Latin version is given. In the latter case, the incipit is of the item itself, not of any introductory comment or attribution. The 'Attribution' column merely repeats the attribution from the text, with suggested identifications generally based on the resemblance of the name to that of an author reputed to have written on the subject in question. An obit or floruit has been provided where the author is either less well-known or late enough to offer possible insights into the text's sources. No systematic attempt has been made to verify whether the item actually appears in anything elsewhere attributed to that author.

Table 15.1. The NLS Adv. 72.1.4 Collection (M).

No.	**Ref.**	**Subject**	**Attribution**
1	26^{r}1–11	'Quem scientia uiuificat…'	Galen
2	26^{r}11–26^{v}1	God	
3	26^{v}1–8	Firmament	
4	26^{v}8–27^{r}13	Sphere	Johannes de Sacrobusco [(d. 1256)]
5	27^{r}13–28^{r}14	Astrology	[Aristotle?][49]
6	28^{r}14–28^{v}6	Element	[Aristotle?]
7	28^{v}6–12	Element	[Aristotle?]
8	28^{v}12–29^{r}1	Fire	[Aristotle?]
9	29^{r}2–29^{r}8	Air	[Aristotle?]
10	29^{r}8–29^{r}12	Water	[Aristotle?]
11	29^{r}12–29^{v}4	Earth	[Aristotle?]
12	29^{v}5–30^{r}1	Clouds	Theodosius
13	30^{r}1–6	Wind	Thaddeus [Florentinus? (d. 1295)]
14	30^{r}6–30^{v}6	Solar eclipse	'lingcol'[50]
15	30^{v}7–31^{v}1	*Materia prima*	[Aristotle?]
16	31^{v}1–5	*Materia prima*	
17	31^{v}5–9	*Materia prima*	
18	31^{v}9–32^{r}9	*Materia prima*	Aristotle

48 The translations of the definienda are approximate and intended as a guide only. For the difficulties of translating pre-modern medical terminology, see: Wallis, *Medieval Medicine*, xxv–xxvii.

49 *In fellsam* (the philosopher) is taken as denoting Aristotle (eDIL s.v. *fellsam*, dil.ie/21558).

50 It is possible that 'lingcol' refers to Robert Grosseteste (d. 1253), Bishop of Lincoln, who was an authority on subjects like light and astronomy, but this is very tentative. I am grateful to the Rev. Thomas Steel for his advice on this identification.

No.	Ref.	Subject	Attribution
19	$32^{r}9$–$32^{v}6$	Substance	Porphyry
20	$32^{v}7$–10	Substance	[Aristotle?]
21	$32^{v}11$–13	Substance	
22	$33^{r}1$–3	Substance	
23	$33^{r}4$–9	Form	[Aristotle?]
24	$33^{r}9$–$33^{v}2$	Form	
25	$33^{v}3$–7	Substantial form	[Aristotle?]
26	$33^{v}8$–11	Privation	[Aristotle?]
27	$33^{v}11$–$34^{r}6$	Privation	
28	$34^{r}7$–10	Privation	
29	$34^{r}9$–$34^{v}11$	Philosophy	[Aristotle?]
30	$34^{v}11$–14	*Scientia*	Avicenna
31	$34^{v}14$–18	'Anima creata est…'	[Aristotle?]
32	$34^{v}19$–$35^{r}3$	'Anima humana est…'	Boethius
33	$35^{r}3$–8	'Cognicon ueri habetur…'	Aristotle
34	$35^{r}8$–12	'Siencia est perfeccon…'	Aristotle
35	$35^{r}12$–15	'Omnis hominis naturaliter…'	Aristotle
36	$35^{r}15$–$36^{r}12$	'Magnum miraculum est homo…'	*The Almagest*, [Pseudo-]Thomas [Aquinas]
37	$36^{r}13$–$36^{v}11$	'Nobilitas scientiarum arguit…'	Aristotle
38	$36^{v}11$–$37^{r}9$	'Omnis medella dependit…'	Arnaldus [de Villa Nova (d. 1311)?]
39	$37^{r}9$–$37^{v}4$	Soul (animal)	
40	$37^{v}5$–12	Soul	Thomas Aquinas
41	$37^{v}12$–$38^{v}5$	Soul	John of Damascus [(d. 749)?]
42	$38^{v}5$–15	Synderisis	Thomas Aquinas
43	$39^{r}1$–9	Soul	Aristotle
44	$39^{r}9$–$39^{v}3$	Soul	Augustine
45	$39^{v}3$–10	Soul	*Liber de Motu Corporis*
46	$39^{v}10$–$40^{r}2$	Soul	Augustine
47	$40^{r}2$–9	Soul	Augustine
48	$40^{r}9$–12	Soul	Regnidus
49	$40^{r}12$–15	Soul	Augustine
50	$40^{v}1$–6	Soul	Augustine
51	$40^{v}6$–11	Soul	Augustine
52	$40^{v}11$–13	Soul	
53	$40^{v}13$–$41^{r}9$	Soul	
54	$41^{r}10$–15	Soul	Boethius
55	$41^{v}1$–16	Body	Guido [de Chauliac (d. 1368)?]
56	$42^{r}1$–17	Nature	Thomas Aquinas
57	$42^{r}17$–$42^{v}10$	Nature	Augustine

No.	Ref.	Subject	Attribution
58	42^{v}11–17	Nature	
59	43^{r}1–10	Nature	[Aristotle?]
60	43^{r}11–14	[illegible]	
61	43^{r}15–43^{v}9	[*Virtus*?]	
62	43^{v}10–44^{r}1	*Virtus*	Albertus [Magnus?]
63	44^{r}1–5	Spirit	Thaddeus [Florentinus?]
64	44^{r}7–13	Spirit	Galen
65	44^{r}14–44^{v}7	Member	Plato
66	44^{v}7–44^{v}14	Humour	Plato
67	44^{v}14–45^{r}11	Humour	Plato
68	45^{r}11–46^{r}1	Natural	Constantine [the African (eleventh cent.)?]
69	46^{r}1–14	Unnatural	Thaddeus [Florentinus?]
70	46^{v}1–14	Contrary to nature	
71	46^{v}15–47^{r}8	Conservation	Francesco di Piedimonte [d. *c.* 1320]
72	47^{r}8–47^{v}2	Prognostication	Francesco di Piedimonte
73	47^{v}3–8	Recuperation	
74	47^{v}9–14	Medicine	Galen
75	47^{v}15–48^{r}7	Medicine	Isaac [Israeli ben Solomon (d. *c.* 932)?]
76	48^{r}7–48^{v}2	Medicine	Augustine
77	48^{v}3–49^{r}3	Understanding	[Aristotle]
78	49^{r}3–49^{r}7	Knowledge	[Aristotle?]
79	49^{r}7–49^{v}4	Wisdom	Aristotle
80	49^{v}4–8	Wisdom	
81	49^{v}8–12	Opinion	
82	49^{v}12–50^{r}6	Theory	Avicenna
83	50^{r}6–9	Speculative knowledge	Aristotle
84	50^{r}9–50^{v}2	Theory	Constantine [the African?]
85	50^{v}3–11	Practice	Constantine [the African?]
86	50^{v}11–51^{r}3	Practice	Avicenna
87	51^{r}4–13	*Doctrina ordinaria*	Thaddeus [Florentinus?]
88	51^{r}13–51^{v}3	Theory	Thaddeus [Florentinus?]
89	51^{v}4–7	Medical speculation	Thaddeus [Florentinus?]
90	51^{v}7–10	'Operacon medecine triplicem …'	
91	51^{v}10–52^{r}2	Putrefaction	Aristotle
92	52^{r}2–9	Putrefaction	Isaac [Israeli ben Solomon?]
93	52^{r}9–52^{v}3	Epidemic	Thaddeus [Florentinus?]
94	52^{v}4–11	Epidemic	Avicenna
95	52^{v}11–53^{r}5	Epidemic	Constantine [the African]
96	53^{r}5–11	Epidemic	Constantine [the African]
97	53^{r}11–53^{v}3	Epidemic	Thaddeus [Florentinus?]

No.	Ref.	Subject	Attribution
98	53^{v}3–10	Exercise	Avicenna
99	53^{v}10–54^{r}2	Nourishment	Thaddeus [Florentinus?]
100	54^{r}2–5	Thirst	
101	54^{r}5–10	'Molle est quod…'	Thaddeus [Florentinus?]
102	54^{r}10–54^{v}5	Sleep	Aristotle
103	54^{v}5–11	Sleep	Aristotle
104	54^{v}12–55^{r}4	Sleep	Thaddeus [Florentinus?]
105	55^{r}4–10	Sleep	Thaddeus [Florentinus?]
106	55^{r}10–55^{v}2	Sleep	
107	55^{v}2–8	Fever	Galen
108	55^{v}8–56^{r}1	Fever	Galen
109	56^{r}1–11	Fever	Isaac [Israeli ben Solomon?]
110	56^{r}11–56^{v}10	Fever	Avicenna
111	56^{v}10–57^{r}3	Fever	Galen
112	57^{r}3–58^{r}1	Fever	Galen
113	58^{r}1–4	Ephemeral fever	Galen
114	58^{r}4–8	Ephemeral fever	Isaac [Israeli ben Solomon?], Galen
115	58^{r}8–58^{v}1	Digestion	Galen
116	58^{v}1–5	Digestion	
117	58^{v}6–9	Aposteme	[John of] Gaddesden
118	58^{v}9–59^{r}3	Wound	Peter [of Spain (fl. thirteenth century)?]
119	59^{r}4–59^{v}3	Bruise	Guido
120	59^{v}4–5	Bruise	Peter [of Spain?]
121	59^{v}6–60^{v}14	Fracture	
122	60^{v}14–61^{r}4	Pain	Gerard [de Solo (d. 1360)?]
123	61^{r}4–10	Pain	Averroes
124	61^{r}10–61^{v}3	Pain	Galen
125	61^{v}3–9	Pain	Avicenna
126	61^{v}10–62^{r}13	Paralysis	Gerard [de Solo?]
127	62^{v}1–5	Paralysis	
128	62^{v}6–63^{r}10	Mania	Gerard [de Solo?]
129	63^{r}10–63^{v}3	Lethargy	Gerard [de Solo?]
130	63^{v}3–12	Lethargy	Bernard de Gordon [(fl. 1270–1330)]
131	63^{v}12–64^{r}5	Frenzy	Gerard [de Solo?]
132	64^{r}6–11	Melancholy	Avicenna
133	64^{r}12–64^{v}7	Epilepsy	Gerard [de Solo?]
134	64^{v}8–65^{r}2	Epilepsy	Gerard [de Solo?]
135	65^{r}3–9	Epilepsy	Gerard [de Solo?]
136	65^{r}10–66^{r}10	Epilepsy	Gilbertinus [Anglicus (1180–1250)?]
137	65^{r}11–66^{v}9	Apoplexy	Avicenna

No.	Ref.	Subject	Attribution
138	66ᵛ10–67ʳ4	Spasm	Gerard [de Solo?]
139	67ʳ4–9	Spasm	Gerard [de Solo?]
140	67ʳ9–68ʳ3	Spasm	Gerard [de Solo?]
141	68ʳ3–13	Congelation	Avicenna
142	68ᵛ1–9	Eye	
143	68ᵛ9–13	Scotoma	Gerard [de Solo?]
144	68ᵛ13–69ʳ4	Scotoma	Gilbertinus [Anglicus?]
145	69ʳ5–13	Cataracts	Avicenna
146	69ᵛ1–6	Ungula	
147	69ᵛ6–12	Macula	[Avicenna?]
148	70ʳ1–5	Sneezing	Gerard [de Solo?]
149	70ʳ6–70ᵛ9	Tongue	
150	70ᵛ9–71ʳ4	Mouth	Gerard [de Solo?]
151	71ʳ5–12	Voice	Peter of Spain
152	71ʳ12–71ᵛ9	'Instrumenta nouem sunt…'	Peter of Spain
153	71ᵛ9–73ʳ7	Uvulua	Gerard [de Solo?]
154	73ʳ7–73ᵛ6	Guta rosacea	Gerard [de Solo?]
155	73ᵛ6–11	Rheum	Gerard [de Solo?]
156	73ᵛ11–74ᵛ7	Rheum	Bernard [de Gordon]
157	74ᵛ8–75ʳ2	Hoarseness	
158	75ʳ2–75ᵛ6	Voice	Gerard [de Solo?]
159	75ᵛ7–13	Heart pain	Gerard [de Solo?]
160	76ʳ1–7	Fainting	
161	76ʳ7–3	Breast	Gerard de Solo?]
162	76ʳ4–9	Indigestion	
163	76ʳ10–77ʳ3	Digestion	Gerard [de Solo?]
164	77ʳ4–7	Digestion	Gerard [de Solo?]
165	77ʳ8–12	Digestion	
166	77ᵛ1–3	Thirst	Gerard [de Solo?]
167	77ᵛ4–78ʳ3	Aversion	Gerard [de Solo?]
168	78ʳ4–8	Aversion	
169	78ʳ9–13	Nausea	
170	78ʳ13–78ᵛ3	Vomiting	
171	78ᵛ4–12	Vomiting	
172	78ᵛ13–15	Anastrophe	
173	79ʳ1–4	Catastrophe	
174	79ʳ5–9	Cholic	
175	79ʳ10–79ᵛ2	Liver	Gerard [de Solo?]
176	79ᵛ3–8	Quinsy	
177	79ᵛ9–13	Coughing	Gerard [de Solo?]
178	79ᵛ14–80ʳ2	Coughing	

No.	Ref.	Subject	Attribution
179	80^{r}3–6	Empyema	Gerard [de Solo?]
180	80^{r}7–11	Empyema	
181	80^{r}12–80^{v}5	Causon fever	Gerard [de Solo?]
182	80^{v}6–15	Causon fever	
183	81^{r}1–81^{v}3	Angel[51]	
184	81^{v}4–82^{r}10	Angel	
185	82^{v}1–5	Lungs	
186	82^{v}6–9	'fantastica .i. sialla na …'	
187	83^{r}1–2	[illegible]	
188	83^{r}3–8	Tertian fever	
189	83^{r}9–14	Hectic fever	Gerard [de Solo?]
190	83^{v}1–8	Hectic fever	Isaac [Israeli ben Solomon?]
191	83^{v}9–84^{r}4	Phthisis	Galen
192	84^{r}5–8	'Longincum est quod…'	Galen
193	84^{r}9–12	Phthisis	
194	84^{r}13–84^{v}4	Pleurisy	Gerard [de Solo?]
195	84^{v}5–10	Pleurisy	Gerard [de Solo?]
196	84^{v}11–85^{r}3	Perplemonia	Gerard [de Solo?]
197	85^{r}3–9	Perplemonia	Avicenna
198	85^{r}9–85^{v}5	Hiccups	Avicenna
199	85^{v}6–86^{r}5	Spleen	Gerard [de Solo?]
200	86^{r}6–11	Stomach	Avicenna
201	86^{r}12–86^{v}7	Kidneys	Gerard [de Solo?]
202	86^{v}8–12	[Kidney?] stones	Gerard [de Solo?]
203	86^{v}13–87^{r}8	Stupefaction	Gilbertinus [Anglicus?]
204	87^{r}9–87^{v}2	*Tortura*	Gilbertinus [Anglicus?]
205	87^{v}3–6	Arthritis	Avicenna
206	87^{v}7–11	Chiragra	
207	87^{v}12–88^{r}4	Podagra	
208	88^{r}4–14	Dropsy	Avicenna
209	88^{v}1–5	Dropsy	Avicenna
210	88^{v}6–11	Dysentery	
211	88^{v}12–89^{r}4	Lientery	
212	89^{r}5–10	Diarrhoea	Bernard [de Gordon?]
213	89^{r}11–89^{v}4	Haemorrhoids	Avicenna
214	89^{v}5–10	Health	Hippocrates
215	89^{v}11–90^{r}3	Health	'ionicius'[52]
216	90^{r}4–9	Illness	'ionisius'
217	90^{r}10–90^{v}3	Neutral	'ionisius'

51 §§ 183–86 are in two different hands and seem to be later additions.

52 The attribution for §§ 215–20 is given at fol. 91^{r}5–7.

No.	Ref.	Subject	Attribution
218	$90^{v}4$–8	Neutral	'ionisius'
219	$90^{v}9$–$91^{r}2$	Neutral	'ionisius'
220	$91^{r}3$–7	Neutral	'ionisius'
221	$91^{r}8$–11	Poison	
222	$91^{r}12$–$91^{v}2$	Poison	The commentator
223	$91^{v}3$–5	Nerves	
224	$91^{v}6$–$92^{r}1$	Muscles	Hugo
225	$92^{r}2$–10	Arteries	The commentator
226	$92^{r}11$–$92^{v}2$	Ophthalmia	Avicenna
227	$92^{v}3$–11	Lacrimal fistula	
228	$93^{r}1$–$93^{v}2$	Subject	
229	$93^{v}3$–7	Form	
230	$93^{v}8$–$94^{r}3$	Accidence	
231	$94^{r}4$–8	Object	
232	$94^{r}9$–$94^{v}2$	Object	
233	$94^{v}6$–9	Object	
234	$94^{v}10$–$95^{r}4$	'Quod prius est…'	
235	$95^{r}5$–9	'Que simul ars…'	
236	$95^{r}10$–$95^{v}1$	'Qulibus pars difiniti…'	
237	$95^{v}2$–$96^{r}12$	Human	
238	$96^{v}1$–13	Balanced complexion	Constantine [the African?]
239	$96^{v}13$–$97^{r}8$	Balanced complexion	Avicenna
240	$97^{r}9$–$97^{v}4$	Proportionally balanced [complexion]	Constantine [the African?]
241	$97^{v}5$–11	Proportionally balanced complexion	Avicenna
242	$97^{v}12$–$98^{v}5$	'Omnis medecina aut[em] est…'	
243	$98^{v}6$–$100^{r}3$	Individual	

Table 15.2. The NLS Adv. 72.1.2 Collection (E).

No.	Ref.	Subject	Attribution
1	$44^{r}1$	[acephalous]	
2	$44^{r}2$–3	Spirit	
3	$44^{r}4$–6	Spirit	
4	$44^{r}5$–7	Pain	
5	$44^{r}8$–9	Pain	Galen
6	$44^{r}9$–10	Pain	
7	$44^{r}11$–14	Medicine	
8	$44^{r}14$–17	Medicine	
9	$44^{r}17$–18	Medicine	
10	$44^{r}19$–20	Speculative knowledge	
11	$44^{r}18$–21	Theory	
12	$44^{v}1$–2	Theory	Avicenna
13	$44^{v}3$–4	Practice	
14	$44^{v}4$–6	Practice	
15	$44^{v}6$–7	Substance	
16	$44^{v}7$–8	Substance	
17	$44^{v}9$–10	Substance	
18	$44^{v}10$–11	'Omnis quod est…'	
19	$44^{v}12$–13	Accidence	
20	$44^{v}13$–15	Accidence	Aristotle
21	$44^{v}16$–18	Hearing	
22	$44^{v}19$–21	Subject	
23	$44^{v}21$–22	Object	
24	$45^{r}1$–2	'Unde illud aicidens…'	
25	$45^{r}2$–5	'Dicendum est quid…'	
26	$45^{r}6$–7	'Non podesta inteligire…'	
27	$45^{r}7$–10	Degree	
28	$45^{r}10$–12	Teaching	Boethius
29	$45^{r}12$–14	Teaching	
30	$45^{r}14$–15	*Doctrina ordinaria*	
31	$45^{r}16$–17	'Natura exindeinte forte…'	
32	$45^{r}17$–20	'Natura exinteinte debele…'	Avicenna
33	$45^{r}20$–22	'Natura non deficit…'	
34	$45^{r}22$–23	'Natura non indigit…'	
35	$45^{v}1$–3	'Natura conuerdit membra…'	
36	$45^{v}4$–6	'Sanguis enem humanus…'	
37	$45^{v}6$–7	White	
38	$45^{v}8$–11	'Est autem sanguinis…'	
39	$45^{v}11$–13	'Quongem in arte…'	

No.	Ref.	Subject	Attribution
40	45^{v}14–17	Organ	Petrus Mustinus
41	45^{v}18–20	Humour	
42	45^{v}20–24	'Nota secundum aseancum…'	
43	45^{v}24–46^{r}2	Crisis	
44	46^{r}2–5	Natural	Constantine [the African?]
45	46^{r}6–9	Unnatural	[Thaddeus Florentinus?]
46	46^{r}8–10	'Res consuetes multo tempore…'	
47	46^{r}10–11	Pestilence	
48	46^{r}12–13	'Aighir himutad corpus nostrum…'	
49	46^{r}12–13	'Malus aer plus aghrauad…'	
50	46^{r}15–16	'Medicus medioris qualitatis…'	Isidore [of Seville? (d. 636)]
51	46^{r}17–18	'Nulla est egritudo…'	Isidore [of Seville?]
52	46^{r}19–21	'Singulis infirmatibus proprio…'	Isidore [of Seville?]
53	46^{r}21–22	'O medidici qudhmodo…'	
54	46^{v}1–2	'Ignorancia medici est…'	
55	46^{v}2–4	'Si medicus non iuuad…'	
56	46^{v}3–4	'Credere expermento absge…'	
57	46^{v}5	'Res sine resione…'	
58	46^{v}6	'Uerecundum est sine…'	
59	46^{v}7–8	'Nemo recti loquitur…'	
60	46^{v}9–10	'Seuius irrant animum…'	
61	46^{v}11–13	'Sicut leccio precedit…'	
62	46^{v}14–15	Eye	
63	46^{v}14–15	'Omnis amans ecus…'	
64	46^{v}16–17	'Omnis parsa corpus…'	
65	46^{v}17–18	'Corpus inseansatum est…'	
66	46^{v}17–19	'Omnia sunt cimila…'	
67	46^{v}20–21	'Duo corpora non…'	
68	46^{v}22–47^{r}3	'Tria fuerint prinsipia…'	Plato
69	47^{r}3–4	Form	
70	47^{r}5–6	Form	[Aristotle?]
71	47^{r}7–9	'Quicumque compitit unum…'	
72	47^{r}9–10	*Materia prima*	[Aristotle?]
73	47^{r}10–11	'Nicil tale est…'	[Aristotle?]
74	47^{r}11–12	*Materia prima*	

No.	Ref.	Subject	Attribution
75	$47^r13–16$	Fever	
76	$47^r16–17$	Fever	
77	$47^r17–20$	Ephemeral fever	
78	$47^r20–22$	Causon fever	
79	$47^r23–24$	Tertian fever	
80	$47^r23–24$	Quartan fever	
81	$47^r25–47^v2$	Quotidian fever	
82	$47^v2–4$	Synochus	
83	$47^v4–7$	Lethargy	
84	$47^v8–9$	Frenzy	Gerard [de Solo?]
85	$47^v9–11$	Paralysis	
86	$47^v12–13$	Epilepsy	
87	$47^v13–15$	Stupefaction	
88	$47^v15–17$	*Macula rubia*	
89	$47^v17–19$	*Tortura*	
90	$47^v19–22$	Insomnia	
91	$47^v22–23$	Coughing	
92	$47^v24–25$	Pleurisy	
93	$47^v25–27$	Aposteme	
94	$48^r1–4$	Wound	Galen
95	$48^r4–6$	Wound	Bernard [de Gordon?]

Appendix 2

Miraculum Magnum Est Homo

The English translation of this passage (**M** § 36) is based on the Gaelic translation, where it departs from the Latin.

> Et is uime sin adubairt Almogestus agus Sanctus Tomas in comento Consolacionis Philosophie.
> Magnum miraculum est homo et animal honorandum. Hic anima intellectiua in natura dei transit quasi ipsę deus sit. Hic per naturam anime diis est coniunctus. Hic demonum genus nouit. Terras colitt. Elementis comicetur acumine mentis. In marís profundum decendit. Celum quod uidetur altisimum animi eius sagacitatę metitur. Intencionem animi eius nulla aeris caligo confunditt, nec terre densitas eius operacionem impedit. Non aque profunditas aspectum eius octumbib [leg. occludit?].
> .i. is mōr in mērbuil duine, agus ainmide inonōrta. Agus is ann so tēit in tanum tuicsinach in nādúir dia, mar bud dia ē fēin. Agus is ann so do cenglad risna dēib é maille re nādūir in anma. Agus is ann so aithniges genus na ndemun agus trebus in talam. Agus cumaiscter é risna dūlib. Agus turlingid le germac na hinntinne a fu[n]domain na mara. Agus tomsid neam do-cīthar co roard le glicus na menman, uair nī buaidrend ceo aeir inntinn anmman. Agus nī tormiscenn dlúithe na talman a hoibriugud. Agus nī maolann doimne na uiscided a radarc.
>
> > (And it is on this matter that the *Almagest* and St Thomas [Aquinas], in a commentary on *De Consolatione Philosophiae*, say:
> > The human is a great miracle, an animal worthy of honour. The rational soul enters into the nature of God, as if it were itself God. By the soul's nature, it is united with the gods. It recognizes demons as a genus, nurtures the earth, intermingles with the elements, descends through mental acuity to the depths of the sea, and, through the mind's ingenuity, measures the heavens that are seen on high, for the mists of the air are no obstacle to the soul's intention. The solidity of the earth does not hinder its work. The depth of the waters does not tire its sight.)

Works Cited

Manuscripts

Dublin, King's Inns Library, MS 15
Edinburgh, Edinburgh University Library, Laing MS III.21
Edinburgh, National Library of Scotland, MS Adv. 72.1.2
Edinburgh, National Library of Scotland, MS Adv. 72.1.4
Edinburgh, National Library of Scotland, MS Adv. 72.1.48

Primary Sources

The Annals of Loch Cé, ed. by William M. Hennessy, 2 vols (Dublin: Longman, 1871)

Asclepius, ed. and trans. [French] by A. D. Nock and A. J. Festugière, *Corpus Hermeticum*, 4 vols (Paris: Société D'édition 'Les Belles lettres', 1944–1945), II (1945); trans. [English] by Brian P. Copenhaver in *Hermetica* (Cambridge: Cambridge University Press, 1992), pp. 67–92

'De febre efemera nó an liagh i n-Eirinn i n-allod', ed. by Winifred Wulff, *Lia Fáil*, 1 (1926), 126–29

ISOS = *Irish Script on Screen* <https://www.isos.dias.ie> [accessed 20 December 2021]

Ptolemy's Almagest, trans. by Gerald J. Toomer (London: Duckworth, 1984)

Rosa anglica seu rosa medicinae: An Early Modern Irish Translation of a Section of the Mediaeval Medical Text-book of John of Gaddesden, ed. and trans. by Winifred Wulff, Irish Texts Society Main Series, 25 (London: Irish Texts Society, 1929)

'Three Irish Medical Glossaries', ed. by Whitley Stokes, *Archiv für celtische Lexikographie*, 1.3 (1900), 325–47

'A Treatise on Fevers', ed. and trans. by Lilian Duncan, *Révue celtique*, 49 (1932), 1–90

Wheatley, William [*recte* Pseudo-Aquinas], 'In Boethii De consolatione philosophiae', ed. by Roberto Busa in *S. Thomae Aquinatis opera omnia*, 7 vols (Stuttgart: F. Frommann-Holzboog, 1980) VII, consulted via <https://www.corpusthomisticum.org/iopera.html> [accessed 30 December 2021]

Secondary Studies

Arlig, Andrew, 'Medieval Mereology', in *The Stanford Encyclopaedia of Philosophy*, ed. by Edward N. Zalta (Stanford: Metaphysics Research Lab, Stanford University, Winter 2021) <https://plato.stanford.edu/archives/fall2019/entries/mereology-medieval/> [accessed 22 December 2021]

Bannerman, John, *The Beatons: A Medical Kindred in the Classical Gaelic Tradition* (Edinburgh: John Donald, 1998)

Barrett, Siobhán, 'Varia I. The King of Dál nAraidi's Salve', *Ériu*, 69 (2019), 171–78

Black, Ronald, *Catalogue of Gaelic Manuscripts in the NLS* (unpublished catalogue, National Library of Scotland, n.d.)

Bronstein, David, *Aristotle on Knowledge and Learning: The Posterior Analytics* (Oxford: Oxford University Press, 2016)

de Brún, Pádraig, *Catalogue of Irish Manuscripts in King's Inns Library, Dublin* (Dublin: Dublin Institute for Advanced Studies, 1971)

eDIL = eDIL 2019: *An Electronic Dictionary of the Irish Language*, based on the Contributions to a Dictionary of the Irish Language (Dublin: Royal Irish Academy, 1913–1976) <www.dil.ie> [accessed 12 June 2022]

Faucher, Nicolas, and Magali Roques, 'The Many Virtues of Second Nature: Habitus in Latin Medieval Philosophy', in *The Ontology, Psychology and Axiology of Habits (Habitus) in Medieval Philosophy*, ed. by Nicolas Faucher and Magali Roques, Historical-Analytical Studies on Nature, Mind and Action, 7 (Cham: Springer, 2018), pp. 1–23

Gupta, Anil, 'Definitions', in *The Stanford Encyclopaedia of Philosophy*, ed. by Edward N. Zalta (Stanford: Metaphysics Research Lab, Stanford University, Winter 2021) <https://plato.stanford.edu/archives/win2021/entries/definitions/> [accessed 22 December 2021]

Harris, Jason, 'Latin Learning and Irish Physicians, *c.* 1350 – *c.* 1610', in *Rosa Anglica: Reassessments*, ed. by Liam Ó Murchú, Irish Texts Society Subsidiary Series, 28 (London: Irish Texts Society, 2016), pp. 1–25

Hayden, Deborah, 'Attribution and Authority in a Medieval Irish Medical Compendium', *Studia Hibernica*, 45 (2019), 19–51

——, '*Auraicept na nÉces* and the *Art of Medicine*', in *Glossing Practice: Comparative Perspectives*, ed. by Franck Cinato, Aimée Lahaussois, and John Whitman (Lanham, MD: Lexington Books, 2023), pp. 113–35

——, 'Observations on the "Doors of Death" in a Medieval Irish Medical Catechism', in *Rosa Anglica: Reassessments*, ed. by Liam Ó Murchú, Irish Texts Society Subsidiary Series, 28 (London: Irish Texts Society, 2016), pp. 26–56

——, 'A Sixteenth-century Irish Collection of Remedies for Ailments of the Male Reproductive Organs', *Celtica*, 33 (2021), 248–77

King, Peter, 'Boethius: The First of the Scholastics', *Carmina Philosophiae*, 16.1 (2007), 23–50

Minnis, Alastair, 'Aspects of the Medieval French and English Traditions of the *De Consolatione Philosophiae*', in *Boethius: His Life, Thought and Influence*, ed. by Margaret Gibson (Oxford: Blackwell, 1981) pp. 312–61

Ní Shéaghdha, Nessa, *Translations and Adaptations into Irish* (Dublin: Dublin Institute for Advanced Studies, 1984)

Novikoff, Alex J., *The Medieval Culture of Disputation: Pedagogy, Practice, and Performance* (Philadelphia: University of Pennsylvania Press, 2013)

O'Boyle, Cornelius, *The Art of Medicine: Medical Teaching at the University of Paris, 1250–1400* (Leiden: Brill, 1998)

Poppe, Erich, 'The Latin Quotations in *Auraceipt na nÉces*: Microtexts and their Transmission', in *Ireland and Europe in the Early Middle Ages: Texts and Trans-

mission, ed. by Próinséas Ní Chatháin and Michael Richter (Dublin: Four Courts Press, 2002), pp. 296–312

Shaw, Francis, 'Irish Medical Men and Philosophers', in *Seven Centuries of Irish Learning 1000–1700*, ed. by Brian Ó Cuív (Dublin: The Stationery Office, 1961), pp. 75–86

——, 'Medieval Medico-Philosophical Treatises in the Irish Language', in *Féil-sgríbhinn Eóin Mhic Néill: Essays and Studies Presented to Professor Eoin MacNeill on the Occasion of his Seventieth Birthday* (Dublin: Three Candles, 1940), pp. 144–57

Wallis, Faith, *Medieval Medicine: A Reader*, Readings in Medieval Civilizations and Cultures, 15 (Toronto: University of Toronto Press, 2010)

Walsh, Paul, *Irish Men of Learning: Studies by Paul Walsh* (Dublin: Three Candles, 1947)

Part III

Charms and Rituals

CAROLINE R. BATTEN

16. Harnessing the Monster

Principles of Similarity and Opposition in the Old English Medical Charms

The Old English vernacular medical corpus contains a notable number of incantations, written amulets, and rituals intended to heal intractable or life-threatening illnesses. These remedies instruct physicians to write Greek letters and saints' names on the arms of a patient with a high fever; to recite psalms, litanies, and the opening lines of the Gospel of John along with an incantation in garbled Irish and another incantation against 'worms'; to speak sixty lines of dramatic verse into a patient's ears and mouth while applying a salve made with a variety of herbs.[1] Such medical rituals contain both Christian and secular elements, and — in addition to being apparently important tools in the physician's arsenal — belong to a vast paraliturgical penumbra of texts permissible in the early medieval English church for practical devotion and pastoral care.[2] We can usefully describe a subset of such remedies as 'charms': texts designed for performance that also include a verbal (spoken or written) incantation, conjuration, or adjuration.[3] Any given charm consists of a different mixture of liturgical, ecclesiastical, or devotional references and ritual actions; herbal prescriptions heavily influenced by classical medicine; traditional incantatory formulae with analogues in other medieval European charm corpora; and, in a very few cases, vernacular poetry with themes both religious and heroic. These remedies are rationally conceived within their early medieval cultural context, indistinguishable from other kinds of medicine within the Old English corpus, and cannot be dismissed as 'superstitious'. Rather, they reflect a holistic approach to bodily and spiritual health that

1 *Lacnunga* 81, 63, 76, respectively; pp. 30–36, 60–68 and 70. All citations of the *Lacnunga* are by remedy number and from *Anglo-Saxon Remedies*, ed. and trans. by Pettit. On medical practice in the early medieval period in England, see Meaney, 'The Practice of Medicine'. For a comprehensive overview of the Old English medical corpus, see Kesling, *Medical Texts*.

2 On this penumbra, see Liuzza, 'Prayers and/or Charms'.

3 Roper, *English Verbal Charms*, p. 15; Olsan, 'The Inscription of Charms'. The word 'charm' is imperfect, though it designates a useful category; see Arthur, *'Charms'*, pp. 8–17.

Caroline R. Batten • University of Pennsylvania; battenc@english.upenn.edu

Medicine in the Medieval North Atlantic World: Vernacular Texts and Traditions, ed. by Deborah Hayden and Sarah Baccianti, KSS, 5 (Turnhout, 2025), pp. 367-388
BREPOLS PUBLISHERS DOI 10.1484/M.KSS-EB.5.143994

can offer insight into early medieval English ideas about the embodied self within the divinely created world.[4]

The Old English medical charms adhere to recognized semiotic principles identified as essential to the performance of any ritual action intended to have a real-world effect, most prominently the three principles derived from the so-called 'law of sympathy': contiguity, similarity, and opposition. Yet these principles are employed in unusual and dramatic ways in Old English medical charms, with narrative and ideological consequences that have not often been explored in previous scholarship.[5] Using two Old English verse charms as case studies, this chapter will argue that the vernacular charm tradition in early medieval English medicine is consistently concerned with figuring and combatting disease as a violent and intentional breaking-open of the body, an intimate colonization of the flesh by a hostile, anthropomorphized agent. In a striking interpretation of the principle of sympathy, the two medical charms examined here combat such violation by harnessing, coercing, and co-opting ambivalent and monstrous forces to operate against one another. Simultaneously, their oppositional use of benevolent Christian symbols and forces to combat disease creatures draws on imagery both eschatological and prelapsarian to temporarily rewrite the relationship between humanity and a dangerous natural world. In the Old English medical charms we can see a culturally specific engagement with profound anxieties over the vulnerability of the human body coupled with the dramatic verbal enactment of a Christian insistence that such vulnerabilities are a temporary state for the faithful.

Principles of Similarity and Opposition in the Old English Medical Charms

Incantatory and ritual acts rely on a presumed relationship of cause and effect between the action and the reality the speaker or practitioner desires to affect. To recite a charm or perform a healing ritual is to assert the semiotic interdependence of the signifier (the ritual act), the signified (the meaning of the ritual act for both practitioner and patient), and the physiological process to which the signified relates.[6] The law of sympathy as a governing principle of 'magic' was first articulated by James Frazer in his 1890 study *The Golden Bough*, in which he suggests that the effectiveness of incantations and ritual actions is predicated on the idea that 'things act on each other at a distance

4 Paz, 'Magic That Works', p. 223; Trilling, 'Health and Healing', pp. 62–64.

5 Previous scholarship on the Old English charms is vast and heterogenous. Representative works that inform the present study include Arthur, *'Charms'*; Garner, *Hybrid Healing* and 'Charms in Performance'; Hindley, *Textual Magic*; Jolly, 'On the Margins', 'Prayers', and *Popular Religion*; Olsan, 'The Inscription of Charms' and 'The Marginality'; Liuzza, 'Prayers and/or Charms'; Paz, 'Magic That Works'.

6 Nöth, 'Semiotics', pp. 59–84.

through a secret sympathy', and that 'like produces like [...] and an effect resembles its cause'.[7] Marcel Mauss later expanded upon this principle, arguing that the law of sympathy generates three sub-laws, 'contiguity, similarity, and opposition: things in contact are and remain the same; like produces like; opposites work on opposites'.[8] The ideas that like produces like and that opposites work on opposites are in fact two sides of the same coin. If a remedy employing holy water is used to cure oedema, the healing water of the remedy works sympathetically on the corresponding fluid in the patient's body, but is also specifically intended to produce the absence of said fluid.

Frazer and Mauss's works include a number of assumptions based in cultural chauvinism that must be abandoned — particularly the idea that ritual and incantatory action is fundamentally 'primitive', an underdeveloped stage in a linear evolutionary progression towards rational scientific practice. Their collective observations on the law of sympathy, however, remain useful tools for describing both the semiotic mechanisms of early medieval English charms and the natural principles of medieval medicine and science. Consider, for example, the tenets of humoral theory, the Galenic medical model popular across medieval Europe.[9] Illnesses were understood to be caused by an imbalance of the four bodily humours — blood, yellow bile, black bile, and phlegm — which each possess a different combination of heat or cold with moisture or dryness. An excess of a hot, dry humour like yellow bile is corrected by the application or ingestion of herbs and foodstuffs with cold, wet properties — thus generating a corresponding increase in cold and wet humours within the patient's body (like produces like) and diminishing the amount of heat and dryness (opposites work on opposites). In the tenth-century Old English medical compendium *Bald's Leechbook*, produced at Winchester and associated with the significant translation projects of Alfred's vernacular renaissance, a remedy for *geal adle* (gall disease) urges the patient to imbibe 'mylsce drincan sio gebet þa biternesse þæs geallan' (mulled or honeyed drinks which will amend the bitterness of the gall).[10] Bitterness is not generally considered a humoral feature, but the assertion that ingesting honey will counter the acidity of bodily fluid resembles the underlying doctrines of that model.

The principle of similarity pervades the Old English medical corpus. The short medical miscellany known as *Leechbook* III, appended to *Bald's Leechbook*

7 Frazer, *The Golden Bough*, pp. 11–12. On the difficulty of describing any text in the Old English medical corpus as 'magic', see Trilling, 'Health and Healing'.

8 Mauss, *General Theory of Magic*, p. 79.

9 For a detailed description of humoral theory and an exploration of its debated role in Old English medicine, see Ayoub, 'Old English *Wæta*'; Batten, *Health and the Body*, pp. 20–23, and also the chapter by Conan Doyle in this volume.

10 *Bald's Leechbook I*, 42, pp. 106–08. All citations of *Bald's Leechbook I* and *II* and *Leechbook III* are by chapter and taken from *Leechdoms*, ed. by Cockayne. All translations from Old English are my own.

by its Winchester scribe, prescribes the following: 'wiþ aswollenum eagum genim cucune hrefn, ado þa eagan of 7 eft cucune gebring on wætre 7 do þa eagan þam men on sweoran þe him þearf sie, he biþ sona hal' (for swollen eyes, take a live crab, remove its eyes and put it back in the water alive, and place the eyes on the neck of a person who has need of it, he will soon be well).[11] The functioning eyesight of the crab is literally transferred to the sick person, with the sheer proximity of the crab's organs apparently sufficient to encourage the patient's own eyes to return to their normal state. The fact that the physician must put the crab back into the water still living suggests that keeping the animal alive somehow exerts a revivifying force on its detached eyes, maintaining their efficacy through an invisible connection based not upon physical contact but on Frazer's 'secret sympathy'. Similarly, multiple remedies for skin ailments and abscesses call for the application of the patient's blood to a carved stick and the casting of the stick into running water, sometimes accompanied by spitting or blowing on the part of the physician.[12] One version of this ritual in *Bald's Leechbook* orders the physician to declare explicitly to the stick and the water: 'hafa þu þas unhæle 7 gewit aweg mid' (you must have this unhealthiness, and go away with it).[13] The sickness, transferred to blood taken from the site of the abscess or scaling, is borne away from the patient in the same way that the stick is carried away by the water. Disease is expelled from the body like spittle or air from the physician's mouth.

Other incantations and prayers refer to narratives of past healing and ask that similar intervention be applied to the present patient.[14] In the eleventh-century medical miscellany referred to by scholars as *Lacnunga*, a Latin prayer for an eye ailment asks God to heal the patient 'sicut sanasti oculos filii Tobi et multorum cecorum quos' (just as you healed the eyes of the son of Tobit and of many blind persons).[15] A Latin charm for toothache in this same text describes an elaborate scenario in which Christ, sitting upon a marble stone, is approached by Saint Peter, who complains that his teeth hurt and is immediately cured by a verbal adjuration from Christ.[16] The invocation of these religious anecdotes as analogues for the present patient or user's condition is predicated on the assumption that events hugely disparate from one another in time and space can be brought into direct relationship by the practitioner's verbal demand, with a point of thematic similarity giving them semiotic contiguity. It also grants the patient protection by integrating them into the order of mythic time; these remedies elevate a single patient's experience of illness into a theatre of war in a greater, cosmic battle to maintain order and health in the face of chaos, disease, and wrongdoing.

11 *Leechbook III*, 11, p. 306.

12 *Bald's Leechbook I*, 32 and 39, pp. 76–80 and 98–104; *Lacnunga*, 63, pp. 30–37.

13 *Bald's Leechbook I*, 32, p. 76.

14 On the function of these 'historiolae' in charms, see Bozóky, 'Medieval Narrative Charms'.

15 *Lacnunga*, 150, p. 104. A similar charm appears in the margins of Cambridge, Corpus Christi College, MS 41, p. 326.

16 *Lacnunga*, 158, p. 108.

This struggle is, in fact, depicted as a battle in the Old English medical texts, between human victims and anthropomorphized disease agents who seek to breach the boundaries of the flesh. In order to understand how the contrasting principle of opposition works in the Old English medical charms, we must examine these concepts in greater detail. Although *Bald's Leechbook* contains passages influenced by humoral theory, another prominent model of illness found in the Old English medical corpus is external–internal: sickness is caused by alien matter or forces entering the body.[17] Worms (*wyrmas*) are named as disease agents more than one hundred and fifty times in the medical texts, including *inwyrmas* (inward-moving worms) and *smeawyrmas* (penetrating worms).[18] Poison or venom (*attor*) is mentioned upwards of thirty times.[19] Disease is also attributed in a notable minority of remedies to adversarial entities. Spasmic and delirious symptoms in Old English medical texts, as well as certain internal pains, are consistently linked with the malevolent influence of nonhuman beings, including *ylfe* (elves) and *deofles* (demons).[20] The fact that these remedies almost always make use of exorcistic elements, liturgical prayers, and ecclesiastical *materia medica* suggests the perceived reality of these beings — as does the *Leechbook* III remedy for *feondes costunge* (the trials of a demon) that encourages the patient to put herbs under their pillow and over their door 'ne mæg þe deofol sceþþan inne ne ute' (so the devil cannot hurt you, within or without), or a remedy a few folios later for *ælfadl* (elf-disease) warning the physician that they may encounter *hwæthwega egeslices* (something terrifying) during the ritualized gathering of elecampane to treat the patient.[21]

This attribution of illness to hostile beings reveals a persistent anxiety over maintaining the boundaries of the human body and preventing incursion, treating illness as a consequence of the breaking-open of the patient's flesh by a nonhuman other. The ailment referred to as *feondseocnes* and *deofolseocnes* (fiend- or devil-sickness) is defined in *Bald's Leechbook* as 'þonne deofol þone monnan fede oððe hine inan gewealde mid adle' (when a devil nourishes a man or controls him within with disease), a quasi-possession suggesting invasion and loss of autonomy over the workings of one's flesh.[22] The metaphors used are various and vivid. A charm for a tumour, for example, addresses the swelling itself as a creature that has built its homestead (*tun*)

17 See for example Barley, 'Anglo-Saxon Magico-Medicine'; Künzel, 'Concepts of Infectious, Contagious, and Epidemic Disease'. For a detailed examination of this model of sickness, see Batten, *Health and the Body*, pp. 23–30.

18 *Dictionary of Old English Corpus* s.v. 'Wyrm', simple search restricted to Cameron Number B21.

19 *Dictionary of Old English Corpus* s.v. 'Attre', 'Attor', simple search restricted to Cameron Number B21.

20 *Bald's Leechbook* I, 63–66, pp. 136–42; *Bald's Leechbook* II, 65, pp. 290; *Leechbook* III 40–41, 54, 58, 61–64 and 67–68, pp. 334–56. See Jolly, *Popular Religion*, pp. 132–68; Dendle, *Demon Possession*, pp. 93–99.

21 *Leechbook* III, 58, 62, pp. 342–52.

22 *Bald's Leechbook* I, 63, pp. 136–38.

under the patient's skin, in an intimate act of colonization.[23] A verse charm in *Lacnunga* attributes a shooting internal pain to an assault on the patient by a troop of spear-wielding female riders. The speaker of the charm describes themselves as standing on the battlefield with a shield, sending another spear flying back at the assailants.[24] Here disease is the result of a martial defeat, a physical submission to a superior opponent who penetrates the body with a weapon. This idea of invasive, assaultive disease can also be inflected with language suggesting sexual violence: *Leechbook* III, for example, contains a remedy for a salve operating 'wið ælfcynne 7 nihtgengan 7 þam mannum þe deofol mid hæmð' (for elf-kind and night-walkers and those people the devil has intercourse with).[25] The medical texts also contain several mentions of a feminine disease agent called a *mære*, which, given its persistent pairing with the Latin lemma *incuba* in early medieval English glossaries, seems to refer to a superhuman sexual predator.[26] Humans are vulnerable to being entered and dominated through symbolically intimate contact with the inhuman: to be diseased, in these remedies, is to submit to the power of another. The Old English adjective *hal* (which is, along with its related noun forms, used more than one hundred and thirty times in the medical corpus) can mean 'healthy, free from disease', but its primary meaning is 'whole, undivided; entire, lacking no part'.[27] Health is the maintenance of the self as a continuous, invulnerable whole, without damage, defect, or point of entry.

It is therefore unsurprising that a number of Old English medical remedies make frequent use of objects, participants, and actions that emphasize or embody wholeness, inviolacy, and a specific quality of purity: the milk of a cow of one colour — described as *unmæle* (unmarked, immaculate) — the participation of virgins of any gender in medical rituals; the use of periods of enforced silence.[28] The principle of opposition evidently dictates that the incursion of disease must be countered by symbols of wholeness, inducing a state of inviolacy in the patient by countering their current, opposite state of vulnerability and openness. The patient's body is made *hal* (healthy) by contact with objects and persons that are also *hal* (whole, undivided). The use of ecclesiastical *materia medica* in remedies for ailments related to elves and demons also, of course, invokes the principle of opposition. The enemies of

23 Metrical Charm 12, in *Minor Poems*, ed. by Dobbie. All citations of Old English verse texts in this chapter, unless otherwise specified, are taken from *Anglo-Saxon Poetic Records*, ed. by Krapp and Dobbie.

24 *Lacnunga*, 127a–b, pp. 90–95.

25 *Leechbook III*, 61, p. 344.

26 See Batten, 'Dark Riders'.

27 *Dictionary of Old English: A to I Online* s.v. 'Hal', 'Hælu'. See also *Dictionary of Old English Corpus* s.v. 'Hal', 'Hælu', simple search restricted to Cameron Number B21.

28 See for example *Lacnunga*, 29, 63–64, 86 and 163, pp. 16, 30–39, 72–75 and 114; *Old English Herbarium*, ch. 104.2, p. 150. All citations are taken from *The Old English Herbarium*, ed. by de Vriend.

mankind and of God are effectively expelled by the material symbols of Christian salvation and purification, and by substances that have been directly imbued with Christ's power. These remedies use holy water, holy salt, eucharistic wafers, patens, portions of the Mass, relevant quotations from the Gospels, and familiar prayers like the *Pater Noster* and *Te Deum* as oppositional correctives.[29] One remedy for *feondseocum men* requires the patient to drink a tonic containing holy water directly out of a church bell.[30] Identifying the principle of opposition in such prominent elements of Old English medicine clarifies the essential link between bodily and spiritual health in these texts, and highlights the ways in which medical practice participates in a wider early medieval cultural narrative about the embattled state of humanity in a hostile world.

It is in the Old English verse charms, however, that the law of sympathy operates as a fundamental principle governing narratives of conflict, destruction, and triumphant survival, turning monstrous forces against one another and asserting the possibility of transcending the limitations of the postlapsarian human body. This chapter now turns to two such charms to examine the ways in which they engage with dynamics of similarity and opposition.

Similarity and Monstrous Coercion in *Wið Dweorh* and the *Nine Herbs Charm*

A particularly dramatic illustration of the law of sympathy can be found in the charm titled *Wið dweorh* (Against a Dwarf) that appears in *Lacnunga* alongside a number of other verse or verse-like incantations.[31] The term *dweorh* likely refers to a high fever (tertian malaria, typhus, or similar), given that it glosses *febris* elsewhere in the medical corpus, but it also very likely refers to a disease-causing being.[32] *Dweorg* glosses the Latin terms *nanus, pigmaeus,* and *pumilio* across three centuries of Old English glossaries — including word-lists contemporary with the copying of the major Old English medical texts — and a suggestive Norfolk lead amulet dated between the eighth and eleventh centuries reads 'Dead is dwerg' (the dwarf is dead), with a scratched drawing of a face.[33] In the context of this charm, which refers to two nonhuman

29 For a variety of examples and discussion, see Kesling, *Medical Texts*, pp. 57–94.

30 *Bald's Leechbook I*, 63, p. 138.

31 This charm has been the subject of a great deal of scholarship; for an overview, see *Anglo-Saxon Remedies*, ed. and trans. by Pettit, II, pp. 171–76. See in particular Hutcheson, '*Wið Dweorh*'; Lynch, '*Wiþ Dweorh* Charms'; Shaw, 'Manuscript Texts'.

32 See *Anglo-Saxon Remedies*, ed. by Pettit, II, p. 174; Meaney, 'Causes', p. 19; Shaw, 'The Manuscript Texts', p. 101. For the connection between *dweorg* and *febris*, see *Peri Didaxeon*, ed. by Löweneck, p. 30; Oxford, Bodl., MS Bodley 130, fol. 86[v], discussed in *The Old English Herbarium*, ed. by de Vriend, pp. 50–51 and 88.

33 *Dictionary of Old English A to I*, s.v. 'Dweorg'. The relevant editions are *An Eighth-Century Latin–Anglo-Saxon Glossary*, ed. by Hessels; *Old English Glosses*, ed. by Pheifer; 'Altenglische Glossen', ed. by Voss; 'The Latin–Old English Glossaries', ed. by Kindschi; *Ælfrics*

creatures in the incantatory verse, a *dweorh* seems to have been a predatory, fever-causing creature. After performing a series of actions involving eucharistic wafers, the practitioner is instructed to speak the following charm into the patient's ears and over the crown of his head:

Hēr cōm ingangan inspidenwiht.
Hæfde him his haman on handa, cwæð þæt þū his hæncgest wǣre.
Leg[d]e þē his tēage an swēoran. Ongunnan him of þǣm lande līþan.
Sōna swā hȳ of þǣm lande cōman þā ongunnan him ðā liþu cōlian.
Þā cōm ingangan dēores sweostar.
Þā geændade hēo, 7 āðas swōr
ðæt nǣfre þis ðǣm ādlegan derian ne mōste,
ne þǣm þe þis galdor begytan mihte,
oððe þe þis galdor ongalan cūþe.[34]

(Here came walking in a creature (?) burning within.
It had its bridle in its hand, said that you were its steed.
It laid its reins on your neck. They began to take themselves from the land.
As soon as they came from the land, then the limbs began to cool themselves.
Then came walking in the beast's sister.
Then she interceded, and swore oaths
that this must never harm the sick person,
nor the one who is able to obtain this incantation,
nor the one who knows how to sing this incantation.)

The text is certainly enigmatic, though several details are immediately apparent. These lines describe an act of animalistic violence and the exertion of physical dominance by one being over another. The assault may well be sexually inflected; the only other disease agent who 'rides' victims in the Old English corpus is the *mære*.[35] The intercession of the beast's sister assures the patient's deliverance from suffering.

Several interpretations are possible, but all operate on a singular and unusual interpretation of the principle of similarity: one or more monstrous creatures are turned against each other to banish disease from the patient. The precise

---

Grammatik und Glossar, ed. by Zupitza. The Norfolk amulet, NMS-63179C, was found in a location disclosed to the public only as 'near Fakenham' and is currently in the possession of its finder, whose identity likewise has not been published. See the object's record under the Portable Antiquities Scheme <https://finds.org.uk/database/artefacts/record/id/751600> for images and discussion of dating. For analysis, see Hines, 'Practical Runic Literacy', pp. 36–40. For a Norse healing charm that likely also names a dwarf as an agent of disease or pain, see Runic Inscription DR EM85; 151B in Samnordisk Runtextdatabas, with discussion in Stoklund, 'Ribe Cranium Inscription'.

34 Text taken from *Lacnunga*, 86, pp. 72–75.

35 *Bald's Leechbook I*, 64, pp. 138–40.

nature of the beings of *Wið dweorh* is elusive, but their danger and inhumanity are obvious. The term *wiht* is used in Old English poetry almost exclusively for monstrous, evil, or bizarre entities, while the word *deor* refers specifically to wild, fabulous, or monstrous animals.[36] The meaning of the compound element *inspiden* is unknown, but metrico-grammatical considerations indicate that it consists of an adverbial prefix and a participle; the likeliest linguistic suggestion to date is that the word is an error for *inswiden*, meaning either 'a creature strengthened within' or 'a creature burning within'.[37] Heat imagery is thematically appropriate for a charm against fever, whether the *inspidenwiht* is the disease agent or an adversary whose burning nature equips it to attack a similarly burning fever. Neither interpretation immediately clarifies what the creature is, but both readings emphasize its strength and chime with the display of inexorable power depicted in the charm's opening lines. Whatever its precise nature, the creature is inhuman, menacing, and violative, with similar connotations of wildness and danger attached to the beast's sister.

If the creature of the first line is the agent of illness, identical with the dwarf of the title, then it rides the patient to cause the ailment in question.[38] In this reading, the opening lines offer a straightforward depiction of disease as violation. Illness is a consequence of being conquered by a malignant creature. The assault of the *wiht* brings the patient close to death: the image of limbs and flesh cooling is used elsewhere in Old English poetry to describe corpses.[39] What is unusual is the sister's intercession. Given that she is evidently an inhuman creature linked to the *inspidenwiht* and the dwarf of the title, she has little reason to intercede on behalf of, or grant protection to, the patient. The sister is somehow turned against her sibling by the charmer, who, rather than employing the principle of opposition and calling on a straightforwardly benevolent force, harnesses or coerces one monster to combat another. The speaker deploys nonhuman creatures against each other rather than against the patient's flesh.

This interpretation does not account for all of the text's elements. If the patient is the creature's victim, the switch from second-person singular (*þu*, l. 2) to third-person plural pronouns (*hy, him*, ll. 3–4) is unaccounted for. There is no obvious reason that the text should suddenly begin to refer to the patient, into whose ears the charm is being spoken, in the third person. Metrically speaking, the phrase *liþu colian* (the limbs [began] to cool) represents the climax of the opening lines, which are a cluster of stylistically dramatic hypermetric verses. The phrase bears the stresses of a light hypermetric

36 *Bosworth Toller Dictionary* s.v. 'Wiht'. For example, see *Beowulf*, ll. 120 and 3038; *Resignation*, l. 51; Charm 2, l. 41. See also *Dictionary of Old English A to I Online*, s.v. 'Deor'.

37 Hutcheson, '*Wið Dweorh*', pp. 185–87.

38 This view is propounded by Skemp, 'Old English Charms', p. 294; Grattan and Singer, *Magic and Medicine*, p. 163; Niles, 'Pagan Survivals', p. 136, among others.

39 For example, *Guthlac B*, ll. 1307–08; *The Rune Poem*, ll. 91–93; *Elene*, ll. 881–82; *The Dream of the Rood*, l. 72.

concluding with a 'D type' rhythm, a pattern consistently used in rhetorically heightened passages in Old English poetry, and is highlighted within the long line by ornamental cross-alliteration ('**l**ande **c**oman [...] **l**iþu **c**olian'). It is incongruous that the (poetic) culmination of a fever-creature's assault should be any kind of cooling. The charm could invoke any number of images to convey mortal danger that were not also reminiscent of an antidote to febrile illness, and the stylistic emphasis given to this image suggests its thematic centrality. Another interpretation, therefore, is that the second-person pronoun refers to the dwarf rather than the patient, and that the burning creature rides the dwarf away from or out of its victim's flesh to cure the patient's disease.[40] In this reading, the sister is forced to intercede by the imminent threat to the dwarf, her sibling, and the image of limbs cooling becomes polysemous, referring to both the death of the dwarf and the breaking of the patient's fever. The dwarf is addressed as *þu* (you) while it is influencing or inside the patient, and in the third person once it has been removed from the patient's body. The ideological mechanism is a plausible one: some early Christian texts refer to exorcists bridling (verb: *compescere*) demons to remove them from a patient.[41] Within the text of the charm itself, the entrances of the 'sister' and the 'burning creature' are described in identical language. The fact that the sister's entrance precedes the procurement of a cure for the patient again suggests that the creature's acts are in some way curative as well, despite its evidently monstrous nature. The charmer thus combats one inhuman, dangerous creature by harnessing or coercing two others. The text operates on the principle that disease agents are most susceptible to assault from similar beings, most easily removed from the human body by other ambivalent forces made to submit to the power of the charmer's incantation. The patient's body is thus exceptionally vulnerable to incursion, but so is the dwarf's. The principle of similarity applies on yet another level: the dwarf's penetration of the patient must be undone through reciprocal violation. The dwarf must be the victim of the same kind of violence that has been visited on the patient to correct the unacceptable breach in the boundaries of the human body.

Previous critics of this charm have not discussed the possibility that *þu* (you) refers to the patient, while the third-person pronouns of ll. 3–4 refer to the creature and the dwarf. In many early Christian exorcistic rituals, the influence of demons is negated by making the patient's body unpleasant or difficult to occupy or control.[42] It is possible that in ll. 2–3a, the burning creature is made to ride the patient, in order to force out the dwarf's influence. In ll. 3b–4, once the dwarf has withdrawn from the patient, the creature forcibly removes the dwarf from the land to destroy it, hence the change of pronouns. Again, the

---

40 As argued by Grendon, 'The Anglo-Saxon Charms', p. 215; Storms, *Anglo-Saxon Magic*, p. 169; and *Anglo-Saxon Remedies*, ed. by Pettit, II, p. 175.

41 Bastiaensen, 'Exorcism', p. 132.

42 Bastiaensen, 'Exorcism', p. 139.

cooling would refer to both the healing of the patient and the death of the dwarf, causing the sister's intercession. As in the other two possible readings of the charm, monsters are made to act against one another; as in the second reading, the dwarf is made to suffer in return for causing suffering; but here the principle of similarity operates in a more profound way. One invasion of the patient is combatted by another. The penetrability of the human body is used to the healer's advantage, and inviting the creature to take control of the patient's flesh removes the dwarf. We lack the cultural and historical context to exactly decipher the action of the charm or precisely identify its characters, but in every reading, the same themes and anxieties recur. The charmer's power derives from their ability to turn malevolent forces against one another, rather than against the patient. Bodies, both human and inhuman, are vulnerable to assault, and the incursion of disease is both reversed by and punished through other violative acts.

Wið dweorh is not the only verse charm to marshal dangerous nonhuman beings to work against disease agents. Several folios earlier in the same manuscript is a long incantatory text usually referred to as the *Nine Herbs Charm*, which commands nine plants to fight against a collection of worms, flying disease agents, a great variety of poisons, and 'þam laþan þe geond lond færeð' (the loathsome one that travels throughout the land, ll. 6, 13, 20), presumably referring to infectious disease — pervasive, permeating, and borne over the earth and through the air.[43] Each plant is addressed in turn, with a description of past events that it participated in or endured. In many of these short narratives, the principle of similarity is immediately apparent. The text declares that these plants have power against poison and pain because they have previously suffered pain themselves: they have been ridden over and trampled, survived in inhospitable environments, been threatened by worms. They are not, however, necessarily heroic allies. The charm commands and demands — rather than supplicating or petitioning, as in other medieval adjurations to named plants.[44] The text nowhere signals that the plants desire to participate in the physician's remedy, and indeed they must be repeatedly ordered to remember their own past declarations of enmity against poison. The charm text claims that these plants are aggressive beings, skilled in conflict — they possess linked capacities for violence and endurance, crashing against (*stunan*) pain, poison, and the archetypal 'worm' — but nowhere does it assert that their nature is inherently benevolent. There is one exception: two of the herbs are described as having been created by Christ 'þa he hongode'

43 Text from *Lacnunga*, 76, pp. 60–69. This charm has also been the subject of much critical attention, described in *Anglo-Saxon Remedies*, ed. by Pettit, II, pp. 98–164. See in particular Banham, 'The Old English Nine Herbs'; Dendle, 'Plants'; Garner, 'Rhetoric'; Weston, 'The Language of Magic'.

44 See for example the *Precatio omnium herbarum* (text in '*Precatio terrae* and *Precatio omnium herbarum*', ed. by McEnerney), and the prayers to castor oil and periwinkle in the *Old English Herbarium*, ed. by de Vriend, chs 176 and 179, pp. 220 and 224.

(while he hung (on the cross), l. 38) as an aid to mankind. Christ himself is not addressed and does not intervene in the present moment of healing, and this short narrative is so different from the others that it throws them into sharp relief. None of the other seven plants are designed for benevolent purposes, or willing to minister to human patients without the charmer's express command and coercion. For example, the description given to nettle marks the plant itself as dangerous:

> Þis is sēo wyrt ðe wergulu hātte;
> ðās onsænde seolh ofer sǣs hrygc,
> ondan āttres ōþres tō bōte. (ll. 27–29)
>
> (This is the plant that is called Evil [*or* Cursed],
> a seal sent this over the surface of the sea,
> as a cure for the harm of another poison.)

Wergulu is a form of *weargol* (evil, malignant); it shares a root with *wearg* (n., villain, criminal, monster; adj., evil, vile, accursed), and is used to describe malevolent spirits, devils, the halls of hell, and Beowulf's famous adversary Grendel.[45] This plant is monstrous, aligned with forces inimical to humanity, and it is itself a poison. The nettle has been made to work against its kin in the past, and the charmer now calls upon it to work against its kin again. The line 'ondan attres oþres to bote' puts alliterative emphasis on *attres* (poison) and *oþres* (other, another), an unusual use of an indefinite pronoun to bear the alliteration of the line. The charm thereby focuses on the fact that *wergulu* is also a poison, drawing attention to its malignant nature and the turning of one monstrous force against another. The phrase 'a cure for the harm of another poison' is the essence of the principle of similarity.

More interesting is the narrative attached to crabapple:

> Wyrm cōm snīcan, tōslāt hē nān,
> ðā genam Wōden VIIII wuldortānas,
> slōh ðā þā nǣddran þæt hēo on VIIII tōflēah.
> Þǣr geændade Æppel 7 āttor
> þæt hēo nǣfre ne wolde on hūs būgan. (ll. 31–35)
>
> (A worm came crawling, it tore apart no one,
> then Woden took up nine glory-sprouts,
> then struck the snake so that it flew apart into nine.
> There Apple and its poison brought it about
> that it [the snake] never wanted to [*or* would never] enter a house.)

Echoes with other language used later in the charm suggest that the nine flying pieces of serpent created by the figure Woden are the source of the nine flying poisons the herbs are said to battle, and that the *wuldortanas* are

45 *Bosworth Toller Dictionary*, s.vv. 'Wergulu', 'Weargol', 'Wearg', and 'Weargolness'.

the herbs themselves.[46] The snake did no harm before its encounter with Woden — here presumably a devil, euhemerized pagan warrior, or malevolent magical practitioner, as in other Old English textual mentions of this figure — so this narrative is in fact the origin story of the diseases the charm seeks to destroy. Woden uses the nine plants to strike the serpent and create nine poisons, which are now best combatted by the same herbs that created them. The implication of the herbs themselves in the creation of the illnesses they are now commanded to fight accords with the principle of similarity, aligns them with the enemies of patient and practitioner, and suggests once again that monsters are best combatted by other monsters. The charm makes it clear that 'Æppel ond attor' (Apple and poison) operated against the snake, joint subjects acting in such concert that they are assigned a singular verb. The anthropomorphized apple may be cooperating in some way with an animate or archetypal poison, but *Æppel* is expanded in the prose as *wudusuræppel*, wild or crab apple. The raw crabapple is, of course, poison-like in its inedibility and astringency. 'Æppel ond attor' may thus be best translated as 'Apple and its poison'.[47] As with *wergulu*, a poisonous plant is turned against an archetypal producer of venom. One source of poison averts another; like affects like. Once again, the plants of the *Nine Herbs Charm* are aligned with the forces they fight.

This narrative also offers some insight into why the Old English verse charms are so interested in harnessing monsters, and why it may be a more dramatic demonstration of power than merely calling upon benevolent (Christian) forces to banish disease agents. The events presented by the charm are difficult to parse, but they bear a resemblance to two Old English narratives about the origin of illness and poison. The first, recounted in the hyper-scholarly religious poem *Solomon and Saturn II*, describes a pagan warrior, Wulf. Wulf goes to the fields of Shinar — the location of the biblical Tower of Babel — kills twenty-five dragons, and subsequently perishes. The text states: 'Đanon atercynn ærest gewurdon, | wide onwæcned' (From there poison-kind first arose, widely spread, ll. 42–43).[48] Wulf's killing of *wyrmas*, like Woden's attack on the snake, leads to the distribution of poisons throughout the world. The Babel narrative is frequently interpreted by early medieval English writers as one of pride, disobedience, and collapse, and indeed the fall of Babel is generally considered to be the origin of widespread pagan wickedness in pre-Conquest English texts.[49] The second narrative invoked by the *Nine Herbs Charm*, of course, is the Fall of Man. Though the charm does not tell the story in a recognizable form, its imagining of the creation and dissemination of illnesses suggestively involves an apple and the banishing

46 *Anglo-Saxon Remedies*, ed. by Pettit, II, pp. 140–45; Skemp, 'The Old English Charms', pp. 300–01. On the nine pieces, see further Chardonnens, 'An Arithmetical Crux'.

47 See further *Anglo-Saxon Remedies*, ed. by Pettit, II, p. 146.

48 Text from *Old English Dialogues*, ed. by Anlezark.

49 On the cultural associations of the Babel narrative in early medieval England, see Major, *Undoing Babel*.

of a serpent. Early medieval English iterations of and commentaries upon Genesis 3 state explicitly that disease was introduced to mankind through the apple Adam consumed, and that poison and poisonous plants were created as a result of the Fall and the newfound hostility between man and nature.[50] The *Nine Herbs Charm* thus draws on various Christian stories about the origin of poison and disease available to an early medieval English audience, and reiterates their central themes, including heathen arrogance, original sin, and the persistence of the devil. To manipulate the enemies of humankind and subject them to the charmer's will — to command poisonous plants to operate against flying venoms, to turn two monsters, one especially associated with wild animals, against a disease-causing threat — is thus to reassert a nearly prelapsarian power over a natural world turned hostile by the events of Genesis. The Fall is momentarily undone: disease is banished, venom driven out, and nature (which included, in the early medieval worldview, the hostile beings we now describe as supernatural)[51] is subordinated to human desires. Using the principle of similarity to harness monsters allows the charmer to restore a fundamentally Christian sense of order in which the surrounding world bows to mankind, not the other way around.

These two charms also, however, achieve this purpose through the principle of opposition. In particular, they use eschatological imagery — the resurrection of body and soul on Judgement Day, the final triumph of Christ over Satan and his forces — to cure a single, individual instance of disease with symbols of the ultimate defeat of all illness. The charms' deployment of both prelapsarian and apocalyptic references within the framework of the law of sympathy reveals their ideological ambition and demonstrates their understanding of the place of humanity in a hostile world: beleaguered and vulnerable in the material present, but assured of ultimate victory.

Eschatology as Opposition

The text of *Wið dweorh* contains the following prose instructions:

> Wið dweorh: man sceal niman VII lytle oflætan swylce man mid ofrað, 7 wri[t]an þas naman on ælcre oflætan: Maximianus, Malchus, Iohannes, Martimianus, Dionisius, Constantinus, Serafion. Þænne eft þæt galdor þæt heræfter cweð man sceal singan, ærest on þæt wynstre eare, þænne on þæt swiðre eare, þænne [b]ufan þæs mannes moldan; 7 ga þænne an mædenman to 7 ho hit on his sweoran, 7 do man swa þry dagas; him bið sona sel.

---

50 See for example *Genesis A*, ll. 936–38; *Guthlac B* ll. 1–875; Bede, *On Genesis*, trans. Kendall, pp. 128 and 135.

51 For the integration of the supernatural and the natural in the early medieval worldview, see Neville, *Representations*.

> (Against a dwarf: a person must take seven little sacramental wafers such as one makes an offering with, and write these names on each wafer: Maximianus, Malchus, Iohannes, Martimianus, Dionisius, Constantinus, Serafion. Then afterwards one must sing the incantation that is said hereafter, first into the left ear, then into the right ear, then above the crown of the person's head; and then let a virgin go to him and hang it on his neck, and let a person do so for three days; he will soon be better.)

The charm calls upon the Seven Sleepers of Ephesus, fifth-century saints who were walled up inside a cave by the pagan emperor Decius. God preserved them by placing them in a deathlike sleep, and the saints awoke hundreds of years later when the stones were removed during the reign of the Christian emperor Theodosius, who declared their survival to be a miracle. The legend circulated in both Latin and the vernacular in early medieval England, and all of these versions emphatically state that the story of the Seven Sleepers is proof of the doctrine of bodily resurrection.[52] This doctrine, articulated by the Old English anonymous prose version of the legend, is 'þæt ealle men on Domes dæg sceolon arisan mid þam ylcan lichaman þe gehwa ær her on life leofode' (that all men on Doomsday must arise with their same bodies, in which each one lived before during (their) life).[53] Not only will the soul be resurrected on Judgement Day, but the body will arise whole and recomposed from the grave. These resurrection bodies are glorified, holy, and perfected. According to Old English verse and prose texts discussing Judgement Day, when the dead rise, their bodies will become like transparent glass, taking on the beauty of roses and lilies, precious metals and jewels, and the moon, sun, and stars, with similar descriptors applied to the Seven Sleepers when they awaken.[54] The verse uses the principle of similarity to counter incursion with incursion, but the prose instructions use the principle of opposition to offer a complete antidote to bodily vulnerability. The charm describes a patient who has been entered, the boundaries of their body incorrectly breached. The prose invokes the symbolic opposite: saints whose bodies are inviolable, indestructible, more like jewels and stars than flesh. The writing of these names on eucharistic wafers — that is, the resurrected, eternal body of Christ, or, if unconsecrated, material with the potential to transmute into Christ's flesh — is a double statement of belief in the perfected immortal body, and the fact that a virgin delivers these twofold

---

52 For editions and source commentary, see *The Anonymous Old English Legend*, ed. by Magennis; Magennis, 'The Anonymous Old English Legend'; and Magennis, 'Ælfric'. For discussion see Honigmann, 'Stephen of Ephesus'; Bynum, *Resurrection of the Body*, pp. 10–11.

53 *The Anonymous Old English Legend*, ed. by Magennis, ll. 326–27.

54 See for example *Christ C*, ll. 1281–82; Blickling Homily X, in *The Blickling Homilies*, ed. by Morris, p. 109; Vercelli Homily IV, ll. 158–60, in *The Vercelli Homilies*, ed. by Scragg, pp. 87–107. For similar language in the Old English Seven Sleepers legends, see for example *The Anonymous Old English Legend*, ed. by Magennis, ll. 717 and 754.

symbols of transcendent flesh to the patient only compounds the effect. The verse charm's anxieties over the violability of the human body are counteracted, and its semiotic mechanisms bolstered, by the reminder that all bodily vulnerability is a temporary state, confined only to the fleeting material world. Postlapsarian suffering is a deviation from the intended natural order, between prelapsarian bliss and eternal life in Heaven after Judgement Day, and may be briefly overcome by a Christian practitioner armed with the correct words. If the appropriate oppositional symbol for the sick body is the perfected, holy one, then the appropriate oppositional symbol for the dangers that threaten human life is the promise of a time when such dangers are permanently defeated.

The *Nine Herbs Charm* similarly calls upon both prelapsarian and eschatological imagery in its closing assertion of healing:

> Crīst stōd ofer alde (*or* adle) ǣngancundes.
> Ic āna wāt ēa rinnende,
> 7 þā nygon nǣdran behealdað;
> mōtan ealle wēoda nū wyrtum āspringan,
> sǣs tōslūpan, eal sealt wæter,
> ðonne ic þis āttor of ðē geblāwe. (ll. 58–63)
>
> (Christ stood over the ancient ones (*or* disease) of every kind (*or* in a unique way).
> I alone know running water,
> and the nine snakes behold it;
> all weeds must now perish from among plants,
> seas must part, all salt water,
> when I blow this poison from you.)

The charmer asserts their ability to command the natural world — parting the seas — and recreate Edenic space — eliminating poisonous or useless plants, leaving only those suitable for human use. The nine snakes, presumably the nine flying poisons derived from the original *nædre* named above, behold the demonstration of the charmer's power and his control over running water, a purifying agent. This ability is presented in the context of Christ standing over his foes. *Alde* may mean 'old or ancient ones', or it may plausibly be an error for *adle* (disease), while the term *ængancundes* may mean 'in a way that is unique' or a 'of any/every kind'.[55] The image is distinctly reminiscent of the well-known motif derived from Psalm 90. 13 of 'Christ treading on the beasts', most often including a serpent or dragon. These beasts traditionally represent sin and the elemental forces of destruction, subjugated by the resurrected redeemer of man through his triumph on the cross and, especially, at Judgement Day. The motif was resonant in early medieval England: it appears in multiple manuscript illuminations, and Christ's feet rest on the heads of two animals

55 *Dictionary of Old English A to I Online*, s.v. 'Ængancundes'.

on both the Ruthwell and Bewcastle Crosses.[56] If previous portions of the charm allude to the Fall and the Passion, this line invokes the Last Judgement, the ultimate defeat of evil and death — and therefore of illness.

Whether Christ stood over 'old ones' or 'disease', he triumphs over the forces that infect the body, including the serpents and worms of the *Nine Herbs Charm*; whether Christ stood over all of these forces of evil, or stood over them in a 'unique way', his triumph at Judgement Day will destroy them permanently. Once again, the principle of opposition is at play, and once again it derives its ultimate power from eschatological imagery specifically. These two charms operate on the premise that the enemies of humanity cannot permanently prevail. They elevate the trials of individuals into struggles for the maintenance of Christian cosmic order, for the restoration of the correct relationships between man, God, and created world. They integrate a single treatment for disease into a schema of creation and salvation history encompassing the entirety of time.

These two verse charms use the law of sympathy not merely as a one-to-one set of correspondences — a hot humour countered by cold food, eyesight restored by the application of a pair of working animal eyes to the patient's flesh — but as a guiding principle governing the manner in which practitioner and patient relate to the world around them. These texts recreate in miniature the final, imminent divine victory anticipated by the Christian faithful. Disease is cured by invoking symbols of its fundamental evanescence: the principle of similarity is used to assert human power over the natural world, turning its creatures against one another, while the principle of opposition is used to remind both speaker and audience that the outcome of the cosmic battle between humanity and the array of hostile (super)natural forces broadly aligned with the demonic is already predetermined. The Old English medical charms make particular use of common semiotic principles to directly access the power of a predetermined salvation history: to assert that their users are — briefly, microcosmically — capable of recreating Paradise on earth.

Works Cited

Manuscripts

Cambridge, Corpus Christi College, MS 41
Cambridge, University Library, MS Ff.I.23
London, British Library, MS Cotton Tiberius C VI
Oxford, Bodleian Library, MS Bodley 130

56 Oxford, Bodl., MS Douce 296, fol. 40r; BL, MS Cotton Tiberius C VI, fol. 126v; Cambridge, University Library, MS Ff.I.23, fol. 195v; BAV, MS Reg. Lat. 12, fol. 98r. On the crosses, see Schapiro, 'Religious Meaning'; Haney, 'The Christ and the Beasts Panel'; Ó Carragáin, 'Christ Over the Beasts'.

Oxford, Bodleian Library, MS Douce 296
Rome, Biblioteca Apostolica Vaticana, MS Reg. Lat. 12

Primary Sources

Ælfrics Grammatik und Glossar: Text und Varianten, ed. by Julius Zupitza (Berlin: Weidmann, 1966)

'Altenglische Glossen aus MS. British Library, Cotton Otho E.i', ed. by Manfred Voss, *Arbeiten aus Anglistik und Amerikanistik*, 21 (1996), 179–203

The Anglo-Saxon Minor Poems, ed. by Elliot van Kirk Dobbie, Anglo-Saxon Poetic Records, 6 (New York: Columbia University Press, 1942)

Anglo-Saxon Poetic Records, ed. by George Krapp and Elliot van Kirk Dobbie, 6 vols (New York: Columbia University Press, 1931–1942)

Anglo-Saxon Remedies, Charms, and Prayers from British Library MS Harley 585, The Lacnunga, ed. and trans. by Edward Pettit, 2 vols (Lampeter: Edwin Mellen, 2001)

The Anonymous Old English Legend of the Seven Sleepers, ed. by Hugh Magennis (Durham: Durham Medieval Texts, 1994)

Bede, *On Genesis (In Genesim)*, trans. by Calvin B. Kendall (Liverpool: Liverpool University Press, 2008)

The Blickling Homilies of the Tenth Century from the Marquis of Lothian's Unique MS AD 971, ed. by Richard Morris (London: N. Trübner & Co., 1880)

An Eighth-Century Latin–Anglo-Saxon Glossary Preserved in the Library of Corpus Christi College Cambridge MS 144, ed. by Jan Hendrik Hessels (Cambridge: Cambridge University Press, 1890)

'The Latin-Old English Glossaries in Plantin-Moretus MS 32 and British Museum MS Additional 32246', ed. by Lowell Kindschi (unpublished doctoral thesis, Stanford University, 1955)

Leechdoms, Wortcunning, and Starcraft of Early England: Being a Collection of Documents, for the Most Part Never Before Printed, Illustrating the History of Science in this Country before the Norman Conquest, ed. and trans. by Thomas Oswald Cockayne, 3 vols (London: Longman, Roberts, and Green, 1864–1866)

The Old English Dialogues of Solomon and Saturn, ed. and trans. by Daniel Anlezark (Woodbridge: Boydell & Brewer, 2009)

Old English Glosses in the Épinal-Erfurt Glossary, ed. by J. D. Pheifer (Oxford: Clarendon Press, 1974)

The Old English Herbarium and Medicina de Quadrupedibus, ed. by Hubert Jan de Vriend (London: Oxford University Press, 1984)

The Old English Medicina de Quadrupedibus, ed. by Hubert Jan de Vriend (Tillburg: H. Gianotten, 1972)

Peri Didaxeon: Eine Sammlung von Rezepten in englischer Sprache aus dem 11/12 Jahrhundert, ed. by Max Löweneck (Erlangen: F. Junge, 1896)

'*Precatio terrae* and *Precatio omnium herbarum*', ed. by John I. McEnerney, *Rheinisches Museum für Philologie*, 126 (1983), 175–87

The Vercelli Homilies and Related Texts, ed. by Donald G. Scragg (Oxford: Oxford University Press, 1992)

Secondary Studies

Arthur, Ciaran, *'Charms', Liturgies and Secret Rites in Early Medieval England* (Woodbridge: Boydell Press, 2018)

Ayoub, Lois, 'Old English *Wæta* and the Medical Theory of the Humours', *Journal of English and Germanic Philology*, 94 (1995), 332–46

Banham, Debby, 'The Old English Nine Herbs Charm', in *Medieval Christianity in Practice*, ed. by Miri Rubin (Princeton: Princeton University Press, 2009), pp. 189–93

Barley, Nigel, 'Anglo-Saxon Magico-Medicine', *Journal of the Anthropological Society of Oxford*, 3 (1972), 67–76

Bastiaensen, A. A. R., 'Exorcism: Tackling the Devil by Word of Mouth', in *Demons and the Devil in Ancient and Medieval Christianity*, ed. by Nienke Vos and Willemien Otten (Leiden: Brill, 2011), pp. 129–42

Batten, Caroline, 'Dark Riders: Disease, Sexual Violence, and Gender Performance in the Old English *Mære* and Old Norse *Mara*', *Journal of English and Germanic Philology*, 120 (2021), 352–80

Batten, Caroline, *Health and the Body in Early Medieval England,* Cambridge Elements. England in the Early Medieval World (Cambridge: Cambridge University Press, 2024)

Bosworth, Joseph, and T. Northcote Toller, *An Anglo-Saxon Dictionary, Based on the Manuscript Collections of the Late Joseph Bosworth and Enlarged by T. N. Toller* (Oxford: Clarendon Press, 1898–1921) <https://bosworthtoller.com> [accessed 27 October 2022]

Bozóky, Edith, 'Medieval Narrative Charms', in *The Power of Words: Studies on Charms and Charming in Europe*, ed. by James Alexander Kapaló, Éva Pócs, and William Ryan (Budapest: Central European University Press, 2013), pp. 101–16

Bynum, Caroline Walker, *The Resurrection of the Body in Western Christianity, 200–1336* (New York: Columbia University Press, 1995)

Cameron, Angus, Ashley Crandell Amos, Antonette diPaolo Healey, and others, *Dictionary of Old English: A to I Online* (Toronto: Dictionary of Old English Project, 2018) <https://tapor-library-utoronto-ca.proxy.library.upenn.edu/doe/> [accessed 27 October 2022]

Chardonnens, László Sándor, 'An Arithmetical Crux in the Woden Passage in the Old English Nine Herbs Charm', *Neophilologus*, 93 (2009), 691–702

Dendle, Peter, *Demon Possession in Anglo-Saxon England* (Kalamazoo: Medieval Institute Publications, 2014)

——, 'Plants in the Early Medieval Cosmos: Herbs, Divine Potency, and the *Scala Natura*', in *Health and Healing from the Medieval Garden*, ed. by Peter Dendle and Alain Touwaide (Woodbridge: Boydell and Brewer, 2008), pp. 47–59

Frazer, James, *The Golden Bough: A Study in Magic and Religion* (London: Macmillan, 1932)

Garner, Lori Ann, 'Anglo-Saxon Charms in Performance', *Oral Tradition*, 19 (2004), 20–42

——, *Hybrid Healing: Old English Remedies and Medical Texts* (Manchester: Manchester University Press, 2022)

——, 'Rhetoric and Remedies: Or, How to Persuade a Plant in Anglo-Saxon England', in *Public Declamations: Essays on Medieval Rhetoric, Education, and Letters in Honour of Martin Camargo*, ed. by Georgiana Donavin and Denise Stodola (Turnhout: Brepols, 2015), pp. 231–52

Grattan, J. H. G., and Charles Singer, *Anglo-Saxon Magic and Medicine: Illustrated Specifically from the Semi-Pagan Text 'Lacnunga'* (London: Geoffrey Cumberlege for the Wellcome Historical Medical Museum, 1952)

Grendon, Felix, 'The Anglo-Saxon Charms', *Journal of American Folklore*, 22 (1909), 105–237

Haney, Kristine Edmondson, 'The Christ and the Beasts Panel on the Ruthwell Cross', *Anglo-Saxon England*, 14 (1985), 215–31

Healey, Antonette diPaolo, John Price Wilkin, and Xin Xiang, *Dictionary of Old English Web Corpus* (Toronto: Dictionary of Old English Project, 2009) <https://tapor-library-utoronto-ca.proxy.library.upenn.edu/doecorpus/> [accessed 27 October 2022]

Hindley, Katherine, *Textual Magic: Charms and Written Amulets in Medieval England* (Chicago: University of Chicago Press, 2023)

Hines, John, 'Practical Runic Literacy in the Late Anglo-Saxon Period: Inscriptions on Lead Sheet', in *Anglo-Saxon Micro-Texts*, ed. by Ursula Lenker and Lucia Kornexl (Berlin: De Gruyter, 2019), pp. 29–60

Honigmann, Ernest, 'Stephen of Ephesus and the Legend of the Seven Sleepers', *Patristic Studies*, 173 (1953), 125–68

Hutcheson, B. R., '*Wið Dweorh*: An Anglo-Saxon Remedy for Fever in its Cultural and Manuscript Setting', in *Secular Learning in Anglo-Saxon England: Exploring the Vernacular*, ed. by László Sándor Chardonnens and Bryan Carella (Amsterdam: Rodopi, 2012), pp. 175–202

Jolly, Karen, 'On the Margins of Orthodoxy: Devotional Formulas and Protective Prayers in Cambridge, Corpus Christi College MS 41', in *Signs on the Edge: Space, Text, and Margin in Medieval Manuscripts*, ed. by Rolf Bremmer and Sarah Larratt Keefer (Paris: Peeters, 2007), pp. 135–84

——, *Popular Religion in Late Saxon England: Elf Charms in Context* (Chapel Hill: University of North Carolina Press, 1996)

——, 'Prayers from the Field: Practical Protection and Demonic Defense in Anglo-Saxon England', *Traditio*, 61 (2006), 95–147

Kesling, Emily, *Medical Texts in Anglo-Saxon Literary Culture* (Cambridge: D. S. Brewer, 2020)

Künzel, Stefanie, 'Concepts of Infectious, Contagious, and Epidemic Disease in Anglo-Saxon England' (unpublished doctoral thesis, University of Nottingham, 2018)

Liuzza, Roy M., 'Prayers and/or Charms Addressed to the Cross', in *Cross and Culture in Anglo-Saxon England: Studies in Honor of George Hardin Brown*, ed. by Karen L. Jolly, Catherine E. Karkov, and Sarah Larratt Keefer (Morgantown: West Virginia University Press, 2007), pp. 276–320

Lynch, Katherine E., 'The *Wiþ Dweorh* Charms in MS Harley 585: A Union of Text and Voice', in *The Genesis of Books: Studies in the Scribal Culture of Medieval

England in Honour of A. N. Doane, ed. by Matthew T. Hussey and John D. Niles (Turnhout: Brepols, 2012), pp. 51–68

Magennis, Hugh, 'Ælfric and the Legend of the Seven Sleepers', in *Holy Men and Holy Women: Old English Prose Saints' Lives and Their Contexts*, ed. by Paul E. Szarmach (Albany: State University of New York Press, 1996), pp. 317–33

——, 'The Anonymous Old English Legend of the Seven Sleepers and its Latin Source', *Leeds Studies in English*, 22 (1991), 43–56

Major, Tristan, *Undoing Babel: The Tower of Babel in Anglo-Saxon Literature* (Toronto: University of Toronto Press, 2018)

Mauss, Marcel, *A General Theory of Magic*, trans. by Robert Brain, 2nd edn (London: Routledge, 2001)

Meaney, Audrey, 'The Anglo-Saxon View of the Causes of Illness', in *Health, Disease, and Healing in Medieval Culture*, ed. by Sheila D. Campbell, Bert S. Hall, and David N. Klausner (Basingstoke: Macmillan, 1992), pp. 12–33

——, 'The Practice of Medicine in England in About the Year 1000', *Social History of Medicine*, 13 (2000), 221–37

Neville, Jennifer, *Representations of the Natural World in Old English Poetry* (Cambridge: Cambridge University Press, 1999)

Niles, John D., 'Pagan Survivals and Popular Belief', in *The Cambridge Companion to Old English Literature*, ed. by Malcolm Godden and Michael Lapidge (Cambridge: Cambridge University Press, 1991), pp. 126–46

Nöth, Winfried, 'Semiotics of the Old English Charm', *Semiotica*, 19 (1977), 59–84

Ó Carragáin, Eamonn, 'Christ Over the Beasts and the Agnus Dei: Two Multivalent Panels on the Ruthwell and Bewcastle Crosses', in *Sources of Anglo-Saxon Culture*, ed. by Paul E. Szarmach and Virginia Darrow Oggins (Kalamazoo: Medieval Institute Publications 1986), pp. 377–403

Olsan, Lea, 'The Inscription of Charms in Anglo-Saxon Manuscripts', *Oral Tradition*, 14 (1999), 401–19

——, 'The Marginality of Charms in Medieval England', in *The Power of Words: Studies on Charms and Charming in Europe*, ed. by James Alexander Kapaló, Éva Pócs, and William Ryan (Budapest: Central European University Press, 2013), pp. 135–64

Paz, James, 'Magic That Works: Performing *Scientia* in the Old English Metrical Charms and Poetic *Dialogues of Solomon and Saturn*', *Journal of Medieval and Early Modern Studies*, 45 (2015), 219–43

Roper, Jonathan, *English Verbal Charms* (Helsinki: Suomalainen Tiedeakatemia, 2005)

Samnordisk Runtextdatabas/Scandinavian Runic-text Database 2020, Department of Scandinavian Languages, Uppsala University <http://www.nordiska.uu.se/forskn/samnord.htm> [accessed 27 October 2022]

Schapiro, Meyer, 'The Religious Meaning of the Ruthwell Cross', *Art Bulletin*, 26 (1944), 232–45

Shaw, Philip A., 'The Manuscript Texts of "Against a Dwarf"', in *Writing and Texts in Anglo-Saxon England*, ed. by Alexander R. Rumble (Cambridge: D. S. Brewer, 2006), pp. 96–113

Skemp, A. R., 'The Old English Charms', *Modern Language Review*, 6 (1911), 289–301

Stoklund, Marie, 'The Ribe Cranium Inscription and the Scandinavian Transition to the Younger Reduced Futhark', *Amsterdamer Beiträge zur älteren Germanistik*, 45 (1996), 199–209

Storms, Godfrid, *Anglo-Saxon Magic* (The Hague: Martinus Nijhoff, 1948)

Trilling, Renée R., 'Health and Healing in the Anglo-Saxon World', in *Studies in Medieval and Renaissance History*, Third Series, vol. 13, ed. by Joel T. Rosenthal and Paul E. Szarmach (Tempe: ACMRS, 2018), pp. 41–69

Weston, Lisa M. C., 'The Language of Magic in Two Old English Metrical Charms', *Neuphilologische Mitteilungen*, 86 (1985), 176–86

DAVID STIFTER

17. Old Irish Healing Charms and Protective Spells

Introduction

Among the written sources that survive from the medieval period and that are associated with medicine and healing, charms are probably the one textual genre that have the least real, practical relevance when viewed in the light of scientific medicine. Their curative effect is akin to that of placebos, and in medical practice they enjoy the same appreciation as homeopathic globuli. The most important aspect from the point of view of medical history, however, is that they can tell us something about how people at the time thought about diseases and what they believed to influence either the emergence or the disappearance of an affliction. But even in this respect we have to approach the matter cautiously and cannot just take the evidence at face value. Given that in the premodern period diseases were classified according to their symptoms rather than by empirical, pathological causes, even this approach tends to yield rather imprecise insights. At the same time, the study of charms is often hampered by the intentional obscurity of their language and by the material difficulties of their transmission.[1] First and foremost, therefore, the study of charms belongs to the fields of philology and religious study. Only when the fundamental philological problems have been solved, does it make sense to proceed to a medical investigation. This is clearly the case for charms in the medieval Irish tradition.

The medieval Irish literary tradition is roughly divided into two periods. Old Irish refers to the Irish language from approximately AD 700-900 and Middle Irish from AD 900-1200. Both of them are grouped together under the name Early Irish, which contrasts with Modern Irish, the language from

1 On the Irish context for this, see Hayden, 'Old English in the Irish Charms' and 'The Context and Obscure Language of Medical Charms'. In the textual editions that follow in this chapter, text between † … † (cruces) indicates passages that are difficult to analyse, understand, and translate.

David Stifter • Maynooth University; david.stifter@mu.ie

Medicine in the Medieval North Atlantic World: Vernacular Texts and Traditions, ed. by Deborah Hayden and Sarah Baccianti, KSS, 5 (Turnhout, 2025), pp. 389-413
BREPOLS PUBLISHERS DOI 10.1484/M.KSS-EB.5.143995

1200 until today.[2] Although the number of extant texts that go back to Old Irish is huge and although they constitute the largest corpus of vernacular writing in Europe from the early Middle Ages, almost the entirety of the written literature survives only in manuscripts that were copied during the Middle or Modern Irish periods and which accordingly display a large amount of linguistic interference from the younger stages of the language. In order to study the Old Irish language undiluted by later influence, we traditionally rely on a small body of texts that survive in contemporary manuscripts from the eighth–tenth centuries. These texts, the Old Irish sources in the strict sense, are collected in the two volumes of the *Thesaurus Palaeohibernicus*.[3] The overwhelming majority of these contemporary Old Irish texts consist of interlinear or marginal glosses to difficult Latin texts. Remarkably, among this material that is mostly concerned with scriptural writing and with Latin grammar, we find nine short magical texts. Old Irish charms fall, roughly speaking, in two groups: protective spells to ward off future harm, and healing charms to cure harm that has already afflicted a person. The former, for which the Latin term *lorica* is often used, are typically very general, whereas the latter often have a specific target.

Because of the manifold problems they pose with regard to reading, translation and content, these texts have experienced much neglect until very recently. However, important progress in their philological interpretation has been achieved in the past years. In this chapter, I will give an overview of all nine magical texts. After a brief introduction to, and an important textual observation about, the four incantations from the monastery of St Gall, I will provide a provisional new edition, based on personal inspection of the manuscript, high-resolution images and multispectral scanning, of the three charms in the Stowe Missal, accompanied by a translation and analysis. The incantation in the Reichenau Primer and the protective spell on a manuscript fragment from Karlsruhe will be subjected to a linguistic and rhetorical-structural analysis.

The St Gall Charms

Four charms are found on a single leaf from around the ninth century, kept in the Stiftsbibliothek of St Gall, Switzerland, and now bound together with other fragments as pages 418–19 of Codex Sangallensis 1395.[4] On its recto, p. 418, the leaf bears an image of the evangelist Matthew. The verso, p. 419, is almost completely filled with four charms, incantations, and instructions how to use them. They are for the removal of a thorn, against urinary disease,

2 Stifter, 'Early Irish', p. 55.

3 *Thesaurus Palaeohibernicus*, ed. and trans. by Stokes and Strachan; henceforth *Thes.*

4 URL: <https://www.e-codices.unifr.ch/de/csg/1395/419/o/>.

against headache, and an omnipotent incantation against various unspecified ailments.[5]

Charms 1, 2, and 4 are in Old Irish, but a line in pseudo-Greek is found at the end of charm 2. Charm 3 is in Latin, but the instructions about its use are in Old Irish. The powers invoked are various Christian figures (charm 1 and especially 3), as well as non-Christian entities (charms 1, 2, and 4). It is likely that Goibniu, who is invoked in charm 1, continues a Celtic god of smithery. His name has close correspondences in the Gaulish theonym dat. *Gobano* <**gobanno-* and especially in the Middle Welsh mythological smith *Gofannon fab Dôn* <**gobannono-*,[6] all derived from Proto-Celtic **gobann-* (smith).

The charms were written by two or three separate hands: the first three charms by Hand 1, the spell of the fourth charm by Hand 2, and the instructions for charm 4 perhaps by Hand 3. The difference between Hands 2 and 3 is first of all that of a text written in majuscule versus one written in minuscule letters. The charm in Hand 2 displays the very unusual feature of separating stressed units by interpuncts, an orthographic feature that I am otherwise unfamiliar with in the Irish manuscript tradition. I will not discuss the contents of the charms here, but I want to raise one issue, the implications of which have not yet been fully appreciated. The texts of Hands 1 and 2 show manifest traces of copying mistakes. Hand 1 has l. 2 *bé ái* for what ought to be <bēaī> = *benaim* (I strike), l. 7 *diangalar* for *din galar* (from the disease), *dunescarat* for *dun·esarcat* (they save), l. 13 dittographic *imduchenn* instead of *imdu da are* (around both your temples), which has been added between the lines, and l. 14 *dogín* for *do·gní* (you make). In l. 7, *eúin* (birds) could be a gloss for *énlaithi* (or vice versa) that was miscopied as if it belongs to the main text. Hand 2 has l. 18 *acuhrú* for *a chrú* (its gore), l. 20 *slānicid* for *slánicid* (remedy) and l. 21 *corops lān* for *corop slán* (may it be whole), where the scribe mistook a length mark for an *n*-stroke. Although one need not make much of the misplaced space in the last phrase, it could be a sign that whoever wrote it did not realize that *slán* was a word. To this we can add the meaningless sequence 'crú ceiti ménn méinni' in l. 2, which looks like textual corruption. For the second charm, and especially for its Latin passage, Tuomi has drawn attention to signs of earlier written transmission.[7]

Not only do these errors prove beyond doubt that the charms were copied from an earlier exemplar, but the nature of the errors even suggests that the

---

5 The St Gall charms are the object of a PhD by Ilona Tuomi in University College Cork. They are edited, translated and discussed in *Thes.*, II, pp. xxvii and 248–49, and Tuomi, 'Parchment, Praxis and Performance'. Charms 1, 2 and 4 are edited, discussed and translated in Carey, 'Magical Texts'; charm 3 is discussed in 'The St. Gall Incantation', ed. by Best, and in Tuomi, 'Nine Hundred Years of the *Caput Christi* Charm'.

6 The Welsh 'divine suffix' *-on* is a functional equivalent to and cognate with the *on*-stem inflection of Old Irish. *Goibniu* must not be confused with *Gobbán Sáer* (*Gobán Saor*), another figure of the Irish mythological tradition. His name is derived from Old Irish *gop* 'muzzle, snout, beak'.

7 Tuomi, 'Nine Hundred Years of the *Caput Christi* Charm', pp. 55–56.

scribes lacked a command of the language they were copying. It is possible that the individual charms were copied from different sources or from a source similar to the Stowe Missal charms written in different graphic styles. The very fact that the St Gall charms are found on the reverse of a portrait of an evangelist is a hint that its practical context is similar to that of the Stowe charms.

The Stowe Missal Charms

The Stowe Missal (Dublin, RIA, MS D ii 3 [1238]) is one of the oldest and most famous manuscripts of Ireland.[8] It is a small book of about 10 × 14 cm, perhaps a pocket reader for the everyday use of an itinerant priest or a monk in a monastery. Of the sixty-seven folios of the manuscript, sixty-five are filled with Latin material: excerpts from the Gospel of John and a missal and other liturgical texts form the main part of the manuscript. Lars Nooij, who conducted a thorough reassessment of the manuscript and its recoverable history, argues that the main part of the Stowe Missal was written after AD 796–798, probably sometime in the first half of the ninth century.[9] It is only on the last pages that we find full-length texts in Old Irish. Immediately after the Latin missal, somebody added a treatise on the Mass in Old Irish (fols 65^{v}–67^{r}).[10] The very last page, folio 67^{v}, must have remained blank originally. At a later stage, this empty space was used to record three magical texts, again in Old Irish. The charms do not fill the entire page, but space remains at the bottom for at least one more short text.

It is immediately noticeable that the three charms differ in their style of writing. However, despite their outward appearance, some letters are highly idiosyncratic and link the three charms not only with each other but also with the main part of the manuscript. For instance, in a practice that is unusual compared with other contemporary manuscripts, the scribe writes capital R in all instances of the letter. Another conspicuous letter form is that of P. It is therefore most likely that the charms were added by the main scribe of the manuscript and thus belong to the same time frame as the rest, i.e. the early ninth century.[11] The visual differences are probably due to circumstantial factors, such as the use of differently shaped quills. If the charms were not written by three different persons, it follows that they must have been written on different occasions. In the absence of manifest copying mistakes, it is likely that they were not copied from another collection, but that they are original autographs. The owner of the manuscript must have jotted them down as

8 Digitized for *Irish Script on Screen* (ISOS) at: <https://www.isos.dias.ie/libraries/RIA/RIA_MS_D_ii_3/english/index.html>.

9 Nooij, 'A New History', pp. 122–23.

10 *Thes.*, II, pp. 252–55.

11 Nooij, 'A New History of the Stowe Missal', pp. 31–35.

he encountered them in his practical pastoral duties, which probably also included the physical treatment of illnesses, defects, and injuries beside spiritual care. One can almost call the charms early, unintentional examples of a medical folklore collection.

The most-commonly used edition of the charms is that in the *Thesaurus Palaeohibernicus*.[12] Based on a black-and-white photograph, it is full of misreadings and only a few isolated lines have been translated. Warner's slightly younger edition offers only minor improvements on the *Thesaurus*.[13] The main recent studies of the charms are several articles by Borsje.[14] That the charms have received so little attention is to no small degree a consequence of the unsatisfactory edition of Stokes and Strachan. The present study distils the central insights of my own research over the past ten years.[15]

The three charms pose countless linguistic and philological challenges, but each in an individual way. The reading of the page is seriously impaired by the wear and tear that it has suffered as the last page of the manuscript. The ink is sometimes faint, almost vanishing, but the worst defect is a large stain in the upper right corner of the page, which covers part of the first charm. The first charm is so damaged that until very recently its content could only be guessed. The second charm's interpretation has been derailed by a century-long misreading of the first word, and the third charm uses rare vocabulary, aggravated by difficult readings that had caused doubt as to whether it contained meaningful language at all.

The present edition is based on an autopsy of the manuscript in the Royal Irish Academy, on the high-resolution images of the *Irish Script on Screen*-project, and on multispectral scans of the page, created in 2020 for Pádraig Ó Macháin's IRC Laureate Award project 'The Materiality of the Late-Medieval Gaelic Vernacular Manuscript (1100–1600)' and kindly put

---

12 *Thes.*, II, p. 250.

13 Warner, *The Stowe Missal*, p. 39.

14 Borsje, *The Celtic Evil Eye*, pp. 204–09; 'The Second Spell'; 'A Spell Called *Éle*', p. 201; and 'Medieval Irish Spells'.

15 I have given the following talks about the Stowe charms: 'Magic in Manuscripts. Towards Decoding an Early Irish Charm', Inaugural Lecture at the National University of Ireland, 2 February 2012; 'Magic Regained. New Readings in the Stowe Missal fol. 67^{v}', 34th *Annual University of California Celtic Studies Conference & Annual Meeting of the Celtic Studies Association of North America*, University of California Los Angeles, 9 March 2012; 'Towards an Understanding of the Early Irish Charms in the Stowe Missal (RIA MS D ii 3 [1238])', *Magic Moments in Maynooth. A Symposium on Charms and Magic in Medieval and Modern Ireland*, National University of Ireland Maynooth, 6 April 2013; 'Coming Full Circle? *c* or *o* in the Second Stowe Missal Charm', *Charms and Magic in Medieval and Modern Ireland 2*, Dept. of Early Irish, National University of Ireland Maynooth, 6–7 June 2014; 'The Old Irish Healing Charms in the Stowe Missal and the Protective Spell in the Karlsruhe Book Cover', *Medicine in the Medieval North Atlantic World*, Maynooth University, 14 May 2021; 'Reading Medieval Irish Charms as Poetic Compositions', *Medieval Medicine Workshop*, Maynooth University, 16 September 2022; 'A Grand Tour of Old Irish Charms and Spells', *Ó Cléirigh Seminar*, University College Dublin, 17 February 2023). A thorough discussion of all problems has to be relegated to a future full new edition of the charms.

at my disposal by Pádraig Ó Macháin. Even with modern technology, the reading of the page remains difficult.[16]

1. aronḍ d{ẹ}ṛ{ç}ṩụịḷ
2. ADmunniur epsc.p nibar iccas {ṣụ́ịḷ}
3. arrár roicca do ṡúil send. ẹṭ c{ạṭḥ.r?.ṣ}
4. gi cr̄ conder^{s}c lais sid cona sellai{ṗṣụạ?ịṣ}
5. rosc slán do sulo:· h̄c̃ dixisset ex pụịṭ
6. ī t̄rã 7 fecit lutũ ex puto et linuit lu[tũ]
7. sup̉ oculos eius 7 dx̄t ei uade et laua *in* na
8. tatoria siloe ꝙ +p̄tat^{ɔ} misus abiit ğ
9. et lauit 7 uenit uidens:~:~ ar delc
10. Mọ saele án tofasci delc nip hon nip anĩ
11. nip at nip galar nip crú c^{u}ach nip loch
12. liach mo aupaith líi grene frisben att
13. benith galar.) ar galar fuel:)
14. Suil suiles camull lind lindas gaine reth rethte
15. srothe telc tuisc lotar teora mucca inanái
16. bethade nethar suil naro suil taber do fual īai
17. tonert 7 toslane roticca ic slane:)

There is nothing in the language and in the orthography of the charms that militates against a date in the ninth century. The feminine nominative of 'three' is the innovatory *teora* (l. 15) instead of the conservative *téoir*. On l. 16, the relative negative *naro·suil* (what has not let flow) with enclitic *ro* is innovatory compared with *nā̆dro·*, which is the predominant form in the Old Irish glosses.[17] The genitive of *súil* (eye) is *sulo* with old-looking *-o*, but this spelling remained an orthographic fossil for centuries after the phonological merger of final *-o* with *-a*.[18] Other archaic-looking features such as *to* for *do* (your) or final *-th* for *-d* (*aupaith, benith*) are in line with common archaizing practices and are not evidence of genuine old age.[19] This practice is also encountered in the Stowe Tract on the Mass: The letters *t* or *th* for *d* are written instead of *d* in *graith, to·ciṅg, aigeth, ngrath, rosaegeth*. Other spelling conventions in the Stowe charms are rare in the extant, contemporary Old Irish corpus. The *punctum delens* occurs twice over *ṡuil*, but not in *mo saele*. It is not used in the early ninth-century Milan glosses, but occurs in the St Gall glosses, which are dated to 851, and becomes commonplace afterwards.

Together with the Tract on the Mass, the Stowe charms belong to a small group of Old Irish texts that follow alternative principles of how to mark

16 Letters that have become visible through Pádraig Ó Macháin's multispectral scans appear in curly brackets.

17 Ó hUiginn, 'Notes', p. 179.

18 Stifter, 'Towards the Linguistic Dating', p. 177.

19 Stifter, 'Towards Linguistic Dating', pp. 173–75.

palatalization orthographically. In the charms' *fúel* and *taber*, the letter *e* is a variant way of representing the vowel schwa after a non-palatalized and before a palatalized sound, instead of usual *fúail* and *tabair*.[20] On the other hand, the conventional spellings with *ai* and plain *i* occur in *sellaip, aupaith* and *benith*. In *reth* for *reith*, the stressed *e* implies the palatalization of the *th*. In *saele* for *saile*, *e* occurs as an orthographic marker of palatalization instead of *i*, while in *slane* for *sláine* no marker is used. The Tract on the Mass contains the examples *cælech, coer*, and *rosaegeth* of this practice, instead of the more conventional *cailech, coäir*, and *ro·saiged*. The fact that such spellings are never used consistently within a text is a sign that these practices developed after the more common orthography had been established, an orthography which the new practice could never supplant.

The First Charm

The three charms are not only distinct through their style of writing, but they are also separated from each other by headings. All three headings contain the preposition *ar* to indicate the object or affliction from which protection or redemption is sought. The heading of the first charm is barely visible at the very top of the page. Visible light and hyperspectral scan combined result in the reading *arond dẹ… ṡuil* (against the … eye). The stretch of text in the middle is a puzzle, even in the hyperspectral scan. Borsje originally thought of *drochṡúil* (evil eye),[21] but there is not enough space for the required letters. Furthermore, the evil eye is not a curable, medical condition. In the case of the evil eye, we would expect a protective spell, but the text has all the hallmarks of a curative spell. I prefer to read *arond dercṡúil* (against a red eye), a possibility more recently also adopted by Borsje.[22] Red eyes are a common consequence of irritations or inflammations of the eye, like conjunctivitis. This must have been a frequent ailment that an early medieval doctor had to attend to. No other symptoms are described in the body of the charm. Despite being so damaged, what is intelligible of the rest of the charm is evidently concerned with curing the ailment of an eye.

The charm consists of two distinct parts, the Old Irish charm or spell proper, followed by a Latin historiola, namely a Biblical act of healing performed by Christ (John 9. 6–7). It follows the Gospel of John closely, but is not exactly the same wording as in the Vulgate. The latter has *uade laua* in verse 7, while our text has an extra *et* between the two verbs, which it shares with the *Vetus Latina* version in the eighth / ninth-century *Codex Usserianus secundus* ('The Garland of

20 See Stifter, 'The Language of the *Cín Dromma Snechtai*'.

21 Borsje, *The Celtic Evil Eye*, p. 206.

22 Borsje, 'Medieval Irish Spells', p. 42. An anonymous reviewer of this chapter mentions that, in addition to red eyes, dry eyes and misty or blind eyes are mentioned frequently in medieval medicine. However, I do not see how a reference to any of those conditions could be linked with the discernible letters of the Old Irish text.

Howth', Dublin, TCD, MS 56 [A 4. 6]). The chief challenge of this charm is the considerable loss of text, especially in the Irish part. Up to approximately twelve or thirteen letters of the Irish text have been blotted out by the stain in the top right corner, and up to six of the Latin text. While the missing Latin portion can be easily reconstructed, the damage to the Irish part is so severe that no reasonable attempt at a reconstruction or translation has been made before. Pádraig Ó Macháin's hyperspectral scanning has revealed fifteen more letters. The new readings are a major progress to everything that went before, but the addition of the hyperspectral letters has also created new problems with the understanding of the text. Although many questions still remain, this is the provisional text:[23]

Arond dercṡúil
Ad·muiniur epscop nIbar íccas súil.
†arrár†ro·ícca do ṡúil.
Sén Dé et †cathr.sgi†Críst
†Conderc lais sid cona sellaip suais†
Rosc slán do ṡúlo.
Haec cum dixisset ex[s]puit in terram
et fecit lutum ex [s]puto et linuit lutum
super oculos eius et dixit ei:
'Vade et laua in natatoria Siloe'
(quod interpretatur misus).
Abiit ergo et lauit et uenit uidens.

(Against a red eye
I invoke Bishop Ibar who heals/healed an eye.
†*arrár*†may he/it heal your eye.
The blessing of God (and?) the battle (?)… of Christ
†*Conderc lais sid cona sellaip suais*†
The healthy sight of your eye.
When he had said this, he spat on the ground
and made clay of the spittle
and rubbed the clay over his eyes
and said to him:
'Go and wash yourself in the pool of Siloam'
(which means 'sent').
He then went away and washed himself and he became seeing.)

The textual comments are restricted to the most salient points:

– 'arrár ro·ícca': I cannot make sense of *arrár*. Borsje understands it as 'in order that [it] may heal'. Although this yields reasonable sense, this ought to be *ara·rícca* in Old Irish, with a prototonic form of the verb and a single *r* in *ara·*.

23 The Latin Gospel text is in italics.

- 'Sén Dé et †cathr.sgi†Críst': The combination of what is visible to the naked eye and what is revealed through hyperspectral imaging renders the first three words 'the blessing of God and' virtually secure, but the manuscript does not allow me at the moment to say more about the precise context. The fourth word begins with *cath* (battle), but the rest of the compound remains obscure. Probably some sort of battle armour or protection is intended. The dictionary has so far not yielded anything that would be reconcilable with the recognizable letters.
- '†Conderc lais sid cona sellaip suais†': Although individual words can be recognized, they do not combine in an overarching sense. *Conderc* is reminiscent of the suppletive augmented preterite stem *ad·condairc* <**ad-con-derc-* of the verb 'to see' or of the noun *derc* (hole; eye), but it cannot be fitted into a meaningful syntactic structure. A variant spelling for the adjective *derg* (red) would be equally possible. The purpose of the superscript *s* over the *r* of *conderc* is obscure. The initial *l-* of *lais* is doubtful, since it is invisible in the hyperspectral image. *Sid* is hardly the noun 'peace' or 'mound', but perhaps rather an error for the anaphoric particle *-side* (the aforementioned). The final *-p* of *sellaip* is very clear in the hyperspectral image, although its function remains mysterious. The letters after *sellaip* are only visible in the hyperspectral image and their reading is very uncertain.

As far as the charm is intelligible, it is concerned with referencing metaphysical authorities and appealing to their powers. The first authority so invoked is Bishop Ibar of Beggerin Island (Co. Wexford), a lesser-known saint of early medieval Ireland, uncle of St Abbán.[24] The Life of St Ailbe relates in an episode how through divine punishment Ibar was once struck by a sudden blindness, but regained his vision after the intervention of St Ailbe. Several key words of the first Stowe charm are mirrored in this episode in the two Latin versions of the *Vita St Albei*. In § 31 of the *Codex Salmanticensis* version (eleventh–twelfth century), Ibar asks Ailbe to bless his eyes (*Benedic oculos*). Ailbe declares: 'Sanet te Deus Pater, sanet te Deus Filius, sanet te Deus Spiritus Sanctus' (May God Father heal you, may God the Son heal you, may God the Holy Spirit heal you).[25] The wording in § 24 of *Vitae sanctorum Hiberniae* (Dublin, TCD, MS 135 [E 3. 11], eleventh–twelfth century) differs slightly. Ibar says to Ailbe: 'Benedic oculos meos et uidebo lumen' (Bless my eyes, and I will see the light). Upon which Ailbe responds: 'Deus unus, Deus trinus, sanet te, et reddet tibi lumen oculorum tuorum' (The one God, the triune God, may he heal you, and he will return you the light of your eyes).[26]

---

24 Culleton, *Celtic and Early Christian Wexford*, pp. 81–96; Ganly, 'The Life and Cult of St Abbán', pp. 64–71.

25 *Vitae sanctorum Hiberniae*, ed. by Heist, p. 125.

26 *Vitae sanctorum Hiberniae*, ed. and trans. by Plummer, I, p. 55.

There is a series of motific parallels and phrasal echoes between the two *Vitae St Albei* and the charm. In both sources, Bishop Ibar is associated with the cure of eyes, even though in the lives he is the patient, whereas in the charm his role seems to be that of the agent. The charm's *sén Dé* (God's blessing) has an equivalent in 'Deus unus' (the one God) (TCD) and *benedic* (bless!). The charm mentions God (*Dé*) and Christ (*cr̄*), the lives refer to the Triune God (TCD) and the Trinity, God Father, Son and Holy Spirit (Salm.). Old Irish 'ro·ícca do ṡúil' (may he/it heal your eye) corresponds to 'reddet tibi lumen oculorum tuorum' (he will return you the sight of your eyes). This Latin phrase also shares three words with the final statement of the charm 'rosc slán do ṡúlo' (the healthy sight of your eye). The meaning of this phrase is straightforward, but it sounds awkward on account of its syntactic isolation. The corresponding words are *rosc* = *lumen* (faculty of sight), *do* = *tuorum* (your), and *súlo* = *oculorum* (eyes). In addition, the Latin formula *sanet te* (may he heal you) has an exact equivalent not in the first, but in the third Stowe Missal charm, namely *rot·ícca* (may it heal you). The close parallels between the two types of texts can be explained by assuming that formulae of the contemporary healing tradition were translated and incorporated into the Latin lives. Less directly comparable, but still noteworthy is the fact that in § 12 of the Bollandist *Vita S. Ibari*, a smith loses his eyes (*oculos amisit*) when he tries to put into the fire a ring that had been stolen from St Ibar.[27]

The occurrence of Bishop Ibar in the charm is meaningful since he is associated with eye disorders, but it does not help in the identification of the disease. There is an ostensible discrepancy within the charm. If my interpretation of the title is correct, the charm is aimed at inflammations of the eye or bloodshot eyes, but the quoted or implied parallels, such as the blind man in the Gospel of John and Bishop Ibar's own condition, have rather to do with blindness. Perhaps the discrepancy is only in our modern eyes. In all likelihood, there is not one specific disease meant at all, but rather a cluster of different afflictions with similar symptoms.

The Second Charm

The second charm is headed *ar delc* (against a thorn). Unlike the other charms, no linguistic difficulty hampers its interpretation, and there is only a small issue with the traditional reading.

Ar delc
Mo saele án to·fásci delc.
Nip hon, nip anim,
nip at, nip galar
nip crú crúach,

27 Grosjean, 'Deux textes', p. 441; Culleton, *Celtic and Early Christian Wexford*, p. 95.

nip loch líach.
Mo aupaith líi gréne.
Fris·ben att, benith galar.

(Against a thorn
My splendid spittle, it presses out a thorn.
May it not be a blister, may it not be a blemish,
may it not be a swelling, may it not be a disease,
may it not be bloody gore,
may it not be a grievous pool.
The splendour of the sun is my charm,
it heals a swelling, smites a disease.)

The first word has been traditionally read as *mc*, an abbreviation for *macc* (son),[28] followed by a variant spelling of *saile* (spittle). The phrase 'son of spittle' used to be understood as an idiom for a salve or ointment, because it was assumed that salves were produced by mixing spittle with other ingredients. The phrase found its way into the *Dictionary of the Irish Language* and has been cited as a particularly quaint example of Irish idiomatic kinship expressions. Borsje's interpretation of the charm built on the premise that a son, namely the son of God, was referenced at the beginning.[29] However, 'son of spittle' is the product of philological imagination and linguistic wishful thinking. Grammatically it is problematic, since the expected genitive of *saile* ought to be *saili*. The manuscript is too early to assume the Middle Irish confusion of final *-i* and *-e*. The correct reading of the manuscript, clearly visible in the ISOS images, is more prosaic. The first word is not *mac* (son), but the possessive pronoun *mo* (my), and the phrase simply means 'my spittle, my saliva'.[30] The phrase has accordingly been removed from the 2019 edition of eDIL. Likewise, in l. 12 *mo aupaith* has to be read instead of *nip aupaith*.[31]

Unlike the first charm, it contains no invocation of metaphysical powers. It consists entirely of the spell, i.e. the words that need to be recited, but has no instruction about the non-verbal components of the healing ritual. The healing power comes from the performer himself, even though he does mention that his charm is equivalent to the light of the sun. The charm is formally very different from the first one in that it employs a plethora of metrical and rhetorical devices. Rhythmically, it can be broken down into short cola of two stresses or, alternatively, into long cola of four stresses. Rhetorical features are repetition (*att* & *galar*), anaphora (*nip*; *mo*), and assonance (*crúach*: *líach*). The first line stands apart as a metrically not strongly integrated prelude, but the rest is bound by a complex alliterative structure. Apart from ordinary narrow

28 E.g., *Thes.*, II, p. 250; Borsje, 'The Second Spell', p. 15.
29 Borsje, 'The Second Spell'.
30 King, 'Ortha na deilge'.
31 Thus *Thes.*, II, p. 250.

alliteration, there is complex alliteration between ***hon anim***, ***crú crúach***, and ***loch líach***. The sequence ***aupaith lii gréne fris·ben att benith galar*** has paired alliteration (***aupaith ... gréne ... att ... galar***) interwoven with 'gaping' alliteration (***líach ... lii***; ***fris·ben ... benith***). One could even say that the consonantal frame of ***galar*** echoes that of ***lii gréne*** – ***lii gréne*** (the splendour of the sun) is thus metrically awarded the role of the remedy of ***galar*** (the illness) because it quite literally inverts it. With the exception of some words in the initial line, every word, including unstressed words, is linked with other elements in the composition. The rhetorical structure can be represented like this:[32]

$\underline{\underline{\mathrm{m}}}$ Ṡ V dF D.
$\underline{\mathrm{n}}\ \mathbf{V}^{\mathbf{n}}\ \underline{\mathrm{n}}\ \mathbf{V}^{\mathbf{n}}$
$\underline{\mathrm{n}}\ \mathbf{V}\ \underline{\mathrm{n}}\ \mathrm{G}$
$\underline{\mathrm{n}}\ \mathbf{C}^{\mathbf{rv}}\ \mathbf{C}^{\mathbf{rv}}$
$\underline{\mathrm{n}}\ \mathbf{L}^{\mathbf{vc}}\ \mathbf{L}^{\mathbf{vc}}$
$\underline{\underline{\mathrm{m}}}\ \mathbf{V}\ \mathbf{L}\ \mathbf{G}^{\mathbf{r}}$
$\underline{\mathrm{f}\mathbf{B}^{\mathbf{vn}}}\ \mathbf{V}\ \underline{\mathbf{B}^{\mathbf{vn}}}\ \mathbf{G}^{\mathbf{lr}}$

The charm has a parallel in a much later Irish manuscript, the fifteenth-century *Leabhar Breac* (Dublin, RIA MS 23 P 16 [1230]), where the chief elements of the spell occur embedded in a wider and rhetorically even more stylized context.[33]

The charm is against a thorn (or some other small, pointed object that can intrude subcutaneously), i.e. against the inflammation and the sepsis that could result from a bacterial infection. This was probably a common medical condition. Some of the words make reference to symptoms: *att* (swelling) and *crú crúach* (bloody gore) probably describe consequences of the infection of the wound. The overt similarity with German *Loch* (hole) makes it subconsciously attractive to understand *loch líach* as referring to a hole that the wound leaves in the skin,[34] but I think it is better understood

32 The words are represented by their initials. Stressed words are in capitals, unstressed elements in lower case. Alliterating words are bold. Superscript letters indicate complex alliteration. The various types of underlining link repeated words. For the conventions of representing alliterative structures, see Stifter, 'An Early Irish Poetic Formula', p. 225.

33 Carey, 'Magical Texts', pp. 13–14, 25–27; Borsje, 'A Spell Called *Éle*', pp. 199–202. This is not the place for an in-depth discussion of this longer charm. I only want to make one textual comment: The phrase ***fuil fletha Flithais*** with complex alliteration has been understood as 'blood of the feast of Flidais' (Carey, 'Magical Texts', p. 26; Borsje, 'A Spell Called *Éle*', p. 200), but the genitive of *fled* (feast) is *fleide* or *flide*, not *fletha* with a non-palatalized consonant (even allowing for the possibility that the lenited voiced dental could be written with *th*). I rather think that *fletha* is a late spelling for *flechtha*, the genitive of *flechad*/*fliuchad* (making wet) with Modern Irish phonetic simplification of *-chth-* to *-th-*. This is the third of a sequence of three references to *fuil* (blood), the other two being bleeding caused by dog bites. It is probable that a realistic condition, such as extraordinary menstrual bleeding, is addressed here, not some vague mythological affliction.

34 So translated by Stokes and Strachan in *Thes.*, II, p. 250; Borsje, 'The Second Spell', p. 16.

literally as a 'lake', i.e. the grievous pool of an oozing wound. In the context of pulmonary diseases, *loch* refers to liquid excretions from the lungs, the 'excessive quantity of liquid or viscous material, such as pus'.[35] This interpretation also suggests itself for the present context. *On* and *anim* (both meaning blemish) give us the further information that the affliction can result in disfigurement. The treatment appears to consist of the healer rubbing his saliva, which has natural antibiotic powers,[36] onto the inflamed spot. However, we must not lose sight of the fact that the spell is in heavily rhetorical, rhythmical style and that some words may be prompted by metrical requirements, not by the desire to accurately describe a medical condition.

The Third Charm

The third charm, headed *ar galar fúel* (against urinary disease), is linguistically the most challenging of the three in the Stowe Missal. In addition to the deterioration of the manuscript, which makes several words difficult to recognize, the charm contains words that are not found anywhere else in Irish literature and which we therefore do not fully understand; it makes reference to beings whose significance is unclear, and the syntax is sometimes ambiguous. This edition presents a major improvement on previous attempts, which abound in misreadings and misunderstandings.[37] However, even though the overall sense is clear, some details remain obscure.

> Ar galar fúel
> Suil suiles camull,
> lind lindas Gaíne,
> reth rethte srothe,
> telc t'uisc[e].
> Lotar téora mucca ina n-aí.
> Beth-ade n-ethar.
> Suil naro·ṡuil.
> Taber do ḟúal i n-aí.
> To nert ocus to ṡláne,
> rot·ícca íc ṡláne.
>
> > (Against urinary disease
> > Let it flow like a camel lets it flow,
> > give a liquid like Gaíne gives liquid,
> > run like streams run.

35 Hayden, 'The Lexicon of Pulmonary Ailment', p. 114. The translation 'liquid excretion' applies likewise to the occurrence of *loch* in the parallel text in the *Leabhar Breac*, which Carey, 'Magical Texts', p. 26, and Borsje, 'A Spell Called *Éle*', p. 200, translate as 'hole'.

36 See Vila and others, 'The Power of Saliva'.

37 E.g., in *Thes.*, II, p. 250.

> Let forth your water.
> Three pigs went into their loo (?).
> May it be that where one goes.
> Let flow what has not flowed.
> Give your urine into a loo (?).
> Your strength and your health,
> may a healing of salvation heal you.)

The first three lines are syntactically parallel: a 2sg. imperative of a simple verb, followed by a third-person relative form of the same verb and its subject. Since relativity is expressed through synthetical endings, the type of relative clause is not formally marked, but I understand it to be for modality (how). *Suilid* (to make flow, let flow) is a causative verb of the W2b type, to *silid* (to drop, flow, drip). In actual fact, despite being able to take in huge volumes of water in a short time, camels are not notable for their abilities in passing water.[38]

It took me nine years to clarify *gaine*. As it turns out, *Gaíne* is the name of a small river of approximately twelve kilometres in length that flows into Lough Derravaragh in Westmeath, today *River Gaine*. The verb *lindaid* is transparently a denominal verb derived from *lind* (liquid), i.e. to give liquid. eDIL records no example of the verb, but it has one instance of the verbal noun under the headword *linnad* (giving milk) (dil.ie/30277). This is highly significant when combined with the only other mention of Gaíne in medieval Irish literature that I am aware of, namely that of a female mythological figure in the *dindṡenchus* (place-name lore) of Mide and the Hill of Uisnech.[39]

> Gaíne ingen Gumóir glain,
> muime Midi midcharthaig,
> ba ferr cach mnaí, cíarbo thuí,
> ba saí, ba fáith, ba prímdruí.
>
> Co·n-erbairt Gaíne co n-úaill
> re Mide cosin mórbúaid:
> 'Is *ós neoch* ro·sníad ar tech
> conid de-seo bías *Uisnech*.'
>
> > (Gaíne daughter of pure Gumór,
> > nurse of mead-loving Mide,
> > surpassed all women although she was silent;
> > she was a sage, she was a seer, she was a chief druid.
> >
> > And Gaíne said with lamentation,

38 For the water-balance of camels and their alleged water-passing powers, see Schmidt-Nielsen and others, 'Water Balance of the Camel'. The motif of the mighty excretions of camels is probably inspired by chapter 1, 1 of Adomnán's *De Locis Sanctis* (Meehan, *Adamnan's De Locis Sanctis*, pp. 40–43; pers. comm. Jean-Michel Picard). It is possible that excretion has been confused with urination by the author of this charm.

39 Text normalized after *The Metrical Dindṡenchas*, ed. and trans. by Gwynn, II, p. 44.

before Mide of the great victory,
'It is *over something* our house was built,
and hence it shall be called *Uisnech*.')

The Hill of Uisnech is a mere twenty kilometres from the River Gaíne. The geographical setting therefore ensures that the figure Gaíne in this snippet of place-name lore must be a personification of the river, even though the river is not mentioned in the poem. What is more significant, however, is that in view of Gaíne's epithet *muimme* (foster-mother) it can be speculated that a myth of a milk-giving figure is hiding behind these references. Probably the charm alludes to the legendary abundance of milk from her breasts rather than to water in the river. The reference to this local fertility figure and/or the tiny course of water that flows right beside Multyfarnham Abbey in Westmeath may be a crucial but hitherto overlooked clue to the question of where the Stowe Missal was originally written.[40]

I interpret *tuisc* as a mistake for *t'uisce* (your water). The omission of the final *-e* finds a possible parallel in *sid* for *-side* in the first charm. The alternative, namely analysing *tuisc* as a spelling for *tóesc* (a gush), faces the problem that *óe* is not expected to be confused with *uí* in the ninth century.

'Lotar téora mucca ina n-aí' (three pigs went into their *aí*): The significance of the three pigs is mysterious, but note that three mysterious boars also occur in the Reichenau incantation. The word *aí* has so far defied any attempt at interpretation. It cannot be any of the otherwise attested words *aí* in the dictionary (1. possessive pronoun, theirs; 2. poetic inspiration; 3. reason; 4. liver), none of which yields any satisfactory sense. The present context requires a word for some sort of locality. *Aí* recurs three lines below, apparently again for a place into which one urinates.[41] Following a suggestion by Sharon Arbuthnot, it seems best to understand *aí* as a colloquial word for 'loo, toilet'.

The phrase *beth-ade n-ethar* is difficult. The suggested analysis indicated by the provisionally placed hyphens seems to be the best way to achieve meaningful words. I analyse *beth* either as a spelling for the 3sg. imperative of the copula or as the subjunctive of the substantive verb *at·tá* (to be), *-ade* as a reduced form of the anaphoric pronoun enclitic *-side*, and *ethar* as the impersonal form of *ethaid* (to go). To account for the nasalization of *n-ethar*, I assume that the unstressed neuter relative pronoun a^{N} (that which) stood in front of it, but was lost through elision after the final vowel of *-ade*.

Although not every last detail of this charm is clear, it permits inferences about the type of affliction. Something is not flowing as it should flow. This points to prostatitis or some other disease of the prostate gland. Images of flowing liquids and water are invoked as analogues of the desired condition.

---

40 See Nooij, 'A New History of the Stowe Missal', pp. 124–40.

41 See Stifter, 'The Gravyty of Dark Matter' for a more detailed discussion of other appearances of words of the shape *aí*.

Summary of the Stowe Missal Charms

From a medical point of view, there is no common theme running through the three charms in the Stowe Missal, except that afflictions such as sore eyes and inflammations caused by subcutaneous foreign bodies were surely common among medieval, and indeed modern, populations. They affected all sections of the population equally. The third charm is more specific in that problems with the prostrate (if that is what it is about) and the ability to pass water are typically a male problem.

Formally and stylistically, the three charms are very diverse. The first seems to consist of a relatively unsophisticated litany of metaphysical powers and statements of efficacy, whereas the second is a finely wrought composition that makes use of a range of rhetorical devices to bind its structural elements together. Some rhythmical parallelism is also found at the beginning of the third charm, but it is not as tightly knit as the second.

All three charms differ decisively from charms known from the modern Gaelic tradition.[42] Those usually have close pan-European parallels, where Christian and biblical figures are invoked to exercise their healing power. This is the case in the first Stowe charm, but its fragmentary character prohibits more detailed insights. On the other hand, the third charm is similar to other Old Irish magical texts like the first and second St Gall charms or the Reichenau incantation, which feature manifestly non-Christian characters. In the second charm, it is explicitly the healer himself who channels the healing power and who frames the treatment as an act of the first person. This is paralleled in the first, second, and fourth St Gall charms, but contrasts sharply with Modern Irish charms where it is always a Christian metaphysical figure that carries out the act of healing.[43]

The Reichenau Incantation

Another magical text, a sort of protective prayer with many opaque mythological allusions, is found in a small ninth-century manuscript, a notebook of a medieval scholar, that is today kept in the Austrian monastery of St Paul im Lavanttal (shelfmark 86a/1). Because the manuscript was in the island monastery of Reichenau on Lake Constance before being brought to St Paul, it is usually called the 'Reichenau Primer'. The manuscript was photographed by Konrad Tristram in 1998;[44] the entire manuscript, which contains several other Old Irish compositions, is discussed as an artefact by Hildegard Tristram.[45] The

42 See, for example, Hillers, 'Towards a Typology', and Wolf, 'Nineteenth-Century Charm Texts'.

43 As an artistic project, the American object artist Allison Kotzig has been turning the Stowe Missal charms into an embroidered tapestry: <https://www.facebook.com/media/set/?vanity=AllisonKotzig&set=a.2652160481499482>.

44 <https://hildegard.tristram.de/schulheft/>.

45 Tristram, 'Die irischen Gedichte'.

incantation on the bottom of fol. 1^{v} can accordingly be called the 'Reichenau Incantation'.[46] Since there are no problems with the manuscript reading, I present here just the slightly normalized text.

> Ad·gúisiu Fid nAllabrach 7 Arggatbrain etir tenid 7 fraig.
> Ad·gúisiu na tri turcu tercu.
> Tairi síabair mo chondáil co n-ith 7 mlicht neich arind·chuiriur.
> Má rom·thoicther-sa in só, rop ith 7 mlicht ad·ceär.
> Manim·rothcaither, ropat choin altai 7 ois 7 imthecht slēbe 7 oäic f̊éne ad·cear.

> (I choose a wood of echoing and a silver raven [or: the wood of Allabair and Argatbran; or: an echoing piece of wood and a silver raven?] between hearth and wall.
> I choose the three lean boars.
> May a spectre come to meet me with corn and milk of somebody for whom I put it (?).
> If this be destined for me, may it be corn and milk that I see.
> If this be not destined for me, may it be wolves and deer and roving the mountains and young *fían*-warriors that I see.)

Ad·gúisiu is the 1st person singular of the W2 verb *asa·gúisi* (to wish, desire; choose). It is one of those compound verbs where the preverbs *ad·* and *as·* appear to occur in free variation. The preverb *as·* is always accompanied by the petrified relative particle *-a*. In eDIL (dil.ie/4368), *asa·gúisi* is lumped together with the H3 verb *asa·gú* of the same meaning.

The polysemy of *fid*, coupled with the reference to unknown entities, is the main reason for the obscurity of the entire text. *Fid* can be 'forest', the material 'wood', 'a piece of wood', or conceivably 'letter', if what is intended is a sortilege with pieces of wood,[47] comparable to Germanic rune sticks. McCone thinks of a wooden board for a game such as *fidchell* or *brandub*,[48] but the board of board games is usually called *clár*. The interpretation of the first line as an allusion to a board game is also strongly advocated by Forsyth: the use of *fid* is reminiscent of *fidchell*, the most prominent of medieval Irish board games, as is the noun *arggatbran* that contains the same element as *branán*, the word for the principal piece in some board games.[49]

There are several formal possibilities for the obscure word *allabrach*, but none is satisfactory. The fact that it is coordinated with the genitive *arggatbrain*

46 It is edited in *Thes.*, II, pp. 293-94, and has been commented on by Stern, 'Über die irische Handschrift', Oskamp, 'The Irish Material'; McCone, *Pagan Past and Christian Present*, pp. 207-09, 'The Celtic and Indo-European Origins', p. 15, Ó Cróinín, *Early Medieval Ireland*, pp. 88 and 99, Carey, 'Magical Texts' pp. 9-13 and 23-24, and Toner, 'Messe ocus Pangur Bán', p. 18.

47 McCone, 'The Celtic and Indo-European Origins', p. 15.

48 McCone, *Pagan Past and Christian Present*, p. 207.

49 Forsyth, 'What Game was *brandub*?'

suggests that it is also a noun in the genitive case, perhaps *allabair* (echo, whisper) with analogical *k*-stem inflection. However, it remains unclear what the echo wood, whisper wood would be.[50] The same is true for the analysis of *allabrach* as an adjective in *-ach* derived from *allabair*, i.e. echoing wood, whispering wood. In addition, this entails the unsyntactical coordination of an adjective with a genitive. In theory, *Allabair* could be a personal name, i.e. wood of Allabair, but no such name or figure are otherwise known. Carey thinks of the herb hellebore.[51] Other options are even less convincing. For instance, the legal text *Bechbretha* § 6 has the hapax *allaibrig* of unknown meaning and analysis.[52]

The significance of 'na tri turcu tercu' (three slender boars) is obscure. If this is meant as a symbol of prosperity, one might rather expect fat boars. Three equally obscure pigs are mentioned in the third Stowe Missal charm. Forsyth suggests that the three slender boars refer to oblong bone dice, which typically come in threes.[53] Before the numeral *tri*, the article appears in the short form *na* as a rule in Old Irish, even in the masculine nominative plural. The ending *-u* of the adjectival accusative plural of *terc* instead of more common *-a* is remarkable and could be triggered by the half-rhyme with the preceding word. Although several scholars interpret the *síabair* as a good fairy that will bring luck, it needs to be borne in mind that this word is usually used in a negative sense.

Condáil can be analysed as a compound of *com-* (together) + *dál* (meeting) or as *con-*, the composition form of *cú* (dog) + *dál*, i.e. meeting of dogs (wolves?). The independent dative *mo chondáil* appears to mean 'to meet me', unless *mo* is for *imo* (in my) with loss of pretonic *i-*. The interpretation of *arind·chuiriur* is difficult. It is probably the dependent form of *fo·ceird* (to put, place) in a prepositional relative clause introduced by *ar* (for, on account of), i.e. for whom/which I put or cast it. McCone tentatively translates 'for which I cast it'[54] with reference to a lot. Carey translates 'on whom I cast it', with self-reference to the spell.[55] The alternative analysis as the compound verb *ar·cuirethar* (to extend, prolong, increase; represent?, advance?; throw), i.e. 'whom/which I throw/increase (?) it', is unlikely, since the neuter infixed pronoun would be superfluous. The genitive *féne*, not recorded in eDIL, is one of the earliest attestations of *fían* (roving warrior-band).

As a rhetorical composition, the incantation is intricately wrought and evenly balanced (Fig. 17.1). It consists of two parts (an initial request and a final contingency clause), separated by a middle part (the desired fulfilment). The two outside parts are characterized by parallel structures and phrasal

50 McCone, *Pagan Past and Christian Present*, p. 207, translates *fid n-allabrach* as 'wood (wooden board?) of notice (?)'.

51 Carey, 'Magical Texts', p. 10.

52 *Bechbretha*, ed. and trans. by Charles-Edwards and Kelly, p. 99.

53 Forsyth, 'What Game was *brandub*?'

54 McCone, 'The Celtic and Indo-European Origins', p. 15. McCone, *Pagan Past and Christian Present*, p. 207, translates 'of whatever I move it for', perhaps with reference to game pieces.

55 Carey, 'Magical Texts', p. 24.

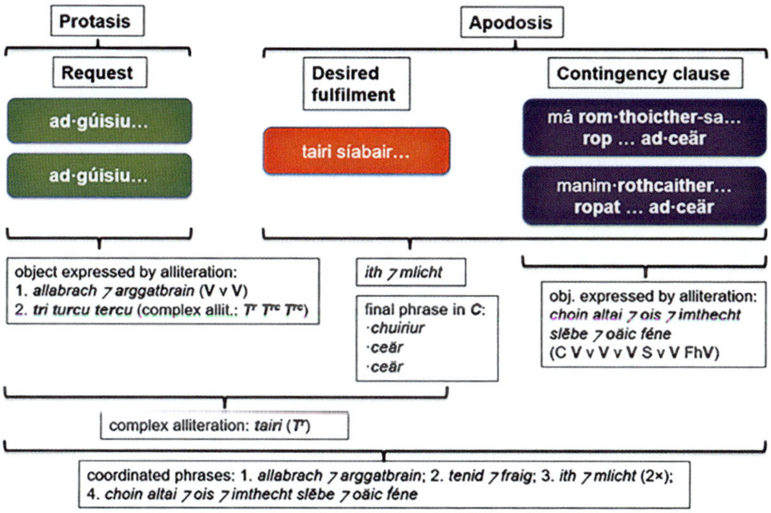

Figure 17.1. Rhetorical-structural analysis of the Reichenau Incantation. Image by author.

repetition: in the request *ad·gúisiu* is repeated; the contingency clause has 'má rom·thoicther-sa ... rop ... ad·ceär' and 'manim·rothcaither... ropat ... ad·ceär'. In the request and the contingency clause, the objects are expressed by alliteration: 1. ***a**llabrach ⁊ **a**rggatbrain* (**V** v **V**); 2. ***t**ri **t**urcu **t**ercu* (complex alliteration: ***T**ʳ* ***T**ʳᶜ* ***T**ʳᶜ*); *choin **a**ltai ⁊ **o**is ⁊ **i**mthecht slēbe ⁊ **o**äic féne* (C **V** v **V** v **V** S v **V** FhV). The clause-final verbs of the middle and final part are bound together through complex alliteration (*arind·**ch**uiriur*: *ad·**ce**är*: *ad·**ce**är*; **vC**ʳ **vC**ʳ **vC**ʳ), as is the initial part with the middle part (***t**ri **t**urcu **t**ercu*: ***t**airi*; ***T**ʳ* ***T**ʳᶜ* ***T**ʳᶜ* ***T**ʳ*).

Coordinated phrases dominate the composition: 1. *allabrach ⁊ arggatbrain*; 2. *tenid ⁊ fraig*; 3. *ith ⁊ mlicht* (2×); 4. *choin altai ⁊ ois ⁊ imthecht slēbe ⁊ oäic féne*. Both *etir tenid ⁊ fraig* (between hearth and wall) and *ith ⁊ mlicht* (grain and milk) are merisms that indicate totalities. The first refers to the entirety of the household, the second one to agriculturalism. Ultimately, however, the purpose of this incantation remains as opaque as its references to concepts and beings that we no longer understand.

The Karlsruhe Prayer

Despite being included in the *Thesaurus Palaeohibernicus*,[56] the Karlsruhe prayer has almost completely escaped the attention of previous scholarship.

56 *Thes.*, II, p. 256.

It is a short prayer for protection, almost a condensed *lorica*, on a fragmentary folio originally from the monastery on the Reichenau, but today kept in the Badische Landesbibliothek in Karlsruhe in Germany (MS Aug. Fr. 18).[57] The fragment contains for the most part Latin text, plus a considerable passage in Old Irish. It has been dated to the beginning of the ninth century.[58]

The folio has been repurposed as a cover for another Karlsruhe manuscript, one with the works of the Venerable Bede (MS Aug. Perg. 167).[59] For that purpose, it had been cut up, which has led to the loss of most of what appears to have been an originally extensive continuous piece of Old Irish prose on the first column. The catalogue calls the Latin part of the fragment a *sacramentarium*; Holder gives a diplomatic edition.[60] From isolated Old Irish words such as *audpairtt* (offering), *turcbail* (raising [of the host]), *sacar[t]* (priest), *aithir[ge]* (penitence), etc.,[61] it can be inferred that the Old Irish prose text may have been of a similar nature to the Stowe Tract on the Mass. The available digital image does not allow a more detailed identification, but a close investigation of the physical manuscript may reveal more text. The second column remains in its entirety, although most of it has been rendered illegible by virtue of having been pasted over with another page. Fortunately, the three lines with the Old Irish prayer on the top have remained intact. The fact that this protective spell had been added to a Christian, liturgical manuscript links this fragment with the Stowe Missal, but also with the St Gall charms. Like those texts, the wider context is not medical.

I provide first a close diplomatic transcription, followed by a normalized edition of the incantation:

> Dithólu æchtrann et námat et gein
> te · et fochide · diphlágaib tened et nói
> ne · et gorte et galræ n̄ile n̄écsāle

> Di thólu æchtrann *et* námat *et* geinte *et* fochide, di phlágaib tened *et* noíne *et* gorte *et* galræ n-ile n-écsamle.

> ([Protect me/us] from a flood of foreigners and foes and heathens and tribulations, from plagues of fire and famine and hunger and of many diverse diseases.)

This is not a healing charm like the ones before, but an almost universal protective spell. The preposition *di*, recognizable as the beginning of the text by its capital letter, depends on an imperative 'protect me/us', e.g. *nom/n·anaich, dom/n·eim, dom/n·essuirc, nom/n·ícc*, which is not expressed. The proposed

---

57 URL: <https://digital.blb-karlsruhe.de/blbhs/content/zoom/26812>. Catalogue information at <https://digital.blbkarlsruhe.de/blbhs/content/titleinfo/21598>.

58 Holder, *Handschriften der Badischen Landesbibliothek*, p. 376.

59 Edited in *Thes.*, II, pp. 10-30.

60 Holder, *Handschriften der Badischen Landesbibliothek*, pp. 376–79.

61 See *Thes.*, II, pp. 252-55.

date of the fragment in the first third of the ninth century conforms with the contents of the incantation. Most of the summarily enumerated afflictions in the incantation are non-medical in nature. The reference to *geinti* (heathens) as an existential threat allows us to read it as a prayer for protection from Viking attacks. The use of this word in the *Annals of Ulster* starts famously with the first Viking attacks in 795 and becomes common after 812. That incursions by 'foreigners and enemies and heathens' are mentioned even before fire and famine reveals what a traumatic experience Viking attacks must have been for people in Ireland at the time. There is no reference to any specific disease in the incantation. Instead, the extremely rare collective noun *galrae* (diseases) is used, a word that, outside the present text, is only attested a single time in a Middle Irish text.[62] It is remarkable that the lenition in *di phlágaib* is graphically expressed through *ph*. Such a spelling is entirely absent from the eighth-century Würzburg and early-ninth-century Milan Glosses, and extremely rare in the mid-ninth-century St Gall Glosses.

Conclusion

Nine short magical texts in the Old Irish language survive in four contemporary manuscript sources, all probably from the ninth century. Although two of those sources, the St Gall folio and the Karlsruhe cover leaf, are fragmentary, it is still evident that in all cases the charms and incantations were added later than the main text of the manuscripts. None of the sources is a dedicated collection of charms, but in each case free manuscript space was repurposed to record the magical texts for the practical daily purposes of the owners of the manuscripts. The charms are preponderantly healing charms, mostly for specific ailments, but in one case also for very general application. One text (the Karlsruhe fragment) is a protective charm, while one appears to be an incantation for luck in life (the Reichenau Primer). Significantly, both are the only magical texts in their manuscripts, while the genuine healing charms occur in groups of three (the Stowe Missal) and four (the St Gall fragment). Furthermore, the latter two occur both together with Gospels or missals. This can be understood as indirect evidence that the healing charms were used by priests in their practical, everyday pastoral activities. The charms may have constituted the last resort where other means of healing had shown no effect.

It is remarkable that in both cases references to Christian saints and other metaphysical entities are found side by side with invocations of clearly non-Christian, possibly pre-Christian figures. It seems that the practitioners, who were using these charms, saw no fundamental conflict between the two worlds. From a stylistic point of view, it is noteworthy that the metrical

62 *The Passions and Homilies*, ed. and trans. by Atkinson, l. 2494.

complexity of the magical texts is inversely proportional to their Christian context, i.e. the fewer overtly Christian references are contained in a charm, the more complex its metrical and rhetorical ornamentation is. This can be taken as an indication that the metrically complex compositions form part of a long oral tradition. Furthermore, in content and form the contemporary Old Irish healing charms are very different from the later Irish charming tradition, especially in the modern period, which largely follows common European trends.

Works Cited

Manuscripts

Carinthia, St Paul im Lavanttal, Stiftsbibliothek, MS 86a/1 ('The Reichenau Primer')

Dublin, Royal Irish Academy, MS D ii 3 (1238) ('The Stowe Missal')

Dublin, Royal Irish Academy, MS 23 P 16 (1230) ('The Leabhar Breac')

Dublin, Trinity College, MS 56 (A 4. 6) ('The Garland of Howth')

Dublin, Trinity College, MS 135 (E 3. 11)

Karlsruhe, Badische Landesbibliothek, MS Aug. Fr. 18

Karlsruhe, Badische Landesbibliothek, MS Aug. Perg. 167

St Gall, Stiftsbibliothek, MS 1395

Primary Sources

Bechbretha. An Old Irish Law-tract on Bee-keeping, ed. and trans. by Thomas Charles-Edwards and Fergus Kelly, Early Irish Law Series, 1 (Dublin: DIAS, 1983)

The Metrical Dindsenchas. Part II. Text, Translation, and Commentary, ed. and trans. by Edward Gwynn, Todd Lecture Series, 9 (Dublin: Royal Irish Academy, 1906)

The Passions and the Homilies from Leabhar Breac: Text, Translation and Glossary, ed. and trans. by Robert Atkinson, Todd Lecture Series, 2 (Dublin: Hodges & Figgis, 1887)

'The St. Gall Incantation against Headache', ed. by Richard I. Best, *Ériu*, 8 (1915), 100

Thes. = *Thesaurus Palaeohibernicus. A Collection of Old-Irish Glosses Scholia Prose and Verse*, ed. and trans. by Whitley Stokes and John Strachan, 2 vols (Cambridge: Cambridge University Press, 1901–1903)

Vitae sanctorum Hiberniae. Ex codice olim Salmanticensi nunc Bruxellensi, ed. by William W. Heist, Subsidia Hagiographica, 28 (Brussels: Société des Bollandistes, 1965)

Vitae sanctorum Hiberniae, partim hactenus ineditae. Vol. 1, ed. and trans. by Charles Plummer (Oxford: Clarendon Press, 1910)

Secondary Studies

Borsje, Jacqueline, *The Celtic Evil Eye and Related Mythological Motifs in Medieval Irish*, Studies in the History and Anthropology of Religion, 2 (Leuven: Peeters, 2012)

——, 'Medieval Irish Spells: "Words of Power" as Performance', in *Words. Religious Language Matters*, ed. by Ernst van den Hemel and Asja Szafraniec (New York: Fordham University Press, 2016), pp. 35–53 and 468–76

——, 'The Second Spell in the Stowe Missal', in *Lochlann. Festskrift til Jan Erik Rekdal på 60-årsdagen. Aistí in ómós do Jan Erik Rekdal ar a 60ú lá breithe*, ed. by Cathinka Hambro and Lars Ivar Widerøe (Oslo: Hermes, 2013), pp. 12–26

——, 'A Spell Called *Éle*', in *Ulidia 3. Proceedings of the Third International Conference on the Ulster Cycle of Tales, University of Ulster, Coleraine, 22-25 June, 2009*, ed. by Gregory Toner and Séamus Mac Mathúna (Berlin: Curach Bhán, 2013), pp. 193–212

Carey, John, 'Chapter One. Magical Texts in Early Medieval Ireland', in *Magic, Metallurgy and Imagination in Medieval Ireland. Three Studies*, Celtic Studies Publications, 21 (Aberystwyth: Celtic Studies Publications, 2019), pp. 1-27 (='Téacsanna draíochta in Éirinn sa mheánaois luath' [aistr. P. Ó Fiannachta], in *Breis faoinár ndúchas spioradálta*, ed. by Ruairí Ó hUiginn, Léachtaí Cholm Chille, 30 [Maigh Nuad, 2000], pp. 98-117)

Culleton, Edward, *Celtic and Early Christian Wexford. AD 400 to 1166* (Dublin: Four Courts Press, 1999)

eDIL = eDIL 2019: *An Electronic Dictionary of the Irish Language*, based on the Contributions to a Dictionary of the Irish Language (Dublin: Royal Irish Academy, 1913–1976) <www.dil.ie 2019> [accessed 18 January 2023]

Forsyth, Katherine, 'What Game was *brandub*?' (forthcoming)

Ganly, Ellen, 'The Life and Cult of St. Abbán: A Dossier Study' (unpublished doctoral thesis, Maynooth University, 2020)

Grosjean, Paul, 'Deux textes inédits sur S. Ibar', *Analecta Bollandiana*, 77 (1959), 426–50

Hayden, Deborah, 'The Context and Obscure Language of Medical Charms in a Sixteenth-century Irish Remedy Book: Four Case Studies', in *Obscuritas in Medieval Irish and Welsh Literature*, ed. by Chantal Kobel (Dublin: DIAS, forthcoming)

——, 'The Lexicon of Pulmonary Ailment in some Medieval Irish Medical Texts', *Zeitschrift für celtische Philologie*, 66 (2019), 105–30

——, 'Old English in the Irish Charms', *Speculum*, 97.2 (2022), 349–76

Hillers, Barbara, 'Towards a Typology of European Narrative Charms in Irish Oral Tradition', in *Charms, Charmers and Charming in Ireland. From the Medieval to the Modern*, ed. by Ilona Tuomi, John Carey, Barbara Hillers, and Ciarán Ó Gealbháin (Cardiff: University of Wales Press, 2019), pp. 79–102

Holder, Alfred, *Die Handschriften der Badischen Landesbibliothek in Karlsruhe. VI. Die Reichenauer Handschriften. Zweiter Band. Die Papierhandschriften. Fragmenta. Nachträge. Nachdruck mit bibliographischen Nachträgen* (Wiesbaden: Harrassowitz, 1971)

ISOS = Irish Script on Screen <www.isos.dias.ie> [accessed 22 January 2023]

King, Dennis, 'Ortha na deilge' (10 June 2009) <http://nimill.blogspot.ie/2009/06/ortha-na-deilge.html> [accessed 21 January 2023]

McCone, Kim, 'The Celtic and Indo-European Origins of the *fían*', in *The Gaelic Finn Tradition*, ed. by Sharon J. Arbuthnot and Geraldine Parsons (Dublin: Four Courts Press, 2012), pp. 14–30

——, *Pagan Past and Christian Present in Early Irish Literature* (Maynooth: Department of Old and Middle Irish, 1990)

Meehan, Denis, *Adamnan's De Locis Sanctis*, Scriptores Latini Hiberniae, 3 (Dublin: Dublin Institute for Advanced Studies, 1983)

Nooij, Lars B., 'A New History of the Stowe Missal' (unpublished doctoral thesis, Maynooth University, 2021)

Ó Cróinín, Dáibhí, *Early Medieval Ireland 400-1200* (Harlow: Longman, 1995)

Ó hUiginn, Ruairí, 'Notes on Old Irish Syntax', *Ériu*, 38 (1987), 177–83

Oskamp, Hans P. A. 'The Irish Material in the St. Paul Irish Codex', *Éigse*, 17.3 (1978), 385–91

Schmidt-Nielsen, Bodil, Knut Schmidt-Nielsen, Thomas R. Houpt, and Stig A. Jarnum, 'Water Balance of the Camel', *American Journal of Physiology*, 185.1 (1956), 185–94

Stern, Ludwig Christian, 'Über die irische Handschrift in St Paul', *Zeitschrift für celtische Philologie*, 6 (1908), 546–55

Stifter, David, 'Early Irish', in *The Celtic Languages*, ed. by Martin J. Ball and Nicole Müller, 2nd edn (Abingdon: Routledge, 2009), pp. 55–116

——, 'An Early Irish Poetic Formula', in *Fír Fesso: A Festschrift for Neil McLeod*, ed. by Anders Ahlqvist and Pamela O'Neill, Sydney Series in Celtic Studies, 17 (Celtic Studies Foundation: University of Sydney, 2018), pp. 223–32

——, 'The Gravyty of Dark Matter. An Edition of *Fil and griän Glinne Aí*', in *Obscuritas in Medieval Irish and Welsh Literature*, ed. by Chantal Kobel (Dublin: DIAS, forthcoming)

——, 'The Language of the *Cín Dromma Snechtai* Texts', in *23 N 10. The Book of Ballycummin*, ed. by Elizabeth Boyle and Ruairí Ó hUiginn, Codices Hibernenses Eximii, 4 (Dublin: Royal Irish Academy, forthcoming)

——, 'Towards the Linguistic Dating of Early Irish Law Texts', in *Medieval Irish Law. Text and Context*, ed. by Anders Ahlqvist and Pamela O'Neill, Sydney Series in Celtic Studies, 12 (Celtic Studies Foundation: University of Sydney, 2013), pp. 163–208

Toner, Gregory, '"Messe ocus Pangur Bán": Structure and Cosmology', *Cambrian Medieval Celtic Studies*, 57 (2009), 1–22

Tristram, Hildegard L. C., 'Die irischen Gedichte im Reichenauer Schulheft', in *Studia Celtica et Indogermanica. Festschrift für Wolfgang Meid zum 70. Geburtstag*, ed. by Peter Anreiter und Erzsébet Jerem (Budapest: Archaeolingua, 1999), pp. 503–29

Tuomi, Ilona, 'Nine Hundred Years of the *Caput Christi* Charm: Scribal Strategies and Textual Transmission', in *Charms, Charmers and Charming in Ireland. From the Medieval to the Modern*, ed. by Ilona Tuomi, John Carey, Barbara Hillers, and Ciarán Ó Gealbháin (Cardiff: University of Wales Press, 2019), pp. 51–64

——, 'Parchment, Praxis and Performance of Charms in Early Medieval Ireland', *Incantatio*, 3 (2013), 60–85 <doi 10.7592/Incantatio2013_Tuomi>

Vila, Taissa, Alexandra M. Rizk, Ahmed S. Sultan, and Mary Ann Jabra-Rizk, 'The Power of Saliva: Antimicrobial and Beyond', *PLoS Pathog*, 15.11 (2019), e1008058 <https://doi.org/10.1371/journal.ppat.1008058>

Warner, George F., *The Stowe Missal: MS. D. II. 3 in the Library of the Royal Irish Academy, Dublin*, 2 vols (London: Henry Bradshaw Society, 1906–1915)

Wolf, Nicholas M., 'Nineteenth-Century Charm Texts: Scope and Context', in *Charms, Charmers and Charming in Ireland. From the Medieval to the Modern*, ed. by Ilona Tuomi, John Carey, Barbara Hillers, and Ciarán Ó Gealbháin (Cardiff: University of Wales Press, 2019), pp. 103–15

DEBORAH HAYDEN

18. Premodern Irish Rituals for Conception and Childbirth in their Insular Context*

Ritual cures relating to fertility, conception, and childbirth occur frequently in the extant written sources for many premodern European medical traditions and reflect the centrality of procreation to religious belief and societal custom of the period. The phrase 'performative rituals' has recently been used by Peter Murray Jones and Lea T. Olsan as a wide-ranging designation for remedies involving verbal charms, prayers, ligatures, amulets, and/or physical gestures or sequences of actions utilizing special objects; such actions might include 'eating or drinking words, and touching, wrapping, or tying things to the body'.[1] As those authors have also pointed out, healing rituals of this kind were often recorded and developed alongside, and sometimes as part of, academic texts on gynaecology that circulated across western Europe. For example, a handful of remedies for difficult birth that are found in the *Trotula* collection of texts on women's medicine and cosmetics, composed in Salerno during the twelfth century, rely on symbolic actions such as drinking a string of letters with the milk of another woman or using the skin of a snake as a birthing girdle.[2] Although some such cures are also attested in earlier sources, they gained popularity by way of their inclusion in the *Trotula* collection, which was translated into numerous European vernaculars during the later Middle Ages.[3]

The aim of this chapter is to discuss the preservation and wider context of some ritual texts relating to fertility and childbirth in the comparatively

* I am grateful to David Stifter and Sarah Baccianti for reading an earlier draft of this paper and for offering several valuable comments. I alone am responsible for any errors or omissions that might remain.

1 Murray Jones and Olsan, 'Performative Rituals', p. 408.

2 Murray Jones and Olsan, 'Performative Rituals', pp. 408–09, citing *The 'Trotula'*, ed. and trans. by Green, pp. 100–03 (§§ 98, 100 and 102).

3 On the transmission of the *Trotula* collection in western Europe, including its vernacular translations, see Green, 'A Handlist [...] Part I' and Green, 'A Handlist [...] Part II'.

Deborah Hayden • Maynooth University; deborah.hayden@mu.ie

Medicine in the Medieval North Atlantic World: Vernacular Texts and Traditions, ed. by Deborah Hayden and Sarah Baccianti, KSS, 5 (Turnhout, 2025), pp. 415-437
BREPOLS PUBLISHERS DOI 10.1484/M.KSS-EB.5.143996

understudied vernacular medical sources from premodern Ireland, focusing primarily on the manuscript transmission of one particular ritual that seems to have been intended either to cause impotence in a man or to test the chastity of a woman.[4] Textual witnesses of the ritual in question are preserved either within remedy collections or as marginal annotations in a handful of late-medieval Irish medical manuscripts, occasionally alongside a so-called 'love charm' that, although apparently intended to serve the opposite purpose of inducing affection, employs similar *voces magicae* or 'words of power' to effect the desired outcome. It is argued that the origins and purpose of these Irish ritual texts can be illuminated by way of comparison with medical and literary sources recorded in other languages of the Insular world, including Latin, English, and Welsh. They also provide insight, however, into the nexus between theoretical medicine, traditional healing practices, and sexual *mores* as they pertained to the mysterious and often perilous matters of conception and childbirth throughout the Middle Ages and into the modern period.

Irish Rituals for Fertility and Childbirth in their European Context

Although the extant Irish-language medical manuscripts that were copied between *c.* 1350–1700 contain a rich array of verbal incantations, textual amulets, and other types of ritual remedies, most of these have never before been published and their relationship to other contemporary vernacular literary traditions has received only limited and sporadic attention in modern scholarship.[5] Other categories of text have, however, been somewhat better served as sources for Irish charms: an example of which is R. I. Best's 1952 edition and translation of nine ritual remedies gleaned from the margins and vacant spaces of certain law tracts in Dublin, Trinity College, MS 1336 (H 3. 17), a composite codex dating to the fifteenth and sixteenth centuries.[6] Among the charms published in Best's edition is the following advice concerning conception, which was written on a slip of vellum (col. 672b of the manuscript) alongside material relating to poetry and the legal compensation due to poets:

> Ben beres ingena iss *ed* foires, fiacail eich do beith fo braigit i n-eill do craicend roin forsa cantar .uii. n-aifrind 7 beraid mac. Maria peperit

4 For a discussion of other Irish remedies intended to cure or cause impotence, several of which involve ritual elements, see 'A Sixteenth-Century Irish Collection', ed. and trans. by Hayden.

5 For a general discussion of this desideratum, see Hayden, 'Old English in the Irish Charms', pp. 351–55, and citations therein. A recent contribution to the subject relevant to the present study is Rempt, 'And Straightaway', which includes an edition of one copy of the charm discussed in the last section of this article; Rempt describes it as a charm for 'conception' (pp. 92–94).

6 'Some Irish Charms', ed. and trans. by Best.

Christum, Anna Maria, Elisabeth Ihoandem, Celina Remigium[7] + n + Sa*tur* 7rl. Ar breith aibeil do mnai.

> (A woman who bears daughters, this is what helps: a horse's tooth to be round her neck in a sealskin thong over which seven masses are sung, and she will bring forth a boy. Mary bore Jesus, Anna Mary, Elisabeth John, Cylinia Remigius. In nomine patris, etc.[8] For a speedy delivery to a woman.)[9]

Although Best offered minimal contextual commentary on the charms that he edited from the H 3. 17 manuscript, he did note a parallel for the above text in Dublin, Royal Irish Academy, MS 24 B 3, p. 77.[10] The latter is a medical manuscript written primarily by the North Connacht medical scribe and doctor Conla Mac an Leagha in the early sixteenth century and the page in question forms part of a collection of cures for various women's ailments, itself contained within a larger remedy book consisting of over 920 remedies and charms arranged in head-to-toe order.[11] The final remedy on p. 77 is a version of a common charm for safe childbirth that reads as follows:

> Ar br*eith* lei*n*im do mnai gan gūas*acht* na[12] brīat*hra* sō sīs do scr*ī*b*ad* a membr*um* 7 a ceng*al* 'ma broi*n*d .i. M[a]ria peperit *Christum*, A*nna* *peperit* Maria*m*, Elizabet*h* <7>[13] Ioh*ann*em, Celi*na* Remegiu*m* + sat*ur* + arepo + ten*et* + o*per*a + rotas no ditan*ntri* do tab*her*t a*r* dig dī 7 bēr*aid* gan gūas*acht.*
>
> (For a childbirth without danger for a woman, these words are written on a parchment and tied around her womb, i.e. Mary gave birth to Christ, Anna gave birth to Mary, Elizabeth [gave birth to] John, Celina [gave birth to] Remigius + sator + arepo + tenet + opera + rotas or put dittany in a drink for her and she will give birth without danger.)[14]

---

7 MS *celuia renui gium*.

8 Best omitted the final part of the charm (*n + Satur*) from his translation here; see further below, pp. 419–20.

9 'Some Irish Charms', ed. and trans. by Best, p. 30.

10 'Some Irish Charms', ed. and trans. by Best, p. 32 (n).

11 On the contents and context of this remedy book, which has been the subject of more extensive investigation since the publication of Best's article, see e.g. Hayden, 'Old English in the Irish Charms'; 'Attribution and Authority'; 'Three Versified Medical Remedies', and 'A Versified Cure for Headache', as well as 'A Sixteenth-Century Irish Collection', ed. and trans. by Hayden; Barrett, 'The King of Dál nAraidi's Salve'; and Nic Dhonnchadha, 'An Irish Medical Treatise'.

12 There appears to be a superfluous punctum delens over the 'n' in this word.

13 The scribe has written the Tironian note for Irish *ocus* ('and') here, but this must be an error, as Elizabeth is the mother of John the Baptist; presumably a repetition of Latin *peperit* is to be understood.

14 Dublin, RIA, MS 24 B 3 (445), p. 77.27–31. A digital facsimile of the manuscript page in question can be viewed on ISOS <https://www.isos.dias.ie/RIA/RIA_MS_24_B_3.html#81> [accessed 28 March 2024]. In this and all following extracts from unpublished manuscript sources, expansions are indicated by italics, missing letters or words are supplied

The use of rubricated initials in Conla Mac an Leagha's manuscript serves to clearly distinguish the above remedy from the cure immediately preceding it in the collection, which corresponds closely to the first part of the charm edited by Best from the vellum slip in TCD MS H 3. 17:

> In ben beris ingena as ē sō a l*eigheas* .i. fīac*al* ei*ch* do ceng*al* a n-eill do *croicend* rōi*n* 7 a *cir*[15] fo 7 n-aiff*renn*aib 7 a cur fo brāgaid.
>
> > (A woman who bears girls, this is its cure, i.e. tie the tooth of a horse in a sealskin thong and sing seven masses over it [lit. 'put it under seven masses'] and put it around the neck.)[16]

On the basis of these comparanda from RIA MS 24 B 3, one might speculate that Best erroneously conflated what were in fact understood to be two separate charms in the H 3. 17 manuscript: one for bearing a son and the other for safe or speedy childbirth. Indeed, not only are the two cures clearly distinguished in Conla Mac an Leagha's remedy book by way of rubricated initials, but their equivalents in the H 3. 17 manuscript are also visually separated on the page, since the scribe has drawn a line around the words '7 beraid mac' and left a slightly larger space between this and the remainder of the charm as it was published by Best.[17]

The ritual for safe childbirth or speedy delivery that forms the second of the two charms attested in the Irish manuscripts noted above is clearly an Irish reflex of the popular ritual motif of the holy mothers, sometimes referred to as the '*peperit* charm', variations of which circulated widely in Europe from the early Middle Ages until at least the beginning of the Renaissance.[18] The core formula of this ritual consists of an enumeration of biblical instances of miraculous childbirth, e.g. Mary, who gave birth to Christ even though she was a virgin; Elizabeth, mother of John the Baptist; and Anna, mother of Samuel, the latter two of which both had children when they were supposedly past childbearing age.[19] As Marianne Elsakkers has noted, the speaker of the charm seems to beg for a miracle analogous to these marvels of conception

---

in square brackets, and erroneous letters to be omitted are indicated using angled brackets. Length-marks, where not found in the manuscript, are marked using a macron over vowels. Word-division and punctuation are editorial. Translations are my own.

15 The MS reading is a 'c' with the typical superscript abbreviation for *-ri* or *-ir* (see <https://codecs.vanhamel.nl/I_(superscript_rounded)>), but the scribe may have intended to write *cur* 'put'; there may also be an instance of dittography here, based on the phrasing of the last part of the text.

16 Dublin, RIA, MS 24 B 3 (445), p. 77.26–27.

17 A digital facsimile of the manuscript page can be viewed on ISOS <https://www.isos.dias.ie/TCD/TCD_MS_1336.html#435> [accessed 28 March 2024].

18 See e.g. Elsakkers, 'In Pain You Shall Bear Children'; the Irish version of the charm is also considered by Barrett, 'Multilingual Medicalese'.

19 For Mary and Christ, cf. Matthew 1. 18, Luke 2. 5, etc.; for Elizabeth mother of John, see Luke 1. 7 and 1. 13; for Anna mother of Samuel, see 1 Samuel 1. 20. Elsakkers, 'In Pain You Shall Bear Children', p. 185, notes that Anna is the only Old Testament mother in the charms.

and birth.[20] Perhaps on account of its frequent use, the '*peperit* charm' was subject to a high degree of variation across languages and time by way of substitution, repetition or expansion and exhibits rhythmic and stylistic features suggestive of orality and practical use.[21] While the earliest known occurrence of the ritual in England is found in an eleventh-century manuscript, the Irish version of the '*peperit* charm' given above from two separate manuscript witnesses of the fifteenth and sixteenth centuries bears a closer similarity to a form transmitted in Latin remedies associated with the Anglo-Norman *Lettre d'Hippocrate*, attested in manuscripts of the thirteenth century. One feature of this later version is that the roster of holy mothers is expanded to include Anna, mother of Mary, and Celina, mother of Remigius.[22]

This later variant of the '*peperit* charm' also instructs the reader to produce a textual amulet on which have been inscribed the words of the so-called '*Sator* square', a palindrome consisting of the five Latin words *sator*, *arepo*, *tenet*, *opera*, and *rotas*, and to place this amulet around the belly. One of the earliest examples of the *Sator* formula was found in the ruins of Pompeii, but it was widely used in the West for healing purposes throughout the Middle Ages and came to be closely associated with childbirth rituals in particular by virtue of its inclusion in the *Trotula* collection of texts on women's medicine. There, it is suggested that a dead foetus might be removed from the womb by consuming cheese or butter on which a series of cryptic letters and the words of the palindrome have been written.[23] This comestible variety of the ritual was evidently known in Ireland, as it was included in the Irish vernacular version of the *Trotula* text that appears to have been made around the mid-fourteenth century.[24] The frequency with which the *Sator* square motif was used in an obstetrical context, moreover, is further illustrated in the charm for safe delivery from TCD MS H 3. 17 given above through the reference to 'Satur, etc.' invoked at the end of the text (albeit omitted from Best's translation). The

20 Elsakkers, 'In Pain You Shall Bear Children', p. 183.

21 Elsakkers, 'In Pain You Shall Bear Children', p. 183.

22 See Murray Jones and Olsan, 'Performative Rituals', pp. 416–18, where subsequent variants of this ritual in remedy collections of the fourteenth and fifteenth centuries are also discussed. For the relevant text in the Anglo-Norman tradition, see Hunt, *Popular Medicine*, p. 133. Both Elsakkers ('In Pain You Shall Bear Children', p. 185 n. 15), and Best ('Some Irish Charms', p. 30, n. on no. V) have observed that *Cilina* (or *Celina*) may refer to the mother of St Remigius, the archbishop of Rheims who baptized Clovis in 497. Skemer, *Binding Words*, p. 239 n. 13, cites another parallel to this version of the text in a fourteenth-century southern French medical miscellany in Limousin dialect (Princeton, University Library, MS Garrett 80), while Hindley, *Textual Magic*, p. 17, notes an English example from Durham, University Library, MS Cosin V. V.13, fols 24^{v}–25^{r} (*c.* 1475–1500), where a drink of dittany is likewise recommended to ease the pain of childbirth.

23 *The 'Trotula'*, ed. and trans. by Green, pp. 100–01; on the *Sator* square, see e.g. Bader, 'Magie in der Volksmedizin', and also the chapter by Conan Doyle in this volume.

24 'A Mediaeval Handbook', ed. by Wulff, p. 40; on the Irish version of the *Trotula*, see also Barrett, 'Multilingual Medicalese', and Arbuthnot, 'Women's Medicine', p. 41.

highly abbreviated nature of this reference suggests that the scribe expected readers to readily understand it without the need for further instruction.

The *Trotula* collection also contains remedies akin to the first of the two (apparently conflated) Irish childbirth rituals included in Best's edition, namely, that concerned with giving birth to a boy. Thus one of the constituent texts of the *Trotula*, known as the *Liber de sinthomatibus mulierum* ('Book on the Conditions of Women'), includes a series of remedies to address impediments to conception, one of which suggests that if a woman wishes to conceive a male, her husband should dry the womb and vagina of a hare and mix the powder with wine, and then give it to her to drink.[25] Although this is the only remedy in the chapter that is explicitly said to be for generating males, Monica Green has suggested that a series of cures immediately following it in the *Trotula* may have been intended to serve the same purpose, since the vast majority of medieval medical texts lack any explicit instructions on how to conceive females.[26] I have not yet identified any parallels for the Irish variant of these cures from the two sources discussed above, which involves wearing an amulet consisting of a horse's tooth in a sealskin thong. The cure clearly belongs to the wider tradition of rituals concerning fertility and conception as exemplified by the *Trotula* collection, however, and demonstrates how such rituals could be repurposed over time to serve distinct communities of readers.

Conversely, some of the remedies included in the *Trotula* reflect the reality that women might wish to prevent conception for various reasons. This is suggested, for instance, by a quotation from Constantine the African (but attributed to Galen) in another section of the *Liber de sinthomatibus mulierum*, according to which 'women who have narrow vaginas and constricted wombs ought not have sexual relations with men lest they conceive and die' (mulieres que habent uuluas angustas et matrices strictas non debent uiris uti, ne concipiant et moriantur). It is also noted in that context that not all such women are able to be continent, and thus require contraceptives.[27] Another constituent text of the *Trotula* collection, *De curis mulierum* ('On Treatments of Women'), offers advice for celibate women and widows 'to whom carnal intercourse is not permitted', noting that 'these women, when they have desire to copulate and do not do so, incur grave illness'.[28] As Monica Green has observed, many such remedies rely on amulets or sympathetic magic rather than the 'many herbs of presumed contraceptive or abortifacient properties

25 *The 'Trotula'*, ed. and trans. by Green, pp. 94–95 (§ 76).

26 *The 'Trotula'*, ed. and trans. by Green, p. 34; Green notes only two exceptions (p. 220, n. 130), one of which appears to be a misinterpretation of a remedy for conceiving males.

27 *The 'Trotula'*, ed. and trans. by Green, pp. 96–97 (§ 83); on this passage, see also the remarks by Green on pp. 34 and 220–21 of her edition.

28 *The 'Trotula'*, ed. and trans. by Green, pp. 120–21: 'quibus non committitur carnale commercium [...] que cum uoluntatem habeant coeundi et non coeunt, grauem incurrunt egritudinem'.

described in a variety of readily available pharmacological texts'.[29] Thus, for example, a woman who does not wish to conceive is advised to carry with her the testicles of a castrated weasel or the nude flesh of the womb of a goat which has never had offspring. A third remedy suggests the following:

> Si autem lesa fuerit in partu et postea pre timore mortis non uult concipere amplius, ponat in secundinam tot grana cathapuciarum uel ordei quot annis uult sterilis permanere. Et si in perpetuum uult sterilis permanere, plenam manum inponat.
>
> > (If she has been badly torn in birth and afterward for fear of death does not wish to conceive any more, let her put into the afterbirth as many grains of caper spurge or barley as the number of years she wishes to remain barren. And if she wishes to remain barren forever, let her put in a handful.)[30]

Here the action of placing grains of spurge or barley inside the afterbirth presumably represents a symbolic transferral of seed, with one grain for every year that the woman wishes to remain protected against pregnancy. This advice was retained in the Irish version of the text, but with the third-person singular of the standardized Latin version sometimes replaced with second-person singular forms — e.g. 'mad āil leat in toirrces do tairmesg' (if you wish to prevent pregnancy) — leading Sharon Arbuthnot to suggest that such cures might have been intended to be 'conveyed directly to the women who had most to gain from it (rather than to medical professionals)'.[31] In this respect, however, the Irish text is typical of many contemporary vernacular renderings of the *Trotula*, and the change of linguistic form may simply reflect wider currents in medical writing of the period that sought to present 'the image of a "female textual community"' as an 'authoritative social voice'.[32]

An Irish Conception Ritual

The remainder of this discussion will consider the transmission and context of one particular Irish ritual that appears to have been intended to cause impotence or to determine that conception has not or will not take place.

---

29 *The 'Trotula'*, ed. and trans. by Green, p. 34; see also the note on pp. 220–21. For the Irish version of this passage, see 'A Mediaeval Handbook', ed. by Wulff, p. 36 (§ 17). On contraception and abortifacients in the pharmacological tradition, see Riddle, *Contraception and Abortion*; on the medical and legislative aspects of abortion the early Middle Ages, see Mistry, *Abortion*.

30 *The 'Trotula'*, ed. and trans. by Green, pp. 96–99 (§ 84–87).

31 Arbuthnot, 'Women's Medicine', p. 41. For the Irish text, see 'A Mediaeval Handbook', ed. by Wulff, pp. 36–37 (§ 17).

32 See the introduction to Michele Savonarola, *A Mother's Manual*, ed. by Zuccolin and trans. by Marafioti, pp. 3–4 and 16–17.

While there is some variation in the text of this charm across the four medical manuscript witnesses of it thus far identified, all surviving copies have in common the instruction to write or recite a series of cryptic words on or over a stick of rowan, which is then to be stepped over by a man or woman. In three manuscript witnesses (one of which is a late transcript of another), the text of the ritual is transmitted alongside another charm that employs similar ritual actions and *voces magicae*, or 'words of power', but seems to have been meant to have the opposite effect of winning a woman's love.

What may be the earliest of the sources in question is Edinburgh, National Library of Scotland, MS Adv. 72.1.21, dated to around the fifteenth century.[33] This manuscript has been tentatively connected with the Irish medical family known by the surname 'Ó Siaghail' and consists of a single gathering of eight folios containing a portion of a commentary on the Hippocratic *Aphorisms*.[34] The elaborate initial on the first page indicates that the beginning of the fragment — which corresponds to Book 5, no. 51 of the Hippocratic text — is complete, but the end of the fragment breaks off mid-sentence on fol. 8^{v} in the middle of a commentary on the ninth aphorism in Book 6. In the lower margins of folios 5^{v}, 6^{r}, and 6^{v} are three entries that are described by the most recent cataloguer of the manuscript, Ronald Black, as 'love-charms, all beginning *Bran ber*'.[35] The following are transcriptions and translations of these marginalia, with each attestation labelled alphanumerically in order to highlight its textual correspondence with copies in the other manuscript witnesses discussed further below:

> **A1** (fol. 5^{v}, lower margin): Bran b*er* beras eo erobi. Cu*r* a slait c*h*áortai*nn*. 7 *dá* nd*e*ca p*er*[36] tairrs[i] nī fuid*h*t*her* pi*t* aici.
>
> > (*Bran ber beras eo erobi.* Put [this] on a stick of rowan and if a woman goes across [it] her vulva will not be obtained [by a man.])
>
> **A2** (fol. 6^{r}, lower margin): Bran b*er* b*er*a ears earb. C*ur* a slait c*h*aort*h*ain*n* 7 dā nd*ech*a f*er* t*h*airsi nī ēirg*h*ean*n* ai*r*.

33 The full manuscript has been digitized on ISOS: see <https://www.isos.dias.ie/NLS/NLS_Adv_MS_72_1_21.html> [accessed 30 March 2024].

34 Black, *Catalogue of Gaelic Manuscripts*. On the Ó Siaghail medical family, see Ó Muraíle, 'The Hereditary Medical Families', pp. 110–11; on the transmission of the Hippocratic aphorisms in medieval Europe, see Kibre, 'Hippocrates Latinus'.

35 Black, *Catalogue of Gaelic Manuscripts.*

36 The MS gives what looks to be the standard abbreviation for *per* or *pro* here (a letter 'p' with a stroke through the descender). This could be taken to stand for *fer* (man), but all other copies of this version of the charm (B1, B1 transcript and C1, discussed below) understand the agent of the ritual to be a woman (*ben*). It may be that the initial *b-* was written as *p-* in the exemplar, perhaps with the form *bé* 'woman, maiden' (see eDIL s.v. 1 bé or dil.ie/5502). It appears, in any case, that there were two variants of the charm in circulation, i.e. one involving the stepping action of a woman and the other that of a man.

(*Bran ber bera ears earb.* Put [this] on a stick of rowan and if a man goes across it, he will not have an erection.)[37]

A3 (fol. 6^{v}, lower margin): Bran b*er* a*r* tela*r* ibe. A *cur* a slait c*h*uill 7 púail trī b*h*uilli ai*r* m*h*naoí d*he* 7 ca*r*fuid*h* t*h*ú.

(*Bran ber ar thelar ibe.* Put it on a stick of hazel and strike three blows on a woman with it and she will love you.)

In addition to the similarity between the first two 'words of power' in each of these examples (*Bran ber*), all involve writing the words on a stick or rod (*slat*). A1 and A2 are clearly variants of a single charm and differ from A3 in that they call for a stick of rowan (*slat cháorthainn*) as opposed to one of *coll* (hazel).[38] The nature of the performative ritual involving this stick also differs across the three texts: in A1 and A2, it is suggested that intercourse might be prevented in some way if a man or woman crosses over the rod, whereas in A3 the woman's love is to be induced by striking (or perhaps merely tapping) a woman with that object.[39] The designation of all three passages as 'love charms' should thus be understood in broad terms as referring to their shared interest in matters concerning sexual relations (a common result, of course, of efforts to arouse desire).

It is unclear whether the copies of these charms in the margins of Edinburgh, NLS, MS Adv. 72.1.21 are contemporary with that text or not. What one can say about this witness, however, is that the inscription of the charms in such a context may have been inspired by the content of the main text with which they are juxtaposed, since a substantial portion of this particular fragment of the Hippocratic *Aphorisms* is specifically concerned with matters relating to fertility and parturition. As already noted, the first aphorism in the fragment (fol. 1^{r}a) corresponds to Book V, no. 51 of the Hippocratic text, which explains that the mouth of the womb is closed when a woman is with child. The following folio (2^{r}a) contains a commentary on Aphorism V.59, which offers advice on how to determine whether or not a woman will be able to conceive a child, suggesting that she be covered with wraps and have perfumes burnt underneath her and arguing that if the smell

37 For the translation of *ní éirgheann air* as 'will not have an erection', see the entry in Dinneen, *Foclóir*, s.v. *éirghim* ('I rise, arise, get up, ascend'), which includes the definition 'of males, in copulation' under examples of the verb followed by the preposition *ar*.

38 Both of these types of wood are portrayed in early Irish literary sources as having magical properties; thus *Vitae sanctorum Hiberniae*, ed. by Plummer, I, pp. cliii–cliv, has noted instances from Irish hagiographical texts where a hazel tree heals all diseases and a stick of rowan is used for divinatory purposes.

39 I have discussed the transmission of A3 in more detail in Hayden, 'The Context and Obscure Language', where I have noted that the 'words of power' in this charm differ substantially across other variant versions. This suggests that the cryptic language used in this particular copy may derive from its association with the text of the otherwise distinct ritual in A1 and A2. It is unclear whether the act of striking three 'blows' (*builli*) over the woman was meant to involve any significant degree of force.

seems to pass through the body to the mouth and nostrils, one could be assured that the woman is not barren through her own physical fault. The verso of this page (fol. 2^{v}a) contains commentary on aphorisms V.61–63, the first two of which explain that suppression of menstruation is a sign that a woman is with child, whereas women who suffer from an imbalance of heat, cold, moisture or dryness will be unable to conceive. Aphorism V.63 then explains that a comparable constitutional imbalance in males will have a similar outcome.[40]

Copies of the three marginal 'love charms' considered above are also found in Dublin, RIA, MS C iv 2 (466), a collection of medical treatises compiled in the sixteenth century by various scribes, among them Niall Ó Cuinn and Brian Mac Maol Tuile.[41] The cataloguer of this manuscript notes that the collection contains 'a calendar, a fragment of a medical treatise, a copy of a *materia medica*, and several poems. It has several curious features [...] and savours somewhat of magic'.[42] Precisely what is meant by 'magic' is not made explicit, but the comment may have been intended to refer to the inclusion of texts such as prognostications from thunder, notes on chiromancy, and charms such as the ones discussed here.[43] The scribe who copied the ritual cures on which this study focuses, Niall Ó Cuinn, refers to them using the term *bricht* (defined in *eDIL*, s.v., as an 'incantation, charm, magic spell').[44] In this case, however, the charms were not added to the manuscript margins, as is the case in Edinburgh, NLS, MS Adv. 72.1.21, but rather were incorporated into a collection of remedies for various bodily ailments that, although somewhat miscellaneous in nature, includes at least one passage of advice for avoiding pregnancy, beg. '*Mad*h *āil le mnaoi gan a* b*heith torrac*' (If a woman wishes to not be pregnant).[45] They also appear in a different order to those in Edinburgh, NLS, MS Adv. 72.1.21, with the first (written near the bottom of fol. 19^{r}) corresponding most closely to A3 above:

> **B3** (fol. 19^{r}17–18): Can i*n* bri*cht* sō a slait cuill 7 būail i*n* ben b*us* āil let<*h*> 7 car*faidh* th*ū* .i. bran. ber. her. he. lar. ibe.

---

40 Cf. Hippocrates, *Aphorisms*, ed. and trans. by Jones, pp. 170–77; the Irish text has not yet been edited.

41 The entry for the manuscript in the *RIA Catalogue*, p. 1217 notes the following dates: 1531 (fol. 1^{r}), 1572 (fol. 8^{r}) and 1535 (fol. 16^{r}). The full manuscript has been digitized for ISOS: see <https://www.isos.dias.ie/RIA/RIA_MS_C_iv_2.html> [accessed 30 March 2024].

42 *RIA Catalogue*, pp. 1217–18.

43 A handful of prognostications from thunder found in the C iv 2 manuscript have been edited in Herbert, 'Some Irish Prognostications', pp. 310–12. Fol. 1^{v} contains a set of verses attributed to returned spirits of the dead, which have been edited and discussed by Simms, 'O'Friel's Ghost'.

44 Ó Cuinn signed his name on fols 13^{r}, 14^{r} and 16^{r}. On the term *bricht*, see eDIL, s.v. 1 *bricht* (dil.ie/6810).

45 Dublin, RIA, MS C iv 2 (466), fol. 18^{v}1–2.

> (Recite this incantation on a hazel stick and strike the woman that you desire and she will love you, i.e. *bran ber her he lar ibe.*)

One might note that here the reader is instructed to 'sing' or 'recite' (*canaid*) the words of the spell, although it is unclear whether the words are supposed to be inscribed on the stick or simply spoken over it. The inspiration for this instruction may have stemmed, however, from the fact that the preceding lines of fol. 19ʳ in the C iv 2 manuscript contain details regarding the appropriate occasions on which to recite certain psalms for protection.[46]

The charm labelled 'B3' is immediately followed on the same page of the C iv 2 manuscript by a copy of the ritual corresponding to A2 above:[47]

> **B2** (fol. 19ʳ19–20): Can i*n* b*richt* ē*tr*esi[48] a fleisg cāortain*n* 7 mā tēid f*er* tai*r*si ni ē*r*gen*n* [air][49] .i. b*r*an. bir. beru. ers. ei*n*rb.
>
> > (Recite this impotence spell on a rowan stick and if a man goes across it he will not have an erection, i.e. *bran bir beru ers einrb.*)

Finally, a copy of the charm labelled 'A1' above is found on the verso of fol. 19 in Dublin, RIA, MS C iv 2:[50]

> **B1** (fol. 19ᵛ7–9): bran. bir. brec. eo. erobi. Can an b*richt* sō a slait cāortuin*n* 7 mā tēid ben tai*r*si nī fuig*h*e en ndui*n*e pit aicce.
>
> > (Recite this incantation over a rowan stick and if a woman goes across it no one will obtain her vulva.)

Transcripts of B1, B2, and B3 were included in a collection of miscellaneous remedies compiled by the nineteenth-century doctor and antiquarian Michael Casey in London, BL, MS Additional 25586.[51] Nic Dhonnchadha described the third of these transcripts (corresponding to B1) as a 'Charm to render a woman impotent', while Robin Flower characterized the first (corresponding to B3) as a 'charm to win a woman's love'.[52] Both scholars

46 Dublin, RIA, MS C iv 2 (466), fol. 19ʳ8–16; cf. the very similar text found on fol. 16ᵛ12–21 of the same manuscript, also in the hand of Niall Ó Cuinn.

47 Dublin, RIA, MS C iv 2 (466), fol. 19ʳ19–20.

48 The manuscript reading of this word is *eesi* with a suspension mark over the first two letters. I am uncertain of the intended expansion, but since the charm seems to have been understood as serving to render a man impotent, I have taken it to be the genitive singular form of the abstract noun *treise* ('strength, vigour, power', dil.ie/41750) with a prefix of negation: cf. eDIL, s.v. *étrén* ('weak, powerless', dil.ie/20909).

49 My reading of this and the preceding word is very tentative, as both are unclear due to fading of the manuscript page.

50 On the gender of the agent performing this ritual, see above, n. 36.

51 See Flower, *Catalogue*, p. 631; the transcripts occur on fol. 179ʳ of London, BL, MS Add. 25586 and their correspondence with the text in Dublin, RIA, MS C iv 2 (466) is noted by Nic Dhonnchadha, 'Michael Casey's Medical Transcripts', pp. 110–11.

52 Flower, *Catalogue*, p. 631; Nic Dhonnchadha, 'Michael Casey's Medical Transcripts', p. 110.

appear to have understood the second of the charm-transcripts in Casey's manuscript (corresponding to B2) to be a love charm comparable to that immediately preceding it on the page (B3), perhaps prompted by the fact that Casey himself had begun it with the words 'mar an gceadna abfleisg caortain' (similarly on a stick of rowan).[53] As demonstrated above, however, the stated purpose of the charms in B2 and B3 is not identical, in that B2 was evidently intended to render a man impotent, whereas B3 sought to arouse feelings of affection in the woman. Casey's comment may thus simply have referred to the instruction to write very similar *voces magicae* on a stick, and it is unclear whether or not he understood them to be two different charms.

At least one further attestation of the ritual to prevent conception (that which corresponds to A1 and B1 above) is found in Section 12 of Edinburgh, NLS, MS Adv. 72.1.2, a composite manuscript dating to the sixteenth and seventeenth centuries and associated with the Beaton family of medical practitioners in Scotland.[54] Section 12 of this codex consists of a gathering of vellum leaves (fols 124–29) that was once the property of a John Beaton (see fol. 124r) and, in contrast to the largely practical orientation of the contents of the manuscript as a whole, its texts are described as being 'almost exclusively scholastic in nature'.[55] The ritual text is written in the lower margin of a page containing a discussion of 'why yew and holly retain their foliage throughout the year'.[56] As has been argued with regard to the marginal copies of the charms in NLS MS Adv. 72.1.21, it may have been the content of the adjacent text that inspired the inscription of the charm at this particular point, since an analogy between female fertility and trees that produce flowers is attested elsewhere in European medical tradition of the later medieval period.[57] The *Trotula* text known as the 'Book on the Conditions of Women', for example, states that 'the common people call the menses "the flowers," because just as trees do not bring forth fruit without flowers, so women without their flowers are cheated of the ability to conceive' (*menstrua, que uulgus appellat flores, quia sicut arbores non afferunt sine floribus fructus, sic mulieres sine suis floribus sue conceptionis officio defraudantur*).[58] Indeed, another section of the 72.1.2 manuscript contains a 'fertility charm for women and trees' that likewise suggests an analogous association between the two objects of the

---

53 Flower, *Catalogue*, p. 631 ('another similar charm follows'); Nic Dhonnchadha, 'Michael Casey's Medical Transcripts', p. 110 ('Idem').

54 On the Beatons, see Bannerman, *A Medical Kindred*. A digital facsimile of Edinburgh, NLS, MS Adv. 72.1.2 is available on ISOS.

55 Black, *Catalogue of Gaelic Manuscripts*.

56 Black, *Catalogue of Gaelic Manuscripts* (fol. 129v).

57 For discussion of this analogy, see *The 'Trotula'*, ed. and trans. by Green, pp. 21–22.

58 *The 'Trotula'*, ed. and trans. by Green, pp. 72–73; for the Irish version of this text, cf. 'A Mediaeval Handbook', ed. by Wulff, pp. 14–15, as well as the discussion in Arbuthnot, 'Medieval Irish Vocabulary of Sex and Reproduction'.

charm. In that context, it is suggested that if a childless woman wishes to bear children, she should write an obscure string of letters on an object and place this around her neck without the knowledge of her husband; it is then stated that the same amulet could also be placed around 'a tree on which fruit never came before' in order to ensure that 'good fruits will come on it from that time on until the death of that same tree'.[59]

Ronald Black described the ritual for preventing conception on fol. 129^{v} — the final words of which are unclear — as a 'charm to protect the vulva' and identified the hand as that of 'Coinneach mac Eoin (Uí Chonchubhair?) [...] Possibly identifiable with "Kenneth Leich", with the father of Domhnall mac Coinnigh [...] and the son of John McConchra of Stronecormick, chirurgeon, 1530':[60]

> **C1** (fol. 129^{v}, lower margin): bir × bran × ar × leor × meor × sgrībh sō an slait caothrainn 7 cuir fo cosibh mnā 7 ní fathar banndacht adi nó g[?] rl[...][61]
>
> > (*bir × bran × ar × leor × meor ×*, write this on a stick of rowan and put it under the feet of a woman and her womanhood [i.e. vulva][62] or a pregnancy(?)[63] is not obtained [?...])

The *voces magicae* in this version of the text differ more substantially from those in other witnesses, although the forms *Bran ber/bir* or *Bir bran* are common across all copies. While 'words of power' in charms are often formulated on the basis of stylistic patterns such alliteration, rhyme and repetition, as is evidenced in the above example, occasionally they include meaningful words that are in some way apposite to the purpose of the charm.[64] It is unclear to me, however, whether or not this can be argued in the case of the ritual texts discussed here.[65]

59 Edinburgh, NLS, MS Adv. 72.1.2, fol. 33^{r}6–7: 'a cur fa bráighid croinn nach tic toradh air roime sin rīam, ticfaidh toradh maith air ō sin amach go bās an croinn cétna sin'. This charm has been edited and translated by Rempt, 'And Straightaway', pp. 80–85.

60 See Black, *Catalogue of Gaelic Manuscripts*, where the association of these figures with two other manuscripts (Edinburgh, NLS, MSS Adv. 72. 1. 3 and 72. 1. 37) is noted.

61 The last letters of the text are difficult to make out in the manuscript.

62 See eDIL, s.v. *bandacht* or dil.ie/5337 for the translation of this term as either 'womanliness, womanhood' or 'female sex, female pudenda'.

63 The word in question is given in the MS as *g* with a suspension mark; I have speculated that it may refer to *géin* 'pregnancy, birth'. My thanks to David Stifter for this observation.

64 For discussion of this phenomenon in relation to Irish charms, see e.g. Hayden, 'Old English in the Irish Charms' and Hayden, 'The Context and Obscure Language'. The stylistic patterns typical of such incantations are discussed at length by Versnel, 'The Poetics of the Magical Charm'.

65 The word *bran*, for example, is defined as both 'raven' and 'bran, chaff' in *eDIL* (see dil.ie/6537 and dil.ie/6538), the latter being an English loanword. It is also attested as a personal name; its equivalent in Welsh (for which see GPC Online, s.v. *brân*) also carries the figurative sense of 'warrior'. David Stifter has pointed out to me a stanza cited in the first and

Comparanda in other Vernacular Medical Texts

The belief that one might exert control over fertility or parturition through the ritual action of stepping over something while reciting powerful words is also evidenced in other Insular literary and folklore traditions of the medieval to modern periods. One of the earliest extant examples is an Old English metrical charm for childbirth from the compilation of remedies, charms and prayers known as the *Lacnunga*, written around the year 1000.[66] This advises a woman who is having difficulty conceiving a child to step three times over a dead man's grave and then recite the following words three times:

> Se wifman se hire cild afedan ne mæg: gange to gewitenes mannes birgenne and stæppe þonne þriwa ofer þa byrgenne, 7 cweþe þonne þriwa þas word:
> Þis me to bote   þære laþan lætbyrde,
> þis me to bote   þære swæran swært-byrde,
> þis me to bote   þære laðan lam-byrde.
>
> (A woman who cannot nourish her child: she should go to a deceased person's grave and then step over the grave three times, and then say these words three times:
> This is my cure for hateful delayed birth,
> this is my cure for grievous black birth,
> this is my cure for hateful lame birth.)

When the woman is pregnant, she is then advised to go to her sleeping husband and say:

> Up ic gonge,   ofer þe stæppe
> mid cwican cilde,   nalæs mid cwelendum,
> mid fulborenum,   nalæs mid fægan.
>
> (Up I go, over you I step
> with a living child, not with a dying one,
> with a child brought to full-term, not with one destined to die.)[67]

second Middle Irish Metrical Tracts (MV I.13 and MV II.57; see 'Mittelirische Verslehren', ed. by Thurneysen, pp. 14 and 43–44, respectively) that contains the line 'Bran berba ball glaine' (Bran of the bright-portioned Barrow), the first two words of which are reminiscent of the initial sounds in some versions of our charm. Although this stanza is invoked in the metrical tracts to illustrate a particular metre, it may have once formed part of a eulogy for the Leinster king Bran who was murdered on 6 May 795: see, for example, the reference to *Bran búadach Berbae* in *The Martyrology of Óengus the Culdee*, ed. and trans. by Stokes, p. 26, as well as the discussion in Charles-Edwards, *Early Christian Ireland*, pp. 469–70.

66 London, BL, MS Harley 585, fols 130r–193r. The most recent edition of the text forms part of *Medical Writings*, ed. and trans. by Niles and D'Aronco.

67 *Medical Writings*, ed. and trans. by Niles and D'Aronco, pp. 510–13 (no. 161).

Although there is a clear parallelism here with regard to the ritual motion of stepping first over the grave and then over a husband, the significance of this symbolism has been variously interpreted. L. M. C. Weston has understood the connection in terms of liminality, arguing that the grave, which 'marks a boundary between the living and the non-living, this human world and the other' might be viewed as akin to the condition of the woman, who bears a not-yet-living child and thus 'embodies a similar boundary within herself'.[68] Marie Nelson has suggested that the act of stepping over a grave signifies a defiance or conquering of death,[69] while Murray Jones and Olsan point out the significance of the woman's agency in this and other metrical childbirth rituals in the *Lacnunga*, noting that the words and bodily acts articulated in them serve to persuade the afflicted individual 'that something not only can be done, but has been done that creates a new reality'.[70]

A similar 'grave-stepping ritual' is also attested in later folklore tradition, albeit sometimes with a different purpose or outcome. Thus Edward Pettit, drawing in part on the work of Gert Sandmann, has cited a number of examples from German, English, and Welsh superstition in which the pregnant woman's act of crossing over a burial place was thought to have the opposite effect of placing the child in mortal danger or of causing the woman herself to become barren.[71] An example of the latter is a legend reported in the eighteenth-century *Statistical Account of Scotland* by John Sinclair (who traced it to the sixteenth-century Scottish historian Hector Boece), according to which the local people of Meigle parish in Perthshire believed that 'if a young woman should walk over the grave of Vanora [the British Helena, identified with Guinevere, wife of the legendary King Arthur], she should entail on herself perpetual sterility'.[72] The outcome of the ritual action in this later account thus appears to be diametrically opposed to that of the Old English metrical charm for conception and resembles more closely the stated purpose of the Irish charm for causing impotence or 'protecting the vulva' considered above. It is noteworthy, however, that Sandmann proposed an alternative reading of the opening line of the charm (*gange... byrgenne*), according to which the form *birgenne* (grave) should be understood as a corruption of the adjective *bircen, beorcen* meaning 'belonging to a birch' (and therefore perhaps 'a birch branch'), and *gewitenes* a word originally intended as *gewittes* (wise). Sandmann thus translated the line in question as '(sie) gehe zum Birkenzweig eines weisen Mannes (wörtlich: eines Mannes von Verstand) und schreite dann

68 Weston, 'Women's Medicine', p. 289.

69 Nelson, 'A Woman's Charm', 3; cf. *Anglo-Saxon Remedies*, ed. and trans. by Pettit, II, pp. 332.

70 Murray Jones and Olsan, 'Performative Rituals', pp. 429–30.

71 *Anglo-Saxon Remedies*, ed. and trans. by Pettit, II, p. 321, citing Sandmann, 'Studien zu altenglischen Zaubersprüchen', pp. 98–99.

72 Boece's account is cited by Sinclair, *The Statistical Account*, p. 507.

dreimal über den Birkenzweig' (let her go to the birch branch of a wise man [lit.: a man of knowledge] and then step over the birch branch three times.)[73]

Sandmann's reading of the Old English passage was firmly rejected by Edward Pettit as untenable,[74] but the act of stepping over a stick rather than a grave in order to exert control over conception is of course reminiscent of the Irish ritual examined above, which unambiguously involves an individual crossing over a stick or rod (*slat*, *flesc*). This act can in turn be compared to other modern folklore beliefs that associate striding over a broom handle not only with pregnancy, but more specifically as a sign of unwanted conception. In the late nineteenth century, for example, the folklore collector Sidney Oldall Addy, writing of the traditional customs of counties in the mid-west of England, reported that:

> If a girl strides over a besom-handle, she will be mother before she is a wife. If an unmarried woman has a child people say 'She's jumped o'er t'besom', or 'She jumped o'er t'besom before she went to t'church.' Mothers used to be particularly anxious that their daughters should not stride over a broom, and mischievous boys have been known to leave brooms on doorsteps and such-like places, so that girls might accidentally stride over them.[75]

There is undoubtedly a connection between such taboos and the widespread marriage-rite in which a couple jump or step over a broom, which is well attested in Wales between the beginning of the eighteenth century and the middle of the nineteenth centuries.[76] Thomas Gwynn Jones has noted that the Welsh phrase 'priodas coes ysgub' or 'priodas coes ysgubell' (broom-stick wedding) was applied to irregular or unlegalized unions, and suggested a connection between the Welsh word for wand (*llath*) and the legal term *llathlud*, which was used in the medieval Welsh law-texts to refer to a marriage involving elopement or abduction without the consent of the girl's kin.[77] It is no doubt significant in this regard that Guinevere, whose supposed burial-place in Meigle parish was believed to cause barrenness in any woman who stepped over it, is a figure widely associated with infidelity (and perhaps also barrenness) in Arthurian literature of the Middle Ages: for although she is not generally depicted as having had children with Arthur himself, her adultery with Mordred forms

73 Sandmann, 'Studien zu altenglischen Zaubersprüchen', pp. 99–100.

74 See e.g. *Anglo-Saxon Remedies*, ed. and trans. by Pettit, II, pp. 321–22.

75 Addy, *Household Tales*, p. 102.

76 Sullivan, '"Jumping the Broom"'; Sullivan's article is a response to the remarks in Dundes, '"Jumping the Broom"'.

77 Gwynn Jones, *Welsh Folklore*, pp. 183–85; on Welsh marriage law and the term *llathlud*, see also Charles-Edwards, 'Naw kynywedi teithiauc', pp. 30–32. It might be noted that Welsh *llath* 'rod, staff, wand, stick' is cognate with Irish *slat*, the term used in most versions of the impotence charm discussed above: see the GPC Online, s.v. *llath* and Stifter, 'Rise of Gemination', § 13.1 (36).

a key element of the king's downfall in Geoffrey of Monmouth's *De gestis Britonum*, while her illicit love-affair with the knight Lancelot is the focus of one the later romances of Chrétien de Troyes.[78]

The Welsh parallels for our Irish 'stepping ritual' are perhaps most vividly illustrated, however, by an episode in the narrative known as *Math uab Mathonwy*, one of the eleven medieval Welsh tales known collectively as the *Mabinogi* or *Mabinogion* and found mainly in two manuscripts dating to the fourteenth and fifteenth centuries.[79] Magic is a recurring theme throughout the plot of *Math*, which revolves around the consequences stemming from three legal violations related to fertility: a rape, a false claim of virginity, and an adultery.[80] As Jane Cartwright has argued, 'virginity and the power associated with virginity are of primary importance' to the events of the tale, which begins with an account of how Math son of Mathonwy, lord of Gwynedd, could only live while his two feet were in the fold of a maiden's lap, with the exception of his being called away to war.[81] The beauty of Math's virgin foot-holder, Goewin ferch Pebin, attracts the unwanted attention of his nephew, Gilfaethwy, whose brother Gwydion arranges for Math to be away from his court so that Gilfaethwy can rape her. Cartwright has pointed out that Goewin's power to protect the king 'is associated exclusively with her virginity', comparing this to the frequent attribution of protective powers or healing properties to virgins (or even chaste wives) in Welsh folk literature and hagiography.[82]

Gwydion and Gilfaethwy are duly punished for their crime when Math uses his magic wand (*hutlath*) to transform them into various types of animals that bring forth offspring. Having served his penance, Gwydion is then consulted regarding a suitable replacement for Math's virgin foot-holder, and suggests his sister Aranrhod, who is subjected to a chastity test that once again involves Math's magic *hutlath*:

> 'A wyr,' heb ef, 'tangneued a gawsawch, a cherennyd a geffwch. A rodwch im kynghor pa uorwyn a geisswyf.' 'Arglwyd,' heb y Guydyon uab Don, 'hawd yw dy gynghori. Aranrot uerch Don, dy nith uerch dy chwaer.' Honno a gyrchwyt attaw. Y uorwyn a doeth y mywn. 'A uorwyn,' heb ef, 'a wyt uorwyn di?' 'Ny wnn i amgen no'm bot.' Yna y kymerth ynteu yr hutlath a'y chamu. 'Camha di dros honn,' heb ef, 'ac ot wyt uorwyn, mi a ednebydaf.' Yna y camawd hitheu dros yr hutlath, ac ar y cam hwnnw, adaw

---

78 On the varying depiction of Guinevere in Arthurian sources, see e.g Samples, 'Guinevere: A Reappraisal'.

79 Namely, the White Book of Rhydderch (Aberystwyth, NLW, MS Peniarth 4–5), dated to *c.* 1350, and the Red Book of Hergest (Oxford, Jesus College, MS 111), dated to between 1382 and *c.* 1410: see *The Mabinogion*, trans. by Davies, p. ix.

80 Valente, 'Gwydion and Aranrhod', p. 332.

81 Cartwright, 'Virginity and Chastity Tests', p. 58.

82 Cartwright, 'Virginity and Chastity Tests', p. 60.

mab brasuelyn mawr a oruc. Sef a wnaeth y mab, dodi diaspat uchel. Yn ol diaspat y mab, kyrchu y drws a oruc hi, ac ar hynny adaw y ryw bethan ohonei. A chyn cael o neb guelet yr eil olwc arnaw, Guydyon a'y kymerth, ac a droes llen o bali yn y gylch, ac a'e cudyawd. Sef y cudyawd, y mywn llaw gist is traed y wely.

> ('Men,' he said, 'you have had peace and you shall have friendship. Now give me advice as to which virgin I should seek.'
>
> 'Lord,' said Gwydion son of Dôn, 'it is easy to advise you — Aranrhod daughter of Dôn, your niece, your sister's daughter.' She was brought to Math. The maiden entered.
>
> 'Maiden,' he said, 'are you a virgin?'
>
> 'That is my belief.' Then he took his magic wand and bent it.
>
> 'Step over this,' he said, 'and if you are a virgin I shall know.'
>
> Then she stepped over the magic wand, and as she stepped she dropped a large, sturdy, yellow-haired boy. The boy gave a loud cry. After the boy's cry she made for the door, but as she went she dropped a small something. Before anyone else could get a second glimpse of it, Gwydion took it and wrapped a sheet of brocaded silk around it and hid it. He hid it in a small chest at the foot of his bed.)[83]

Here we find a performative ritual nearly identical to that articulated in the Irish texts discussed above. A key difference, however, is that the purpose of the 'stepping' exercise in the Welsh source is clearly to test the chastity of the woman rather than to prevent conception or cause impotence in a man. Arguing in favour of the phallic imagery of Math's magic wand, which serves to demonstrate not only that Aranrhod is not a virgin but also that she has concealed two pregnancies, Jane Cartwright has suggested that 'the fact that Aranrhod steps over the wand, and, in the process, opens her legs as she straddles the phallic symbol, is important to the sexual imagery of the test'.[84] Following in this vein, one might wonder whether the narrator's passing comment that Math 'bent' his wand before placing it on the ground was understood to symbolize the fact that the man for whose benefit the chastity test was being performed — in this case, Math himself — was not responsible for any offspring that might result from the woman's performance of the ritual act. Such an interpretation recalls the sexually explicit reference in the A2/B2 version of the Irish impotence charm discussed above, where stepping over a stick seems to have been understood as a means of preventing a man from engaging in intercourse.

Similar imagery of procreation is evidenced in other parts of *Math uab Mathonwy*. For example, Roberta Valente has pointed out that the 'small

---

83 *Math uab Mathonwy*, ed. by Hughes, p. 9 (text); *The Mabinogion*, trans. by Davies, p. 54 (translation).

84 Cartwright, 'Virginity and Chastity Tests', p. 61.

something' (*y ryw bethan*) that dropped from beneath Aranrhod and caused her to flee in shame when she stepped over Math's wand is evidently a foetus, and Gwydion's concealment of it in a chest at the foot of his bed, from which it later emerges as a child who is subsequently raised by Gwydion himself, serves to mimic the process of birth from the womb.[85] Prior to this episode, moreover, Math had used his *hutlath* to transform Gwydion and Gilfaethwy into female animals who give birth to offspring as a punishment for a rape. The very public and shame-inducing nature of their punishment, as well as of Aranrhod's chastity test, underlines the power of the narrative's pervasive sexual symbolism, and of performative rituals more generally, as a means of articulating the *mores* of a society in which the kin-group formed an important legal unit and an inability to identify the father of a child could have serious social and economic consequences. As Cartwright notes, 'Ultimately [...] the message implicit in this branch of the *Mabinogi* is that virginity and fertility were not personal, private matters, for they were of extreme importance to the kin group as a whole.'[86]

The Irish version of this 'stepping ritual', as it appears in the handful of late-medieval medical manuscripts discussed above, can similarly be situated in relation to questions concerning fertility and conception, but it is unclear whether the ritual act was intended in that context as a chastity test or as a means of preventing a future conception. The occurrence of the motif in sources from other linguistic traditions of the Insular world suggests, moreover, that comparable 'stepping rituals' could be interpreted as a means of ensuring successful conception and birth. It is possible, however, that the symbolism of crossing a stick in order to prevent or determine the absence of a pregnancy, as appears to be conveyed in the Irish sources, might have been viewed as a defiance or resistance of conception, on analogy with the aforementioned interpretation of the grave-crossing, in the Old English metrical charm for a difficult birth, as a 'conquering or defiance of death'.[87]

Such observations are necessarily of a somewhat speculative nature, and one should perhaps be wary of drawing firm conclusions regarding a ritual of which the form and stated purpose varied so considerably across time and space. It is clear, however, that the handful of Irish 'performative rituals' for conception and childbirth considered in this study provide insight into the relationship between learning and texts recorded in the various vernacular medical, literary and folklore traditions of the premodern Insular world. They also attest to the value of the comparatively neglected corpus of Irish medical manuscripts as a source for a wide spectrum of gynaecological and obstetrical practices in the premodern period — one that can contribute significantly to work currently ongoing in relation to other medieval European traditions.

85 Valente, 'Gwydion and Aranrhod', p. 339.
86 Cartwright, 'Virginity and Chastity Tests', p. 63.
87 See above, pp. 428–29.

Works Cited

Manuscripts

Aberystwyth, National Library of Wales, MS Peniarth 4–5
Dublin, Royal Irish Academy, MS C iv 2 (466)
Dublin, Royal Irish Academy, MS 24 B 3 (445)
Dublin, Trinity College, MS 1336 (H 3. 17)
Durham, University Library, MS Cosin V. V.13
Edinburgh, National Library of Scotland, MS Adv. 72.1.2
Edinburgh, National Library of Scotland, MS Adv. 72.1.21
London, British Library, MS Additional 25586
London, British Library, MS Harley 585
Oxford, Jesus College, MS 111
Princeton, University Library, MS Garrett 80

Primary Sources

Anglo-Saxon Remedies, Charms, and Prayers from British Library MS Harley 585: The Lacnunga, ed. and trans. by Edward Pettit, Mellen Critical Editions and Translations, 6A–6B, 2 vols (Lewiston: Edwin Mellen Press, 2001)

Hippocrates, *Aphorisms*, ed. and trans. by W. H. S. Jones, Loeb Classical Library, 150 (Cambridge, MA: Harvard University Press, 1931)

The Mabinogion, trans. by Sioned Davies (Oxford: Oxford University Press, 2007)

The Martyrology of Oengus the Culdee: Félire Óengusso Céli Dé, ed. and trans. by Whitley Stokes, Henry Bradshaw Society, 29 (London: Harrison and Sons, 1905)

Math uab Mathonwy: The Fourth Branch of the Mabinogi, ed. by Ian Hughes, Mediaeval and Modern Welsh Series, 13 (Dublin: DIAS, 2013)

'A Mediaeval Handbook of Gynaecology and Midwifery…', ed. by Winifred Wulff, *Irish Texts*, 5 (London: Sheed and Ward, 1934)

Medical Writings from Early Medieval England, Volume I. The Old English Herbal, Lacnunga, and Other Texts, ed. and trans. by John D. Niles and Maria A. D'Aronco, Dumbarton Oaks Medieval Library, 81 (Cambridge, MA: Harvard University Press, 2023)

Michele Savonarola, *A Mother's Manual for the Women of Ferrara: A Fifteenth-Century Guide to Pregnancy and Pediatrics*, ed. by Gabriella Zuccolin and trans. by Martin Marafioti, The Other Voice in Early Modern Europe: The Toronto Series, 89 (New York and Toronto: Iter Press, 2022)

'Mittelirische Verslehren', ed. by Rudolf Thurneysen, in *Irische Texte mit Wörterbuch*, ed. by Rudolf Thurneysen and Ernst Windisch, 3rd series, vol. 1 (Leipzig: S. Herzel, 1891), pp. 1–182

'A Sixteenth-Century Irish Collection of Remedies for Ailments of the Male Reproductive Organs', ed. and trans. by Deborah Hayden, *Celtica*, 33 (2021), 248–76

'Some Irish Charms', ed. and trans. by R. I. Best, *Ériu*, 16 (1952), 27–32

The 'Trotula': A Medieval Compendium of Women's Medicine, ed. and trans. by Monica Green (Philadelphia: University of Pennsylvania Press, 2001)

Vitae sanctorum Hiberniae, ed. and trans. by Charles Plummer, 2 vols (Oxford: Clarendon Press, 1910)

Secondary Studies

Addy, Sidney Oldall, *Household Tales with Other Traditional Remains, Collected in the Counties of York, Lincoln, Derby, and Nottingham* (London: D. Nutt, 1895)

Arbuthnot, Sharon, 'The Medieval Irish Vocabulary of Sex and Reproduction. Insights from the *Trotula* and Other Medical Texts', *Kelten*, 89 (2021) <https://kelten.vanhamel.nl/k89-2021-arbuthnot-irish-literature-medieval-medicine> [accessed 9 May 2023]

——, 'Women's Medicine in Late Medieval Ireland: The *Trotula* Texts', in *Birth and the Irish: A Miscellany*, ed. by Salvador Ryan (Dublin: Wordwell, 2021), pp. 40–44

Bader, Richard-Ernst, 'Magie in der Volksmedizin', *Medizinhistorisches Journal*, 22.2–3 (1987), 115–34

Bannerman, John, *The Beatons: A Medical Kindred in the Classical Gaelic Tradition* (Edinburgh: John Donald, 1986)

Barrett, Siobhán, 'The King of Dál nAraidi's Salve', *Ériu*, 69 (2019), 171–78

——, 'Multilingual Medicalese', in *Medieval Multilingual Manuscripts: Texts, Scribes and Patrons*, ed. by Nike Stam (forthcoming)

Black, Ronald, *Catalogue of Gaelic Manuscripts in the National Library of Scotland* <https://www.isos.dias.ie/libraries/NLS/english/index.html> [accessed 3 August 2022]

Cartwright, Jane, 'Virginity and Chastity Tests in Medieval Welsh Prose', in *Medieval Virginities*, ed. by Anke Bernau, Ruth Evans, and Sarah Salih (Cardiff: University of Wales Press, 2003), pp. 56–79

Charles-Edwards, Thomas, *Early Christian Ireland* (Cambridge: Cambridge University Press, 2000)

——, 'Naw kynywedi teithiauc', in *The Welsh Law of Women*, ed. by Dafydd Jenkins and Morfydd E. Owen (Cardiff: University of Wales Press, 1980), pp. 23–39

Dinneen, Patrick S., *Foclóir Gaedhilge agus Béarla. An Irish-English Dictionary* (Dublin: Irish Texts Society, 1927)

Dundes, Alan, '"Jumping the Broom": On the Origin and Meaning of an African American Wedding Custom', *The Journal of American Folklore*, 109, no. 433 (1996), 324–29

eDIL = eDIL 2019: *An Electronic Dictionary of the Irish Language*, based on the Contributions to a Dictionary of the Irish Language (Dublin: Royal Irish Academy, 1913–1976) <www.dil.ie> [accessed 3 August 2022]

Elsakkers, Marianne, '"In Pain You Shall Bear Children" (Gen. 3: 16): Medieval Prayers for a Safe Delivery', in *Women and Miracle Stories: A Multidisciplinary Exploration*, ed. by Anne-Marie Korte (Leiden: Brill, 2001), pp. 179–209

Flower, Robin, *Catalogue of Irish Manuscripts in the British Library* [formerly *British Museum*], *Volume* 2 (London: British Museum, 1926; repr. Dublin: DIAS, 1992)

GPC Online = *Geiriadur Prifysgol Cymru. A Dictionary of the Welsh Language* (Cardiff: University of Wales, 2014) <www.geiriadur.ac.uk> [accessed 3 August 2022]

Green, Monica, 'A Handlist of Latin and Vernacular Manuscripts of the So-called *Trotula* Texts, Part 1: The Latin Manuscripts', *Scriptorium*, 50 (1996), 137–75

——, 'A Handlist of Latin and Vernacular Manuscripts of the So-called *Trotula* Texts, Part 2: The Vernacular Translations and Latin Re-writings', *Scriptorium*, 51 (1997), 80–104

Gwynn Jones, Thomas, *Welsh Folklore and Folk-Custom* (Cambridge: D.S. Brewer, 1979)

Hayden, Deborah, 'Attribution and Authority in a Medieval Irish Medical Compendium', *Studia Hibernica*, 45 (2019), 19–51

——, 'The Context and Obscure Language of Healing Charms in a Sixteenth-century Irish Remedy Book: Four Case Studies', in *Obscuritas in Medieval Irish and Welsh Literature*, ed. by Chantal Kobel (Dublin: DIAS, forthcoming)

——, 'Old English in the Irish Charms', *Speculum*, 97.2 (2022), 349–79

——, 'Three Versified Medical Recipes Invoking Dían Cécht', in *Fír Fesso: A Festschrift for Neil McLeod*, ed. by Anders Ahlqvist and Pamela O'Neill, Sydney Series in Celtic Studies, 17 (Sydney: Celtic Studies Foundation, University of Sydney, 2018), pp. 107–23

——, 'A Versified Cure for Headache and Some Lexicographical Notes', *Keltische Forschungen*, 8 (2019), 7–22 <https://doi.org/10.25365/kf-8-2019-7-22>

Herbert, Máire, 'Some Irish Prognostications', *Éigse*, 14.4 (1972), 303–18

Hindley, Katherine Storm, *Textual Magic. Charms and Written Amulets in Medieval England* (Chicago: University of Chicago Press, 2023)

Hunt, Tony, *Popular Medicine in Thirteenth-century England* (Cambridge: D. S. Brewer, 1990)

ISOS = *Irish Script on Screen – Meamrám Páipéar Ríomhaire* (School of Celtic Studies, Dublin Institute for Advanced Studies) <www.isos.dias.ie> [accessed 3 August 2022]

Kibre, Pearl, 'Hippocrates Latinus: Repertorium of Hippocratic Writings in the Latin Middle Ages (II)', *Traditio*, 32 (1976), 257–92

Mistry, Zubin, *Abortion in the Early Middle Ages, c. 500–900* (York: York Medieval Press, 2015)

Murray Jones, Peter, and Lea T. Olsan, 'Performative Rituals for Conception and Childbirth in England, 900–1500', *Bulletin of the History of Medicine*, 89.3 (2015), 406–33

Nelson, Marie, 'A Woman's Charm', *Studia Neophilologica*, 57 (1985), 3–8

Nic Dhonnchadha, Aoibheann, 'An Irish Medical Treatise on Vellum and Paper from the 16th Century', in *Paper and the Paper Manuscript: A Context for the Transmission of Gaelic Literature*, ed. by Pádraig Ó Macháin (Cló Torna: Department of Modern Irish, University College Cork, 2019), pp. 111–25

——, 'Michael Casey's Medical Transcripts in Gilbert MS 147', *Éigse*, 40 (2019), 43–114

Ó Muraíle, Nollaig, 'The Hereditary Medical Families of Gaelic Ireland', in *Rosa Anglica: Reassessments*, ed. by Liam P. Ó Murchú, Irish Texts Society Subsidiary Series, 28 (London: Irish Texts Society, 2016), pp. 85–113

Rempt, Menna, '"And Straightaway the Fountain of Her Blood Dried Up" (Mark 5:29): Constructing a Template for Late Medieval Irish Obstetric Charms' (Unpublished RMA thesis, Utrecht University, 2019)

RIA Catalogue = *Catalogue of Irish Manuscripts in the Royal Irish Academy*, ed. by T. F. O'Rahilly and others, 8 vols (Dublin: Royal Irish Academy, 1926–1970)

Riddle, John M., *Contraception and Abortion from the Ancient World to the Renaissance* (Cambridge, MA: Harvard University Press, 1992)

Samples, Susan, 'Guinevere: A Reappraisal', *Arthurian Interpretations*, 3.2 (1989), 106–18

Sandmann, Gert, 'Studien zu altenglischen Zaubersprüchen' (unpublished doctoral thesis, Westfälischen Wilhelms-Universität zu Münster, 1975)

Simms, Katharine, 'O'Friel's Ghost', in *Sacred Histories. A Festschrift for Máire Herbert*, ed. by John Carey, Kevin Murray, and Caitríona Ó Dochartaigh (Dublin: Four Courts Press, 2015), pp. 401–08

Sinclair, John, *The Statistical Account of Scotland, Drawn up from the Communications of the Ministers of the Different Parishes, Vol. 1* (Edinburgh: William Creech, 1791)

Skemer, Don C., *Binding Words. Textual Amulets in the Middle Ages* (University Park, PA: Pennsylvania State University Press, 2006)

Stifter, David, 'The Rise of Gemination in Celtic', *Open Research Europe. Linguistic Diversity Collection*. Version 1: 2.2.2023. Version 2: 8.2.2024 <https://doi.org/10.12688/openreseurope.15400.2> [accessed 30 March 2024]

Sullivan, C. W. III, '"Jumping the Broom": A Further Consideration of the Origins of an African American Wedding Custom', *The Journal of American Folklore*, 110.436 (1997), 203–04

Valente, Roberta L., 'Gwydion and Aranrhod: Crossing the Borders of Gender in *Math*', in *The Mabinogi: A Book of Essays*, ed. by C. W. Sullivan III (New York and London: Garland, 1996), pp. 331–45

Versnel, H. S., 'The Poetics of the Magical Charm: An Essay in the Power of Words', in *Magic and Ritual in the Ancient World*, ed. by Paul Mirecki and Marvin Meyer, Religions in the Graeco-Roman World, 141 (Leiden, 2002), pp. 105–58

Weston, L. M. C., 'Women's Medicine, Women's Magic: The Old English Metrical Childbirth Charms', *Modern Philology*, 92.3 (1995), 279–93

KATHERINE LEACH

19. Conformity and Innovation in Premodern Welsh Medical Charms

At some point in later sixteenth-century Wales, a biblical soldier (Longinus) became identified with a medieval Arthurian character (Lancelot), at least in the eyes of one scribe. Longinus, whose lance pierced Christ's side at the crucifixion, was commonly invoked in blood-staunching charms. Lancelot (or Lawnslot in Welsh), the Arthurian character of the Grail Cycle, hardly needs introduction. Although Longinus' transformation into Lawnslot was fleeting and is attested in just one blood-staunching charm text, it is a noteworthy example of the ways in which Welsh charm texts rely on certain shared European traditions while also shaping the text to specific cultural preferences. This chapter will consider how Welsh healing charms conformed to a wider, shared European tradition while also allowing for various adaptations and innovations unique to the Welsh corpus.

Healing charms exist in many languages and cultures.[1] They can be understood as ritual means of addressing situations of sickness and anxiety through a combination of specific language and actions, often augmented with herbal medical prescriptions. As texts, charms enjoy a particular flexibility, belonging at once to the realms of both the formal (book knowledge) and the informal (practical, everyday practice), while also occupying an ambiguous — and often contested — space in the domains of medicine, religion, and popular magic or superstition.[2] Healing charms are found in a variety of Welsh manuscripts, often alongside works of medicine, religious texts, and poetry. Typically, they are found in Welsh, or they are dual-language charms in Welsh and Latin, although English and (less frequently) French examples

1 On medical charms from other Insular linguistic traditions, see the chapters in this volume by Caroline Batten, David Stifter, Deborah Hayden and Sarah Baccianti.

2 For more on the interplay between science, magic, and religion see Kieckhefer, *Magic in the Middle Ages*.

Katherine Leach • Dartmouth College; kate.leach-2@dartmouth.edu

Medicine in the Medieval North Atlantic World: Vernacular Texts and Traditions, ed. by Deborah Hayden and Sarah Baccianti, KSS, 5 (Turnhout, 2025), pp. 439-462
BREPOLS PUBLISHERS DOI 10.1484/M.KSS-EB.5.143997

exist in Welsh manuscripts.[3] The earliest Welsh healing charms are found in manuscripts dating to around the end of the fourteenth century and many of the earliest extant Welsh charm types display a remarkable continuity throughout the Middle Ages and into the Early Modern era.

Charms typically contain verbal formulae meant to be spoken, written, worn, or enacted in some way.[4] Charms can consist of short verbal formulae in which the efficacy relies on the recitation of various words of power. Similarly, written charms rely on strings of efficacious writing and instruct that the text be written upon a specified material and hung about the patient, in a dwelling, or even burned or ingested.[5] The performative action and the power inherent in the words themselves constitute the efficacious element of the charm. One fever charm instructs that three liturgical phrases be written on three communion wafers over three days and then the sacred words and the objects upon which they are written are to be ingested by the patient. This charm, which was popular in medieval English manuscripts, can also be found in several Welsh manuscripts:

> Rhag yr Acses. Kym*er* dair Arlladen, ac yscrivena arnyn Pater est alpha et o ar un o honyn, ai rhoi ir kalf oi bwytta, a doeded i pater noster kyn i bwyta / ar ail dydd ysgrivena ar yr ail filius est vita et veritas, a gwna iddo i bwyta a doydyd 2. paternoster kyn i bwyta ar trydydd dydd kymered y drydedd afrlladen ac ysgrivened arni spiritus sanctus est et domini a gwna dri ffwynt fal hyn ••• a ffar ir klaf i bwytaf a doydyd tri Paternoster kyn i bwytaf ac ef a fydd iach drwy ras Dyw Amen.
>
> > (Against the fever. Take three hosts and write on them: 'the Father is the Beginning and the End' on one of them and give it to the patient to eat, and say one Our Father before eating. On the second day write on the second [host], 'The Son is the way and the truth' and make him eat it and say two Our Fathers before eating. On the third day take the third host and write on it, 'The Holy Spirit is and of the Lord' and make three marks like this ••• and make the patient eat it and say three Our Fathers before eating and he will be healthy through the grace of God, Amen.)[6]

---

3 Although my focus here is on medieval and the earliest early modern charms, Welsh charms are also found in manuscripts of the seventeenth–twentieth centuries. Owen Davies has published prodigiously on charms, magic, and cunning folk in Britain from the later seventeenth century onward: see Davies, 'Healing Charms'; Davies, 'Charmers and Charming in England and Wales'; Davies, 'Cunning-Folk in England and Wales'; and Davies, *Popular Magic*. See also Bosse-Griffith, *Byd y Dyn Hysbys*.

4 For discussion concerning the semantic range of the word 'charm', see Olsan, 'Charms in Medieval Memory', p. 60, and Skemer, *Binding Words*, p. 18.

5 Olsan, 'Writing on the Hand'. See also Hindley, 'Eating Words and Burning Them'.

6 London, MS Wellcome 417, fol. 31^{v}. This is a manuscript from the second half of the sixteenth century, though it is itself a compilation of medical texts likely copied from a fifteenth-century exemplar. Unless otherwise noted, all dates in this chapter are taken from Huws, *A*

The instruction to make three marks upon the wafer could signify the order in which to eat the wafers, or it could have been conceived of as symbolic of the wounds of Christ.[7] Olsan understands the wafers in the Middle English charms to be consecrated hosts, given the efficacy ascribed to them in healing, due to their consecration by a priest in preparation for the Eucharist.[8] Communion wafers had long been regarded for their powers of miraculous healing, and the use, or rather, misuse of hosts was a source of anxiety within the medieval Church, as is made evident at the Fourth Lateran Council of 1215, at which decrees were passed to protect consecrated hosts from being stolen for magical purposes.[9] Despite the theological issues regarding this practice, charms of this group flourished in English manuscripts over the whole of the medieval period. A similar medieval English version can be found in Oxford, Bodl. Lib., MS Add. B.1:

> for ye feuer: Take 3. obleyes & wright on ye first pater est apha et ω & gyue ye sike to eate ye first daye, on ye second wright filius est vita & make 2. crosses & gyue ye sicke to eate on ye seconde day, & on ye 3 wright sp˜s sc˜tus est benedictum & make 3 crosses & kneele downe & say wth good devotion .5. pr nr & 5 a & a creede & thow shalt be hole.[10]
>
> > (For the fever: Take three obleys and on the first, write pater est alpha et omega and give (it to) the sick to eat the first day. On the second, write filius est vita and make two crosses and give (it to) the sick to eat on the second day. On the third, write spiritus sanctus est benedictum and make three crosses and kneel down and say with good devotion five Our Fathers and five Hail Marys and a Credo and you shall be whole.)

The precise rationale for the substitution of apples for wafers remains uncertain, although several plausible explanations exist. Due to increasing anxiety within the Church regarding misuse of the host, access to the communion wafers was impeded and fever charms of this type were adapted, allowing for the charm to be written on leaves, apples, or parchment. Lea Olson highlights Adolf Franz's observation of a tenth-century benediction performed over apples or cheese to bring about healing from chills and fevers. She also notes that the substitution of an apple for wafers was used early in the English charm corpus, possibly because the alternative might be necessary in situations where access to a priest was limited, such as in female orders or in the home

---

Repertory of Welsh Manuscripts and Scribes. I am grateful to Daniel Huws for making available a draft version of the work prior to publication. Unless otherwise noted, all transcriptions and translations are my own. I have left the Welsh largely unedited.

7 See Olsan, 'Writing on the Hand', p. 18 for a fifteenth-century Middle English charm that gives similar instructions.

8 Olsan, 'Writing on the Hand', p. 18.

9 See Browe, 'Die Eucharist als Zaubermittle' and Browe, *Die eucharistischen Wunder des Mittelalters.*

10 Oxford, Bodl. Lib., MS Add. B.1, as presented in Klaassen, *Making Magic*, p. 49.

of a layman.[11] Several such charms were copied into Welsh manuscripts as well. An early Welsh fever charm (late fourteenth or early fifteenth century) instructs users to write on apples over three days. This charm is found within a larger section of medicine that is, overall, noticeably lacking in charms.

> Rac pob teirton. Yscriuenner y my6n tri aual yn tri diwarna6t. Yn yr aual kyntaf. + on agla pater. Yn yr eil aual. + on agla filius. Yn y trydyd aual. + On agla spiritus sanctus. A'r tryded dyd ef a uyd iach.
>
> > (Against all fevers. Let three apples be written upon in three days: In the first apple + On agla Pater. In the second apple + On agla Filius. In the third apple + On agla Spiritus Sanctus. And on the third day he will be healthy.)[12]

Overall, although fever charms specifying that the words of power should be written and ingested in a pattern of threes were popular in England, they do not seem to have resonated with a Welsh audience to quite the same degree. Much more popular in the Welsh tradition were fever charms that relied on a divine narrative for their power.

The *Super Petram* Charm Type in the Welsh Corpus

While some charms rely on efficacious written and verbal elements and ritual, as we have seen above, other charms are longer and feature *historiolae*: short narratives about Christ, saints, biblical characters, or events from religious or mythological cycles. According to Olsan, narrative charms enable the simultaneous representation of a sacred past, living predicament and future expectation.[13] Such texts create a connection between the biblical past and the situation of the patient or charm user in the present. The power of a narrative charm lies partly in this perceived link between past and present, and the virtue of the charm is in its ability to break down the boundaries between narrative past and present reality, bringing the patient closer to the divine narrative and thus the divine power.[14] In other words, the circumstances of the narrative parallel the situation in the present, and affect the present

---

11 Olsan, 'Writing on the Hand', pp. 17 and 19. Olsan references Franz, *Die kirchlichen Benedictionen*.

12 Oxford, Jesus College, MS 111, fol. 233r, col. 937. A similar example exists in a sixteenth-century manuscript, Oxford, Bodl. Lib., MS Add. B.1: 'Pro febribus medicina probata. Take an apple & cutt it in 3 peeces & on ye first part wright these wordes Ihs̄ ageos dn¯s78 & on ye .2. part wright xp¯s otheos dn¯s .3. on ye 3 part wright resur- rexit a mortuis dn¯s79 & gyue him to eat & he shall be holl by gods grace .3 pr nr 2 a. 1 c' (as printed in Klaassen, *Making Magic*, p. 45).

13 Olsan, 'Charms in Medieval Memory'. See also Olsan, 'Latin Charms of Medieval England'.

14 For more on the structure and function of narrative charms, see Waller, 'Echo and the *Historiola*'. I am grateful to Katherine Hindley for this reference. See also Hindley, 'Eating Words and Burning Them', and Frankfurter, 'Narrating Power'.

through a sort of homeopathic magic, or the principle of *similia similibus*.[15] One common narrative charm type was included in a Welsh manuscript from the mid-fifteenth century:[16]

> Petrus aute*m* iacebat febritans sup*er* petra*m* mermoria*m*[17] et uenit ei ihc + ait illi. Petre quid iaces hic Respondens petrus + ait ille. domine iaceo hic in mala febre. Tu*n*c ait ihc ad petru*m*, surge + dimitte illam + co*n*tinuo surrexit + dimisit ill [...] tu*n*c ait petrus ad ihm d*omi*ne rogo te ut que*m*cu*m*que hoc su*per* se portauerit ut dicerit no*n* noceat ei febres frigide nec calide cotidiana n*ec* biduana nec triduana nec quartuana. tu[n]c ait ihc ad Petru*m*, Petre fiat tibi sicut petisti fiat fiat. In no*mine* pa*t*ris. Jh*esus* nazareus crucifixus rex iudeo*rum* miserere mei in manus tuas.
>
>> (Peter was lying with a fever on a rock of marble and Jesus came to him and said, 'Peter why are you lying here?' Peter, answering, + said, 'Lord I am lying here because of a bad fever.' Then Jesus said to Peter, 'Arise + cast it out'. + He rose immediately and cast it out [...] then Peter said to Jesus, 'Lord I ask you that whosoever shall carry this on them and say it shall not be harmed by cold fevers nor hot [nor] quotidian, nor biduan nor tertian nor quartan.' Then Jesus said to Peter, 'Peter, let it be for you as you have asked. Let it be, let it be.' In the name of the father. Jesus of Nazareth, crucified King of the Jews, have mercy on me in your hands.)[18]

This charm features a narrative motif commonly found in the charms of medieval Europe, and early Latin versions of the charm exist from at least the tenth and eleventh centuries.[19] The hallmark feature of this charm type — labelled by scholars as the *Super Petram* — is the dialogue between Christ and Peter, usually while Peter is lying or sitting upon a rock, suffering from an ailment. Sometimes Peter is placed before the gates of a city (usually Jerusalem) and often he is suffering from a toothache rather than a fever. The Welsh-manuscript charm above is not the only example of a *Super Petram* charm being used to heal a fever rather than a toothache. Similar charms have been discovered in English manuscripts.[20] In the Welsh corpus, *Super Petram*

---

15 For more on narrative charms see Bozóky, 'Medieval Narrative Charms', p. 101.

16 Huws, *A Repertory*, p. 60.

17 *marmoream.*

18 Aberystwyth, NLW, MS Llanstephan 2, p. 348.

19 Roper, *English Verbal Charms*, p. 122. Roper also gives an example of an eleventh-century example, found in an English manuscript: 'Christus super marmoreum sedebat petrus tristes ante eum stabat manum ad maxillum tenebat et interogebat eum dominus dicens: quare tristis es petre? Respondit Petrus et dixit: domine dentes me dolent. Et dominus dixit: adiuro te migranea uel gutta maligna per patrem et filium et spiritum sanctum'.

20 Olsan, 'Latin Charms of Medieval England', gives an example (p. 132) from London, BL, MS Sloane 122 (fol. 163^{r}): 'Pro Febrebus. In nomine Patris et Filij et Spiritus Sancti Amen. Petrus autem iacebat febricitantibus super petram mormoriam. Et super veniens illi Iesus

charms were much more commonly used as a fever charm, although there are instances of this charm being employed against a toothache, as was common in other European traditions. One of the earliest, if not the earliest, collection of Welsh medical charms includes a *Super Petram* charm for toothache that also references Susanna, who, along with Apollonia, was commonly invoked in medieval toothache charms:[21]

> Contra dolorem dentium. In nomine patris + *et* filii. *et* spiritus sancti. + amen + Qui liberauit susanam de falso crimine libera istum famulum tuum N. de dolore dentium. Petrus sedebat super petram *et* maria uirgo deum tenebat caput suum *in* manu sua superueniens dominus dixit ei qualem tristiciam habes respondens petrus dixit. dentes mei dolent vermiculi deuoratur carnem meam *et* ossa mea. Respondens dominus dixit. Signate eos + In nomine patris + *et* filii. *et spiritus sancti*. amen. + *christus* vincit + *christus* uincit. *christus* regnat + *christus* imperat + *christus* ab omni malo hunc famulum dei defendat. amen.
>
> > (Against a toothache. In the name of the Father + and the Son + and the Holy Spirit + Amen + He who liberated Susana from false judgement, liberate your servant N. from toothache. Peter sat on a stone. And while the Virgin Mary held his head in her hand, God approached and said to him, 'why do you have such sorrow?' Responding, Peter said, 'my teeth hurt, worms devour my flesh and my bones.' The Lord said, 'Mark them with a sign + In the name of the Father + and the Son + and the Holy Spirit + Amen. Christ conquers + Christ conquers + Christ reigns + Christ commands + Let Christ defend this servant of God from all evil. Amen.')[22]

While this is a standard *Super Petram* dialogue between Peter and Christ, this charm is interesting for its inclusion of the Virgin Mary. It appears that this charm has merged at least two charm types into one, as Tony Hunt records a toothache charm in an Anglo-Norman manuscript that also places the Virgin Mary upon a stone, complaining of a worm called *migranea* that has penetrated her teeth.[23]

---

dixit, "Petre quid iacis?" Et respondit ei Petrus, "Domine iaceo de febre mala." Et dixit Iesus, "Surge et dimitte illam, et continuo surrexit et dimisit." Et dixit Petrus, "Domine, rogo te vt quicumque haec verba super se portaverit scripta quod non n[o]ceat ei febres frigide nec calide, cotidiane, biduane, triduane, nec quartane." Et ait Iesus, "Petre, Fiat tibi sicut petisti nomine meo." Amen.'

21 Divine narratives common in medieval European toothache charms include *historiolae* relating to Saint Apollonia, whose teeth were pulled out by her torturers, and Saint Susanna, who is more commonly found in charms to cure headache and alleviate other general pains, and whose narrative usually refers to her being wrongfully accused of and judged for promiscuity, and then beheaded.

22 Cardiff, Card. Lib., MS 3.242, p. 53.

23 Charme ad dentz: sancta Maria supra petram sedevat, Spiritus Sanctus superveniebat et dicebat 'Quid tristaris Maria?' et dicebat 'Dolent dentes mei. Venit [vermis] migraneus et me mordit'. 'Adiuro te migranea [fol. 14^r] gutta per Patrem et Filium et Spiritum Sanctum …' (*Anglo-Norman Medicine II*, ed. by Hunt, p. 232).

Lea Olsan has pointed out that healing charms in medieval Christianity are most often found when a primary feature or symptom of an ailment coincided with a culturally charged image that could be effectively expressed as a charm: a specific charm motif is associated with its symptom by a specific image or word.[24] Olsan further argues that the existence of a medieval charm often probably depends less on the inherent nature of the medical condition than on the cultural perceptions of the disease or symptom.[25] Although, to my knowledge, there are no biblical or apocryphal traditions in which Christ cured Peter of a toothache (or a fever), the medieval association of Saint Peter with toothache is likely rooted in his name and the potential for a play on the words *Petrus/petram*, as he is most commonly said to be sitting upon a rock when he encounters Christ. W. F. Ryan argues that Peter became identified with toothache charms because of the 'quality of rock hardness and marble whiteness that is sought for the tooth', as well as on account of the renaming of Simon as Peter in the '*Tu es Petrus*' episode in the Gospel of Matthew 16.18: 'Tu es petrus, et super hanc petram aedificabo ecclesiam meam' (You are Peter, and upon this rock I will build my church).[26]

Although the *Super Petram* type was one of the most frequently copied charms in medieval Europe, and was also exceedingly popular in Ireland,[27] it was not used as frequently as a toothache charm in Wales, at least not as far as the extant manuscript evidence shows. Thus far I have uncovered only twelve toothache charms in the medieval and early modern Welsh corpus, though there are undoubtedly more. Fewer than half of the Welsh toothache charms are of the *Super Petram* charm type popular elsewhere in Europe. Barbara Hillers notes the popularity of *Super Petram* toothache charms in Ireland, in English and in Irish-language versions and she has demonstrated that English versions of this type are found in all provinces of Ireland but display a remarkable homogeneity and similarity to English versions collected in England. The Irish-language versions, however, demonstrate much more variance, and Hillers suggests that these charms developed out of Latin versions of the *Super Petram* charm that would have reached Ireland through monastic networks.[28] Charms recorded in Scotland also feature the invocation of Peter in a toothache charm, as well as the motif of the marble stone upon which he sat.[29] In the Welsh corpus, this charm type was always copied in Latin, which may suggest that it found its way into Wales either through early

24 Olsan, 'Latin Charms of Medieval England', p. 130 and Olsan, 'Charms in Medieval Memory', pp. 66–67.

25 Olsan, 'Latin Charms of Medieval England', p. 130.

26 Ryan, *Bathhouse at Midnight*, p. 154.

27 Hillers, 'Towards a Typology of European Narrative Charms', p. 86.

28 Hillers, 'Towards a Typology of European Narrative Charms', pp. 87–88.

29 Such charms are not commonly found in Scottish Gaelic but rather were circulated in English and Latin, and with a great emphasis placed on the written word. For more, see Mackenzie, *Gaelic Incantations*.

Latin manuscripts that circulated through monastic networks, or from Latin charms included in medical books produced elsewhere that circulated and were accessed and used as source texts for our Welsh manuscripts. Overall, toothache and fever charms in Welsh manuscripts are fairly representative of common European charming practices and, unsurprisingly, many have direct parallels in the English corpus of charm texts.

The *Longinus* Charm Type in the Welsh Corpus

Charms for staunching blood and healing general wounds make up the largest percentage of healing charms in the Welsh corpus. Such texts are found in Welsh, Latin, and English. I have thus far discovered fifty-one charms for staunching blood, healing general wounds, and curing animal bites (mostly rabid dogs or snakes). Jonathan Roper's database of English charms, which includes texts from the Old English period up through the twentieth century, suggests that the most popular use of healing charms in England was for staunching blood, and this is true of the Welsh corpus as well. Of the fifty-one Welsh wound charms, thirty-six are for staunching blood. Roper notes that of the 311 healing charms in his English charm database, sixty-three (or, roughly twenty per cent) were used for staunching blood.[30] In Roper's English collection, the most common blood-staunching charm was the *Flum Jordan*, which relied upon an extra-biblical narrative about the river Jordan coming to a halt at Christ's baptism. *Flum Jordan* charms have also been collected in modern Ireland, though Barbara Hillers has argued that the charm type belongs more firmly to an English tradition.[31] *Flum Jordan* charms are not popular in the pre-modern Welsh corpus, which favoured the *Longinus* charm type for stopping blood flow.

The *Longinus* charm type was especially common in the medieval West and continued to be used well into the modern period.[32] Versions have survived in Latin and in various vernaculars, including Old High German, Russian,

30 Roper's work relies heavily on secondary scholarship and printed works, and though it is a monumental source of scholarship, it does not consider a great number of medieval charms that remain known but unpublished. One scholar, Katherine Hindley, is in the early stages of compiling a database of medieval English charms. Once her database is complete, the total number of charms (and the types to which they belong) will no doubt be drastically altered. The second most popular category of charms, according to Roper, was for the general healing of wounds, with thirty-four examples (or ten per cent): see Roper, *English Verbal Charms*, p. 62.

31 Hillers, 'Towards a Typology of European Narrative Charms', pp. 79–102.

32 For a foundational comparative study of blood-loss charms, see Ebermann, *Blut- und Wundsegen*. While my focus is on Welsh healing charms up to around the mid-seventeenth century, Davies, 'Healing Charms in Use in England and Wales', pp. 19–32, has presented some fascinating charms circulating in Britain in later eras, including Longinus charms for stopping blood.

French, Norse, Italian, Swedish, Byzantine Greek, and Irish.[33] The efficacy of the charm relies upon a narrative based on the account of Christ's crucifixion in the Gospel of John, as well as the mid-fourth-century apocryphal Gospel of Nicodemus, which names the soldier who pierced Christ's side when he was on the cross. The *Legenda Aurea* also relates that Longinus was blind until he pierced the side of Christ, whose blood came into contact with Longinus's eyes, miraculously restoring his vision.[34] It seems a bit of a paradox that a charm for *stopping* blood would rely so heavily on this episode of blood *flowing*, but the charms suggest a parallel between Longinus being cured by the power of Christ's blood and the patient being cured through invocation of the same redeeming blood.[35] Although the Welsh charms do not narrate that his blindness was healed through contact with the blood of Christ, many refer to him as being blind.

An examination of the development of Welsh *Longinus* charms from the earliest examples (late fourteenth and early/mid-fifteenth centuries) to the later sixteenth century and beyond provides a fascinating insight into the ways in which a charm type can both conform to the standard European tradition while also sustaining subtle but unique innovations. *Longinus* charms were included in the earliest Welsh collections of healing charms:

> Rac g6aetlin o wythien mal o le arall: ysgriuenna y geireu hynn. Longeus miles latus d*omini* p*er*foraui*t* *et* continuo exiuit sanguis *et* aqua + In n*omine* p*atris* stet sa*n*guis + In no*mine* filii restet sanguis + In no*mine* sp*iritus* *sancti* non exeat gutta. Ter fiet ista benediccio *et* restet sanguis.
>
> > (For bleeding from a vein or another place, write these words: Longinus the soldier pierced the side of the Lord and immediately blood and water flowed out + in the name of the Father let the blood stop + in the name of the Son let the blood stand firm + in the name of the Holy Spirit let a drop not escape. Let this blessing be done three times and let the blood stop.)[36]

This charm generally conforms to the standard Latin versions in manuscripts of other traditions.[37] Another early Welsh version reads:

---

33 Roper, *English Verbal Charms*, p. 113.

34 *The Golden Legend*, trans by. Ryan, p. 202.

35 For more on water and flowing liquids in blood-staunching charms, see Fisher, 'The Anglo-Saxon Charms', pp. 111–16.

36 Cardiff, Card. Lib., MS 3.242, p. 1.

37 A standard Latin version of this charm type might run: 'A charm for to stau*n*che blod. Longin*us* miles lat*us* do*minii* *nostri* + Iesu Ch*risti* la*n*cea p*er*foraui*t* et *con*tinuo exiuit sa*n*guis et aq*ua* i*n* redempcionem i*nostram*. *Adiuro te sanguis* p*er* ipsum + Ch*ristum* p*er* latus ei*us* p*er* sangui*nem* eius + sta + sta + sta. + Ch*ristus* et Ioh*annes* descen*derunt* i*n* flume*n* iordanis. aq*ua* obstipuit et stetit, sic faciat sa*n*guis isti*us* corp*oris* [fol. 35f] In + Ch*risti* no*mine* et *sancti* Joh*annis* bap*tiste* ame*n*. Et dica t*er* p*ater* noste*r* et t*er* Aue Ma*ria*.' The charm, from Cambridge, Univ. Lib., MS Add. 9308, is printed in Olsan, 'The Corpus of Charms', pp. 218–19.

> rac gwaetlin. Longius Ebreus miles latus d*omini* nos*t*ri ihesu xr*ist*i p*er*forauit *et* continuo exiuit sanguis *et* aqua, sanguis redempconis *et* aqua baptismatis. In no*min*e pa*t*ris + cessat sanguis + in no*min*e filii restat sanguis + in no*min*e sp*iritus sanc*ti amplius no*n* exeat sanguis.
>
> > (against bleeding. Longi[n]us the Hebrew soldier pierced the side of our Lord Jesus Christ and immediately blood and water ran out: the blood of redemption and the water of baptism. In the name of the Father the blood stops + in the name of the Son the blood stands firm + In the name of the Holy Spirit let the blood not run out.)[38]

The *Longinus* charms above represent two of the earliest attested Welsh manuscript examples of this charm type. In general, the earliest Welsh-manuscript versions of the *Longinus* charm type tend to privilege Latin over Welsh, using Welsh only to provide brief practical instructions regarding the enactment of charm. However, the *Longinus* charm type was quickly assimilated into the Welsh tradition, almost always appearing as a vernacular Welsh charm from the later fifteenth century onwards and also remaining fairly consistent within the corpus. They also soon begin to exhibit a distinct literary flair that versions from other linguistic and cultural traditions lack:

> Llyma swyn y stobio gwaed o brathnev i ddynion. Gwnaf i iti, waed, fal ir agores lonsivr y marchog vrddol dall o wlad yr Ebriw ar gwaiw ruddefvdd yn ystlyss Iesu Grist yn harglwydd ni yni ddoeith dwy ffrwd vn o waed er yn pryni ni ag vn o ddwr er yn golchi ni. Gorchymvn iti waed estobio yn enwr dad yn enw y mab. Na cherdda di, waed, yn [enw]yr ysbryd duw glan. Nac ysgog di, waed, nag o gig nag o gnawd nag o ie nag o with. Yn enw dad, yn enw ar mab ar ysbryd dyw glan. A dowed y swyn yma deir gwaith a he[n]war dyn y bor swyn iddo y waed yn kolli. A dyrro dy law ar i ben o byddi di yn gallu krydda[39] ef a dowaid v bader a ffumb afi meria er anrydedd yr v archoll llydan a ddioddefodd yn harglwydd y ni iesv grist er brynv yr holl cristynogion y byd amen.
>
> > (Here is a charm to stop blood from wounds to people. I will do to you, blood, just as Lonsiur the blind, dubbed knight from the land of Israel, pierced the side of Jesus Christ our Lord with the red-bronze lance, and there came two streams: one of blood in order to redeem us and one of water in order to cleanse us. I command you, blood, stop in the name of the Father. In the name of the Son, do not flow, blood. In [the name of] the Holy Spirit of God. Do not move, blood, not from meat nor from flesh nor from tendons nor from veins. In the name of

---

38 Aberystwyth, NLW, MS Peniarth 47, part IV, p. 31 (in a mid-fifteenth-century hand).

39 Another possibility is to read this verb as *ceryddaf* (to amend, make good). A variant reading might be: 'Place your hand on his head until you can make him good.' My thanks to Diana Luft for this suggestion (email communication, 18 February 2020).

> the Father, in the name of the Son, and the Holy Spirit of God. Say this charm three times and name the man to whom the charm is for and who is losing blood. Put your hand on his head until you can lessen it [i.e., the blood flow]. And say five Our Fathers and five Ave Marias in honour of the five extensive wounds that our Lord Jesus Christ suffered in order to redeem all the Christians of the world, Amen.)[40]

From the later fifteenth century onwards, most Welsh-manuscript *Longinus* charms include the description of Longinus as a Hebrew knight and refer to him as blind. This is quite different to the English-manuscript charms (in Latin and in English), where he is rarely described as being blind, and is usually simply called a Hebrew and/or a soldier (*miles*). Later Welsh versions of the *Longinus* charm are more likely to feature an augmented characterization of Longinus, identifying him by an expanded Welsh epithet 'Longinus marchoc evrddol ebrv' (Longinus the noble Hebrew knight).[41]

One manuscript from the late sixteenth century includes two charms representative of the standard development of later *Longinus* charms:

> (a.) Llyma sswyn i stopio gwaed brath nai ddyrnod. Mi a y swyna y ty waed val yr ygorodd Longys farychoc yrddol o Ebriw ar gwayw ryddefydd ar ysdlys jesu grist yn harglwydd ni oni a ddeth or brath ddwy frwd un o waed er yn prynu ni ac un o ddwfwr er yn golychi ni. Yr wy yn gorychymyn iti waed ystopo yn enw y tad ar mab. Na cherdda di, waed, yn enw yr ysbryd glan. Nag ystoc, waed, yn enw y tad ar mab ar ysbryd glan. A dwaid swyn hwnn tair gwaith, a henwa y dyn i bo y waed yn kerdded a dod dy law ar y ben a dowaid v pader a ffymp afi mareia a chredo er ynrydedd yr pymp archoll prynysinal a ddioddefodd yn harglwydd ni jesu grist er tyny enaid tyn o kaethiwed yffern.
>
> > ([a.] Here is a charm to stop blood from a bite or wound. I charm you, blood: just as Longys [Longinus] the dubbed knight from Israel pierced the side of our Lord Jesus Christ with his red-bronze lance, until two streams came from the wound: one of blood in order to redeem us and one of water in order to cleanse us. I command you, blood, to stop in the name of the Father and of the Son. Do not flow, blood, in the name of the Holy Spirit. Do not stir, blood, in the name of the Father and of the Son and of the Holy Spirit. Say this charm three times and name the man whose blood is flowing. Put your hand upon his head and say five Our Fathers and five Ave Marias and a Credo in honour

40 Aberystwyth, NLW, MS Peniarth 204, p. 1. The charm is written in a poor, mid-sixteenth-century hand.

41 *Evrddol* can mean dignified or noble, but when used referring to a knight, also means dubbed. It is not problematic that the texts assign to him an epithet that connotes such respect and nobility, as he was said to have converted to Christianity after the crucifixion and his legend grew to the extent that he became venerated as a saint.

> of the five redeeming wounds that our Lord Jesus Christ suffered in order to draw out (the) soul(s) of mankind from the bonds of hell.)[42]

> (b.) Llyma swyn ysdopio gwaed dyn. Mi a swyna i ti, waed. Val yr acores Lownyslo farchoc yrddol or briw ar gwayw ryddefydd ar ystlys jesu grist yn harglwydd. Afone a ddoeth or brat[h]ay ddwy ffrwd un o waed er yn pryny ar un llall er yn golychi. Mi a orychmyna iti waed ystopio yn enw y tad ar mab ar ysbryd glan. Nac ystoc wayd yn enw y tad ar mab ar ysbryd glan. A dowaid y swyn yma dair gwaith a henwi y dyn y bo y waed yn kolli. A rhoi i law ar y ben a dwedyd v. pader a ffym afi mareai er anrydedd yr v.arycholl pena oedd ai gorff yn harglwydd ni jesu grist er tyny enaid dyn o yffern.

> ([b.] Here is a charm to stop a person's blood. I charm you, blood. Just as Lownyslo the dubbed knight from Israel pierced the side of our Lord Jesus Christ with his red-bronze lance. Rivers came from the wounds, two streams: one of blood to redeem us and the other to cleanse us. I command you, blood, stop in the name of the Father, and the Son, and the Holy Spirit. Do not stir, blood, in the name of the Father, and the Son, and the Holy Spirit. And say this charm three times and name the man whose blood is flowing. And put your hand on his head and say five Our Fathers and five Ave Marias in honour of the five chief wounds that were upon the body of our Lord Jesus Christ in order to draw out (the) soul(s) of mankind from hell.)[43]

In the second charm above, Longinus is referred to as Lownyslo, a variant of Lawnslot, the Welsh version of Lancelot, demonstrating an interesting conception of the character of Longinus. In addition to expanded and innovated descriptions of Longinus, the vernacular Welsh versions of the charm in this period typically describe his lance as being ruddy or red-bronze in colour: a feature that, to my knowledge, is unattested in other traditions but seems natural in the Welsh corpus. Welsh poetry is replete with descriptions of reddened, bloody spears, so it is unsurprising that Welsh scribes would seize the opportunity to style Longinus in the manner of the warriors and lords of Welsh poetry. The medieval Welsh poem *Y Gododdin* contains lines such as: 'With huge dark-socketed crimson spears' (stanza IX); 'They stained their spears ruddy with blood' (Stanza X); 'Three spears stained with blood' (Stanza XVIII); 'a red spear before Eidin's lord' (Stanza C).[44] Additionally, in medieval Welsh poetry patrons were complimented in terms of their prowess in battle. The poet Guto'r Glyn, for example, refers to one of his patrons as 'a badger with his red spear overthrowing a hundred men' (Poem 3.9).[45] It

---

42 Aberystwyth, NLW, MS 873B, p. 35.

43 Aberystwyth, NLW, MS 873B, p. 251.

44 Translations from Clancy, *The Earliest Welsh Poetry*.

45 The poems of Guto'r Glyn can be found at <http://www.gutorglyn.net/gutoswales/index.php>.

seems, then, that it would be a natural impulse for Welsh scribes to model Longinus on standard Welsh poetic conventions. Indeed, the character of Longinus (and his association with healing) was so deeply embedded in the cultural consciousness that in the mid-fifteenth century, Guto'r Glyn composed a poem to a patron suffering with an arrow embedded in his thigh, where Longinus is referred to in the opening stanza:

> Christ was given of the Virgin Mary
> to carry a heavy cross so as to die for us.
> Yesterday I wept for your suffering,
> your breast and crown and agony.
> A blind man took his spear to pierce you
> into the fresh blood with the bitter pain.[46]

Overall, the *Longinus* motif for stopping blood is well attested throughout Europe, and the Welsh corpus of charms demonstrates that it was used in Wales from the time of the earliest extant books of medicine and healing charms (the later fourteenth century). Extant sources point to the *Longinus* charm type as having entered the Welsh tradition via Latin but by the later fifteenth century, vernacular versions were almost always preferred. The use of the *Longinus* motif continued in the Welsh tradition well beyond the date of the latest charms that I have collected from Welsh manuscripts (seventeenth century). On the surface, the Welsh *Longinus* charms share several features with *Longinus* charms of other traditions, in Latin and in the vernacular. However, the vernacular Welsh *Longinus* charms tend to feature more detailed and elaborate narrative, such as descriptions of Longinus and his lance, along with the general narrative describing the blood and water flowing from the wound. They are, on the whole, indebted to the Welsh poetic tradition in a way that no other charm type in the Welsh corpus has thus far demonstrated and they exhibit a distinct literary flair unattested elsewhere.

An Outlier in the Welsh Corpus: A Charm Against Scrofula

The charms discussed thus far in this chapter represent standard shared European charming traditions, with the *Longinus* charm type both conforming to, yet also showing unique innovations in, these traditions over the course of the fifteenth and sixteenth centuries. Yet there are a small number of charms in the Welsh corpus for which I have been unable to find a single analogue. The most striking is perhaps a charm for scrofula, found in at least two manuscripts.[47] This charm is among one of the more astounding examples of the performative,

46 Translated by Eurig Salisbury at <http://www.gutorglyn.net/gutorglyn/poem/?poem-selection=069>.

47 And found in a third manuscript as a fragment.

verbal power of a charm, and is to my knowledge unparalleled in any other linguistic or cultural tradition.

Scrofula refers to a tumour or swelling in the neck, now associated with tuberculosis.[48] The disease was often referred to as the 'King's evil' due to the widespread belief that the monarchs of England and France were endowed with a divine ability to lay hands on scrofula patients and cure the disease. During these touching ceremonies, which were introduced in England by Edward the Confessor, passages from the Gospels of Mark and John were read over the sick.[49] This ritual was supposedly continued up into the eighteenth century, and its popularity was captured in medical descriptions and treatises as well as literature, such as Shakespeare's *Macbeth*.[50]

I am unaware of a particularly strong tradition of healing charms for scrofula in England. Perhaps the seeming lack of popularity is due to the popularity of the royal touch ceremony, and the fear of promoting a cure that would have been a threat to its legitimacy. I have thus far uncovered two complete Welsh scrofula charms, both of the same variant. Their overarching theme focuses on the exorcism of nine disease-causing worms. Lea Olsan has noted that worms are commonly associated with diseases of the flesh, and that such charms also feature verbal rituals that enact the killing or diminishing of the worms, usually in the form of counting them away.[51] The earliest example is from the early sixteenth century and is also one of the longest Welsh-language charms thus far uncovered:

> Llyma swyn rrac y manwnnion Mi a swyna y ti rrac y manwynion trwy awdryrdawd yr Arglwydd Jessu Grist ar Arglwyddes Fair y Fam. A thrwy ath awdyrdawd y pedwar peroffwyd ar hygain. A thrwy awdyrrdawd yr holl gonffessoriaid saint. A thrwy awdyrdawd yr holl ferthyrri o saint a santesav. A thrwy yr holl werryddon o santesav. A thrwy awdyrdod yr holl engylion ar holl archengylion. Mi ath dystrywa: mi ath [d]ysdrywais mi ath diwraidda mi ath ddiwreiddaiss. Mi ath differewythaf mi ath differwythais. Dros ix mor, dros ix mynydd, dros ix tiwarchen elfydd hyt na bo ynoch na chwydd nac adwyth na chlwyf na chlefyd na gwayw na gwyn na ffryf gwryw na ffryf benyw, nac yth waed nac yth weli nac yth wythi nac yth lythni nac yth fer nac yth es[g]yrn nac yth kac[52] nac yth knawd nac yth

48 Grzybowski and Allen, 'History and Importance of Scrofula', p. 1472.

49 William of Malmesbury recorded the first known instance of this 'royal touch', in which a young woman with swollen glands was healed by the king after washing and rubbing the afflicted areas. William attributed this healing (more likely due the clearing, opening, and draining of the lesions) to divine miracle and the power became associated with the monarchy. For more on this see Turrell, 'The Ritual of Royal Healing', p. 6.

50 In Act IV, Scene 3, Malcom describes the ritual he observed at the court of Edward the Confessor.

51 Olsan, 'The Worm in the Worm Charms' (paper given at the International Society for Folk Narrative Research – Committee on Charms, Charmers and Charming and Belief Narrative Network Committee, Three Day Conference, Budapest, Dec. 2017).

52 Likely meant to be *kic*, as in another version, and as would be more expected as a doublet with *knawd*.

bedwar aelawd. Dy holl korff yn iach i gyd o wartha dy pen hyd yn gwadne dy draed. Amen. Patter noster ac Afi Maria. *Kwm gelon Crist ymresebion dragendi fal y dragon*[53] aethon fal y daython ni lwyddo Duw y manwynion mwy no naw merched brenin Rriallon or ix ir viii or viii ir vii or vii ir vi or vi ir v or v ir iiii or iii ir iii or iii ir ii or ii ir i or i heb i yn y byd. Ymaeith; ymaeith ir mor diffaith ymaith bryfyn ir mor sygyn. Mi ach gorchmyna chwi ych naw ir ddaiar ddyddgwy ddyddgofwy ddyddgain ddydd glwy gwallgofwy gwallgain cyrgwy cyrgofwy cyrgain yr ddayar ych ix yn ych cyfair. A dwaid gwaith pob pryd a thre prryd porre annos, a ffater ar ol pob gwaeith ac y swynych.

> (Here is a charm against scrofula. I charm you against scrofula through the power of the Lord Jesus Christ and the Lady Mary his mother. And through the power of the twenty-four prophets. And through the power of all the holy confessor saints. And through the power of all the holy martyrs, male and female. And through all the holy virgins. And through the power of all the angels and archangels. I will destroy you, I have destroyed you I will uproot you, I have uprooted you. I will weaken you, I have weakened you. Across nine seas, across nine mountains, across nine sods of earth until there not be within you swelling nor harm nor disease nor illness nor agony, nor pain nor any worm, male or female in your blood nor your wound nor your veins nor your appetite nor your marrow nor your bones nor your meat nor your flesh nor your four limbs. Your whole body healthy from the top of your head to the soles of your feet. Amen Pater noster and Ave Maria. *Kwm gelon Crist ymresebion dragendi* like the dragon they went away as they came. May God not allow the scrofula to prosper any more than the nine daughters of King Rhiwallon. From nine to eight, from eight to seven, from seven to six, from six to five, from five to four, from four to three, from three to two, from two to one, from one to not a single one. Away, Away to the uninhibited sea, away worm to the undertow of the sea. I command you nine to the earth *ddyddgwy ddyddgofwy ddyddgain ddyddglwy gwallgofwy gwallgain cyrgwy cyrgofwy cyrgain* into the earth all nine of you directly. And say [it] once at every meal & 3 days morning and night, and a Pater after every time that you recite the charm.)[54]

The charm consists of several components, beginning with a formulaic invocation of a wide-ranging cast of divine characters. The text then launches into a highly performative series of threats to the disease or the disease-causing agent(s). This section is one of, if not *the*, most highly dramatized sections of any Welsh charm. The power of the words to destroy the disease or its cause

53 An ambiguous phrase, perhaps purposefully so, that resists translation.

54 Aberystwyth, NLW, MS Peniarth 204, pp. 10–12.

is strengthened in the performative, ritual utterances that depict completion of the threatened act: 'I will destroy you, I have destroyed you', etc. Following this highly effective series of threats, the charm then exorcises the disease and its cause out of the patient's body and into a series of liminal spaces: nine seas, nine mountains, nine sods of earth (or, mounds). The use of the number nine here foreshadows the counting down and expelling and naming of the nine disease-causing agents, apparently nine sister-worms. The folkloric elements in this section of the charm are strong. The reference to nine seas is reminiscent of the 'ninth wave' tradition in Irish literature and legend.[55] In addition to the nine seas as a place of banishment, the charm also later commands the agents of the disease to the wild, or uninhibited wasteland of a sea. Many narrative charms use the motif of space, presented in terms of divine power and demonic power. Such charms often feature a divine character juxtaposed with the demon or disease-agent, often a worm. Éva Pócs has noted that in many modern Eastern European charms, the dwelling place of the demons and demonic disease-causing agents is often a barren stone desert, which she describes in terms of opposition: human/non-human or demonic; divine/satanic.[56]

The charm's banishments in general, and their verbal formulae, are vaguely reminiscent of liturgical rituals to banish demons in several rituals for blessing holy water, salt, and honey, and sanctifying the boundaries of a church or parish. In the tradition of Latin benedictions, demons are also banished to places such as 'profundum desertum, ut nominibus nihil noceant or ubi nec aratur nec seminatur'.[57] In the Welsh scrofula charm, the nine disease worms are banished in a series of adjurations. After the first of the exorcisms, the charm enumerates the body parts of the patient, so that the demon will be unable to remain hidden within the patient.[58] This litany of body parts is common in charms of various traditions and most often begins at the head and works down the body.

The charm then uses a countdown motif to exorcise the worms from the patient's body. Diminishing charms that feature such counting down, often from nine or seven, are common in the wider, shared European charming tradition. One Old English charm features the very similar motif of counting down the sisters in a charm for a glandular swelling, scrofula, worms, or general evil:

55 Note, for example, in *Lebor gabála Érenn*, when the sons of Míl must remain at sea, beyond nine waves from the shore: see *Lebor gabála Érenn*, ed. and trans. by Macalister.

56 Pócs, 'Miracles', p. 36.

57 Pócs, 'Miracles', p. 36. Here she cites Weinreich's Latin benediction text and offers her translations of the above as 'a deserted depth, so that may harm nothing by means of names' and 'which is not ploughed nor sown'. Pócs also notes that the motif of banishing the demon or disease-agent into rocky, barren deserts or marshes was popular throughout Europe, but was more predominant in Eastern and South-Eastern Europe.

58 Pócs, 'Church Benedictions', p. 187.

> Wiþ cyrnel. Neogone wæran Nodþæs sweoster. þa wurdon þa nygone to VIII. and þa VIII to VII and þa VII to VI and þa VI to V and þa VI to V and þ V to IIII and þa IIII to III and þa III to II and þa II to I and þ I to nanum. þis þe lib be cyrneles and scrofelles and weormes and æghwylces yfeles. Sing Benedicte nygon siþum.
>
> (For glandular swelling: Nine were the sisters of Nođ [i.e. (?) Node]: Then nine became eight and the eight (became) seven, and the seven (became) six, and the six (became) five, and the five (became) four, and the four (became) three, and the three (became) two, and the two (became) one, and the one (became) none. May this be your remedy for glandular swelling and scrofula and 'worm' and for every evil; sing the *Benedicite* nine times.)[59]

Here the kernel refers to a swelling or tumour of the flesh. Storms asserts that, 'the monotonous repetition of the same formula gives it an intensity and a weight that leaves no room for embellishments'.[60] A much earlier analogue can be found in the works of Marcellus Empiricus, a fourth- and fifth-century medical writer from Gaul who included in his medical work, *De medicamentis*, several charms and other material that are often called 'popular' or 'superstitious'. In one instance, Marcellus gives a charm against swollen glands in which the 'gland sisters' are counted down from nine until no more are left:

> Glandulas mane carminabis si dies minuetur, si nox ad vesperam, et digito medicinali ac pollice continens eas dices: Novem glandulae sorores, octo glandulae sorores, septem glandulae sorores, sex glandulae sorores, quinque glandulae sorores, quattor glandulae sorores, tres glandulae sorores, duo glandulae sorores, una glandula soror. Novem fiunt glandulae ... una fit glandula, nulla fit glandula.
>
> (You shall sing on the swollen glands in the morning when the day is shortening, and towards evening when the night is shortening, and holding between your healing finger [i.e. the fourth finger] and thumb you shall say 'the nine swollen glands are sisters, the eight swollen glands are sisters, the seven swollen glands are sisters, the six swollen glands are sisters, the five swollen glands are sisters, the four swollen glands are sisters, the three swollen glands are sisters, the two swollen glands are sisters, the one swollen gland is sister. There were nine glands ... There was one gland, there was no gland'.)[61]

---

59 London, BL, MS Harley 585 (*s.* x–xi), as translated in *Anglo-Saxon Remedies*, ed. and trans. by Pettit, I, p. 107.

60 Storms, *Anglo-Saxon Magic*, p. 150.

61 This charm curiously restarts the count at one gland-sister, beginning at nine and counting down to zero, but dropping the reference to the glands as sisters in the second part of the charm. As published and translated in Storms, *Anglo-Saxon Magic*, pp. 151–52.

Although Storms did not consider this Latin version to have been a source for the Old English charm (rather, he posited that the source of the Old English charm was Germanic; an argument based solely, it would seem, on the name Noththe [= Nođ]), there are fascinating parallels to the Welsh scrofula charm found in both the Old English and Latin charms. There is no reason not to suppose that multiple layers of influence, over several centuries, influenced the formation of the Welsh scrofula charm.

The diminishing gland-sisters charm is not the only parallel to be found in earlier traditions. One German charm presents other parallels to the Welsh scrofula charm:

> Contra vermes. Gang ut nesso mid nigun nessiklinon, ut fana themo marge an that ben, fan themo bene an that flesg, ut fan demo flesge an thia hud, ut fan thera hud an thesa strala. Druhtin werthe so.
>
> > (Go out, worm, from your nine little ones, out from the marrow to the bone, from the bone to the flesh, out from the flesh to the skin, out from the skin to this arrow. Lord, may it happen thus.)[62]

A. A. Barb believed this charm, as well as the Noththe charm, to have unquestionably developed out of the apocryphal Coptic text, 'Book of the Resurrection of Christ', attributed to the Apostle Bartholomew. In this text, 'Death' or the 'Destroyer' descends into the underworld with six sons in order to enter Christ's tomb and take possession of his body. They are, of course, defeated, and the seven demons are described as 'wriggling' like worms. To back up this claim, Barb cites a German charm that features Peter lying in his tomb, eaten up with worms, which gradually diminish, from nine to zero.[63] In most European worm charms, Job eventually became the main character of the diminishing worm charm type, logically because of his connection with worms and disease in several biblical and extra-biblical traditions.[64]

---

62 As presented and translated in Storms, *Anglo-Saxon Magic*, p. 149.

63 Barb, 'Animula Vagula Blandula', pp. 26–28.

64 For example, Hunt, *Popular Medicine*, p. 81, prints the earliest Anglo-Norman example of a Job charm, from the twelfth century (London, BL, MS Sloane 84, fol. 40^{v}). The charm is for gout, though it was also used for farcy and diseases resulting in swelling, as in scrofula. 'Carmen Contra guttam: In nomine Patris et Filii et Spiritus Sancti. Jop vers hout. Quanz en hout? .IX en hout, de IX. . VIII., de VIII. . VIIe [*sic*], de. Vii> .Vi., de VI. .V., de .V. .IIII., de .IIII. .III., de III. .II., de .II. .I. de .I. nul. Si verreiment cum Deus uuarit seint Job, si uuarisse il icest hume vel ista mulier de cest enfermete u de festre hu de gute. In nomine Patris et Filii. Christus natus, Christus passus, et Christus resurectus a mortuis. Ego sum Alfa et Omega, primus et novissimus, initium et fin[is] mundi et consumacio seculi et vita et pax + In nomine Patris et Filii et Spiritus Sancti'. Another French charm of the fifteenth century uses the Job and worm motif in a remedy for farcy (Exeter, Ex. Cath., MS 3519): 'Charme de seint Job pur lez vermez ou [e]lez sount; "Com a Dieu ployt par la volunte de Dieu et par la grace de Dieu et par la creaunce de luy, si en garist et auxi garisez tu de tez mayus et de tez dolours, de ceo en avant ja mal te ne facent." In nomine Patris et Filii et Spritus Sancti trois foitz soit dit ove .iii. Pater Noster et .iii. Ave Maria et .iii. Credo'.

The Welsh scrofula charm exists in two almost identical versions, which present nearly identical names for the nine disease-causing worms. The reference to the 'nine daughters of King Rhiwallon' is strange and unattested elsewhere in the Welsh tradition. Traditionally Rhiwallon was not a king, but a physician in the court of a Welsh ruler, and the progenitor of the line of renowned Welsh physicians known in later lore as the *Meddygon Myddfai* (Physicians of Myddfai). Several medieval and early modern Welsh medical texts feature colophons that reference Rhiwallan and his three sons. In these charms, it seems that the semi-legendary healing sons of Rhiwallon have been conflated with the tradition of the fever demons, usually sisters, of older traditions. Lea Olsan notes the prevalence of demon sisters found in fever charms of medieval England and Germanic traditions, but the 'gland sisters' of Marcellus Empiricus demonstrate that this was not solely a Germanic tradition.[65] This charm is a fascinating and so far uniquely Welsh example of a diminishing charm, featuring several motifs common in the wider, shared tradition but patently demonstrating a high level of unique innovation, adaption, and expansion of these shared motifs into a distinct and unparalleled charm. The direct adjurations to the disease and banishing the disease-causing worms to liminal places is common in nearly all charming traditions. That the cause of the disease is a group of worms is not entirely surprising either, given that there were many diseases thought to be the result of worms. Although this charm contains several individual elements found in various earlier Latin and Germanic traditions, it is unlike any charm of other traditions, as far as I am aware. It is possible that this text features commonalities found in charms of Scotland, Ireland, or another Celtic tradition whose corpus of charms is not yet as easily accessible as those of England and other European traditions. One nineteenth-century charm from Brittany contains a curious parallel to the two fuller versions of scrofula given above, in that it refers to the banishment of the disease over nine seas and nine mountains. The charm, which is for shingles, reads:

65 One charm invokes seven divine figures (the Seven Sleepers) against the seven evil fever sisters (see Franz, *Die kirchlichen Benediktionen*, II, pp. 482–83 for the text). The charm is found in London, BL, MS Sloane 389, fols 91^{v}–92^{r}. The relevant excerpt reads: 'coniuro vos quo septem estis sorores prima daliola secunda vestulia tercian fugaliaquarta suferalie quinta affrecta sexta lilia septema luc/talia per patrem + et filiumet spiritum sanctum + et per diem in diebus et per misericordiam domini nostri Ihu xpi + per omnes angelos + archangelos + per apostolos + martires + confessores atque virgines + omnes sanctos dei per omnes virtutes celorum et per celum et terram + mare et omnes que in eis sunt' (I conjure you who are seven sisters, the first Daliola, the second Vestulia, the third Fugalia, the fourth Suferalie, the fifth Affrecta, the sixth Lilia, the seventh Luctalia through the Father and Son and Holy Spirit and through the day of days and through the mercy of our Lord Jesus Christ and through all the angels, archangels and through the apostles, martyrs, confessors and virgins and all the saints of God through all the powers of heaven and earth and sea and all that are in them). See Olsan, 'Writing on the Hand', p. 12.

> Pass your hand over your chest several times, at the ailing area, in a clockwise direction, while saying 'Shingles, go away! This is not your place here nor elsewhere. Between nine seas and nine mountains, there is your lodging.'[66]

A similarly worded charm for shingles was used in Wales even into the nineteenth century. Elias Owen collected a charm that was performed only in the morning, and only after both the patient and the charmer had fasted. The charmer would blow on the inflammation nine times, spit upon it, and rub it in while saying the following:

> Yr Eryr Eryres
> Mi a'th ddanfonais
> Dros naw mor a thros naw mynydd
> A thros naw erw o dir anghelfydd
> Lle na chyfartho ci, ac na frefo fuwch
> Ac na ddelo yr byth yn uwch.
>
> > (Male eagle, female eagle,
> > I send you
> > Over nine seas, and over nine mountains,
> > And over nine acres of unprofitable land,
> > Where no dog shall bark, and no cow shall low,
> > and where no eagle shall higher rise.)[67]

Conclusion

One of the most striking elements of the genre of healing texts is the extent to which healing customs associated with different traditions share many common elements while at the same time shaping certain conventions of the genre to specific cultural values and needs. In general, the corpus of Welsh charms conforms to those of England and Europe. Nearly all of the Welsh charms find some analogue in the charms circulating in England and on the Continent. Even the major outliers, such as the scrofula charms, are evocative in some small way of other traditions, usually in the use of a specific motif or phrase. Yet, while the Welsh corpus of charms does demonstrate an active participation in wider trends, many of them show evidence of unique Welsh innovation and adaptation, such as the poetic and highly stylized Welsh *Longinus* charms, or the scrofula charms that likely developed out of various early Latin and Germanic diminishing charms for scrofula and swollen nodes.

66 Lecouteux (trans. Graham), *Traditional Magic Spells*, p. 143.

67 Text and translation from Owen, *Welsh Folklore*, p. 264. Note that the Welsh word *eryr* has a secondary meaning of shingles or herpes.

My aim in this chapter was to demonstrate the similarity of the Welsh-manuscript charm corpus to that of England and Europe, while at the same time highlighting the ways in which Welsh scribes adapted certain conventions of the genre based on specific cultural needs and factors. There is much work to be done on the corpus of charms in premodern Welsh manuscripts. Work of this kind is inherently interdisciplinary. Textually, the healing charms operated across linguistic, religious, and cultural boundaries as they were copied, disseminated, and adapted. The healing charms of the Welsh-manuscript corpus display an enduring adaptability and degree of continuity across centuries. The Welsh charms are multi-faceted and complex, and a thorough analysis of this corpus can unearth nuanced insights into not only sociolinguistic developments, but also developments in popular culture, popular religious practice, book and manuscript production, and the dissemination of knowledge between northern Atlantic and European networks in the late-medieval and early modern periods. The corpus of healing charms, and the corpus of medical writing more broadly, can help illuminate rich networks of information exchange and collaboration, and these texts can highlight the rich and varied linguistic and cultural history of premodern Wales.

Works Cited

Manuscripts

Aberystwyth, National Library of Wales, MS Llanstephan 2
Aberystwyth, National Library of Wales, MS Peniarth 47
Aberystwyth, National Library of Wales, MS Peniarth 204
Aberystwyth, National Library of Wales, MS 873B
Cambridge, University Library, MS Additional 9308
Cardiff, Cardiff Library, MS 3.242
Exeter, Exeter Cathedral, MS 3519
London, British Library, MS Harley 585
London, British Library, MS Sloane 84
London, British Library, MS Sloane 122
London, British Library, MS Sloane 389
London, Wellcome Library, MS 417
Oxford, Bodleian Library, MS Additional B.1
Oxford, Jesus College, MS 111

Primary Sources

Anglo-Norman Medicine: Volume II, ed. by Tony Hunt (Cambridge: D. S. Brewer, 1997)

Anglo-Saxon Remedies, Charms, and Prayers from British Library MS Harley 585: The Lacnunga, ed. and trans. by Edward Pettit (Lewiston.: E. Mellen Press, 2001)

Jacobus de Voragine, *The Golden Legend: Readings on the Saints*, trans. William Granger Ryan, 2 vols (Princeton: Princeton University Press, 1993)

Lebor gabála Érenn : The Book of the Taking of Ireland, ed. by Robert Alexander Stewart Macalister, 5 vols, Irish Texts Society, 34, 35, 39, 41, and 44 (Dublin: Irish Texts Society, 1932–1942)

Secondary Studies

Barb, Alphons Augustinus, 'Animula Vagula Blandula', *Folklore*, 61.1 (1950), 15–30

Bosse-Griffith, Kate, *Byd y Dyn Hysbys: Swyngyfaredd yng Nghymru* (Talybont: Y Lolfa, 1977)

Bozóky, Edina, 'Medieval Narrative Charms', in *The Power of Words: Studies on Charms and Charming in Europe*, ed. by James Kapaló, Éva Pócs, and William Ryan (Budapest, New York: Central European University Press, 2013), pp. 101–15

Browe, Peter, 'Die Eucharist als Zaubermittle in Mittelalter', *Archiv für Kulturgeschichte*, 20.2 (1930), 134–54

——, *Die eucharistischen Wunder des Mittelalters* (Breslau: Verlag Müller & Seiffert, 1938)

Clancy, Joseph P., *The Earliest Welsh Poetry* (London: Macmillan, 1970)

Davies, Owen, 'Charmers and Charming in England and Wales from the Eighteenth to the Twentieth Century', *Folklore*, 109 (1998), 41–52

——, 'Cunning-folk in England and Wales during the Eighteenth and Nineteenth Centuries', *Rural History*, 8.1 (1997), 91–107

——, 'Healing Charms in Use in England and Wales 1700–1950', *Folklore*, 107 (1996), 19–32

——, *Popular Magic: Cunning-folk in English History* (London and New York: Hambledon, 2003)

Ebermann, Oskar, *Blut- und Wundsegen in ihrer Entwicklung dargestellt* (Berlin: Mayer, 1903)

Fisher, Rebecca M. C., 'The Anglo-Saxon Charms: Texts in Context', *Approaching Methodologies*, 4 (2012), 108–26

Frankfurter, David, 'Narrating Power: The Theory and Practice of the Magical *Historiola* in Ritual Spells', in *Ancient Magic and Ritual Power*, ed. by Marvin Meyer and Paul Mirecki, Religions in the Graeco-Roman World, 129 (Brill: Leiden, 1995), pp. 451–70

Franz, Adolf, *Die kirchlichen Benediktionen im Mittelalter*, 2 vols (Freiburg: Herder, 1909)

Grzybowski, Stefan, and Edward A. Allen, 'History and Importance of Scrofula', *The Lancet*, 346.8988 (1995), 1472–74

Hillers, Barbara, 'Towards a Typology of European Narrative Charms in Irish Oral Tradition', in *Charms, Charmers, and Charming in Ireland: From the Medieval to the Modern*, ed. by Ilona Tuomi, John Carey, Barbara Hillers, and Ciarán Ó Gealbháin (Cardiff: University of Wales Press, 2019), pp. 79–102

Hindley, Katherine Storm, 'Eating Words and Burning Them: The Power of Destruction in Medieval English Charm Texts', *Zerstörung von Geschriebenem:*

Historische und transkulturelle Perspektiven, ed. by Carina Kühne-Wespi, Klaus Peter Oschema, and Joachim Friedrich Quack (Berlin: De Gruyter, 2019), pp. 359–72

Hunt, Tony, *Popular Medicine in Thirteenth-century England* (Cambridge: D. S. Brewer, 1990)

Huws, Daniel, *A Repertory of Welsh Manuscripts and Scribes* (Aberystwyth: National Library of Wales, 2022)

Kieckhefer, Richard, *Magic in the Middle Ages* (Cambridge: Cambridge University Press, 2014)

Klaassen, Frank, ed., *Making Magic in Elizabethan England. Two Early Modern Vernacular Books of Magic* (University Park, PA: Penn State University Press, 2019)

Lecouteux, Claude, *Traditional Magic Spells for Protection and Healing*, trans. by Jon E. Graham (Rochester, VT: Inner Traditions, 2017)

Mackenzie, William, *Gaelic Incantations, Charms, and Blessings of the Hebrides: With Translations, and Parallel Illustrations from Irish, Manx, Norse, and Other Superstitions* (Inverness: Northern Counties Newspaper and Printing and Pub., 1895)

Olsan, Lea, 'Charms in Medieval Memory', in *Charms and Charming in Europe*, ed. by Jonathan Roper (Houndmills, Basingstoke, Hampshire and New York: Palgrave Macmillan, 2004), pp. 59–88

——, 'The Corpus of Charms in the Middle English Leechcraft Remedy Books', in *Charms, Charmers and Charming: International Research on Verbal Magic*, ed. by Jonathan Roper, Palgrave Historical Studies in Witchcraft and Magic (London: Palgrave Macmillan, 2009), pp. 214–37

——, 'Latin Charms of Medieval England', *Oral Tradition*, 7.1 (1992), 116–42

——, 'The Worm in the Worm Charms' (paper given at the International Society for Folk Narrative Research – Committee on Charms, Charmers and Charming and Belief Narrative Network Committee, Three Day Conference, Budapest, Dec. 2017

——, 'Writing on the Hand in Ink: A Late Medieval Innovation in Fever Charms in England', *Incantatio. An International Journal on Charms, Charmers and Charming*, 7 (2018), 9–45

Owen, Elias, *Welsh Folk-lore. A Collection of the Folk-tales and Legends of North Wales* (Oswestry and Wrexham: Woodall, Minshall, and Co., 1896; repr. Somerset: Llanerch Press, 1996) <https://www.gutenberg.org/files/20096/20096-h/20096-h.htm>

Pócs, Éva, 'Church Benedictions and Popular Charms in Hungary', in *The Power of Words: Studies on Charms and Charming in Europe*, ed. by James Kapaló, Éva Pócs, and William Ryan (Budapest, New York: Central European University Press, 2013), pp. 165–98

——, 'Miracles and Impossibilities in Magic Folk Poetry', in *Charms, Charmers and Charming: International Research on Verbal Magic*, ed. by Jonathan Roper, Palgrave Historical Studies in Witchcraft and Magic (London: Palgrave Macmillan, 2009), pp. 27–53

Roper, Jonathan, *English Verbal Charms*, Folklore Fellows Communications, 136, no. 288 (Helsinki: Suomalainen Tiedeakatemia, 2005)

Ryan, William Francis, *Bathhouse at Midnight: An Historical Survey of Magic and Divination in Russia*, Magic in History (University Park, PA: Pennsylvania State University Press, 1999)

Skemer, Don C., *Binding Words: Textual Amulets in the Middle Ages* (University Park, PA: University of Pennsylvania Press, 2006)

Storms, Godfrid, *Anglo-Saxon Magic* (Dordrecht: Springer Netherlands, 1948)

Turrell, James F., 'The Ritual of Royal Healing in Early Modern England: Scrofula, Liturgy, and Politics', *Anglican and Episcopal History*, 68.1 (1999), 3–36

Waller, Daniel James, 'Echo and the *Historiola*: Theorizing Narrative Incantation', *Archiv für Religionsgeshichte*, 16.1 (2015), 263–80

SARAH BACCIANTI

20. *Kveisustrengurinn*

An Old Norse Charm*

As has been explored in several other chapters in this volume, ritual cures and healing charms are often found in the extant written medical sources across medieval western Europe, emphasizing the overlap between medical knowledge and religion in the *materia medica* circulating in the Middle Ages. In discussion of healing charms, both in this volume and in the scholarship on medieval medicine and charm tradition, the analysis of their content and writing systems draws attention to the fluidity of the boundaries between religion, medical knowledge and folk belief, or even magic. As suggested by Kieckhefer, 'magic is a crossing-point where religion converges with science, popular beliefs intersect with those of the educated classes',[1] and, as convincingly posited by Bauer, it is the intersection between religion and magic that should be the focus on any discussion about (healing) charms.[2] Healing charms are a unique tradition that moves back and forth from aural to written to performative culture, as extensively discussed by Olsan,[3] and thus in using ritual words (or *voces magicae*) and ritual actions, as I will discuss below, they highlight the importance of their power and efficacy in the moment of performance. As Murray Jones and Olsan have argued in relation to charms for conception and childbirth, the purpose of verbal charms is 'to bring about a desired result'.[4] Skemer has noted that written amulets in the late Middle Ages included a variety

* The initial work of this research was supported by the British Academy Newton International Fellowship [NF170760] and the Snorri Sturluson Icelandic Fellowship (2019) at Stofnun Árna Magnússonar á Íslandi. I am grateful to Deborah Hayden and Jonas Wellendorf for offering several valuable comments on this chapter. Any remaining errors or omissions are entirely my responsibility.
Unless otherwise noted, translations from Old Norse in this chapter are my own from the manuscripts and/or editions cited. In all manuscript transcriptions, abbreviations have been expanded and are presented in *italic*.

1 Kieckhefer, *Magic in the Middle Ages*, p. 1.

2 Bauer, 'Biblical Magic'.

3 Murray Jones and Olsan, 'Performative Rituals'.

4 Murray Jones and Olsan, 'Performative Rituals', p. 409.

Sarah Baccianti • National Museums NI, sarah.baccianti@nationalmuseumsni.org

Medicine in the Medieval North Atlantic World: Vernacular Texts and Traditions, ed. by Deborah Hayden and Sarah Baccianti, KSS, 5 (Turnhout, 2025), pp. 463-485
BREPOLS PUBLISHERS DOI 10.1484/M.KSS-EB.5.143998

of different types of texts, from scriptural quotations, Biblical names, litanies and prayers, to the names of unknown deities, symbols, cryptic combinations of letters or numbers, magic squares, and palindromes: 'a patchwork of sources that could either be quoted or paraphrased from memory or scribally copied verbatim from written exemplars'.[5] Bauer, relying on Braavig and Schreirner, further expands the role of words of power, suggesting that 'both religion and magic were based on the belief that through the use of certain, mostly hidden and occult, knowledge — or at least an elitist knowledge that was not manifest to everybody — the real world could be influenced'.[6] Taking into consideration the existing scholarship on charms, the present chapter focuses on one Scandinavian healing charm in particular, Reykjavík, Landsbókasafn Íslands, MS Lbs fragm. 14, 1^{r}–1^{v}, commonly known as *Kveisustrengurinn* or *Kveisublaðið* (which is often referred to in English as Colic String / Colic Leaf).[7] This charm is considered in parallel with other healing charms in circulation in medieval Scandinavia, primarily medieval Iceland, providing an opportunity to read them within the tradition of medical practice in medieval western Europe.

Kveisustrengurinn, written around the year 1600 in Iceland,[8] is made of a single strap of vellum measuring 584 mm long and 108 mm wide. It is written on both sides by an unknown scribe in a late cursive hand. Black ink is used throughout, and in places it is faint and partially illegible; some dots and illegible words in red ink can be noted at the margin of the text. On the recto of the strip there are ninety-six lines of text, and at the top there is a nine-centimetre space left blank; on the verso there are 108 lines. The strip has two holes and is dark and worn-out, with visible folding, and in some places crumpling signs (Figs 20.1 and 20.2). At the two extremities there are other, smaller holes to which there were strings attached,[9] which were used to wrap it around the patient's body. The manuscript has been in The National and University Library of Iceland's special collections since 1902, after it had been found accidentally in the archives of the Bishopric of Hólar, hidden among other documents.[10] No other records of *Kveisustrengurinn*

5 Skemer, 'Amulet Rolls', pp. 197–98.

6 Bauer, 'Biblical Magic', pp. 271–72.

7 Unlike previous and current scholarship, I do not refer to the charm as a charm against colic, as the term *kveisa* covers several types of diseases which also include colic. The last adjuration in the charm specifies one ailment, gout, along with the general term *kveisa*: 'Ég særi þig gigt z kveisa burt að flýja, / ég mana þig, ég deyfi þig, ég drep þig kveisa' (ll. 194–95) (I adjure you gout and inflammation/boil to flee, I dare you, I subdue you, I kill you, inflammation/boil).

8 The electronic catalogue handrit.is dates the manuscripts 1590–1610, and Magnús Már Lárusson ('Eitt gamalt kveisublað') provides the approximate date of *c.* 1600.

9 In personal conversation, Gunnar Marel Hinriksson, special collections librarian at Landsbókasafn Íslands, has noted that the strings attached to the strip were lost in more recent archival practice.

10 See the information relating to the strip in handrit.is (Lbs fragm. 14) and in Magnús Már Lárusson, 'Eitt gamalt kveisublað'. The manuscript fragment was catalogued with the other documents from Hólar (fasc. VI, no. 2) on 24 July 1902.

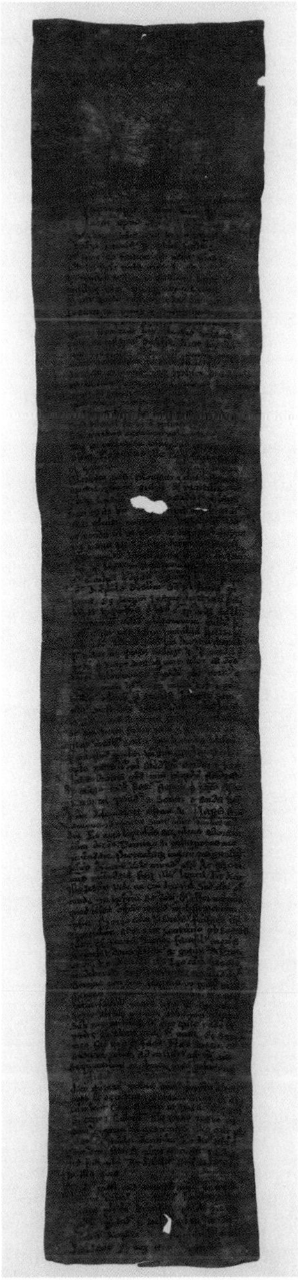

Figure 20.1. Reykjavík, Landsbókasafn Íslands, MS Lbs fragm. 14, fol. 1r. Courtesy of National and University Library of Iceland, Manuscript Collection.

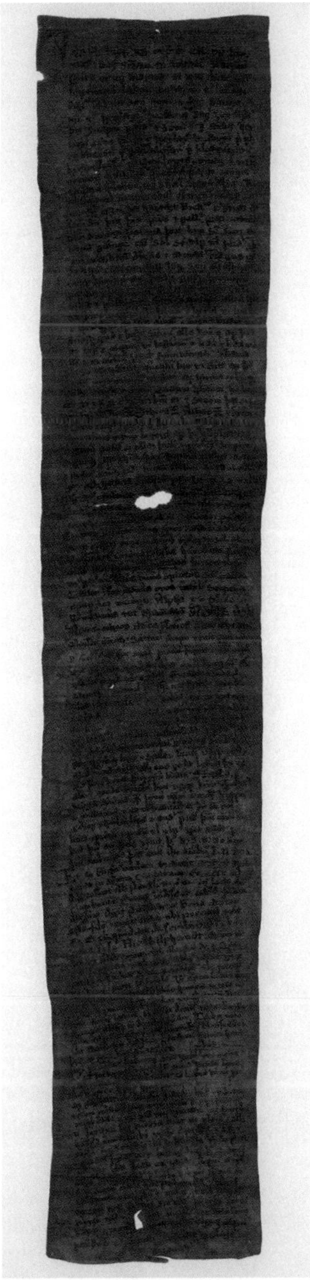

Figure 20.2. Reykjavík, Landsbókasafn Íslands, MS Lbs fragm. 14, fol. 1v. Courtesy of National and University Library of Iceland, Manuscript Collection.

have been found that date prior to 1902. Even though we do not have much evidence for the life of the strip, its survival provides clues about healing and religious practices in Iceland in the late-sixteenth century. As demonstrated in the preceding chapters, healing charms and healing amulets were already common cures in antiquity and their popularity continued into the Middle Ages. Parchment leaves like the one of *Kveisustrengurinn* were common healing artefacts, and a few prayer rolls that were used as wearable charms have survived from the Middle Ages. *Kveisustrengurinn* is the only example still extant from medieval Iceland.

The text, which is written in Old Norse with passages in Latin and a handful of words in Greek and Hebrew, is a charm that offers protection against various ailments. Linguistically, as mentioned above, many words are difficult to recognize because of the deterioration of the vellum, and throughout the charm, the use of the three languages highlights the different elements of the text and the power of words, such as in the invocation to earthly elements and the invocation to God and Jesus Christ as the ultimate healers.[11] This charm, unlike other healing charms found in Norse medical manuscripts, relies solely on the power of words and scriptural writings. For instance, unlike the healing charms in Dublin, RIA, MS 23 D 43, where the preparation of drinks and poultices — together with the carving of words on wood, leaves, apples or body parts — is part of the ritual of the charm, *Kveisustrengurinn* does not offer any herbal prescriptions.[12]

The charm begins with the Prologue of the Gospel of John (John 1. 1–14):[13]

11 Indeed, the tradition of *Christus medicus* (Christ the Physician) stresses the importance of healing the body and the soul, an image that is often used also in the healing miracles of the *Biskupa sögur* (Bishops' Sagas). See Arbesmann, 'The Concept of "Christus Medicus"'. The metaphor of *Christus medicus* first occurred in the letter to the Ephesians attributed to bishop Ignatius of Antioch (d. in the second century), and it was later consolidated in the fifth century by Augustine, who advances a soteriological reading of the trope. In *Mǫrtu saga ok Maríu Magðalenu*, we find the following statement, taken from Pope Gregory I's *Homily XXXIII*: 'En várr herra sannr læknir' (*The Saga of the Sister Saints*, ed. and trans. by Van Deusen, p. 122) (But our Lord the true physician); see also Van Deusen, 'Old Norse-Icelandic Legend' as well as Baccianti, 'Guaritori, acqua santa e latte materno' and 'Healing Hands, Holy Water, and Hellish Diseases'.

12 See Baccianti, 'Guaritori, acqua santa e latte materno'. For instance, a blood-staunching charm in Dublin, RIA, MS 23 D 43, fol. 2r states: 'W*ið* alls kyns blóðras: Tak hi*ar*tar horn b*r*ent, z stapa m*eð* vín z gef at d*r*ecka. […] Sic*ut* *vere* c*r*edim*us* q*uod* bea*t*a vi*r*go ma*r*ia pepe*r*it d*eu*m o*mn*ium infante*m*' (For all kinds of bleeding, take burned hart's horn and crush it with wine and give to drink. […] Sicut vere credimus quod beata virgo Maria peperit deum omnium infantem).

13 The text of the *Kveisustrengurinn* is taken from Magnús Már Lárusson's edition (1951) [Magnús Már Lárusson, 'Eitt gamalt kveisublað'] with manuscript abbreviations expanded in *italic*. However, I have changed word division and punctuation to follow modern convention, and I have added corrections and improvements where appropriate. Ellipsis is used to indicate illegible or lost letters; words in square brackets are words no longer legible on the manuscript but present in Magnús Már Lárusson's edition.

In principio erat uerbum, z verbu*m*
erat apud deum z deus erat ver-
bum.[14] Hic erat in principio apud
deum. Omnia p*er* ipsum facta svnt:
et sine eo factum est nihil, quod factu*m*
est. In ipso vijta erat, et vijta erat lux
hominum, et lux in tenebris lucet,
et tenebræ eam non apprehenderunt.
Erat homo missus a deo, cui nomi*ne*
Ioan*nes*. Hic venit ad testificandum, vt
testaret*ur* de luce, vt omnes crederent p*er*
ipsu*m*. Non erat lux ille,[15] sed missus
erat, vt testaret*ur* de luce. Erat lux illa,
lux vera: quæ illuminat omne*m* homi-
nem venientem in mundum. In mun-
do erat, et mund*us* per Ipsum factus
est, et mund*us* eum non Cognouit. In propria[16]
venit, et sui eum non receperunt. [Quo]t-[17]
quot autem receperunt eum, dedit eis
vt liceret filios dei fierij, videlicet his qui
credidissent in no*m*ine[18] ipsius, Qju[19] non ex
Sanguinibus, neque ex voluntate carn*is*,
neq*ue* ex voluntate viri, sed ex deo nati
sunt. Et Sermo ille caro factus est,
et habitauit in nobis: et conspeximus
Glorijam eius, Glorijam velut vnigeniti
a patre,[20] plenus gratia et veritate —[21]

(In the beginning was the word, and the word
was with God and God was the word.
This was in the beginning with
God. All things were made by Him: and without
Him was made nothing, that was made. In Him

---

14 Erasmus's post-1516 Latin translation has the following wording: 'In principio erat sermo, et sermo erat / apud deum, et deus erat ille sermo' (*Novum Testamentum*, p. 13).

15 'Non erat ille lux illa' in Erasmus' Gospel of John (*Novum Testamentum*, p. 14).

16 The letters in the manuscript are illegible. Following the 1516 version of Erasmus' Latin translation, the illegible word could be *propria*, or following the 1535 version it could be *sua*. Magnús Már Lárusson transcribes it as 'propria'.

17 The letters are partially illegible: only the letter 't' is visible, hence the addition of *Quot* following Erasmus's 1535 Latin translation. Magnús Már Lárusson transcribes it as *Quotquot*.

18 Here the charm follows the 1516 Latin translation, whereas the 1535 version has *in nomen*.

19 Scribal error; it should read *Qui*.

20 Magnús Már Lárusson wrongly transcribes it as 'aparte'.

21 Lbs fragm. 14, fol. 1r (ll. 1–27).

was life, and life was light
of men, and light shines in darkness,
and darkness did not grasp it.
A man was sent from God, who is named
John. This man came to testify, to give testimony
of the light, that all may believe through him.
He is not the light, but was sent
to testify about the light. It was that light,
the true light: which enlightens every man
who comes into the world. He was the world,
and the world was made by Him
and the world did not know him. He
came unto His own, and His own did not receive him.
But as many as received Him, He gave them the
power to become sons of God, that is to those
who had believed in His name. Those who are
born not of blood, nor of the will of the flesh, nor
of the will of man, but of God.
And that Word became flesh,
and dwelt among us: and we beheld
His glory, the glory of the only begotten
of the Father, full of grace and truth —)

The source of the Prologue of the Gospel of John used in the charm is that of Erasmus of Rotterdam's Latin translation of the New Testament. The original source for this charm, which combines both Erasmus' 1516 and 1535 Latin translations of the Gospel of John, is so far unknown. Interestingly, despite the majority of the prologue reflecting Erasmus' 1535 translation, the opening lines still use the word *verbum* instead of *sermo*,[22] most probably because it was a commonly used formula in charms. Prayers, liturgical phrases, and biblical *historiolae* were often used in protective charms. Karen Jolly observes 'the thoroughly Christian character of the bulk of charm formulas and their closeness to liturgical prayers', arguing that 'many so-called charms employ Scripture and prayers found in the liturgy while liturgical prayers often function rhetorically in the same way as charms, as effective means of cure'.[23] It is indeed reductive to read *Kveisustrengurinn* and other Norse healing charms only through the lens of magic,[24] as has been done

22 See Brown's edition of Erasmus' Latin translation of the Gospel of St John for an explanation of the change from *verbum* to *sermo* (*Novum Testamentum*, p. 13).

23 Jolly, 'Medieval Magic', p. 36.

24 For a discussion of healing charms and medical knowledge in medieval Iceland and Denmark see Baccianti, 'Guaritori, acqua santa e latte materno' and 'Healing Hands, Holy Water, and Hellish Diseases'. See also the work of Alessia Bauer, who has discussed some healing charms in the context of the use of biblical texts for magical purposes.

in much past scholarship.[25] The use of the apotropaic prologue of the Gospel of John (1. 1–14)[26] is relatively common in healing charms, often quoting only the very beginning of the Gospel, 'In principio erat verbum' (In the beginning was the word), stressing both the power of the word of God and its truth.[27] Don Skemer has observed, in his discussion of amulets in roll format in the late Middle Ages, that 'The prologue to the Gospel of St John, whether used orally or in writing, had a legendary association with divine protection from demons and evil since the early centuries of the Christian era.'[28] In subsequent studies, Skemer further argued that 'It is probably significant that in Christian iconography John was the Evangelist most closely associated with Christ. Perhaps the apocryphal Acts of John helped promote his reputation for healing through the power of God.'[29] Moreover, the *In principio erat verbum* formula was also used in the medical manuscripts circulating in Iceland and Denmark, as in Dublin, RIA MS 23 D 43, where the opening lines of the Gospel are used in a charm against fever (fol. 1^{r}) and one for blood staunching (fol. 1^{v}).

Following the apotropaic Latin Prologue of the Gospel of John (1. 1–14), the charm continues in Old Norse with an adjuration to rid the patient from all inflammation/boil ailments (*kveisu meinsemdir*):

25 See e.g. Dillmann, *Les magiciens dans l'Islande ancienne*; Maraschi, '*Similia similibus curantur*', pp. 269–86 and 'Sympathetic Graphophagy'; and Mitchell, *Witchcraft and Magic in the Nordic Middle Ages*, 'Leechbooks, Manuals, and Grimoires' and 'Faith and Knowledge in Nordic Charm Magic'. In this latest study, whilst still centring his argument on magic, Mitchell offers a more nuanced approach to the topic, which considers the role played by 'foreign' scientific and medical learning in the transmission of charms.

26 The reading of the Prologue was introduced in the Catholic mass liturgy in the thirteenth century and used until the Second Vatican Council (1962) and was often referred to *Ultimum Evangelium* (Last Gospel) as it was read at the end of the Tridentine Mass. The use of the Prologue is mentioned in the *Rituale Romanum* for the care of the sick (*de visitatio et cura infirmorum*) and exorcism (*Ritus exxorcizandi obsessos a dæmonio*) (*Rituale Romanum*, pp. 152 and 586).

27 Examples of the use of the Gospel of John can be found in vernacular charms in Scandinavia, England, Wales, France, etc. as it was a common trope associated with protective and therapeutic charms. See e.g. Gierløw, 'In principio'; Svanhildur Óskarsdóttir and Árni Heimir Ingólfsson, 'Dýrlingar og daglegt brauð í Langadal'; Storms, *Anglo-Saxon Magic*; Sims-Williams, *Religion and Literature*; Arthur, '*Charms*', *Liturgies, and Secret Rites*; Kesling, *Medical Texts*; Leach, 'Healing Charms and Ritual Protection'; Hindley, *Textual Magic* and 'The Power of Not Reading'.

28 Skemer further identifies a series of references to the use of the Gospel's opening verses, for instance 'In the early sixteenth century the English reformer William Tyndale complained about people who "hang a piece of St John's gospel about their necks"' (Skemer, 'Amulet Rolls', p. 212; see also Skemer, *Binding Words*, pp. 87–89). Maguire has noted that Christian imaging used as charms on clothing was often condemned, for example by Bishop Asterius of Amasea (d. 410) and Jerome (d. 420). Augustine (d. 430) criticized the custom of using the book of John's Gospel for the cure of headache and fever by placing it on someone's head; however, he preferred this use to the one of amulets (Maguire, 'Magic and the Christian Image', p. 65; see also Montesano, '*Supra acqua*', pp. 55–56).

29 Skemer, *Binding Words*, p. 87.

J nafni faud*ur*, [son]ar[30] z anda heijlags
særi eg af þeim ... Gudz ... aa sier
allar queijsu meijnsemd*er*. Ieg særi hi*er* allt
et vonda til at flyia, at dofna, at duyna,
jeg mana, jeg særi, jeg deyfi, ieg stefni
aullu*m* vondu*m* hlutu*m* huort þ*eir* eru vr jau*rdu*
eda af lopti vr skyum e*dur* af dupti Iardar
e*dur* aalfa e*dur* ofann z g … nga … e*dur* af hu*e*riu*m*
diaufuls dijkjum Sem til ku*n*na at
koma.[31]

> (In the name of the Father, the Son and the Holy Spirit
> I adjure you from them […] of God […] on
> him all boil/inflammation ailments. I adjure here all
> evil to flee, to die out, to dwindle away,
> I dare, I adjure, I subdue, I summon all evil
> things whether they are from the earth
> or from the air from the clouds or from the dust of the earth
> or from elves or above […] or from every
> devil's ditch that may
> come.)

The repetition of *Ég særi* occurs in three different passages of the charm (ll. 28–37, 114–23, and 192–99). The first adjuration begins with the *In nomine Patris*[32] formula in Old Norse (l. 28), to free the patient from all boil/inflammation ailments (l. 30) and to drive away and vanquish the evil spirits that cause the disease.[33] A similar prayer to banish disease can be found in eleventh-century London, BL, MS Cotton Caligula A XV, fols 123^{v}–124^{r}, which invokes the Norse god Thor as a godly help in healing the sick: 'Kuril sárþvara far þú nú, fundinn ertu. Þórr vígi þik þursa dróttin, Iuril (leg. Kuril) sárþvara. Viðr áðravari (leg. -vara)' (Kuril of the wound-spear, go now, you have been found. May Þórr consecrate you, lord of þursar, Kuril of the wound-spear. Against? vein-pus).[34] Two Old English charms in the *Lacnunga*, known as 'Wið færstice' ('for sudden stabbing-pain') and 'Nine Herbs Charm'[35] seem to suggest that certain ailments, especially sudden ones and those that were

30 Letters are missing as there is a hole in the manuscript.

31 Lbs fragm. 14, 1^{r} (ll. 28–37).

32 The formula is used in several healing charms in the Norse *materia medica*. *In nomine Patris* was used interchangeably in Latin (L) and Old Norse (ON), e.g. Dublin, RIA, MS 23 D 43, fols 2^{r} and 3^{r} (L); Dublin, RIA, MS 23 D 43, fols 2^{v} and 3^{r} (ON); Copenhagen, AM 434a 12mo, fols 1^{r}, 3^{r} and 37^{r} (ON); and Copenhagen, AM 434a 12mo, fols 2^{v}, 5^{v} and 36^{v}.

33 Note the use of verbs such as *flýja* and *dvína* (l. 31) and the wording in the second adjuration (ll. 115–23).

34 Edition and translation in Hall, 'Þur sarriþu þursa trutin', p. 201.

35 Respectively, *Anglo-Saxon Remedies*, ed. and trans. by Pettit, I, pp. 88–89 and 60–69 (*Lacnunga* CXXVII and LXXVI).

invisible, were often defined as *onflyge* (flying disease) and *fleogendum attre* (flying venoms).[36] As remarked by Cameron and reinforced by Jolly and Kesling, diseases were thought to be airborne, especially those sudden ones 'caused by elves or witches shooting arrows at the sufferer'.[37]

The use of *álfr* (elf) is not uncommon in healing charms and it is often linked to the Christian demonic tradition. For instance, there is a charm against elves in the Norse corpus that forms part of the Icelandic medical manuscript Copenhagen, AM 434a 12mo (*c.* 1500): 'Vid alfa-volkun: In nomine patris Samuel et filii Misael et spiritus sancti Raguel'[38] (for misery [illness] caused by elves: In nomine patris Samuel et fili Misael et spiritus sancti Raguel). On the Bergen rune stick (N B257; *c.* 1380), moreover, runes are said to be carved to protect against supernatural beings:

> Rist ek bótrúnar, / rist ek bjargrúnar, / einfalt vid álfum, / tvifalt við trollum, / þrifalt við þu [...] / vi ð inni skœ ðu / skag-valkyrju / svát ei megi / þótt æ vili / lævis kona /
>
> > (I cut runes of help; I cut runes of protection; once against elves, twice against trolls, thrice against [...] against the harmful 'skag'-valkyrie, so that she never can, though she may always want to — evil woman!)[39]

Just as in the Anglo-Saxon medical tradition, it is not possible to ascertain a specific ailment (either physical or mental) caused by elves. *Alfa-volkun* could hence have a similar meaning to the Old English *ælf-sogoða* (internal pain/ illness caused by elves) or *ælf-adle* (elf-illness) found in *Leechbook* III, which portrays afflictions that require the use of liturgical formulae of adjuration or the utterance/inscriptions of names of God or holy words.[40]

The combination of apotropaic and religious elements, such as the cross, holy water, *nomina sacra*, *historiolae*, and prayers, along with ingredients, both indigenous and exotic, such as herbs, eggs, salt, and spices, is a common feature of other charms in Scandinavian medical manuscripts. For instance, the charm against fever mentioned above incorporates all these elements: 'Þetta e*r* got*t* vi*d* ridu. ath rista a epli e*d*a lauki hasis eos trema neos salvator

---

36 See Caroline R. Batten's chapter in this volume for a discussion of internal ailment linked with supernatural beings, such as elves and demons, in Old English medical texts.

37 Cameron, *Anglo-Saxon Medicine*, p. 142; Meaney, 'The Anglo-Saxon View of the Causes of Illness'; Jolly, *Popular Religion*; Kesling, *Medical Texts*.

38 *Den islandske lægebog*, ed. by Kålund, p. 11. *Alfa-völkun* is a *hapax legomenon*: *álfr* (elves) & *völkun* (mysery, hardship); a possible translation could be disease caused by elves (see *The Dictionary of Old Norse Prose* <https://onp.ku.dk/onp/onp.php?o1692>).

39 Edition and translation of the runic instruction in Lozzi Gallo, 'On the Interpretation of *ialuns*', pp. 135–36; see also MacLeod and Mees, *Runic Amulets*, pp. 34–35.

40 For a more in-depth discussion of elves in (healing) charms see, Cameron, *Anglo-Saxon Medicine*, pp. 130–58; Meaney, 'The Anglo-Saxon View of the Causes of Illness'; Jolly, *Popular Religion*; Hall, *Elves in Anglo-Saxon England*; Hall, '"Þur sarriþu þursa trutin"'; Simek, 'Elves and Exorcism'; Kesling, *Medical Texts*.

emanuel' (For a fever it is good to cut this on an apple or onion: *hasis eos trema neos salvator Emanuel*).[41] One of the entries in the Old English *Lacnunga* calls for the writing and utterance/singing of prayers and scriptural passages for a remedy against an elf-disease, showcasing the array of prayers and formulae that could be used in charms and rituals to heal patients, some of which are found also in *Kveisustrengurinn*:

> Þis is se halga drænc wið ælfsidene ond wið eallum feondes costun- gum: Writ on husldisce: 'In principio erat uerbum' usque 'non conpre- henderunt', et plura 'Et circumibat Ihesus totam Galileam docens' usque 'et secuti sunt eum / turbe multe'; 'Deus in nomine tuo' usque in finem; 'Deus misereatur nobis' usque in finem; 'Domine Deus in adiutorium' usque in finem. [...] Sing ðas gebedsealmas: 'Miserere mei Deus', 'Deus in nomine tuo', 'Deus misereatur nobis', 'Domine Deus', 'Inclina Domine', ond 'Credo', ond 'Gloria in excelsis Deo', ond letanias, 'Pater noster'
>
> > (This is the holy drink for elfish magic and for all the temptations of the Devil: Write on a paten: 'In the beginning was the word' as far as 'comprehended it not', and furthermore 'And Jesus went about all Galilee teaching' as far as 'and great crowds followed him'; 'God in your name' until the end; 'May God have mercy on us' until the end; 'Lord God to my aid' until the end. [...] Sing these precatory psalms: 'God have mercy on me', 'God in your name', 'May God have mercy on us', 'Lord God', 'Turn, Lord', and the Creed, and 'Glory to God in the highest', and litanies, the 'Our Father')[42]

In *Kveisustrengurinn*, the *In nomine Patris* invocation in Old Norse appears four times (ll. 28, 55, 103 and 203), and the invocation that closes the charm is followed by *Amen*. As I will show below, the invocations to expel the disease are in Old Norse, and the scriptural passages, together with prayers, *nomina sacra*, or the *Trisagion* are in either Latin or Greek, underlining the authority of the sacred word. As Olsan has noted, 'names (known and unknown) call for and bespeak power, functioning variously as invocations, declarations of divine presence, word magic, or as signs of authority like seals attached to documents'.[43] Notably, one invocation combines Latin and Old Norse, using the former for calling on the Holy Trinity, and Old Norse to beseech Heaven, the Earth and the Sun: 'Jaurd kref eg orda en*n* vp*p* him-/ins, Sol, Sa*n*ctam trijnitate*m*'[44] (Earth, I call the words, high Heaven, Sun, Sanctam Trinitatem).

The other two *historiolae* from Erasmus's translation of the New Testament are, just like the Prologue to the Gospel of John, often used in healing charms.

41 RIA, MS 23 D 43, fol. 1^{r}; see Baccianti, 'Guaritori, acqua santa e latte materno' for a discussion of the charm. Manuscript abbreviations are expanded in *italic*.

42 *Anglo-Saxon Remedies*, ed. and trans. by Pettit, I, pp. 16–17 (*Lacnunga*, XXIX).

43 Olsan, 'Writing on the Hand', p. 15.

44 Lbs fragm. 14, 1^{r} (ll. 97–98). *Upphiminis* is an errouneous rendition by the scribe of *uphimæn*.

The first one is from the Gospel of Matthew 8. 1–13,[45] which narrates how Jesus healed a leper and the servant of a centurion.[46] The passage is followed by an adjuration in Old Norse:

Siaalfuan
Gud er eg bidiandi at han*n* liaae mi*er*
lijftungu læknis orda, nu e*r* lijkn*ar*-
dag*ur*, læknis dag*ur* heylsu dag Biargar z
nu e̲r̲ heilagr*ar* þren*n*ingar dag*ur* Jeg sig*ne*
þig j nafni faud*ur*, z Sonar og anda heij-
lags eijns Gudz j heijlag*re* þrenningu *fyrir* fl-
og kueijsu, *fyrir* faar kveijsu, *fyrir* blóð queysu,
beijn qeijsu, jardar, lopts, vindz og vatnz
queijsu z allz kon*ar* queijsu[47]

(I beg God Himself to grant me
a healing-tongue and medical words, now is a favourable
day, a doctor's day, a health day to help and
now is Holy Trinity day I bless
you in the name of the Father, and son and holy
spirit of one God in the Holy Trinity, for
shooting pain, for severe pain, for bloody boil)[48]
bone disease, earth, air, wind and water
disease and all kinds of disease)

Echoing the preceding scriptural passage, the charm invokes God the healer, but also God as the provider of healing powers. This passage is reminiscent of other healing charms, such as the Bergen rune stick discussed above, that predate *Kveisustrengurinn*. For example, the Ribe healing stick (DR EM85; 493, *c.* 1300) invokes the power of the earth, universe, and the sun, together with Christian powers, such as Mary and God, to grant the healer 'læknæs hand / ok līf-tungæ at livæ' ('leech-hands and a healing tongue to heal') against the trembler (*bivindnæ*)—possibly a fever with shivers:

Iorð biðak varðæ   ok uphimæn,
sōl ok santæ Marīa   ok sialfæn Guð drōtæn,
þæt han læ mik   læknæs hand
ok līf tungæ   at livæ bivindnæ
þær bōtæ þarf.
Ōr bak ok ōr bryst,   ōr lækæ ok ōr lim,
ōr øvæn ok ōr øræn,   ōr allæ þe þær ilt kanīat kumæ.

---

45 Lbs fragm. 14, 1^r (ll. 56–90).
46 The second *historiola*, which occurs towards the end of the charm (ll. 167–84), is also from the Gospel of Matthew (9. 1–8) and tells of paralysed man forgiven and healed by Jesus.
47 Lbs fragm. 14, 1^v (ll. 98–107).
48 *fyrir blóð queysu* could also be a haemorrhage.

Svart hetær stēn, han stær ī hafæ ūtæ.
þær ligær ā þe nī nouðær, þær [...] þen [...] þæ þes skulæ hværki,
skulæ hværki søtæn sofæ æþ varmnæn vakæ,
førræn þū þæssæ bōt bīðær þær ak orð at kvæðæ rōnti.
Amæn ok þæt sē.

(I pray earth to guard and high heaven,
the sun and holy Mary and the lord God himself,
that he grant me leech-hands
and a healing tongue to heal the trembler
when a cure is needed.
From back and from breast, from body and from limb,
from eyes and from ears; from wherever evil can enter.
A stone is called Svart (i.e. 'black'), it stands out in the sea,
there lie upon it nine needs, who [...] then [...] should,
shall neither sleep sweet nor wake warm,
until you pray this cure which I have proclaimed in runic words.
Amen, and so be it.)[49]

The listing of the various body parts that could be affected by a disease is also present in *Kveisustrengurinn* in the second adjuration, in Old Norse, which occurs halfway through the charm:

Særi Eg allz haat-
tada kueijsu af þ*es*sari gudz þionustu
kuin*n*u [...] mz Ih*es*u Chr*is*ti
vilia z fulltijngi. Særi Eg queysu allra h*a*n-
da kins vr haufdi þijnu z heijla, vr haalsi
z herdu*m*, vr andliti, augu*m* z augna braam, vr
Briosti, quid z baki. Særi ec alls kon*ar* q[50] af þi*er*
vr m*er*g z mæni, vr leggjum z lidu*m* z lida mó-
tu*m* z vr aullu*m* þinu*m* Samteijngdu*m* lijkama.[51]

49 MacLeod and Mees, *Runic Amulets*, pp. 123–24. See also Jesch and Lee, 'Healing Runes' for more on healing runes, and Moltke, 'Runepindene fra Ribe'. This characteristic is also mentioned in stanzas 4 and 11 of the eddic poem *Sigrdrífumál*: 'Heilir æsir, / heilar ásynjur, / heil sjá in fjölnýta fold, / mál ok mannvit / gefið okkr mærum tveim / ok læknishendr, meðan lifum. / Limrúnar skaltu kunna, / ef þú vilt læknir vera / ok kunna sár at sja; / á berki skal þær rísta / ok á baðmí viðar, / þeim er lúta ausr limar' (*Sigrdrífumál*, 313–21) (Hail to the Æsir! / Hail to the goddesses! / Hail to the mighty, fecund earth! / May you give eloquence and native wit to this glorious pair / And healing hands while we live! / Limb-runes you must know if you want to be a healer / and know how to see to wounds; / on bark they must be cut and of the tree of the wood, / on those whose branches bend east.) (*The Poetic Edda*, pp. 163 and 164). Stanza 9 of *Sigrdrífumál* mentions *bjargrúnar* (helping runes) for childbirth.

50 Most probably an abbreviation of *queisu*.

51 Lbs fragm. 14, 1ᵛ (ll. 115–23).

(I adjure every kind of
inflammation/pain from this God's servant
woman [...] with Jesus Christ's
will and help. I adjure all kinds of pain/inflammation
from your head and brain, from the neck
and shoulders, from the face, eyes and eyebrows from
the chest, stomach and back. I adjure you of every kind [pain?]
from you
from marrow and spinal cord, from legs and limbs and
joints, from all your joined [whole?] body.)

The charm enumerates the various body parts, starting from the head and moving down to the legs, to exorcise the evil spirit causing the ailment to leave the body, even when hidden in the brain, marrow, or stomach. Both the Ribe rune stick and *Kveisustrengurinn* bear a resemblance to the charms found in the Leofric Missal, in the section *item super energumino baptizato* ('In the same way over a baptized demoniac'), and the exorcism of body parts titled *alia* ('other'). Kesling has discussed the tradition of the body part exorcism in relation to the *Lacnunga* charm against *aelf-sogoþa*, and has suggested, following Sims-Williams's argument,[52] that this type of exorcism most probably has Irish origins.[53]

This passage also provides clues on the patient affected (or the owner of the charm) who is described as a servant of God (guðs þiónustu kuin*nu*), most probably a humility topos to show respect towards God 'the Physician'. The information about the owner of the charm/amulet is reiterated in two other instances: 'lækna þu ég bíð þessa þína þiónustu kuin*nu*. S ✠ n ✠ a. *fra*'[54] (Heal, I wait for this, your female servant S ✠ n ✠ a. *fra*); and a third time, towards the end of the charm, in an adjuration that lists and emphasizes the healing powers of God:

52 Sims-Williams, 'Thought, Word, Deed', pp. 88–91.

53 Kesling, *Medical Texts*, pp. 86–92; see also Jolly, *Popular Religion*, p. 163 and David Stifter's chapter on the Irish charms in this volume, especially his discussion of the Stowe Missal. 'Domine sancte pater omnipotens aeterne deus, per impositionem scrip- ture huius et gustum aquae, expelle diabolum ab homine isto. De capite, de capillis, de uertice, de cerebro, de fronte, de oculis, / de auribus, de naribus, de ore, de lingua, de sublingua, de gutture, de collo, de corpore toto, de omnibus membris, de compaginibus membrorum suorum, intus et foris, de ossibus, de uenis, de neruis, de sanguine, de sensu, de cogitationibus, de omni conuersatione, et operetur in te uirtus christi, in eo qui pro te passus est, ut uitam aeternam merearis. Per.' (Lord, holy father, all-powerful eternal God, through the imposition of this writing [or scripture] and taste of water, expel the devil from this man, from the head, from the hair, from the top, from the brain, from the forehead, from the eyes, from the ears, from the nostrils, from the mouth, from the tongue, from under the tongue, from the throat, from the neck, from the whole body, from all the limbs, from the joints of all his limbs, internal or external, from the bones, from the veins, from the tendons, from the blood, from the senses, from the thoughts, from every habit, and let Christ's virtue work in you, who died for you, that you may merit life eternal. Through.) (As quoted in Kesling, *Medical Texts*, pp. 88–89).

54 Lbs fragm. 14, 1^{v} (ll. 158–59).

Þu ed san*n*a lios Guddo*m*zins
ih*es*us þu e*r*t vor læknijng Sem græd*er* vor meijn
So se*m* þu lijfgad*er* z heijlan*n* giord*er* þen*n*an*n* lima
fallz siuka ed*ur* kueijsu Siuka. So lækna þu nu *fyrir*
þin*n* krapt z ord þ*es*sa þijna þionustu kuin*n*u. S ✠ n[55]

(You that are the true light of Divinity,
Jesus, you are our cure that heals our wounds
Just as you called this paralysed person back to life
And healed this person afflicted by boils. Heal now,
by your power and word this servant woman of yours. S ✠ n)

Interestingly, in the last two passages, after the mention of the sick woman, two letters divided by a cross follow the word *kuinnu*: S ✠ n. I am uncertain whether these stand for the initials of the woman or are part of the combination of repeated letters that appear in the second half of the charm. In this section of the charm there is a prayer that includes, just as at the end of the lines quoted above, a series of crosses and letters, along with a list of *nomina sacra*, invocations to the Holy Trinity and other apotropaic elements. This is the only section of the charm that combines Latin, Hebrew, and Greek, resembling textual amulets circulating elsewhere in Europe in the late Middle Ages that combined a mix of languages, images, and magical traditions. A few lines before the prayer there is an incomplete *Trisagion* (Thrice Holy), a Greek chant typically used in the Orthodox liturgy, as well as in Byzantine charms: 'AGios ✠ Otheos ✠ AGios ✠ ysteros / AGios athanaatos'[56] (Holy God ✠ Holy Mighty ✠ Holy God ✠ Holy Immortal). The prayer to Jesus Christ begins with a list of divine names, beginning with *Jesus Christ, Messiah, Emmanuel, Sabaoth, Adonay,* which are commonly found in healing charms. It also includes the divine name AGLA[57] and the palindrome SATOR AREPO TENET OPERA ROTAS:[58]

55 Lbs fragm. 14, 1^{v} (ll. 185–89).

56 Lbs fragm. 14, 1^{v} (ll. 128–29).

57 AGLA is a divine name for God and stands for a Hebrew benediction 'Atta gibbor leolam adonai' (You are mighty forever, Lord).

58 This palindrome was usually configured as a magic square, however in charms found in manuscripts (medical or prayer books) it was often written on a line. Skemer offers a concise and clear explanation of the five-line Roman magic square SATOR AREPO: 'Many imaginative interpretations have been posited for this magic square, including the literal translation, "Arepo the sower guides the wheels by his work." The possibility of rearranging the letters of the palindrome to spell out PATER NOSTER in cruciform may help explain the popularity of this bit of ancient magic in the medieval Christian imagination' (Skemer, *Binding Words*, p. 116). The SATOR formula is used in linear form also in Norse medical manuscripts, for instance in AM 434a 12mo, fol. 1^{r} (in order to cure a headache, the entry instructs the reader to carve the words on wood and in RIA, MS 23 D 43, fol. 2^{r}: 'Ef kona hefir of m*i*cit blóðlat þa rist þu fyr*ir* nefnda bloðstem*mu* fimbra x*risti* at kefli z þar me*ð* verssit. Sator arepo tenet op*er*a rotas' (If a woman is a great blood flow, carve the appellation (charm?) above for blood

J*hesus* chr*istus*, Messias, [E]maanuel, saabaaoth ad-
o*n*aj, vnitas. S[ancta] trijnitas, vija, vitja,
virtus. Omnipote*ns* ho*m*ousion Saluator. pij*us* [...]
[...] Creator rede*m*ptor, fons, spes, saalus, sac*er*dos
Imas otheos origo maanus splendor Sol. Gloria
Lux, p*ara*clet*us*, Córóná, Colu*m*ba, humilitas, fortiss-
imus, latissimus, athanathos kirios theos
vn*us* pat*er* vn*us* filius vnus Spiritus. *Sanctus* panton
Craaton ysos aGnus oves uitul*us* Serpens
aries leo vermis: Alpha z o P*ri*mus et
tet*ra* Gram*m*ato*n* AGla ☩ AGla[59]
AGios. otheos AGios yscyros AGios athanaatos eleyson ymas.
Satior[60] Arepo tenit op*er*a rotas
p*er* Crucidis hoc Signu*m* procul fugiat omne*m* maal-
ignu*m* z p*er* idem Signum [saluet*ur*] [omn*e*][61] benignu*m* Eli
heli heleij helioa*m*[62] lux t[etra][63] Gram*m*aton. Sodaael.
adonajj Emanuel jh*esus* Ih*esus* nazarenus rex judeoru*m*
filij dei [...] [Miser*ere*] me Salua me et Sana me
z Custodi m[e quia opera][64] iuram [...]
te[65]

(Jesus Christ, Messiah, Emanuel, Sabaoth, Saviour,
unity. Holy Trinity, way, life,
virtue. Omnipotent, same saviour being. Pious [...]
[...] Redeemer, Creator, source, hope, health, priest,
Imas otheos (Mighty on us), origin, hands, Sun's splendour. Glory,
light, Holy Spirit/helper, halo, dove, humility, very strong,
very tall, immortal, Lord God,
one father, one son, one spirit. Holy Pantokrator,
just, lamb, sheep, calf, serpent
ram, lion, worm: Alpha and Omega, First/Beginning and
Last/End tetragrammaton, AGla ☩ AGla

staunching, fimbria Christi on stick and also the verse Sator Arepo Tenet Opera Rotas). On the *SATOR* square, see also Conan T. Doyle's and Deborah Hayden's chapters in this volume.

59 Magnús Már Lárusson wrongly transcribes it as AGia ☩ AGia.

60 Scribal error; it should read *Sator*.

61 The words *saluetor* and *omne* are no longer legible on the manuscript, but present in Magnús Már Lárusson's transcription.

62 Most probably a reference to the last word spoken by Christ on the cross.

63 The word *tetra* is no longer legible on the manuscript, but present in Magnús Már Lárusson's transcription.

64 The words *Misesere* and *me quia opera* are no longer legible on the manuscript, but present in Magnús Már Lárusson's transcription.

65 Lbs fragm. 14, 1^{v} (ll. 135–54).

AGios. otheos AGios yscyros AGios athanaatos eleyson ymas[66]
Sator Arepo Tenit Opera Rotas
through this sign of the cross let every evil flee
and by the same sign save all that is good. Eli
heli heleij heliam, light, tetragrammaton, Sodaael,
Saviour, Emanuel, Jesus, Jesus Nazarene, King of the Jews,
Son of God […] Have mercy on me, save me, heal me,
and protect me I swear on the works I do
for you)

This prayer in *Kveisustrengurinn* can be categorized as a 'Heavenly Letter' type of charm. These charms, which were already circulating in the fourth century, were popular throughout the Middle Ages.[67] Indeed, other charms in England, Wales and on the continent include similar lists of divine names (*De nominibus Dei*) that were invoked for protection, as in the protection prayer, *Domine Ihesu Christi fili dei vivi miserere* in Edinburgh, University Library, MS 66, fols 43^{v}–44^{r}, a sixteenth-century prayer book:[68]

> Domine Ihesu Christi fili\ dei vivi miserere mei et defende me\ famulum tuum, N,[69] hodie et cotidie\ omni nocte et omni tempore ab omnibus adversita\tibus et de omnibus inimicis meis et ab omnibus malis\ dampnis et prodicionibus, Messyas, soth, ema\nuel, sabaoth, adonay, panton, craton, tetra\gramaton, yskiros, agyos, ymas, eleyson\ o theos, athanatos, alpha et omega, vermis, vi\tulus, leo, ovis, aries, agnus homo, usion\ serpens, primus, novissimus filius pater, filius\ spiritus sanctus, trinus, creator omnium rerum deus mi\sericors eternus principium finis. Salva me et de\fende me ab omnibus malis.[70]
>
> (Lord Jesus Christ, so of the living God, have mercy on me and protect me, your servant, N, today and every day, every night and every time from all adversities and from all my enemies and from all evil, damages and betrayals, Messiah, Sother, Emmanuel, Sabaoth, Adonay, Pantokrator, Tetragramaton, Ischyros, Hagios, Ymas Eleyson, Theos,

---

66 Trisagion: Holy God, Holy Mighty, Holy Immortal, Have mercy on us.

67 For more on the Heavenly Letters Charm tradition, see Skemer, *Binding Words*, 96–107; Hebing, '"Allmygti god this lettyr sent"' and 'The Textual Tradition of Heavenly Letter Charms'.

68 See e.g. the Welsh Heavenly Letter charm in Cardiff, NLW, MS Sotheby C.2 (transcribed and discussed in Leach, 'Healing Charms and Ritual Protection') and the English one in Oxford, Bodl. Lib., MS 850, fols 93^{v}–94^{r} (transcribed and discussed in Hebing, '"Allmygti god this lettyr sent"').

69 *N* stands for *nomen*. Charms and prayers often included the name of the owner, however, just as in this prayer, the name has been substituted with *N*, so that when recited the personal name could be added aurally.

70 <www.abdn.ac.uk/burnet-psalter/text/043v.htm> and www.abdn.ac.uk/burnet-psalter/text/044r.htm [accessed 16 June 2023].

> Athanatos, Alpha (the Beginning), Omega (the End), the Worm, the Calf, the Lion, the Sheep, the Ram, the Lamb, the Serpent, the First, the Last, Son, Father, Son, Holy Spirit, the Threefold, the Creator of All things, God, the Merciful, the Eternal, the beginning of the end, save me from all evil.)

Hebing has observed that the Heavenly Letter charm 'is a type of charm that is inextricably linked with the physicality of the written word'.[71] The list of divine names and the use of liturgical/exorcism formulae, as I have highlighted above, demonstrate that *Kveisustrengurinn* and other medical charms in the corpus of Scandinavian medical texts have analogues in the charm tradition of medieval Western Europe. Indeed, these charms were often adapted for an indigenous audience or for a specific patient, but one can generally trace a specific tradition or trope, underlining the movement, reception and transmission of medical and liturgical knowledge in the medieval North Atlantic.

One cannot draw firm conclusions about the sources of *Kveisustrengurinn* and its owner, but what I hope to have shown here is that this charm belongs the learned tradition of healing charms circulating together with medical manuscripts in medieval western Europe. As discussed in the preceding chapters, reading and analysing healing charms separately from their manuscript context and from the corpus of medical texts associated with them is problematic. How, when and why *Kveisustrengurinn* ended up in the archives of the Bishopric of Hólar is a question to which there is no definitive answer, so far. However, I believe that discussing it within the frame of medical knowledge in medieval Iceland is important in order to understand the role played by scholars and clerics in the reception and transmission of medical and liturgical/biblical knowledge in medieval Scandinavia. I agree with Ciaran Arthur, who, in relation to Anglo-Saxon charms, has argued that:

> These texts are Christian rituals that developed from learned traditions and that were components of new liturgies for the sick, the possessed, travellers, political leaders, monastic communities, and lay people. They frequently incorporate prayers, formulas, and objects from other liturgies, and many seem to employ complex strategies of textual concealment, indicating that only highly skilled ecclesiastics could read and perform them.[72]

---

71 Hebing, '"Allmygti god this lettyr sent"', p. 723.

72 Arthur, *'Charms', Liturgies, and Secret Rites*, p. 215; see also Svanhildur Óskarsdóttir and Árni Heimir Ingólfsson, 'Dýrlingar', who discuss the importance of the religious context and the use of liturgical texts in everyday life of those who used the codex Reykjavík, AM 461 12mo. Hebing has also stressed the importance of considering charms in their context, arguing that 'Charms were not out place among religious texts — at least, not according to the average medieval charm user. Whether or not charms were recognized as different from prayer is irrelevant in that respect, as most contemporaries would not have been preoccupied with labelling a text as either one or the other' (Hebing, '"Allmygti god this lettyr sent"', p. 726).

Conclusion

Healing charms that contain similar wording and formulae as the in *Kveisustrengurinn* were already circulating in Icelandic medical manuscripts in the fourteenth century, combining Christian, classical, and pagan lore.[73] However, after the Reformation (mid-sixteenth century), which reinforced Danish rule in Iceland and ultimately outlawed Catholicism, the Church and local authorities started condemning any healing charms, as they were considered witchcraft.[74] This could be one of the possible reasons why *Kveisustrengurinn* was found in the archives of the Bishop of Hólar, as it was probably confiscated by the Church or given to the Bishop in order to be investigated. Witch trials started post-Reformation, and the laws against witchcraft were further enforced in 1617 with King Christian IV of Denmark's Witchcraft Act. This Act echoed what Martin Luther wrote about the use of amulets and liturgical texts in the popular religious practices at the time, including healing charms:

> Aber ein greulicher misbrauch und zeuberen ist es auch gewesen, das man dis Euangelium Johannis 'In principio erat Verbum' auff ein klein zeddelin geschrieben, [...], an hals oder anders wo him henget. Item wider den Donner und Wetter lieset, wie das in Bapsthum ist gebreuchlich gewesen, wie denn auch die Zeuberer derer namen: Jhesus, Maria, der vier Euangelisten, Mattheus, Marcus, Lucas, Joannes, der heiligen dreier Könige, item der Wörter: Jhesus Nazarenus Rex Judeorum, pflegen zu misbrauchen und treibens in irer bösen büberen und buleren. Das ist daher komen, das die Gottlosen gesehen haben, das die Apostel, ire Jünger und nach inen viel fromer Bischofe und Heiligen wunder und Zeichen gethan, wenn sie nur etliche Wort aus dem Euangelio gesprochen. Da namen sie auch die Wörter und wölten als balde dergleichen Zeichen dar nach thun.[75]
>
> > (But a frightful misuse and a piece of witchery to write the words *in principio erat verbum* on a slip of paper [...] and hang it around one's neck or somewhere else; or to read these words as a protective charm against thunder or storm, as was customary in the papacy. Sorcerers also have the habit of misusing the names of Jesus, Mary and the four evangelists, Matthew, Mark, Luke and John; of the holy three kings; also the words *Jhesus Nazarenus Rex Judeorum* in connection with their knavery and hatemongering. The godless do this in imitation of the apostles, their disciples, and many pious bishops and saints of a later day, who performed signs and wonders if they spoke only a few words from the Gospel.)

---

73 See e.g. MacLeod and Mees, *Runic Amulets*; Jolly, 'Anglo-Saxon Charms' and 'Medieval Magic'; and Bauer, 'Biblical Magic'.

74 See e.g., Ohrvik, *Medicine, Magic and Art*.

75 Luther, *Martin Luthers Werke: Kritische Gesamtausgabe*, vol. 46, p. 628; English translation: Luther, *Sermons on the Gospel of St John*, chs 1–4, ed. by Pelikan, vol. 22, pp. 106–07.

Recently, Viðar Hreinsson has suggested, based on palaeographical and literary evidence, that Jón lærði Guðmundsson (1574–1658) might have written *Kveisustrengurinn*. Jón, an Icelander from the Westfjords, was a poet, naturalist, and healer with an interest in medicinal herbs, runes, and supernatural beings, and throughout his life he was known for his teaching and healing skills. In 1631, he was convicted for witchcraft because his writings did not comply with the new laws; he was then exiled and outlawed in 1637. It is indeed possible that Jón lærði Guðmundsson copied the charm, but he was definitely not the author, as similar charms had been circulating in Iceland and the North Atlantic for several centuries. *Kveisustrengurinn* is the work of a cleric, familiar with scriptural texts, protection prayers and exorcism.

No real conclusive narrative can be drawn about the origin and story of *Kveisustrengurinn*. We cannot confirm who copied it, who owned it, or why it was in the archives of the Bishopric of Hólar. Yet, it is a text that combines and blurs medicine, magic, and religion; that provides a glimpse into sixteenth- and seventeenth-century Iceland; and that reveals the relationships between its readers and users. The circulation, or lack thereof, of the strip offers a portrayal of its social life and how it served different audiences. As Kathryn Kerby-Fulton has pointed out, 'Once a text has left its author's hands, reception is everything'.[76] The life of this strip shows that it is not just a charm, but a continuum of materiality and text. As Jude Hill argues, using Edward Lovett's collection of early twentieth-century amulets and charms at the Wellcome Historical Medical Museum, not having any documented evidence about the life of an object does not prevent interpretation; rather, 'gaps in biographies, raise important research questions in their own right'.[77] *Kveisustrengurinn* holds within itself traces of its relationships with its users and readers. Not only is it a text that was read or touched, but it was also worn on the body. Today, it is an object devoid of touch or closeness to skin; thus its function changes, and so does its meaning. By researching and engaging with the charm, we create and interact with a new layer of its story. At first glance, the manuscript is simply a strip of vellum with words in Latin, Greek, and Old Norse, but when we look into its history we can unfold the history of Iceland, as well as the history of medicine, of magic, of religion, and of archival practices. *Kveisustrengurinn* thus bridges the manifold boundaries of space and time, becoming associated with the places and people it has encountered, or has been linked to, whilst connecting different societal practices and fields of knowledge.

76 Kerby-Fulton, *Books under Suspicion*, p. 159.

77 Hill, 'The Story of the Amulet', p. 77.

Works Cited

Manuscripts

Cardiff, National Library of Wales, MS Sotheby C.2
Copenhagen, Den Arnamagnæanske Samling, MS AM 434a 12mo
Dublin, Royal Irish Academy, MS 23 D 43
Edinburgh, University Library, MS 66 ('Prayer Book')
London, British Library, MS Cotton Caligula A XV
Oxford, Bodleian Library, MS 850
Reykjavík, Landsbókasafn Íslands, MS Lbs fragm. 14
Reykjavík, Stofnun Árna Magnússonar á Íslandi, MS AM 461 12mo

Primary Sources

Anglo-Saxon Remedies, Charms and Prayers from British Library MS Harley 585: The Lacnunga, ed. and trans. by Edward Pettit (Lewiston: Edwin Mellen Press, 2001)

The Dictionary of Old Norse Prose (ONP) <https://onp.ku.dk/onp/onp.php?> [accessed 28 March 2023]

Den islandske lægebog: Codex Arnamagnæanus 434 a, 12 mo, ed. by Kristian Kålund (D. Kgl. Danske Vidensk. Selsk. Skr. 6. Række, historisk og filosofisk Afd. VI.4) (Copenhagen: HHøst/Bianco Lunos Bogtrykkeri, 1907)

Lbs fragm. 14 <https://handrit.is/manuscript/view/is/LbsFragm-0014/0#mode/2up> [accessed 10 June 2022]

Martin Luther, *D. Martin Luthers Weke. Kritische Gesamtausgabe*. Weimar Ausgabe, Abteilung Schriften, 46 (Weimar: Hermann Böhlaus Nachfolger, 1912–1921)

——, *Sermons on the Gospel of St. John / [Martin Luther]* (vol. 22), ed. by Jaroslav Pelikan, American edn (Saint Louis: Concordia, 1957)

Novvm Testamentvm ab Erasmo Recognitvm II. Evangelivm Secvndvm Iohannem et Acta Aposolorum, ed. by Andrew J. Brown, in *Opera Omnia Desiderii Erasmi Roterodami. Recognita et adnotatione critica instrvcta notisque illvstrata* (tom. VI, vol. 2), ed. by F. Akkerman and others (The Hague: Elsevier Science, 2001)

Rituale Romanum: Pauli V Pontificis Maximi Iussu Editum Aliorumque Pontificum Cura Recognitum Atque Ad Normam Codicis Iuris Canonici Accomodatum Ssmi. D. N. Pii Papae XII Auctoritatae Ordinatum Et Auctum, Cum Textu Psalmorum E Vulgata Bibliorum Editione. Ed. prima iuxta typicam cum textu psalmorum e vulgata bibliorum edition (Bonn: nova et vetera, 2012)

The Poetic Edda, trans. by Carolyne Larrington (Oxford: Oxford University Press, 2014), pp. 163–64

The Saga of the Sister Saints. The Legend of Martha and Mary Magdalen in Old Norse-Icelandic Translation, ed. and trans. by Natalie M. Van Deusen (Toronto: The Pontifical Institute of Mediaeval Studies, 2019)

Sigrdrífumál, in *Eddukvæði II. Hetjukvæði*, ed. by Jónas Kristjánsson and others (Reykjavík: Hið islenzka fornritafélag, 2014), pp. 313–21

Secondary Studies

Arbesmann, Rudolph, 'The Concept of "Christus Medicus" in St. Augustine', *Traditio*, 10 (1954), 1–28

Arthur, Ciaran, *'Charms', Liturgies, and Secret Rites in Early Medieval England* (Woodbridge: Boydell & Brewer, 2018)

Baccianti, Sarah, 'Guaritori, acqua santa e latte materno: alcuni resoconti di pratiche e incantesimi medici nell'Isalanda medievale', *Filologia Germanica-Germanic Philology*, Supplemento, 3 (2022), 33–52

——, 'Healing Hands, Holy Water, and Hellish Diseases: Some Accounts of Medical Performance in Medieval Iceland', in *The Medieval North and its Afterlife: Essays in Honor of Heather O'Donoghue*, ed. by Siân Grønlie and Carl Phelpstead (Berlin: Medieval Institute Publications, 2024), pp. 67–77

Bauer, Alessia, 'Biblical Magic as a Manifestation of Folk Belief in the North', in *Faith & Knowledge in Late Medieval & Early Modern Scandinavia*, ed. by Karoline Kjesrud and Mikael Males, Knowledge, Scholarship, and Science in the Middle Ages, 1 (Turnhout: Brepols, 2019), pp. 269–96

——, *Laienastgrologie im nachreformatorischen Isald. Studien zu Gelehrsamkeit und Aberglauben* (Münchner Nordisticsche Studien 21) (Munich: Herbert Utz Verlag, 2015)

Braavig, Jens, 'Magic: Reconsidering the Grand Dichotomy', in *The World of Ancient Magic: Papers from the First International Samson Eitrem Seminar at the Norwegian Institute in Athen, 4–8 May 1997*, ed. by David R. Jordan, Hugo Montgomery, and Einar Thomassen (Bergen: Paul Astroms, 1999), pp. 21–54

Cameron, Malcolm L., *Anglo-Saxon Medicine* (Cambridge: Cambridge University Press, 1993)

Dillmann, François-Xavier, *Les magiciens dans l'Islande ancienne: Études sur la représentation de la magie islandaise et de ses agents dans les sources littéraires norroises*, Acta Academiae Regaise Gustavi Adolphi, 92 (Uppsala: Swedish Science Press, 2006)

Gierløw, Lilli, 'In principio', in *Kulturhistorisk leksikon for nordisk middelalder* (Copenhagen: Rosenjilde og Bagger, 1956–1978; repr. 1982), XVIII, cols 670–74

Hall, Alaric, *Elves in Anglo-Saxon England. Matters of Belief, Health, Gender and Identity* (Woodbridge: Boydell & Brewer, 2007)

——, '"Þur sarriþu þursa trutin": Monster-Fighting and Medicine in Early Medieval Scandinavia', *Asclepio: Revista de Historia de la Medicina y de la Ciencia*, 61 (2009), 195–218

Hebing, Rosanne, '"Allmygti god this lettyr sent": English Heavenly Letter Charms in Late Medieval Books and Rolls', *Studies in Philology*, 114.4 (2017), 720–47

——, 'The Textual Tradition of Heavenly Letter Charms in Anglo-Saxon Manuscripts', *Amsterdamer Beiträge Zur Alteren Germanistik*, 69 (2012), 203–22

Hill, Jude, 'The Story of the Amulet: Locating the Enchantment of Collections', *Journal of Material Culture*, 12.1 (2007), 65–87

Hindley, Katherine Storm, 'The Power of Not Reading: Amulet Rolls in Medieval England', in *The Roll in England and France in the Late Middle Ages. Form and*

Content, Materiale Textkulturen, 28, ed. by Stefan G. Holz, Jörg Peltzer, and Maree Shirota (Berlin and Boston: De Gruyter, 2020), pp. 289–306
——, *Textual Magic: Charms and Written Amulets in Medieval England* (Chicago: University of Chicago Press, 2023)
Jesch, Judith, and Christina Lee, 'Healing Runes', in *Viking Encounters*, ed. by Anne Pedersen and others (Aarhus: Aarhus University Press, 2020), pp. 386–98
Jolly, Karen, 'Anglo-Saxon Charms in the Context of a Christian World View', *Journal of Medieval History*, 11 (1985), 279–93
——, 'Medieval Magic: Definitions, Beliefs, Practices', in *Witchcraft and Magic in Europe: The Middle Ages*, ed. by Karen Jolly, Edward Peters, and Catharina Raudvere (London: Athlone, 2002), pp. 1–26
——, *Popular Religion in Late Saxon England: Elf Charms in Context* (Chapel Hill: University of North Carolina Press, 1996)
Kerby-Fulton, Kathryn, *Books under Suspicion: Censorship and Tolerance of Revelatory Writing in Late Medieval England* (Notre Dame, IN: University of Notre Dame Press, 2006)
Kesling, Emily, *Medical Texts in Anglo-Saxon Literary Culture* (Woodbridge: Boydell & Brewer, 2020)
Kieckhefer, Richard, *Magic in the Middle Ages* (Cambridge: Cambridge University Press, 2014)
Leach, Katherine, 'Healing Charms and Ritual Protection in Premodern Wales' (unpublished doctoral thesis, Harvard University, 2020)
Lozzi Gallo, Lorenzo, 'On the Interpretation of Ialuns in the Norwegian Runic Text B257', *Arkiv för nordisk filologi* 116 (2001), 135–51
MacLeod, Mindy, and Bernard Mees, *Runic Amulets and Magic Objects* (Woodbridge/Rochester, NY: Boydell and Brewer, 2006)
Magnús Már Lárusson, 'Eitt gamalt kveisublað', *Árbók Hins íslenzka fornleifafélags*, 51 (1951–52), 81–90
Maguire, Henry, 'Magic and the Christian Image', in *Byzantine Magic*, ed. by Henry Maguire (Washington, DC: Dumbarton Oaks Research Library and Collection, 1995), pp. 51–71
Maraschi, Andrea, *Similia similibus curantur. Cannibalismo, grafofagia e "magia" simpatetica nel Medioevo (500–1500)* (Spoleto: Cisam, 2020)
——, 'Sympathetic Graphophagy in Late Medieval Scandinavian Leechbooks and Collections of Charms', in *Civilizations of the Supernatural: Witchcraft, Ritual, and Religious Experience in Late Antique, Medieval, and Renaissance Traditions*, ed. by Fabrizio Conti (Budapest: Trivent Publishing, 2020), pp. 247–64
Meaney, Audrey L., 'The Anglo-Saxon View of the Causes of Illness', in *Health, Disease and Healing in Medieval Culture*, ed. by Sheila Campbell, Bert Hall, and David Klausner (London: Palgrave McMillan, 1992), pp. 12–33
Mitchell, Stephen A., 'Faith and Knowledge in Nordic Charm Magic', in *Faith and Knowledge in Late Medieval Scandinavia*, ed. by Karoline Kjesrud and Mikael Males, Knowledge, Scholarship, and Science in the Middle Ages, 1 (Turnhout: Brepols, 2020), pp. 193–211

——, 'Leechbooks, Manuals, and Grimoires. On the Early History of Magical Texts in Scandinavia', *ARV. Nordic Yearbook of Folklore*, 70 (2014), 57–74

——, *Witchcraft and Magic in the Nordic Middle Ages* (Philadelphia: University of Pennsylvania Press, 2011)

Moltke, Erik, 'Runepindene fra Ribe', *Fra Nationalmuseets Arbejdsmark 1960* (Copenhagen: Nationalmuseet, 1960), pp. 122–36

Montesano, Marina, *"Supra acqua et supra ad vento": "Superstizioni", maleficia e incantamenta nei predicatori francescani osservanti (Italia, sed. XV)*, Istituto Storico Italiano per il Medio Evo, Nuovi Studi Storici, 46 (Rome: Istituto Storico Italiano, 1999)

Murray Jones, Peter, and Lea T. Olsan, 'Performative Rituals for Conception and Childbirth in England, 900–1500', *Bulletin of the History of Medicine*, 89.3 (2015), 406–33

Ohrvik, Ane, *Medicine, Magic and Art in Early Modern Norway. Conceptualizing Knowledge* (London: Palgrave, 2018)

Olsan, Lea, 'Writing on the Hand in Ink: A Late Medieval Innovation in Fever Charms in England', *Incantatio*, 7 (2018), 9–45

Schreiner, Klaus, 'Volkstumliche Bibelmagie und volkssprachliche Bibellekture: Theologische und soziale Probleme mittelalterlicher Laienfrommigkeit', in *Volksreligion im hohen und späten Mittelalter*, ed. by Peter Dinzelbacher and Dieter R. Bauer, Quellen und Forschungen aus dem Gebiet der Geschichte, n.s., 13 (Paderborn: Schoningh, 1990), pp. 329–73

Simek, Rudolf, 'Elves and Exorcism: Runic and Other Lead Amulets in Medieval Popular Religion', in *Myths, Legends, and Heroes: Essays on Old Norse and Old English Literature in Honour of John McKinnell* (Toronto: University of Toronto Press, 2011), pp. 25–52

Sims-Williams, Patrick, *Religion and Literature in Western England 600–800* (Cambridge: Cambridge University Press, 1990)

——, 'Thought, Word, Deed: An Irish Triad', *Ériu*, 29 (1978), 78–111

Skemer, Don C., 'Amulet Rolls and Female Devotion in the Late Middle Ages', *Scriptorium*, 55.2 (2001), 197–227

——, *Binding Words. Textual Amulets in the Middle Ages* (University Park, PA: Pennsylvania State University Press, 2006)

Storms, Godfrid, *Anglo-Saxon Magic* (The Hague: Martinus Nijhoff, 1948)

Svanhildur Óskarsdóttir, and Árni Heimir Ingólfsson, 'Dýrlingar og daglegt brauð í Langadal. Efni og samhengi í AM 461 12mo', *Gripla*, 30 (2019), 107–53

Van Deusen, Natalie M., 'The Old Norse-Icelandic Legend of Saints Mary Magdalen and Martha' (unpublished doctoral thesis, University of Wisconsin– Madison, 2012)

Manuscript Index

General Index

Knowledge, Science, and Scholarship in the Middle Ages

All volumes in this series are evaluated by an Editorial Board, strictly on academic grounds, based on reports prepared by referees who have been commissioned by virtue of their specialism in the appropriate field. The Board ensures that the screening is done independently and without conflicts of interest. The definitive texts supplied by authors are also subject to review by the Board before being approved for publication. Further, the volumes are copyedited to conform to the publisher's stylebook and to the best international academic standards in the field.

Titles in Series

Faith and Knowledge in Late Medieval and Early Modern Scandinavia, ed. by Karoline Kjesrud and Mikael Males (2020)

Travelling Wisdom: Medieval Science in the North, c. 1000–1500, ed. by Christian Etheridge and Michele Campopiano (2021)

Michael Schonhardt, *Mit Sphaera und Astrolab: ‚Die Entdeckung der Natur' in süd-ostdeutschen Klöstern im hohen Mittelalter* (2022)

Antoni Grabowski, *The Craft of History: Turning History into a Discipline in the Twelfth and Thirteenth Centuries* (2024)